SCHEIN'S COMMON SENSE EMERGENCY Abdominal Surgery

Fifth Edition

Danny Rosin MD FACS

Attending General and Advanced Laparoscopic Surgeon,

Sheba Medical Center, University of Tel Aviv, Israel

Paul N. Rogers MB ChB MBA MD FRCS (Glasgow)

Consultant General and Vascular Surgeon, Department of Surgery,

Queen Elizabeth University Hospital, Glasgow, UK

Mark Cheetham MB BS BSc MSc MD FRCS (Gen)

Consultant General and Colorectal Surgeon, Department of Surgery,

Royal Shrewsbury Hospital, Shrewsbury, UK

Moshe Schein MD FACS FCS (SA)

Attending Surgeon, Marshfield Clinic,

Ladysmith and Rice Lake, Wisconsin, USA

tfm Publishing Limited, Castle Hill Barns, Harley, Nr Shrewsbury, SY5 6LX, UK
Tel: +44 (0)1952 510061; Fax: +44 (0)1952 510192
E-mail: info@tfmpublishing.com;
Web site: www.tfmpublishing.com

Editing, Design & Typesetting: Nikki Bramhill BSc (Hons) Dip Law
Fifth edition: © 2021
Cartoons: © 2016, 2021 Evgeniy E. (Perya) Perelygin, MD
Front cover painting: © 2020 Dan Schein (E-mail: danschein@gmail.com)

Paperback ISBN: 978-1-910079-87-4

E-book editions: © 2021
ePub ISBN: 978-1-910079-88-1
Mobi ISBN: 978-1-910079-89-8
Web pdf ISBN: 978-1-910079-90-4

Printed by Gutenberg Press Ltd., Gudja Road, Tarxien, PLA 19, Malta
Tel: +356 21897037; Fax: +356 21800069

Contents

Contributors

Roland E. Andersson MD PhD Associate Professor, Department of Clinical and Experimental Medicine, Linköping University, Linköping, Sweden; Consultant, Department of Surgery, County Hospital Ryhov, Jönköping, Sweden (➲ Chapter 21)
rolandersson@gmail.com

Ahmad Assalia MD Associate Professor of Surgery, Chief of Advanced Laparoscopic and Bariatric Surgery, Rambam Health Care Campus, Haifa, Israel (➲ Chapter 29)
assaliaa@gmail.com

Jack Baniel MD Head, Urology Institute, Rabin Medical Center, Petach Tikva, Israel (➲ Chapter 35)
baniel@netvision.net.il

Mark Cheetham MB BS BSc MSc MD FRCS (Gen) Consultant General and Colorectal Surgeon, Royal Shrewsbury Hospital, Shrewsbury, Shropshire, UK (➲ Chapters 1, 3-7, 9-14, 16, 18-20, 24-28, 33, 36-47)
markcheets@aol.com

Harold Ellis CBE MCh FRCS Professor, Applied Biomedical Research Group, Hodgkin Building, Guy's Campus, London, UK (➲ Chapter 2)
harold.ellis@kcl.ac.uk

Adam L. Farquharson MB ChB MEd MFSTEd FRCS (Gen Surg) Consultant General and Colorectal Surgeon, Training Programme Director — Professional Development HEE (WM), Educational Lead — General Surgery HEE (WM), Department of Surgery, Royal Shrewsbury Hospital, Shrewsbury, Shropshire, UK (➲ Chapter 25)
adam.farquharson@nhs.net

Wojciech J. Górecki MD PhD Associate Professor, Jagiellonian University Medical College; Chief, Department of Pediatric Surgery, University Children's Hospital, Kraków, Poland (➲ Chapter 34)
migoreck@cyf-kr.edu.pl

Ghaleb Goussous MB BS MSc FRCS Senior Colorectal Surgery Fellow, Royal Derby Hospital, Derby, Derbyshire, UK (➲ Chapter 27)
ghaleb.goussous@nhs.uk

Anat Ilivitzki MD Department of Radiology, Rambam Medical Center, Haifa, Israel (➲ Chapter 29)
a_ilivitzki@rambam.health.gov.il

Rifat Latifi MD FACS FICS Professor and Chairman of Surgery, New York Medical College, School of Medicine; Director, Department of Surgery; Chief, General Surgery, Westchester Medical Center Health, Valhalla, New York (➲ Chapter 31)
rifat.latifi@wmchealth.org

Ari Leppäniemi MD Chief of Emergency Surgery, Abdominal Center, University of Helsinki, Finland (➲ Chapters 17 and 31)
ari.leppaniemi@hus.fi

Evgeniy E. Perelygin MD Attending Surgeon, Department of Urology, Perm Clinical Center, Perm, Russia (➲ All chapters)
perya70@gmail.com

Paul N. Rogers MB ChB MBA MD FRCS (Glasgow) Consultant General and Vascular Surgeon, Department of Surgery, Queen Elizabeth University Hospital, Glasgow, UK (➲ Chapters 1, 3-7, 9-14, 16, 18-20, 22, 32, 33, 36-47)
pn.rogers@btinternet.com

Danny Rosin MD FACS Attending General and Advanced Laparoscopic Surgeon, Department of General Surgery and Transplantation, Sheba Medical Center, Tel Hashomer; The Faculty of Medicine, Tel Aviv University, Israel (➲ Chapters 1, 3-7, 9-16, 18-20, 33, 36-47)
drosin@mac.com

James C. Rucinski MD FACS Attending Surgeon, Director of Surgical Education, New York Methodist Hospital, Brooklyn, New York, USA (➲ Chapters 6 and 8)
jcrucinski@gmail.com

Roger Saadia MD FRCS(Ed) Professor of Surgery (retired), University of Manitoba and Health Sciences Centre, Winnipeg, Canada (➲ Chapter 30)
rsaadia@shaw.ca

Contributors

Erik Schadde MD FACS Director HPB Fellowship, Swiss HPB Center, Department of Surgery, University Hospital Zurich, Zurich, Switzerland (➲ Chapter 23)
erik.schadde@uzh.ch

Moshe Schein MD FACS FCS (SA) Attending Surgeon, Marshfield Clinic, Ladysmith and Rice Lake, Wisconsin, USA (➲ Chapters 1, 3-7, 9-14, 16, 18-20, 33, 36-47)
mosheschein@gmail.com

Simon Shaw BSc (Hons) MB BS FRCS Consultant General and Colorectal Surgeon, Department of Surgery, Conquest Hospital, East Sussex, UK (➲ Chapters 24-26, 28)
simon.shaw7@nhs.net

Wesley P. Stuart MB ChB MD FRCS (Ed) Chief of Medicine, Consultant Vascular Surgeon, Queen Elizabeth University Hospital, Glasgow, UK (➲ Chapter 22)

Editors' note

This book has been assembled — in pieces — during long years of intensive personal involvement, clinical and academic, urban and rural, with emergency abdominal surgery in many countries across the continents.

A long line of good old friends from all around the world were helpful in generating this book and its four preceding editions. For the foundations in this noble surgical field Moshe is indebted to the late **George G. Decker** of Johannesburg. Drs. **Asher Hirshberg** and **Adam Klipfel** contributed to the *first edition*. Dr. **Robert Lane**, Ontario, Canada, helped us with the three first editions. Professor **Ahmad Assalia** has been part of this book from its early days; he co-edited the *third edition* and continues to share with us his wisdom. Thanks also to **Roger Saadia**, **Wojciech Górecki**, **Jim Rucinski**, **Jack Baniel Ari Leppäniemi**, **Roland Andersson** and **Erik Schadde** who continue supporting this project.

Dr. **Alfredo Sepulveda** of Santiago, Chile, edited the Spanish translation (*first edition*); Dr. **Francesco Vittorio Gammarota** of Rome, Italy, edited the Italian translation (*second edition*); Professor **Wen-hao Tang**, China, edited the Mandarin translation (*third and fourth editions*); Drs. **Alexander Ferko, Leo Klein**, **Eduard Havel**, **Dušan Šimkovic**, **Karel Šmejkal**, Czech Republic, edited the Czech translation (*second edition*); Dr. **Wojciech Górecki**, Poland, edited the Polish translation (*third edition*); Dr. **Teimuraz Kemoklidze**, Georgia, edited the Georgian translation (*third edition*); Dr. **Slava Ryndine**, South Africa, helped to organize the Russian translation (*third edition*); Dr. **Bogibek Rakhimov** produced an online Uzbekistani edition. And we will always remember with affection the late Professor **Boris Savchuk** of Moscow who edited the first Russian translation (*first edition*).

We are grateful to the many members of **SURGINET**, who over the years have stimulated our brains with their constant international feedback. Thanks to Dr. **Evgeniy (Perya) Perelygin** who drew many new caricatures for this edition and to **Dan Schein** who painted the image on the front cover.

Special thanks go to **Nikki Bramhill** who continues, single-handedly to produce this book (the first three editions were published by Springer) — no one does it better than Nikki!

Editors' note

Many of the aphorisms and quotations used to decorate this book were retrieved from *Aphorisms & Quotations for the Surgeon* (2002) and *A Companion to Aphorisms & Quotations for the Surgeon* (2008), edited by Moshe Schein and published by Nikki Bramhill's tfm Publishing Ltd, Shrewsbury, UK.

The reader will find that there are not a few duplications scattered throughout the book. We did this on purpose, as repetition of important points is crucial in adult education.

Any reader who has a question or a comment about anything to do with this book is invited to email any of us directly:

- drosin@mac.com;
- pn.rogers@btinternet.com;
- markcheets@aol.com;
- mosheschein@gmail.com.

We will reply!

Finally, we are indebted to our loving wives, Gilly, Jackie, Julia and Heidi, for their patience and sacrifice.

The Editors

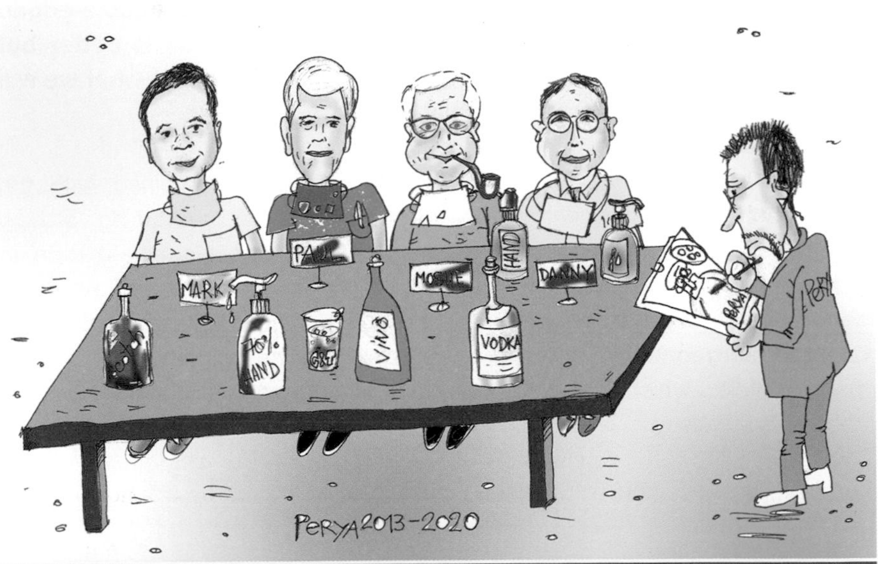

The Editors.

Preface

Common things are common except common sense.

Yasser Mohsen

Congratulations! You bought a book. This is a remarkable achievement!

The mere fact that you are now reading this page, nay, that you have actually picked this book up... means that you belong to an endangered species — steadily dwindling — of young surgeons who actually read real books. Not only lecture notes or clips on YouTube — but books!

We are pleased to present the *fifth edition* of this book, which, since it first appeared 20 years ago, has become popular with surgeons having to deal with emergency abdominal surgery.

Is there anything new in this field that merits the revision and update of such a book every 4-5 years? Yes. The way we practice emergency surgery is constantly evolving. With almost unlimited access to abdominal imaging, we can rapidly pinpoint the diagnosis and avoid an unnecessary operation, or perform an indicated operation instead of engaging in a prolonged period of uncertainty. We are gradually becoming more selective and cautious — understanding that **everything we do involves wielding a double-edged sword and that in emergency surgery usually doing less is better but occasionally doing more may be life-saving. At least — this is what we will want you to believe after reading this book...**

At the same time, changes in surgical education combined with the exaggerated obsession with modern technology are producing a new generation of general surgeons. **In the new era, super-specialization in 'advanced lap' procedures is considered profitable and 'sexy' whereas general surgical emergencies are left to the juniors or the allegedly 'less talented' surgeons**. So, in many places emergency surgery is considered a 'bastard' field , which everybody can do... usually in the late hours when the 'robots' go to sleep.

In this brave new world we need to constantly update ourselves. We have to relearn how to deal with the old s**t — which is becoming rare — even when its odor is masked by the perfume of modern practice. And this is what we continue to do in this new edition — reciting the written-in-stone sacred, old basics but also showing how to integrate them with the evolving modern world.

What is new in the fifth edition?

Ari Leppäniemi (University of Helsinki) is busy retiring and thus resigned as a co-editor; but he continues to provide a few excellent chapters. **Mark Cheetham** (Shrewsbury, Shropshire, UK) joined us and took it on himself to produce a completely new section on colorectal emergencies.

All the contributors are well known to us personally as experts in their field. All existing chapters have been revised, expanded or rewritten by the old or new contributors and/or the Editors. Each chapter has been carefully scrutinized by us, its style and tone tuned to conform to the overall 'voice' of the book. In this edition we have eliminated or combined together a few old chapters in order to produce a somewhat more compact volume.

From the beginning we knew that a book like this — written in a practical, colloquial, and direct in-your-face style will be either loved or hated. And indeed, a few reviewers (of the first edition) — appalled by dogmas that clashed with their own, and language not exactly conforming to Strunk and White's *The Elements of Style* — almost killed it. But many more loved it. Previously we have cited from the many complimentary reviews and the enthusiastic feedback we have received — and still do — from numerous readers around the world; we won't cite these here.

Motivated by the enthusiasm with which the book is being received around the world — particularly among those practicing 'real surgery' in the 'real world' — we set about enhancing it to produce a text that should be palatable to all of you — wherever you try to save lives — be it in Mumbai, Karachi, Cairo, Belgrade, Soweto, Mexico City, Kiev, Copenhagen, Philadelphia, Glasgow, Krakow and, yes — even in Paris (we hope there are a few French surgeons who can, and want to, read English…).

Dr. Anton Chekhov said: "Doctors are just the same as lawyers; the only difference is that lawyers merely rob you, whereas doctors rob you and kill you too." **Our chief aim in writing this book was to help you not kill your patients.** This non-orthodox book is not yet another tedious, full-of-details textbook. We do not need more of these. It's aimed at you, the young practicing surgeon (by young we mean someone who is not frozen in his own dogmas) who desires a focused and friendly approach to emergency abdominal surgery. We hope and believe that this modest book will be of some value to you.

André Maurois said: "In literature, as in love, we are astonished at what is chosen by others." We hope you chose this book.

Cheers! (■ See photos on the facing page.)

The Editors
Tel Aviv, Glasgow, Shrewsbury, Northern Wisconsin

P.S.: Please note that Danny has taken over from Moshe the role of leading editor. As Paul and Moshe are aging, this surely is their last edition. They hope that Danny and Mark will carry the torch into the next few editions!
P.P.S.: As this edition was written during the unprecedented days of the Coronavirus pandemic, when elective surgery was limited and the 'robots' were asleep, it's clear that emergency surgery will always remain a necessity.

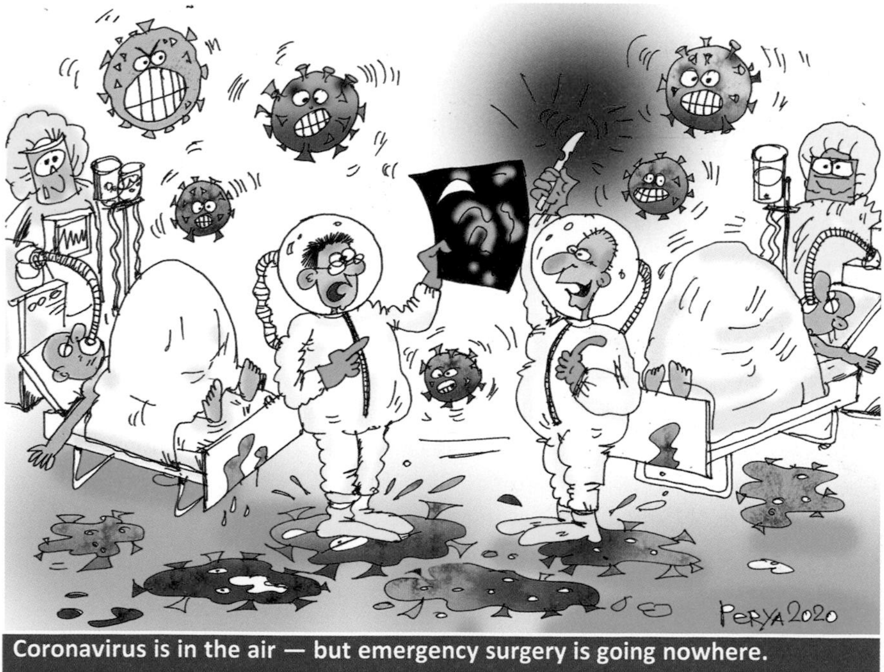

Coronavirus is in the air — but emergency surgery is going nowhere.

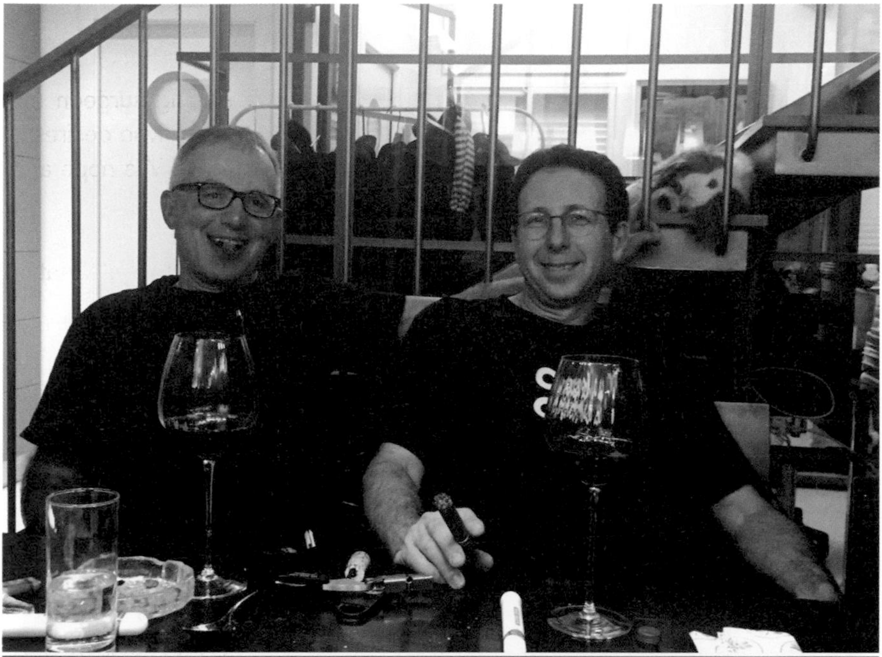

Danny and Moshe in a typical biliary debate, with the late Pushkin (2006-2019) snoozing on the stairs.

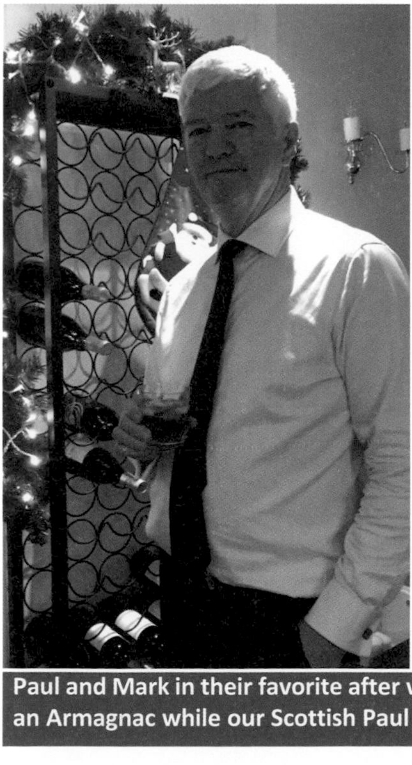

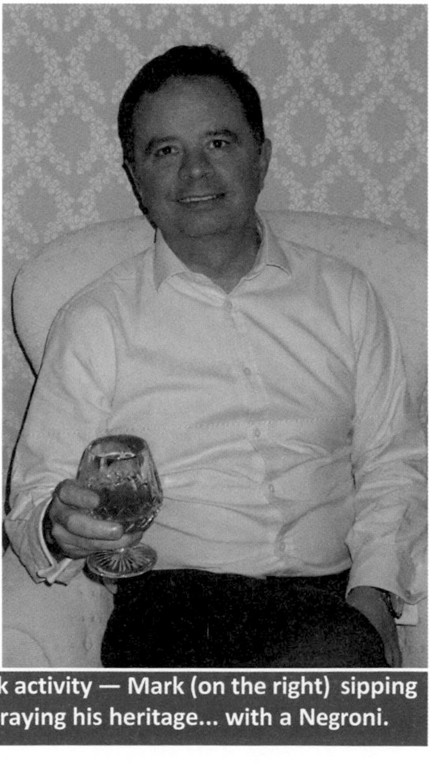

Paul and Mark in their favorite after work activity — Mark (on the right) sipping an Armagnac while our Scottish Paul betraying his heritage... with a Negroni.

PART I

General considerations

Chapter 1

General philosophy

The Editors

> *Good judgment comes from experience, experience comes from bad judgment.*
>
> **Rita Mae Brown**

> *Wisdom comes alone through suffering.*
>
> **Aeschylus, Agamemnon**

> *Fools say that they learn by experience. I prefer to profit by others' experience.*
>
> **Otto von Bismarck**

> *Surgeons are internists who operate...*

At this moment — just as you pick up this book and begin to browse through its pages — there are many thousands of surgeons around the world facing a patient with an abdominal catastrophe. The platform on which such an encounter occurs differs from place to place — a modern emergency department in London, a noisy and crowded casualty room in the Bronx, or a doctor's tent in the African bush. But the scene itself is amazingly uniform. It is always the same — you confronting a patient; he suffering, in pain, and anxious. And you too are anxious: anxious about the diagnosis, concerned about choosing the best management, troubled about your own abilities to do what is correct.

We are in the 21st century but this universal scenario is not new. It is as old as surgery itself. **You are perhaps too young to know how little some things have changed — or how other things have changed, and not always for the better — over the years**. Yes, your hospital may be in the forefront of modern medicine; it has a team of subspecialists on call to provide advice (it has an even larger administrative team of functionaries to monitor you...), its emergency room has standby, state-of-the-art spiral computed tomography and magnetic resonance imaging machines, but, practically, something has not changed: **it is the patient and you (often with the entire 'system' against you) — you who are duty bound to provide a correct management plan and execute it**. And it often feels lonely out there; even we, experienced old farts, can feel the loneliness.

The 'best' management of an abdominal emergency

It is useful to compare the emergency abdominal surgeon to an infantry officer (■ Figure 1.1). Away from the limelight and glory that surrounds cardiac or neurological surgeons, emergency abdominal surgery is closer to infantry engagements than it is to airborne action. **You cannot win a war by**

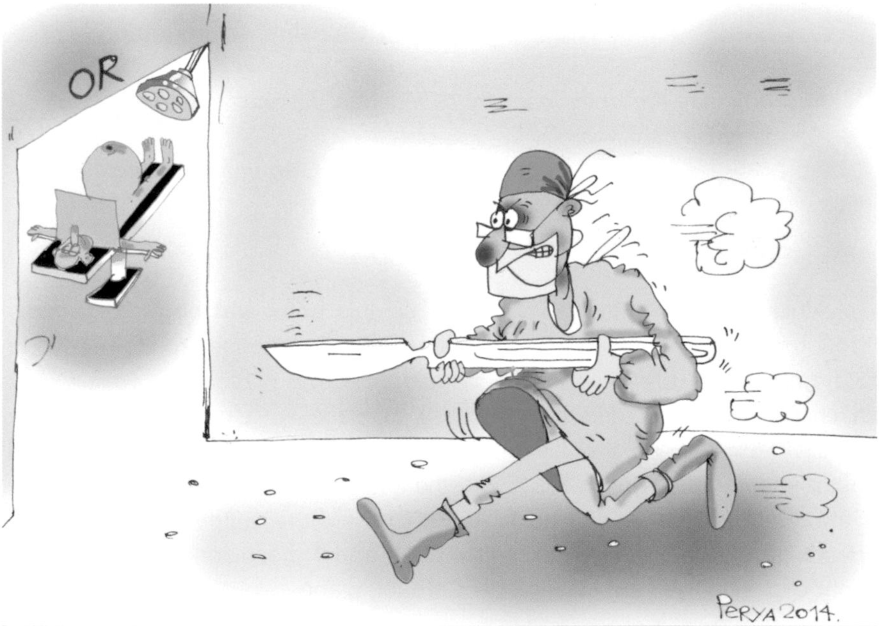

Figure 1.1. "Think as an infantry soldier..."

remote control with cruise missiles or robots alone; you need infantry on the ground. Likewise, technological gimmicks have a limited place in emergency abdominal surgery, which is principally the domain of the surgeon's brain and hands. **To achieve the final 'victory' someone must agonize, sweat, bleed, and wet his hands — remember the bad smell from your hands after operating on a perforated colon?** Some readers may struggle with this military metaphor but the truth of the matter is that emergency abdominal surgery shares a few simple rules with infantry action — developed in the trenches and during offensives — rules that are the key to survival and victory (■ Table 1.1). Such a code of battle echoes the 'best management' of abdominal emergencies.

There are many ways to skin a cat and you know from your various surgical mentors that different clinical pathways may arrive at a similar outcome. However, one of the diverse pathways is the 'best' — thus, the 'correct' one! **To be considered as such, the preferred pathway has to save life and decrease morbidity in the most efficient way**.

The 'best' management in each section of this book is based on the following elements:

- Old-established principles (don't reinvent the wheel).
- Modern-scientific understanding of inflammation and infection.
- Evidence-based surgery (see below).
- Personal experience.

Today many options exist to do almost anything. Any search on Google or PubMed will overwhelm you with papers that can justify almost any management pathway, with people practicing *surgical acrobatics* for the mere sake of doing so. Data and theory are everywhere: the sources are numerous but what you really need is *wisdom* — to enable you to apply correctly the knowledge you already have and constantly gather. **And wisdom is what we are trying to provide. So please open your mind**.

Table 1.1. The surgeon as an infantry soldier.

Rule	Infantry action	Emergency abdominal surgery
Rule 1	Destroy your enemy before he destroys you	Outmaneuver death (save a life)
Rule 2	Spare your own men	Reduce morbidity (handle tissues gently)
Rule 3	Save ammunition	Use resources rationally (every stitch must count) and avoid unnecessary tests
Rule 4	Know your enemy	Estimate the severity of disease (think how organs and cells are doing)
Rule 5	Know your men	Understand the risk-benefit ratio of your therapy (don't try to do too much in one operation, if the patient will not tolerate it)
Rule 6	Attack at 'soft' points	Tailor your management to the disease and the patient (mild disease, definitive surgery; severe disease, damage control)
Rule 7	Do not call for air force support in a hand-to-hand battle	Do not adopt useless gimmicks — use your mind and hands (and sutures)
Rule 8	Conduct the battle from the front line — not from the rear	Do not take and accept decisions over the phone (when you are in charge, you are in charge)
Rule 9	Take advice from the generals but the decision is yours	Procure and use consultation from 'other specialties' selectively (if the consultant gives a wrong answer, change the consultant)
Rule 10	Avoid friendly fire	Reduce iatrogenesis (don't overdo it)
Rule 11	Consider using the drones	Avoid suicidal missions (e.g. when interventional radiology can help you in difficult anatomic locations)
Rule 12	Maintain high morale among your troops	Be proud in providing the 'best' management (but give the anesthetists and nurses some credit)
Rule 13	Say "follow me!"	Lead by example!

Factors affecting decision making (■ Figure 1.2)

"There is nothing new in the story...," Winston Churchill said, "want of foresight, unwillingness to act when action would be simple and effective, lack of clear thinking, confusion of counsel until the emergency comes, until self-preservation strikes its jarring gong..." How true is this Churchillian wisdom when applied to emergency surgery. How often do we forget old — written in stone — principles while reinventing the wheel?

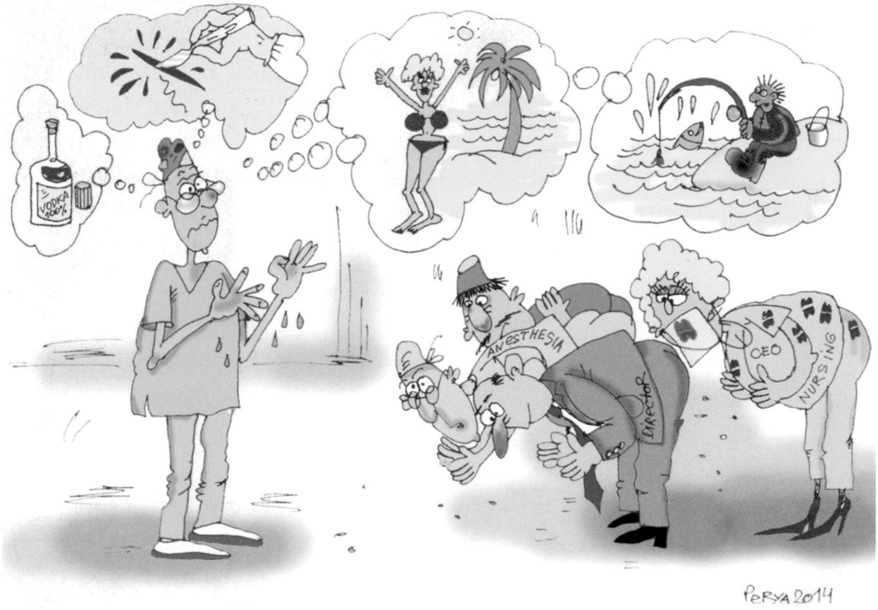

Figure 1.2. "Each of us has a different 'general philosophy'..."

The inflamed patient

Think about your patient as being INFLAMED by myriad inflammatory mediators, generated by the primary disease process, whether inflammatory, infectious or traumatic — so if you measure C-reactive protein (CRP) in these patients, in most it will be elevated! Local inflammation (e.g. peritonitis) and the systemic response may lead to organ dysfunction or failure, and the eventual demise of your patient. **The greater the inflammation — the sicker the patient and the higher the expected morbidity and mortality. Consider also that anything you do in attempting to halt your patient's inflammation**

may in fact contribute to it — adding fuel to the inflammatory fire. Excessive surgery, inappropriately performed, and too late, just adds nails to your patient's coffin.

The philosophy of treatment that we propose maintains that in order to cure or minimize the inflammatory processes and the anti-inflammatory response, **management should be accurately tailored to the individual patient's disease — as the punishment fits the crime, so should the remedy fit the disease**. A well-trained foot soldier does not fire indiscriminately in all directions. These days he can summon the drones for a surgical strike!

This means that during emergency operations you should avoid unnecessary steps as much as you can. This implies not escalating the procedure and not adding anything 'incidental'. So when resecting a perforated colon you should not add an 'incidental' cholecystectomy only because the pre-op CT showed gallstones; or at the end of a tedious procedure for adhesive small bowel obstruction you don't want to chop out the harmless appendix only because it happened to appear in the operative field.

- If you do too much some people would always say that doing less could have saved the patient.
- If you do too little some people would always say that doing more could have saved the patient.
- How much to do in the emergency situation requires common sense.
- Common sense requires knowledge and experience and... common sense!

Evidence

Economic considerations sometimes motivate the physician to accept that part of the scientific evidence that best supports the method that gives him the most money.

George Crile

A few words about what we mean when we talk about 'evidence'. Many formal classifications of scientific evidence are in circulation. Here is one version along with what some people think about it (■ Table 1.2).

Table 1.2. An example of a formal classification of scientific evidence.

Level of evidence	Description	Comments
Ia	Evidence from meta-analysis of randomized controlled trials	*Meta-analysis is to analysis as metaphysics to physics.* **H. Harlan Stone**
Ib	Evidence from at least one randomized controlled trial	*Is it really randomized? Sometimes it is hard to believe...*
IIa	Evidence from at least one well-designed controlled trial which is not randomized	*Statistical numbers are like prisoners of war — torture them enough and they will admit to anything.* **Basil Pruitt**
IIb	Evidence from at least one well-designed experimental trial	*Hard to believe but humans are a little different from rats!*
III	Evidence from case, correlation, and comparative studies	*As a general rule, results of observational studies should be taken with a grain of salt. Otherwise, one might conclude that gray hair causes heart attacks.* **Edward H. Livingstone**
IV	Evidence from a panel of experts	*An expert surgeon: someone more than fifty miles from home with a Powerpoint presentation.*

To the above 'official' classification we wish to add a few more categories frequently used by surgeons around the world.

- V — "In my personal series of X patients (never published) there were no complications."
- VI — "I remember that case... forty years ago..."
- VII — "This is the way I do it and it is the best."
- VIII — "My grandmother thinks this is a good idea."

Note that level III retrospective case series form the main bulk of surgical literature dealing with abdominal emergencies, whereas levels V-VIII (also called by some as 'anecdata'), are the main forms of evidence used by surgeons in general — think about your own departmental meetings! And level VIII evidence may remind you of your chairman! To paraphrase a quote from *Memoirs of Hadrian* by Marguerite Yourcenar: **"In any combat between fanaticism (dogmatism) and common sense the latter has rarely the upper hand."**

We want to show you that this should not be the case! You should educate yourself to think in terms of levels of evidence and resist local dogmas. We believe that support for much of what we write here is available in the published literature (the 'real' one — not the 'fake'), but we choose not to cite it because this is not that kind of book. When high-level evidence is not available, we are forced to use an individual approach and common sense, and that is much of what this book is about.

> *Evidence is the base of medicine but common sense is the salt of it.*
>
> **Slava Ryndine**

> *The absence of evidence isn't the evidence of absence.*
>
> **Henry Black**

> *As far as the surgical literature goes, use the 'Texas mockingbird approach': eat everything in sight and vomit what you can't use.*
>
> **Lew Flint**

Remember: You can get away with a lot... but not always. The following pages will help you to develop your own judgment — pointing to the correct/preferred pathway in any situation. This is obviously not a bible but it is based on a thorough knowledge of the literature and vast personal experience. So wherever you are — in India, Pakistan, Norway, Chile, Botswana, Canada or Palestine, and whatever your resources are — the general approach to emergency abdominal surgery should be the same. **So come and join us: to do it well, decrease morbidity, save lives, have fun — and attain glory!**

"The glory of surgeons is like that of actors, which lasts only for their own lifetime and can no longer be appreciated once they have passed away. Actors and surgeons... are all heroes of the moment."

Honoré de Balzac

"The operation is a silent confession to the surgeon's inadequacy."

John Hunter

Chapter 2

A brief history of emergency abdominal surgery

Harold Ellis

We are proud to offer this chapter by Professor Ellis of London: a renowned surgeon, educator, writer, editor, anatomist, and surgical historian. Among his many books, we would particularly recommend *Operations That Made History* and *A Brief History of Surgery*. The Editors.

> *In the study of some apparently new problems we often make progress by reading the work of the great men of the past.*
> **Charles H. Mayo**

From the earliest days until comparatively modern times, surgeons were ignorant about the causes of the vast majority of acute abdominal emergencies and equally ineffectual in their treatment. They were, of course, well familiar with abdominal trauma and the dire consequences of perforating injuries of the belly, the great majority of which would be fatal. Thus, in the Bible we read in the Book of Judges:

> But Ehud made him a dagger, which had two edges of a cubit length, and he did gird it under the raiment of his right thigh. And he brought the present unto Eglon, King of Moab. And Eglon was a very fat man... And Ehud put forth his left hand and took the dagger from his right thigh, and thrust it into his belly. And the haft went in after the blade and the fat closed over the blade, so that he could not draw the blade out of his belly; and the dirt came out... And behold their Lord was fallen down dead on the earth.

Occasionally, a fecal fistula would form, and the patient survived. That great 16th century French military surgeon, Ambroise Paré, recorded in his *Case Reports and Autopsy Records*:

> In time I have treated several who recovered after having had wounds by sword or pistol pass through their bodies. One of these, in the town of Melun, was the steward of the Ambassador of the King of Portugal. He was thrust through with a sword, by which his intestines were wounded, so when he was dressed a great deal of fecal matter drained from the wound, yet the steward was cured.

Occasionally, a prolapsed loop of bowel, projecting through a lacerated abdominal wound, might be successfully reduced. Still less often, an enterprising surgeon might suture a laceration in such a loop and thus save the patient's life.

In 1676 Timothy Clark recorded the case of a butcher who attempted suicide with his butcher's knife in the village of Wayford in the country of Somerset, located in the southwest corner of England. Three days later, a surgeon who Clark does not name replaced the prolapsed gut, removed extruded omentum and prolapsed spleen, and the patient recovered. Clark, himself, in 1633 had removed the spleen of a dog with survival, thus showing that the organ was not essential to life and confirming an observation made by Vesalius a century beforehand.

Strangulated hernias were also well known to ancients. Treatment usually consisted of forcible manipulative reduction, which was aided by hot baths, poultices, and the use of the head-down, feet-up position. Sometimes their efforts succeeded, but there was, of course, a dire risk of rupture of the gut, especially in advanced cases. William Cheselden in 1723 reported the case of a woman in her 73rd year with a strangulated umbilical hernia. At operation, he resected 26 inches of gangrenous intestine. She recovered with, of course, a persistent fecal fistula. The extreme danger of strangulated hernia is well demonstrated by the fact that Queen Caroline, wife of George II of England, died of a strangulated umbilical hernia at the age of 55 in 1736.

Acute abdominal emergencies have no doubt affected humankind from its earliest existence, yet it has only been in comparatively recent times — the past couple of hundred years — that the pathology and then the treatment of these conditions were elucidated. This is because over many centuries post-mortem examinations were either forbidden or frowned upon in most societies.

Operations on the abdomen were performed rarely, if at all, until the beginning of the 19th century. So, what Berkeley Moynihan called "the pathology of the living", the pathology of the abdominal cavity as revealed in the operating theater, awaited to a large extent the development of anesthesia in the 1840s and antiseptic surgery in the 1870s.

Knowledge of the causes of the acute abdomen advanced little in the 2000 years following the days of Hippocrates in the 5th century BC. The Greek and Roman doctors were keen clinical observers. They recognized that, from time to time, a deep abdominal abscess might discharge spontaneously or be amenable to surgical drainage with recovery of the patient. Every other serious abdominal emergency was given the name of 'ileus' or 'iliac passion' and was considered to be due to obstruction of the bowels. Of course, the fatal abdominal emergencies they were seeing were indeed due either to mechanical obstruction or to the paralytic ileus of general peritonitis. Thus in Hippocrates we read:

> In ileus the belly becomes hard, there are no motions, the whole abdomen is painful, there are fever and thirst and sometimes the patient is so tormented that he vomits bile... Medicines are not retained and enemas do not penetrate. It is an acute and dangerous disease.

Over the centuries there was little to offer the patient beyond poultices to the abdomen, cupping, bleeding, purgation and enemas, all of which probably did more harm than good. It was not until 1776 that William Cullen, of Edinburgh, coined the term 'peritonitis' for inflammation of the lining membrane of the abdominal cavity and its extensions to the viscera. However, he did not think the exact diagnosis of great importance since "when known, they do not require any remedies besides those of inflammation in general".

Appendicitis

Lorenz Heister, of Helmstadt in Brunswig, must be given credit for the first description of the appendix as the site of acute inflammation, reporting this at an autopsy in 1755. For more than a century after this there were occasional autopsy reports, but most cases were unrecognized or labelled 'typhlitis', 'perityphlitis' or 'iliac passion'.

In 1848, Henry Hancock, of Charing Cross Hospital, London, reported the drainage of an appendix abscess in a young woman who was 8 months pregnant. She recovered, but in spite of Hancock's plea, so fixed was the idea that it was useless to operate once peritonitis was established that his advice was ignored for some 40 years. Indeed, it was a physician, not a surgeon, who advised appendicectomy and early diagnosis. This was Reginald Fitz, Professor of Medicine at Harvard, who, in 1886, published a review of 257 cases, which clearly described the pathology and clinical features and advised removal of the acutely inflamed organ or, in the presence of an abscess, surgical drainage. Fitz's advice was taken up rapidly in the United States. Thomas Morton of Philadelphia was the first to report, in 1887, the correct diagnosis and successful removal of a perforated appendix (although Robert Lawson Tait as early as 1880 had a similar case, he did not report this until 1890). The surge in early diagnosis and operative treatment was particularly pioneered by Charles McBurney of the Roosevelt Hospital, New York, who described 'McBurney's point' and devised the muscle split incision, and J.B. Murphy of Chicago, who emphasized the shift in pain in 'Murphy's sequence'. In 1902, Fredrick Treves, of the London Hospital, drained the appendix abscess of King Edward VII, 2 days before the coronation, and did much to raise the general public's awareness of the disease.

The ruptured spleen

The spleen is the most commonly injured viscus in closed abdominal trauma, yet there was surprising diffidence among the pioneer abdominal surgeons to perform a splenectomy on these exsanguinating patients — in spite of the fact that Jules Péan of Paris had performed a successful splenectomy on a girl with a massive splenic cyst in 1867. Two unsuccessful attempts to save life in splenic rupture were reported in 1892 by Sir Arbuthnot Lane of Guy's Hospital, London, and three more fatal cases were recorded by Friedrich Trendelenburg in Leipzig the following year. The wording of these case reports strongly suggests that had blood transfusion been available, the patients might well have survived.

It fell to Oskar Riegner in Breslau to perform the first splenectomy for a pulped spleen with survival in 1893. The patient, a lad of 14, was found to have the spleen completely severed and there was 1.5L of blood in the abdomen. Normal saline was given subcutaneously into all four limbs. His recovery was complicated by gangrene of the left foot, which required amputation, but he left the hospital, complete with artificial limb, 5 months after his splenectomy.

Intestinal obstruction

Not surprisingly, early attempts to deal with large bowel obstruction (usually due to a left-sided colonic cancer) comprised performance of a colostomy. The first attempt to do this was made by Pillore of Rouen in 1776. He actually carried out a cecostomy on a wine merchant with gross abdominal distension due to a rectosigmoid growth. The operation produced great relief, but the patient died on the 28th day because of necrosis of a loop of jejunum, brought about by the large amounts of mercury given in the pre-operative attempts to overcome the obstruction. It remained for Pierre Fine of Geneva, in 1797, to perform a successful transverse colostomy. The patient, a lady of 63 with an obstructing sigmoid growth, died 14 weeks later with ascites.

Not until the introduction of anesthesia and antisepsis could routine resection of bowel cancers be performed, the first success in this era being reported by Vincent Czerny in Heidelberg in 1879. It was soon realized that resection of the obstructed colon was very likely to result in a fatal anastomotic leak. Exteriorization of the growth, with formation of a double-barrelled colostomy and its subsequent closure was introduced by Frank Thomas Paul of Liverpool in 1895, and by Johannes von Mikulicz-Radecki of Breslau a little later. This procedure, the Paul-Mikulicz operation, was shown by the latter to reduce mortality in his own cases from 43% with primary resection to 12.5% with the exteriorization method.

With its vivid clinical features of intestinal obstruction in a baby, passage of redcurrant jelly stools, a palpable abdominal mass and sometimes a prolapsing mass to be felt per rectum or even seen to protrude through the anal verge, it is not surprising that intussusception in children was one of the earliest specific pathologies of the acute abdomen to be recognized. Treatment was expectant, with the use of enemas or rectal bougies, in attempts to reduce the mass. Surgeons were encouraged to do this by very occasional reports of success and still rarer accounts of recovery following the passage of the sloughed gangrenous bowel per rectum. The first operative success was reported by Sir Jonathan Hutchinson, of the London Hospital, in 1871. His patient, a girl aged 2, had her intussusception reduced through a short midline incision, the operation requiring just a few minutes. Hutchinson's meticulous report tabulated 131 previously recorded cases, which make sad reading indeed.

There was a downside to this new abdominal surgery. It was not long after this new era commenced that the first reports appeared of small bowel obstruction due to postoperative adhesions. Thomas Bryant of Guy's Hospital recorded the first example in 1872 — a fatal case following an ovariotomy. A second fatality, 4 years after removal of an ovarian mass, was reported in 1883 by William Battle of London. Today, postoperative adhesions and bands account for some three-quarters of all cases of small bowel obstructions in the Western World.

Perforated peptic ulcer

Untreated, a perforated peptic ulcer nearly always results in fatal peritonitis. Unsuccessful attempts at repair were made by Mikulicz-Radecki in 1884 and by Czerny in 1885 and subsequently by a number of other surgeons. This depressing series came to an end under most difficult circumstances. In 1892, Ludwig Heusner of Wuppertal, Germany, repaired a perforated gastric ulcer high up on the lesser curve in a 41-year-old businessman with a 16-hour history; the operation was performed in the middle of the night by candlelight! The convalescence was complicated by a left-sided empyema, which required drainage. Two years later, Thomas Morse, in Norwich, published the successful repair of a perforation near the cardia in a girl of 20. With these two successes, operation for this condition became routine. Interestingly, gastric ulcer at the turn of the 20th century was far commoner than duodenal ulcer and was especially found in young women.

Ruptured ectopic pregnancy

Until 1883 a ruptured ectopic pregnancy was a death sentence. This is surprising because the early pioneers of abdominal surgery, going back to pre-anesthetic era, were, in the main, concerned with removal of ovarian masses. Indeed, the first elective abdominal operation for a known pathology was the removal of a massive ovarian cyst by Ephraim McDowell in Danville, Kentucky, in 1809. Yet, for some inexplicable reason, the surgeon would stand helplessly by the bedside and watch a young woman, in the most useful time of her existence, exsanguinate from her ruptured tube. The first surgeon to perform successful surgery in this condition was Robert Lawson Tait, of Birmingham, whom we have already mentioned performing a successful appendicectomy in 1880. Tait was asked to see a girl with a ruptured ectopic pregnancy by Dr. Hallwright, a general practitioner. Hallwright suggested that Tait should remove the ruptured tube. Tait recorded the following:

> The suggestion staggered me and I am afraid I did not receive it favourably. I declined to act and a further haemorrhage killed the patient. A post-mortem examination revealed the perfect accuracy of the diagnosis. I carefully inspected the specimen that was removed and found that if I had tied the broad ligament and removed the tube I should have completely arrested the haemorrhage, and I now believe that had I done this the patient's life would have been saved.

Eighteen months later, Tait operated on a clearly dying patient, the first occasion in which such an operation was performed. The patient, in those pretransfusion days, died of exsanguination. Finally, in March 1888, Tait performed a successful salpingectomy on such a case, who survived even though, at operation, the abdomen was full of clot. Years later, he was able to report 39 cases, with but two deaths, including the first.

Envoi

Even today, the acute abdomen presents a diagnostic and therapeutic challenge to the surgeon. This is in spite of the fact that we have the ancillary aids of radiology and other imaging, biochemical and haematological studies to help the diagnosis and blood transfusion, fluid replacement, nasogastric suction, antibiotics and skilled anesthetists to assist with therapy.

The study of surgical history shows that, occasionally, like the frog — we go one step forward, two steps back... (■ Figure 2.1).

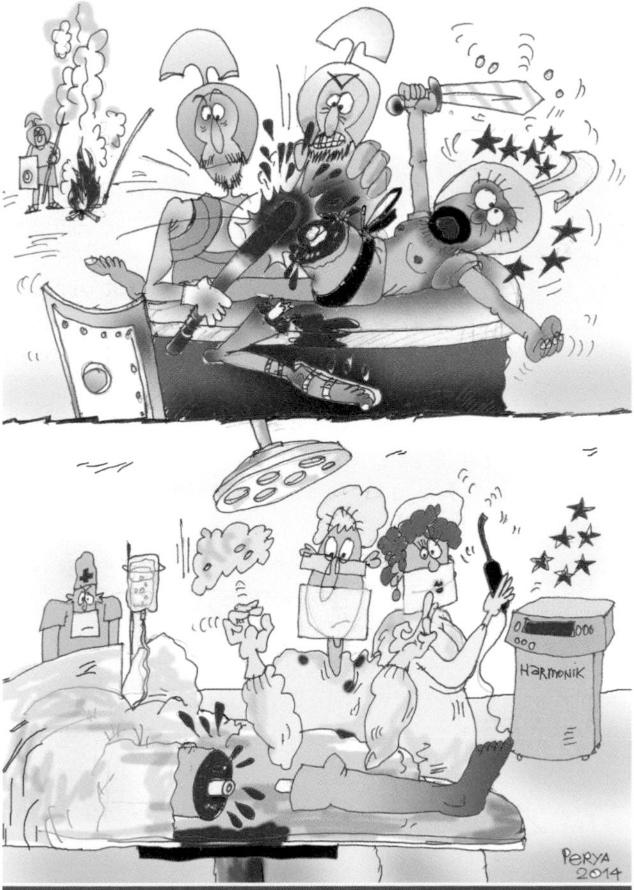

Figure 2.1. Great advance in surgery!

"Let us therefore look back with a mélange of amazement, pride, and humility at the efforts of our surgical forefathers as they paved the way for us in the management of this fascinating group of diseases!"

Harold Ellis

PART II

Before the operation

Chapter 3

The acute abdomen

The Editors [1]

For the abdominal surgeon it is a familiar experience to sit, ready scrubbed, and gowned, in a corner of the quiet theatre, with the clock pointing midnight. ...In a few minutes the patient will be wheeled in and another emergency laparotomy will commence. This is the culmination of a process which began a few hours previously with the surgeon meeting with and examining the patient, reaching a diagnosis, and making a plan of action.

Peter F. Jones

The general rule can be laid down that the majority of severe abdominal pains which ensue in patients who have been previously fairly well, and which last as long as six hours, are caused by conditions of surgical import.

Zachary Cope

Simply stated, the term 'acute abdomen' refers to abdominal pain of short duration that requires a decision regarding whether an urgent intervention is necessary. This clinical problem is the most common cause for you to be called upon to provide a surgical consultation in the emergency room, and serves as a convenient gateway for a discussion of the approach to abdominal surgical emergencies.

It is as much an intellectual exercise to tackle the problems of belly ache as to work on the human genome.

Hugh Dudley

---

[1] Asher Hirshberg, MD, contributed to this chapter in the first edition of this book.

The problem

Most major textbooks contain a long list of possible causes of acute abdominal pain. These 'big lists' usually go from perforated peptic ulcer down to such esoteric causes as porphyria and black widow spider bites. The lists are popular with medical students and residents in internal medicine, but are useless for practical guys like you.

The experienced surgeon called upon to consult a patient with acute abdominal pain in the emergency room (ER) in the middle of the night simply doesn't work this way. He or she doesn't consider the 50 or so 'most likely' causes of acute abdominal pain from the list, attempting to rule them out one by one. **Instead, the intelligent surgeon tries to identify a clinical pattern, and to decide upon a course of action from a limited menu of management options.** Below we will demonstrate how the multiple etiologies for acute abdominal pain actually converge into a small number of easily recognizable clinical patterns. Once recognized, each of these patterns dictates a specific course of action.

The acute abdomen: management menus and clinical patterns

The management options

Seeing a patient with an acute abdomen in the ER (■ Figure 3.1), you have only a few **management options** to choose from the following menu:

- **Immediate operation** ("surgery now... now... by now I mean now!"), e.g. gunshot wound, patient unstable.
- **Emergency operation** ("surgery within 2-3 hours... no need to run!"), e.g. perforated appendicitis.
- **Urgent operation** ("let us take some time and optimize the patient and operate tomorrow morning"), e.g. acute calculous cholecystitis.
- **Invasive non-surgical treatments** ("let's embolize the bleeder").
- **Conservative treatment — in the ICU if necessary** ("we plan to admit and treat with intravenous fluids, antibiotics, possibly image again. We may still decide to operate later").
- **Observation** ("we're not yet sure what's going on, might be medical. Let's watch").
- **Discharge home**.

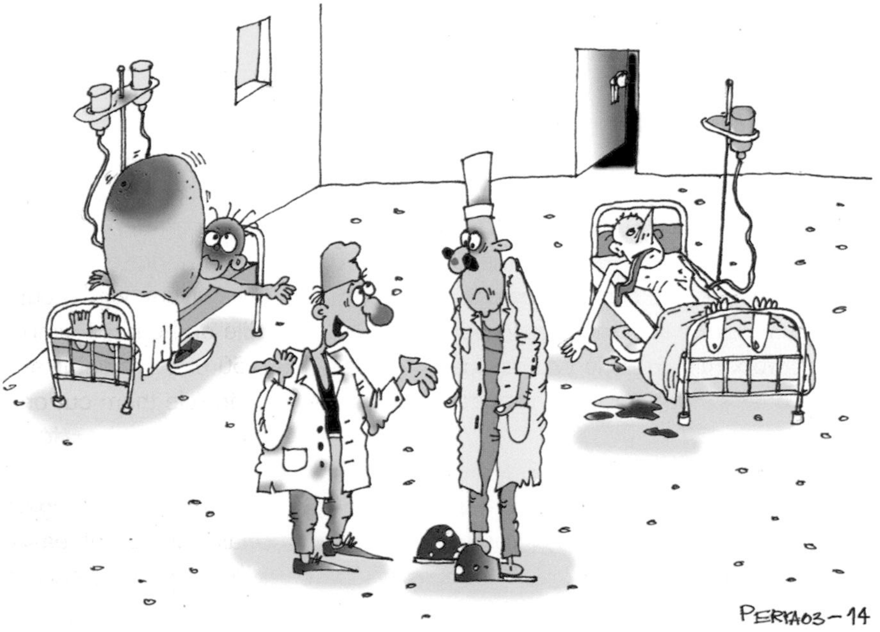

Figure 3.1. "Which of them has an 'acute abdomen'?"

The clinical patterns

The acute abdomen usually presents as one of the well-defined clinical patterns listed below:

- Abdominal pain and shock.
- Generalized peritonitis.
- Localized peritonitis (confined to one quadrant of the abdomen).
- Intestinal obstruction.
- Waste basket ('non-specific' abdominal pain or due to 'medical causes').
- Gynecological.
- Trauma.

The last two patterns (gynecological and trauma) are addressed elsewhere in this book. Occasionally a **mixed picture of obstruction/peritonitis** may present. For each of these clinical patterns you have to choose a management option from the aforementioned menu — **but your first task is to identify the specific pattern in order to know how to proceed!**

Abdominal pain and shock

This is the most dramatic and least common clinical pattern of the acute abdomen. The patient typically presents pale and diaphoretic, hypotensive and in severe abdominal pain, the so-called **abdominal apoplexy**. The two most common etiologies of this clinical pattern are a **ruptured abdominal aortic aneurysm** and a **ruptured ectopic pregnancy** (➲ Chapters 32 and 33). **For these two conditions the only management option is immediate surgery (or, in the case of a ruptured aneurysm, endovascular intervention) NOW!** No time should be wasted on 'preparation' and on ancillary investigations. Losing a patient with abdominal apoplexy in the CT scanner is a cardinal, and unfortunately not too rare, sin.

Note, however, that other abdominal emergencies may also present with abdominal pain and shock due to fluid loss into the 'third space'. This may occur for example in patients with **intestinal obstruction** (➲ Chapter 19), or **severe acute pancreatitis** (➲ Chapter 17) — particularly if neglected or superimposed on a deficient cardiovascular system. In many of these situations an emergency operation is not necessary; and — as we will be nagging you over and over again — **operating on a poorly resuscitated patient is like skating on thin ice**.

Generalized peritonitis

The clinical picture of generalized peritonitis consists of diffuse, severe abdominal pain in a patient who looks sick and toxic. The patient typically lies motionless, and has an extremely tender abdomen with 'peritoneal signs' consisting of board-like rigidity, rebound tenderness, and voluntary defense-guarding. **Surprisingly enough, less experienced clinicians occasionally miss the diagnosis entirely**. This is especially common in the geriatric patient who may have weak abdominal musculature or may not exhibit the classical peritoneal signs. Peritoneal signs are also difficult to elicit in the very obese patient where layers of fat are interposed between your hands and the intra-abdominal pathology.

The most common error in the physical examination of a patient with acute abdominal pain is rough and 'deep' palpation of the abdomen, which may elicit severe tenderness even in a patient without any abdominal pathology. Palpation of the abdomen should be very gentle, and should not hurt the patient. We appreciate that at this stage of your surgical career you do not need a detailed lecture on examination of the acute abdomen. Forgive us, however, for emphasizing that the absence of rebound tenderness means nothing and that a good way to elicit peritoneal irritation is by asking the patient to cough or by shaking (gently) his bed, or by very gentle percussion of the abdomen — starting away from the painful area and slowly moving towards it. **Deliberate demonstration of the clinical sign of rebound tenderness is cruel, unnecessary and to be deplored.**

The three most common causes of generalized peritonitis in adults are a perforated ulcer (➲ Chapter 16.2), **colonic perforation** (➲ Chapter 26), and **perforated appendicitis** (➲ Chapter 21). Classically, with exceptions listed below and in the individual chapters, the management of a patient with diffuse peritonitis is an emergency operation within a few hours (*surgery tonight*), after a brief period of pre-operative optimization as outlined in ➲ Chapter 6.

An important exception to this management option is the patient with acute pancreatitis. While most patients with acute pancreatitis present with mild epigastric tenderness, the occasional patient may present with a clinical picture mimicking diffuse peritonitis (➲ Chapter 17). **As a precaution against misdiagnosing these patients, it is essential practice always to measure the serum amylase (or lipase) in any patient presenting with significant abdominal symptoms** (➲ Chapter 4). Note, however, that amylase/lipase levels are not completely reliable but abdominal CT would establish the diagnosis in doubtful cases. **An exploratory laparotomy in a patient suffering from severe acute pancreatitis may lead to disaster; believe us — as we discovered in the pre-imaging era, when we were young and aggressive. Remember: God put the pancreas in the back because he did not want surgeons messing with it.**

Localized peritonitis

In the patient with localized peritonitis, the clinical signs are confined to one quadrant of the abdomen. Once you have decided which quadrant is the problem, there are only a few possible diagnoses from which to choose. Like the French Chief of Police said in the movie *Casablanca*: "Round up the usual suspects."

In the **right lower quadrant (RLQ)** the most common cause of localized peritonitis is **acute appendicitis** (➲ Chapter 21). In the **right upper quadrant (RUQ)** it is **acute cholecystitis** (➲ Chapter 18.1). In the **left lower quadrant (LLQ)** it is **acute diverticulitis** (➲ Chapter 26). What about the **left upper quadrant (LUQ)**? Peritonitis confined to this quadrant is uncommon, making this quadrant the 'silent one'. Well, not always so silent: you can see the occasional colonic diverticulitis or tumor perforation with an abscess high in the descending colon, or 'funny' splenic problems such as a splenic infarct, but usually these are only discovered with CT.

As a general rule, localized peritonitis is rarely an indication for an emergency operation — 'tonight'! As you will learn from the relevant chapters most episodes of **acute diverticulitis** can be managed without an operation (➲ Chapter 26). The majority of patients with **acute cholecystitis** will benefit from early cholecystectomy 'tomorrow', or within 72 hours, even though 'cooling' the gallbladder, followed by delayed surgery, is widely practiced (➲ Chapter 18.1). Even **acute appendicitis** is no longer considered a dire emergency — in most cases the operation can be postponed until the morning (➲ Chapter 21). Buy a copy of this book as a gift to your ER docs so that they too will understand...

What to do if the diagnosis is uncertain? Yes, even in this era of instant US or CT imaging this can happen! And, obviously, this situation is not so rare if you practice away from modern imaging technology. You should then admit the patient for observation, hydrate him with intravenous fluids, give antibiotics (e.g. if the diagnosis of acute cholecystitis or diverticulitis is entertained), and conduct serial physical exams. **Do not omit analgesia! Condemning the patient to suffer long periods of untreated pain in order "not to mask signs and symptoms of an undiagnosed abdominal disaster" is an outdated practice**. Instead, provide small doses of the good old (and cheap) morphine.

REMEMBER: ailments get better with time, <u>true</u> surgical problems get worse with time. Thus time is a superb diagnostician; when you return to the patient's bedside after a few hours you may find all the previously missing clues. Of course, after you have consulted the relevant chapters in this book...

In **women of fertile age**, lower abdominal peritonitis, on either side, tends to be gynecological in origin, and is commonly managed conservatively (➲ Chapter 33).

Intestinal obstruction

The clinical pattern of intestinal obstruction consists of central, colicky abdominal pain, distension, vomiting and constipation (➲ Chapters 19 and 25).

As a general rule the earlier and more pronounced the vomiting, the more proximal the site of obstruction is likely to be; on the other hand, the more marked the distension, the more distal is the site of obstruction. Thus, vomiting and colicky pain are more characteristic of small bowel obstruction, whereas constipation and gross distension are typical of colonic obstruction. However, the distinction between these two kinds of obstruction usually hinges on the plain abdominal X-ray — that is, if your ER doc still bothers obtaining it prior to the 'obligatory CT'.

There are two management options for these patients: a trial of conservative treatment, or operative treatment after adequate preparation. The major problem with intestinal obstruction is not in making the diagnosis but in deciding on the appropriate course of action. If the patient has a history of previous abdominal surgery and presents with small bowel obstruction but without signs of peritonitis, the working diagnosis is 'simple' adhesive small bowel obstruction. The initial management of these patients is conservative, with intravenous fluids and nasogastric tube decompression. In the presence of clinical features of **intestinal compromise** — fever, peritonitis, suggestive lab tests — the indication for operation is more persuasive. But, as always, in real life things are much more complicated so please read ➲ Chapter 19.

There are a few classic pitfalls with small bowel obstruction:

- The **'virgin' abdomen** (no previous abdominal surgery). Here, typically adhesion may not be the underlying cause. **Get a CT**. In these cases there is often a treatable cause for the obstruction, and it makes you feel good during the operation to have found it.
- The **missed groin hernia**. The elderly lady with no previous surgical history who presents with small bowel obstruction due to an *incarcerated femoral hernia*. **Always examine the groin!** Insist on patients having their pants and underpants off. The fact that modern ER docs tend to diagnose incarcerated inguinal hernias only on CT is sad. But we want you to detect such hernias on examination, prior to CT, which then becomes unnecessary.
- The **silent cecal cancer**. The patient with alleged 'simple' adhesive small bowel obstruction who improves on conservative treatment and is discharged, only to come back later with a large tumor mass in the right colon. **These cancers can act as a ball valve, causing intermittent obstruction of the ileocecal valve**.
- The **gallstone ileus**. The elderly lady whose partial small bowel obstruction resolves and recurs intermittently and is finally diagnosed as *gallstone ileus*. **Always look for air in the bile ducts on plain abdominal X-rays. If you don't think about it you will miss it!**

- The **post-gastric surgery patient**, who presents with intermittent episodes of obstruction originating from a *bezoar* in the terminal ileum.

Unlike small bowel obstruction, colon obstruction is almost always an indication for surgery — 'tonight' or 'tomorrow' but usually 'tomorrow'. A plain abdominal X-ray cannot make the diagnosis as functional **colonic pseudo-obstruction** (Ogilvie's syndrome) or chronic megacolon cannot reliably be distinguished from a mechanical obstruction. Thus, these patients need additional imaging (contrast enema, CT) or fiberoptic colonoscopy to clinch the diagnosis (➲ Chapter 25).

The abdominal 'waste basket'

- **Non-specific abdominal pain (NSAP).** Many patients with acute abdominal pain undergo a clinical examination and a limited 'negative' work-up — which today in many centers may include a CT scan — only to be labeled as "non-specific abdominal pain" (NSAP), and then discharged. **It is important to keep in mind that in an ER setting, more than half of patients presenting with acute abdominal pain have NSAP, with acute appendicitis, acute cholecystitis and 'gynecological causes', being the commonest 'specific' conditions.** But the exact pathology you see depends of course on your geographical location and pattern of practice. Just remember that patients discharged home labeled with a diagnosis of NSAP have an increased probability of a subsequent diagnosis of abdominal cancer or other lingering pathologies. Therefore, try to follow-up these patients and re-investigate if indicated.
- **Non-abdominal conditions can present with acute abdominal pain.** While most cases of inferior wall MI, lower lobe pneumonia, ketoacidosis and even the notorious porphyria will probably be diagnosed by the ER docs before they call you for 'surgical clearance', be aware not to fall into this dangerous trap.

Exploratory laparotomy or laparoscopy for the acute abdomen?

Many of us, old farts, were raised on the dictum that clinical peritonitis is an indication for abdominal exploration. Many of you, promising emerging stars, are nurtured with the concept of "let us insert a camera and see what's going on".

The notions that "peritonitis is an indication for operation" and that "only skin separates us from the diagnosis" developed before the days of modern abdominal imaging; but is this still true today, justifying opening the abdomen or inserting a scope, without resonable evidence of a surgical pathology necessitating an operation?

We do not think so. **We believe that modern abdominal imaging has revolutionized emergency abdominal surgery, and that if you have immediate access to abdominal CT and/or ultrasound you have to use it. This, as will be discussed in many of the following chapters, will avoid an operation in many patients, or make operative treatment less invasive and more specific. Thanks to CT the abdomen is no longer a black box**. Use abdominal imaging liberally for the benefit of your patients — especially when the diagnosis is not clearly evident. It is OK to operate on a young man with classicial features of acute appendicitis without a pre-operative CT; but a woman of child-bearing age needs abdominal imaging (probably US) to exclude gynecological conditions and so do elderly patients in whom other pathologies are more likely. **This is all just common sense really**.

The surgeon who strives for perfection
Needs some basis for patient selection
He would like to be sure
There's a good chance for cure
Before he begins the resection.

Elwood G. Jensen

Yes, what's common is common and what's rare is rare, but rare things can be lethal — always keep them in mind!

Who should look after the 'acute abdomen' and where?

Everybody's business is nobody's business.

Many patients suspected of having an acute abdomen or other abdominal emergencies do not require an operation. **Nevertheless, it is you — the surgeon — who should take, or be granted, the leadership in assessing, excluding or treating this condition, or at least play a major role in leading the managing team**. To emphasize how crucial this issue is, we dedicate an entire section of this chapter to it — although its scope would fit into a paragraph.

Unfortunately, in real life, surgeons are often denied the primary responsibility. Too often we see patients with **mesenteric ischemia** rotting away in medical wards, the surgeon being consulted "to evaluate the abdomen", only when the bowel is dead, and the patient is soon to be. A characteristic scenario is a patient with an abdominal surgical emergency, admitted under the care of non-surgeons who undertake a series of unnecessary, potentially harmful and expensive diagnostic and therapeutic procedures. Typically, internists, gastroenterologists, infectious-disease specialists and radiologists are involved, each prescribing his own wisdom in isolation (many treating the patient for '**CRPitis**' or **ECOUO** — elevated CRP of unknown origin...) (■ Figure 3.2). When, finally, the surgeon is called in, he finds the condition difficult to diagnose, partially treated or maltreated. Eventually, the indicated operation is performed, but too late and with a consequent higher morbidity and mortality. The etiology of such chaos is not entirely clear. **Motives of power, ego and financial opportunity are surely involved; it is politically correct to call this a 'system failure'.**

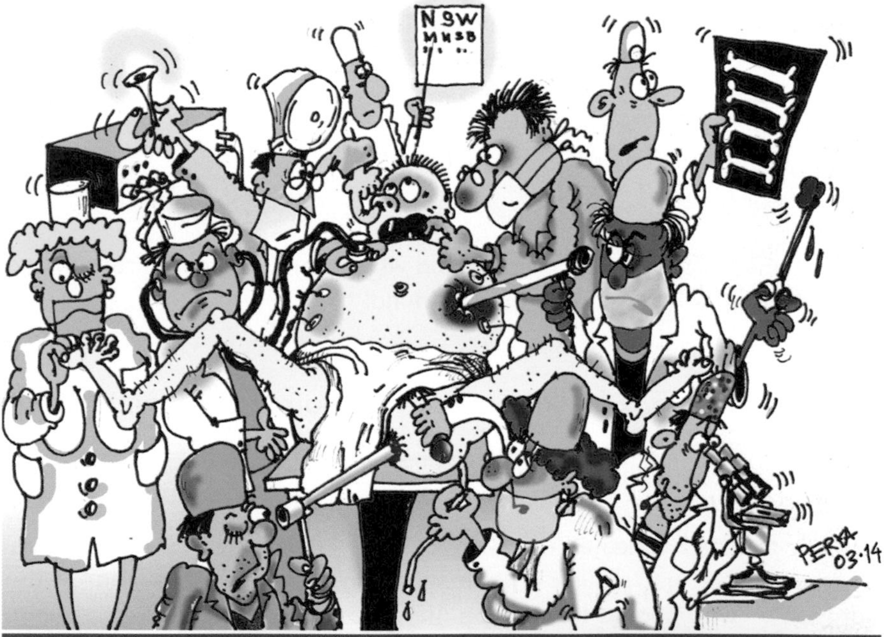

Figure 3.2. "Who is responsible?"

The team approach to the acutely ill surgical patient should not be discarded. The team, however, should be led and coordinated by a general surgeon. He is the one who knows the abdomen from within and without. He is the one qualified to call in consultants from other specialties, to order valuable tests, to veto those that are superfluous and wasteful. And, above all, he is the one who will eventually decide that enough is enough and the patient needs to be taken to the operating room.

When you decided to become a general surgeon you became the captain of the ship, navigating the deep ocean of the abdomen. Do not abandon your ship while the storm rages on!

Continuity of care is a *sine qua non* in the optimal care of the acute abdomen as the clinical picture, which may change rapidly, is a major determinant in the choice of therapy and its timing. Such patients need to be frequently reassessed by the same clinician, who should be a surgeon. Any deviation from this may be hazardous to the patient; this is our personal experience and that which is repeated *ad nauseum* in the literature. Why don't we learn? The place for the patient with an acute abdominal condition is on the surgical floor, surgical intensive care unit (ICU), or in the operating room and under the care of a surgeon — yourself. Don't duck your responsibilities!

The key for the 'best' outcome of the acute abdomen is:

- Operate only when necessary, and do the minimum possible.
- Do not delay a necessary operation, and do the maximum when indicated.

"The concept that one citizen will lay himself horizontal and permit another to plunge a knife into him, take blood, give blood, rearrange internal structures at will, determine ultimate function, indeed, sometimes life itself — that responsibility is awesome both in true and in the currently debased meaning of that word."

Alexander J. Walt

Chapter 4

Rational diagnostic procedures

The Editors [1]

To open an abdomen and search for a lesion as lightly as one would open a bureau drawer to look for the laundry, may mean lack of mental overwork to the surgeon, but it means horror to the patient.

J. Chalmers Da Costa

To see what is in front of one's nose needs a constant struggle.

George Orwell

The 21st century brought bad news to the surgical cowboys. In the good old days you examined the patient, observed the systemic signs of infection or inflammation, poked the abdomen with your delicate hands and noted "peritonitis" and hurrah — "take him to the OR", you exclaimed with gusto, bathing in the admiration of the nurses and the envy of the non-surgeons — *Gee, what a clinician!* But these days even the born cowboys must feign being tame farmers: in almost all cases one can now only go to the OR with an established, at least a strongly suspected, diagnosis!

When treating a patient with acute abdominal pain it is tempting to make extensive use of ancillary investigations. This leads to the emergence of 'routines' in the emergency room (ER) whereby every patient with acute abdominal pain undergoes a series of tests, which typically includes a complete blood count, blood chemistry and serum amylase and/or lipase, plus

1 Asher Hirshberg, MD, contributed to this chapter in the first edition of this book.

or minus whatever is fashionable, the *soup de jour* if you like; and such soup, it seems, is getting as thick as a minestrone, when eager young docs add to it bizarre ingredients such as D-dimer, calcitonin, and a plain X-ray of the abdomen (AXR). As you know, in many centers the latter has been replaced with the knee jerk of a CT. Many of these tests have a very low diagnostic yield and are not cost effective. **However, they are also an unavoidable part of life in the ER and are often, if not usually, obtained before the surgical consultation.**

For some surgeons the clinical finding of clear-cut *diffuse peritonitis* is still an indication to proceed with laparotomy or laparoscopy with no further imaging. But what appears clear-cut to the experienced surgeon — and remember that he too may be wrong — may be less so for you. **And please note the following caveats**:

- **Intestinal distension**, associated with obstruction or inflammation (e.g. enteritis or colitis) may produce diffuse abdominal tenderness — mimicking 'peritonitis'. The *whole* clinical picture along with the AXR will guide you toward the proper diagnosis (➲ Chapters 19 and 25).
- **Acute pancreatitis** may present with clinical acute peritonitis. You should always obtain a serum *amylase* or *lipase* level in any patient with significant abdominal pain to avoid falling into the **not uncommon trap of an unnecessary and dangerous operation** (➲ Chapter 17).
- ***Clostridium difficile* enterocolitis** should be considered in any patient who receives, or has recently received, any quantity of antibiotics. This may present — from the beginning — as an acute abdomen **without diarrhea**. Here, the optimal initial management is medical and not a laparotomy. Sigmoidoscopy and/or computed tomography (CT) may be diagnostic (➲ Chapter 24).

Blood tests

As stated above, 'routine labs' are of minimal value. In addition to amylase level the only 'routines' that can be supported are white cell count, hematocrit and baseline evaluation of renal function. An *elevated white cell count* denotes an inflammatory response. Be aware that acute cholecystitis or acute appendicitis can be present even when the white cell count is within the normal range. Its elevation, however, supports the diagnosis. Many surgeons are now convinced that *C-reactive protein (CRP)* levels are more sensitive in the diagnosis of an inflammatory response. It has entered most 'lab routines', but elevation may be delayed, and specificity is low. A low *hematocrit* in the emergency situation signifies a chronic or subacute anemia; it poorly reflects the magnitude of any acute hemorrhage. **However, in patients receiving i.v. fluids, a low hematocrit commonly indicates hemodilution**. *Liver function tests* are of value in patients with right upper quadrant pain, diagnosed to have acute cholecystitis (note: liver function tests may be normal or nearly normal in acute cholecystitis; rely on clinical examination and ultrasound) or cholangitis (➲ Chapter 18). **Low serum *albumin* on admission is a useful marker of the severity of the acute, or acute-on-chronic disease, and is also of proven prognostic value**. When operating, for example, on someone with albumin levels of 1.5g/dL you know that you have to do the minimum and to expect trouble after the operation; and, as you will hear repeatedly below, to avoid an intestinal anastomosis.

Remember: Whichever tests are ordered, either by you or by someone else on your behalf (usually the ER doctor), be aware that the significance of the results should never be judged in isolation but considered as part of the whole clinical picture.

Radiological studies

Chest X-ray (CXR)

An erect CXR is routinely obtained to search for **free air under the diaphragm**, as this is demonstrated in the majority of patients with perforated peptic ulcer (➲ Chapter 16). With **colonic perforation**, the amount of free air seen on an upright CXR can range from none to huge, from a few bubbles of localized perforation of diverticulitis to the abdominal ballooning after a colonoscopic tear — ➲ Chapters 26 and 29. Remember that free air is better seen on an erect CXR than an abdominal one. **Free intraperitoneal air is not always caused by a perforated viscus and it is not always an indication for an operation**. There is a long list of 'non-operative' conditions that may produce free intraperitoneal air, such as a tension pneumothorax or even vigorous *cunnilingus* (oral sex). So, don't diagnose in haste, look at the whole clinical picture.

Any textbook tells you that lower lobe pneumonia may mimic an acute abdomen, so think about it. Obviously, findings such as lung metastases or pleural effusion may hint at the cause of the abdominal condition and influence treatment and prognosis. Pneumothorax, pneumomediastinum or pleural effusion may be associated with spontaneous esophageal perforation —

Boerhaave syndrome, which can present as an acute abdomen. **The value of a CXR in blunt or penetrating abdominal injury is obvious — a chest tube inserted before the operation for a small pneumothorax would prevent a life-threatening tension pneumothorax during the operation; you surely understand why (yes, we know there are myth-hunters that challenge even that...).** A pre-operative CXR may also be requested by the anesthesiologists, especially after you have inserted a central venous line, or indeed for no reason at all.

Finally, and rarely, be aware that what looks to you on chest radiography like free air under the right diaphragm is not free air but bowel (usually the hepatic flexure of the colon) interposed between the liver and diaphragm. This entity is named after the Austrian radiologist who described it: Dr. Chilaiditi. If asymptomatic it is termed the "**Chilaiditi sign**". When symptoms are attributed to it (subcostal pain, constipation, respiratory distress), it becomes the "**Chilaiditi syndrome**". We have never encountered this 'syndrome', but others claim (please don't believe them) an occasional need for its operative treatment with 'colopexy' or colectomy! In uncertain cases abdominal CT shows the 'free air' to be in the colon.

Plain abdominal X-ray (AXR)

This is the classical surgeon's X-ray, as only surgeons know the true value of these simple and cheap radiographs. Radiologists can look at and talk about AXRs forever, searching for findings that could justify additional imaging studies. We surgeons need only a few seconds to decide whether the AXR is 'non-specific', namely, does not show any obvious abnormality, or shows an **abnormal gas pattern** or **abnormal opacities**. Unfortunately, in many of today's 'modern' ERs the humble AXR is bypassed in favor of the CT. In fact now, for many (but we hope not for you), the CT supplants not only the AXR but also proper history taking and physical examination. **Do not forget that we operate on patients and not only on CT abnormalities**. Go to ➲ Chapter 5 to read about AXRs in detail.

Abdominal ultrasound (US)

Abdominal US is a readily available diagnostic modality in most places. Its reliability is operator-dependent; the ideal situation is when the US is performed and interpreted by an experienced clinician — a surgeon. And, in fact, many surgeons are trained to use US as part of the physical examination (Point-of-care US, POCUS). We recommend you become a wizard by attending a (Hocus) POCUS course. US is very accurate in the diagnosis of acute cholecystitis (➲ Chapter 18); it is also used by gynecologists to rule out acute pelvic pathology in female patients (➲ Chapter 33), and to demonstrate urological pathologies such as hydronephrosis (➲ Chapter 35). A non-compressible tubular structure (a 'small sausage') in the right lower quadrant may be diagnostic of acute appendicitis, but as will be discussed in ➲ Chapter 21, there are more accurate modes to reach this diagnosis. US is useful in demonstrating intra-abdominal fluid — be it ascites, pus, or blood, localized or diffuse. In blunt abdominal trauma, FAST (focused abdominal sonography for trauma) has almost replaced the use of diagnostic peritoneal lavage. An US-guided aspiration of unexplained intraperitoneal fluid can clarify the diagnosis: is it bile or pus or feces? What is the level of amylase, bilirubin and creatinine in the fluid? This gives you an idea of what's going on (see ➲ Chapter 30).

Abdominal computed tomography

The use of the CT scan in the acute abdomen remains a subject of some controversy. While it is true that a CT scan should *not* be part of the management algorithm in *all* patients with acute abdominal pain, **the existing spiral CT technology is nevertheless immediately available and very powerful. The temptation to use it is strong, especially among less experienced clinicians and those who are more experienced but wish to achieve an early and accurate diagnosis and avoid unnecessary procedures**.

The major role of CT, where it can really make a critical difference, is with 'clinical puzzles'. Not infrequently, the surgeon encounters a patient with acute abdominal pain that does not fit any of the clinical patterns described in ➲ Chapter 3. Under these circumstances, CT is very helpful in identifying a significant intra-abdominal problem. **It is even better in *excluding* the latter by being absolutely normal** — letting you go home and pour an inch or so on the rocks. Know the feeling? Finally, the indispensable role of CT in abdominal trauma is discussed later (➲ Chapter 30).

The use of CT may help in avoiding surgery altogether — where previously 'negative', 'exploratory' or 'non-therapeutic' operations would have been performed. It may suggest that alternative percutaneous treatment is possible and, even if an operation is still required, it may indicate the best incision and approach (➲ Chapter 10). CT has a definite role in the post-laparotomy patient as discussed in Part IV — "After the operation". For a detailed discussion on the interpretation of abdominal CT go to ➲ Chapter 5.

Contrast studies: barium vs. water-soluble contrast

In previous editions we elaborated about barium and its risks as a contrast medium in emergency situations, but luckily it is now hardly available, and anyway most radiologists hate the messy fluorography and prefer CT, being a little away from the patient.

A GI contrast study in the emergency situation has only two queries to answer:

- **Is there a leak and, if so, where?** (Remember that the absence of a contrast leak does not completely exclude a bowel perforation.)
- **Is there an obstruction and, if so, where?** (Do realize that a contrast CT is much more accurate in defining the site and cause of any obstruction and in addition gives other useful information about the condition of the bowel.)

For these purposes **Gastrografin®** (or any water-soluble agent) is adequate. Use Gastrografin® in upper gastrointestinal studies to document or exclude gastric outlet obstruction, treat small bowel obstruction or postoperative ileus (➲ Chapters 19 and 41) or instil as an enema to diagnose colonic obstruction or perforation. Unlike barium, water-soluble contrast is harmless should it leak into the peritoneal cavity.

A piece of general advice: do communicate with the radiologists and radiographers. As Leo Gordon says: "**The quality of the X-ray ordered is directly proportional to the specificity of the clinical information supplied to the radiologist**." Talk to your radiologist, in person or on the phone; often, once your questions and worries are expressed he or she would suddenly see what was previously missed.

We deplore (the word 'despise' may be not too strong) residents, or doctors in general, who cite from radiological reports without ever seeing the actual images. **Our method: check the images first, make a conclusion, and then check the radiology report to see if the radiologist agrees with your diagnosis**. Viewing the images together with the radiologist is often a surprisingly productive exercise — even on the phone with a radiologist sitting in Mumbai or Hawaii.

Unnecessary tests

Dr. Lope Estevez Schwarz of Berlin shared with us this attractive German phrase: "Wer viel misst, misst viel Mist" — **free translation: people who test too much tend to get bullshit...** Amen!

Unnecessary testing is plaguing modern medical practice (■ Figure 4.1). Look around you and notice that the majority of investigations being ordered do not add much to the quality of care. These unnecessary tests are expensive and potentially harmful. In addition to the therapeutic delay they may cause, be familiar with the following paradigm: **the more non-indicated tests you order, the more false-positive results are obtained, which in turn compel you to order more tests and lead to additional, potentially harmful, diagnostic and therapeutic interventions. Eventually, you lose control... and, sadly, you create VOMIT (victims of modern imaging technology)**.

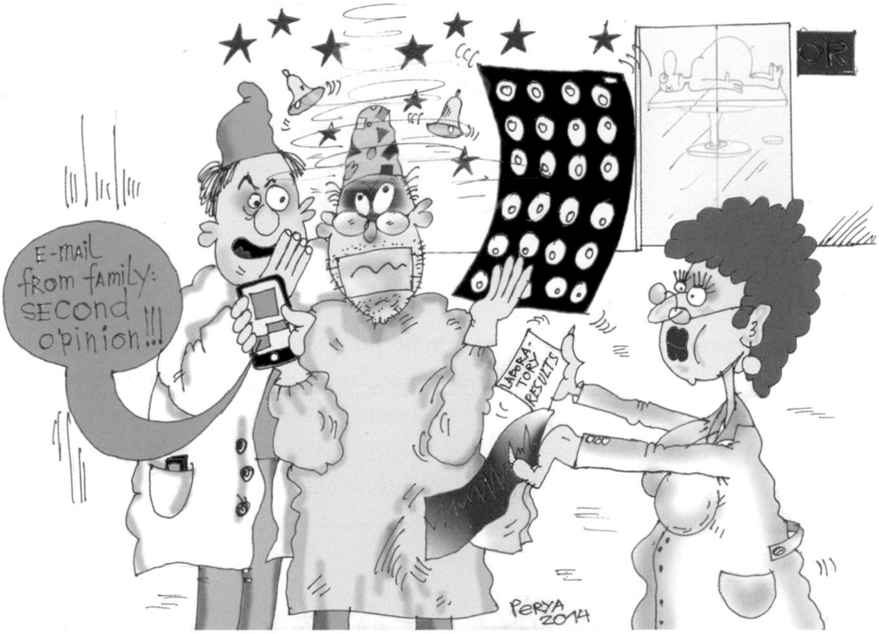
E-mail from family: SECOND opinion!!!
LABORA-TORY RESULTS
OR
PERYA 2014

Figure 4.1. Rational diagnostic procedures. "Boss, get an MRI!"

What are the reasons for unnecessary tests? The etiology is a combination of ignorance, lack of confidence, and laziness. When abdominal emergencies are initially assessed by non-surgeons who do not 'understand' the abdomen, unnecessary imaging is requested to compensate for ignorance. Junior clinicians who lack confidence tend to order tests "just to be sure — not to miss" a rare disorder. And experienced clinicians occasionally ask for an abdominal CT over the phone in order to procrastinate. Isn't it easier to ask for a CT rather than to drive to the hospital in the middle of the night, or to interrupt the golf game, and examine the patient? ("Let's do the CT and decide in the morning...").

An occasional surgical trainee finds it difficult to understand "what's wrong with excessive testing?" "Well," we explain, "Why do we need you at all? Let us all go home instead, and instruct our ER nurses to drive all patients with abdominal pain through a predetermined line of tests and imaging modalities." But patients are not cars on a production line. They are individuals who need your continuous judgment and selective use of tests.

Perhaps the day is near when all patients on their way from the ambulance to the ER will be passed through a total body CT scanner — read by a computer. But then luckily we will not be practicing surgery and this book will be long out of print. We do not believe, however, that patients will fare better under such a system.

Believe nobody — question everything... the more the noise — the less the fact.

Diagnostic laparoscopy

This is an invasive diagnostic tool (some call it "controlled penetrating abdominal trauma") to be used under anesthesia in the operating room, after the decision to intervene has been already taken. It has a selective role as discussed in ➲ Chapter 12. Yes, frequently, it is tempting "just to have a peek" and solve the diagnostic dilemmas, at the small price of a few small scars and the advantage of avoiding the radiation associated with a CT scan. For some, diagnostic laparoscopy is seen as an extension of the imaging effort, and not as 'real' surgery.

Remember: **We should not forget that this is indeed a surgical procedure, for which we need a sound indication. Complications, as well as unnecessary interventions (like removing a normal appendix), are part of the package deal.**

Before ending we wish to cite yet again Leo Gordon: "The emergency room is the best place to evaluate an emergency." Think about what investigations you wish to order while the patient is still in the ER; logistically, in most hospitals, it will be more difficult to obtain all these tests after the patient has been admitted.

"God gave you ears, eyes, and hands; use them on the patient in that order."

William Kelsey Fry

Chapter 5

Abdominal imaging

The Editors [1]

The diagnostic problem of today
Has greatly changed — the changes have come to stay;
We all have come to confess, though with a sigh
On complicated tests we much rely
And use too little hand and ear and eye.

Zachary Cope, *The Acute Abdomen in Rhyme*

Armed with a good understanding of the natural history of disease processes, and able to correlate radiological imaging with the clinical scenario, or previous operative observations, we surgeons should be well positioned to interpret abdominal imaging — at least as well as the radiologists. We have already discussed (➲ Chapter 4) the role of abdominal imaging in the evaluation of the patient with an acute abdomen. In this chapter we will try to provide you with practical tips on **how to look at the images and what to look for.**

To save space (we have laboured to reduce the bulk of this book) we decided to eliminate a few radiological images from this edition. **Instead, we suggest that you go to Google Images, enter the type of study and the presumed diagnosis and view the numerous examples of what you want to see.**

---

[1] Hans Ulrich Elben, MD, contributed to this chapter in the previous editions of this book.

Plain abdominal X-ray (AXR)

Tragically, this simple, cheap and safe X-ray is increasingly bypassed in favor of an immediate computed tomography (CT) scan — which delivers a much greater radiation dose. This is a pity because there is so much that you can learn from a quick glance at the AXR.

Look for abnormal gas patterns

Gas outside the lumen of the bowel:

- **'Free air'** (pneumoperitoneum) is best seen on an erect chest X-ray (CXR; ➲ Chapter 4) but may also be seen on an AXR. If the CXR and AXR are 'normal' and you suspect perforation of a viscus, a **left lateral decubitus** abdominal film may show free gas in the peritoneal cavity.
- Make a habit of always looking for **atypical gas patterns** — occasionally you may be rewarded with an eye-popping diagnosis: **gas in the biliary tree** (pneumobilia) implies either a cholecysto-enteric fistula (see gallstone ileus; ➲ Chapter 19), a previous enterobiliary bypass or, more commonly, a sphincterotomy of the sphincter of Oddi (via endoscopic retrograde cholangiopancreatography [ERCP]). Note that gas in the intrahepatic biliary ducts is seen *centrally*, while gas in the *periphery* of the liver suggests **portal vein gas**. The gas finds its way into the portal venous system through a breach in the bowel wall — usually associated with **mesenteric ischemia** or **severe colitis** — and rarely with *pylephlebitis*. Commonly, gas in the portal vein as a result of ischemic small or large bowel is associated with **pneumatosis intestinalis**, i.e. the presence of gas within the bowel wall.
- **Gas in the gallbladder wall** signifies a necrotizing infection (➲ Chapter 18). A **soap-bubble appearance** signifies free gas in the *retroperitoneum*; in the epigastrium this is associated with *infected pancreatic necrosis* (➲ Chapter 17), in the right upper quadrant with a retroperitoneal *perforation of the duodenum*, and in either gutter it is associated with retroperitoneal *perforation of the colon.*

Note that all these types of pathological air pattern are much easier to detect on CT images.

Gas pattern within the lumen of the bowel:

- Abnormal gaseous distension/dilatation of **small bowel loops**, with or without fluid levels, implies a small bowel process — be it *obstructive* (small bowel obstruction, ➲ Chapter 19), *paralytic* (ileus), ➲ Chapter 41) or *inflammatory* (e.g. Crohn's disease, ➲ Chapter 24). **Remember — *acute gastroenteritis* may produce small bowel air-fluid levels; the diarrhea hints at the diagnosis.**
- Abnormal gaseous distension/dilatation of the **colon** denotes colonic *obstruction* or *volvulus* (➲ Chapter 25), colonic *inflammation* (inflammatory bowel disease, ➲ Chapter 24) or colonic *ileus* (pseudo-obstruction, ➲ Chapter 25).

Distinguishing small bowel from colon on an AXR is easy: the 'transverse lines' go all the way across the diameter of the small bowel (the *valvulae conniventes*) and only partly across the colon (the *haustra*). In general, loops of small bowel are situated centrally while large bowel occupies the periphery. Well, we will let you see these images here — ■ Figure 5.1.

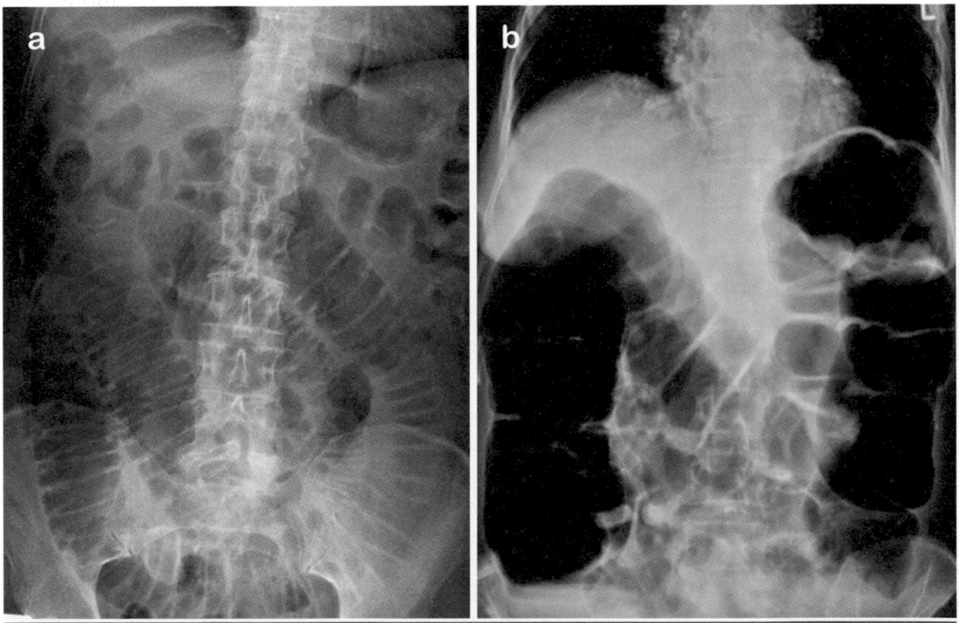

Figure 5.1. Abdominal X-ray: small bowel vs. large bowel. a) Small bowel obstruction. Note the valvulae conniventes crossing the whole width of small bowel. b) Distal obstruction of the colon. Note the haustra crossing a portion of bowel width.

Useful hints:

- Gaseous distension of small bowel + no gas in the colon = **complete small bowel obstruction**.
- Gaseous distension of small bowel + minimal quantity of colonic gas = **partial small bowel obstruction**.
- Significant gaseous distension of both the small bowel and the colon = **paralytic ileus**.
- Significant gaseous distension of the colon + minimal distension of the small bowel = **colonic obstruction or pseudo-obstruction**. (The magnitude of small bowel distension proximal to large bowel obstruction depends on the competence, or incompetence, of the ileocecal valve.)

Abnormal opacities

The opacities which you are able to spot on the AXR are the **calcified ones**: *gallstones* in the gallbladder (visible in about one-fifth of patients with cholelithiasis), *ureteric stones* (visible in some patients with ureteral colic), *pancreatic calcifications* (seen in some patients with chronic pancreatitis), and *appendicular fecaliths* (occasionally seen in patients with appendicitis). Clinically irrelevant calcified lesions that are common include *phleboliths* in the pelvis and calcified lymph nodes in the right iliac fossa, usually associated with previous tuberculosis. *Fecal matter* may opacify the rectum and colon to a variable degree — achieving extreme proportions in patients with fecal impaction. Note that a moderate amount of fecal material in the right colon is normal, while a column of feces on the left implies some abnormality, ranging in severity from simple constipation to early malignant obstruction. Another opacity, which may surprise you, is a forgotten surgical instrument or gauze swab. Also, **massive ascites** has a typical picture on AXR (■ Figure 5.2).

The simple abdominal X-ray is an extension of your clinical evaluation, which is not complete without it.

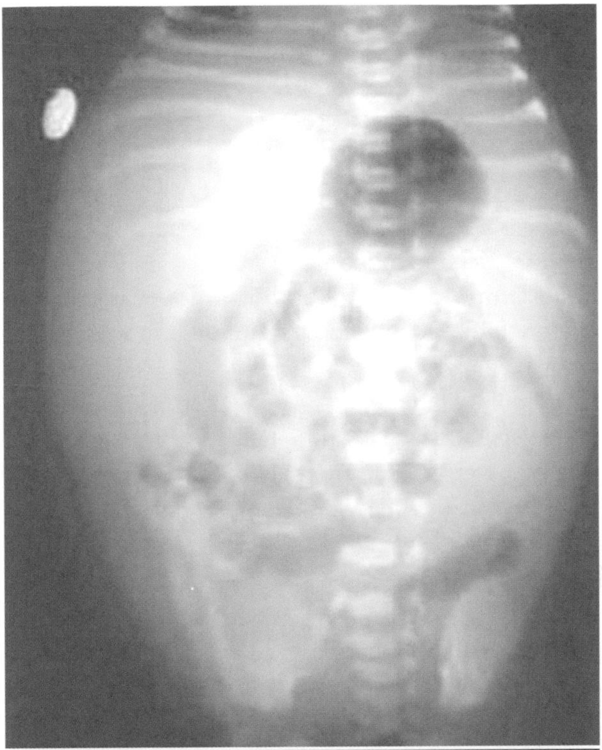

Figure 5.2. Abdominal X-ray demonstrating massive ascites. In the supine position the bowel gas lies centrally and there is nothing peripherally. The lighter bowel loops are practically floating on a lake of ascites in the abdominal cavity.

Computed tomography in abdominal emergencies

The road to the operating room does not always have to pass through the CT scanner but an appropriately indicated CT may obviate the need for a surgical journey.

The supremacy of CT in the imaging of the abdomen is not in dispute. CT shows details that no other diagnostic method does: free gas, fluid, masses, tissue planes, inflammatory changes, opacities, blood vessels and organ perfusion. **So why should we object to the indiscriminate use of CT as practiced today in many countries around the world?**

We object for the simple reason that in many patients the diagnosis can be established without CT — the obtaining of which can delay treatment, and confuse the picture by showing non-significant findings (see ➲ Chapter 4).

Typically, whenever radiologists publish papers on the use of CT in various abdominal emergencies they always declare sensitivity and specificity rates approaching 100%. When surgeons, however, look objectively at the overall impact of CT on the diagnosis and treatment of specific conditions, the real impact of CT tends to be less impressive.

In addition, remember that the radiation exposure of one abdominal CT examination can be several hundred times that of a chest X-ray. **According to the US Food and Drug Administration this amount of radiation exposure may be associated with a small increase in radiation-associated cancer in an individual.** This is particularly relevant if people were to receive this examination repeatedly, starting at a young age — as in the young lady presenting with lower abdominal pain to an ER in Brooklyn, where CT shows an ovarian cyst. Two weeks later she shows up at another ER in the Bronx where another CT shows (surprise!) the same cyst. And of course, somebody has to pay for the CT...

> **The key word in the effective use of abdominal CT is 'selectivity'.** Rather than indicating a need for exploration, CT is more useful in deciding when NOT to operate — avoiding unnecessary 'exploratory' laparotomies or 'diagnostic' laparoscopies. Also, a 'normal CT' can exclude surgical abdominal conditions — allowing the early discharge of patients without the need for admission for observation.

The introduction of fast scanners that image the abdomen from the diaphragm to the pubis in a single breath has greatly improved the image quality and reduced the time required to obtain the images. However, it does require that patients be transported to the CT suite and exposes them to the risks of aspiration of oral contrast media and adverse reactions to intravenous (i.v.) contrast media such as anaphylaxis and **nephrotoxicity**. Unenhanced (no i.v. contrast) helical or spiral CT scans are being increasingly used in suspected appendicitis, while CTs without oral contrast have been reported as accurate in patients suffering from blunt abdominal trauma. **Whatever the CT methodology in your hospital, you — who knows the abdomen inside out and understands the natural history of abdominal diseases — have to be able to analyze the CT images better than the radiologist.**

As is the case with all imaging studies, interpretation of CT scan images requires a systematic approach, and it takes plenty of practice to become confident in one's own ability. One also needs to spend time, and the more time you spend the more findings — both negative and positive — you pick up. We are going to describe the way we look at a CT scan of the abdomen; it is not 'ideal' or 'perfect' but it works for us, especially in the middle of the night when senior radiologists are hard to find. In the morning they will, with *latte* in hand, dictate detailed reports. **This is when you have to go over the images with them — you will be surprised how often, now, equipped with the accurate clinical information you provide, they will see something that was missed at night**. Just think how often the final report dictated in the morning differs from the preliminary one penned at night...

Spend a few hours on YouTube where you will find excellent clips on how to look at abdominal CT studies.

It is important to pay attention to a few technical aspects of the study before beginning to interpret it. While there is a lot of literature to support the notion that there is no need for oral or intravenous contrast material, the use of contrast improves *your* own diagnostic yield. One exception to this is when *ureteric calculi* are at the top of the differential diagnosis list and a non-contrast study gives almost all the information required.

Contraindications to intravenous contrast medium:

- **Impaired renal function** (consult your hospital protocol, remember the importance of pre-CT hydration).
- **History of prior allergic reaction** to iodinated contrast medium.
- **Severe asthma** or congestive heart failure.
- **Diabetic patient** on metformin (if renal function is normal you can use intravenous contrast but metformin should be stopped for 2 days thereafter).
- **Multiple myeloma** or **sickle-cell anemia**.
- **Pheochromocytoma** — i.v. contrast may precipitate a hypertensive crisis.

Reviewing the abdominal CT

- It is important to note the **distance between two CT 'slices'**. Usually the technologists use 5mm intervals between the slices but it is sometimes helpful to request 3mm cuts of the appendiceal area in a clinically difficult case. Most hospitals nowadays have done away with hard copies and introduced instead Picture Archiving and Communication Systems (PACS), which make access to images easier. In the latter case, scrolling through the scan gives information that is much easier to interpret than if individual films are examined.

- We always begin with a good look at the **scout film**; it provides similar information to a flatplate of the abdomen and provides a 'global view'.
- The visualized portions of the **lower lung fields** should also be looked at in both *mediastinal* and *lung windows*. Pulmonary infiltrates and pleural effusions can be easily identified and at times are a reflection of an acute sub-diaphragmatic process. An unsuspected pneumothorax in a trauma patient will also be obvious in the lung windows.
- Whilst it is easier to concentrate on the **area of interest** (e.g. the right lower quadrant in a patient with suspected appendicitis) and look for findings to support or exclude the diagnosis, **it is essential to look at the rest of the abdomen**. One needs to look specifically for the presence of free gas and free fluid, and to see all the solid organs (liver, spleen, kidneys, pancreas), the hollow ones (stomach, small and large bowel), and blood vessels. **One key point is to follow the structure in question in serial images (stacking) to obtain as much information as possible**.
- It is important to visualise the abdominal contents both in the **transverse-axial** (up-down) as well as the **vertical-coronal** plane (front-back), as the images tend to supplement each other. The sagittal-lateral cuts (from left to right) have their uses as well — for example, helping the location of abdominal wall hernias, or visualising the mesenteric vessels emerging from the aorta.
- Viewing the images with the PACS you can calculate the **Hounsfield Units** (HU) for the various structures you see. To remind you take a look at ■ Table 5.1 overleaf.

A few additional tips:

- **Pneumoperitoneum**. While an erect chest film can identify a straightforward case of pneumoperitoneum, a CT scan is the most sensitive means available for its detection. On a CT scan, gas collects beneath the two rectus muscles around the falciform ligament. It also collects between the liver and anterior abdominal wall and within the 'leaves' of the mesentery. The findings are at times very subtle and only a few bubbles of extraluminal gas are all that is required to make the diagnosis of pneumoperitoneum. **The key to the identification of extraluminal gas is inspection of all the scans of the abdomen in *lung windows***. It is easier with PACS as we can manipulate the window settings. Even if your hospital belongs to the dark ages and

Table 5.1. CT Hounsfield Units (HU) for various structures.

Structure	HU
Bone	1000
Liver	40-60
Blood#	40
Muscle	10-40
Kidney	30
Water	0
Fat	-50-100
Air	-1000

A fresh clot could measure over 70 Hounsfield Units; fresh blood measures about 40 HU, but if you come back the next day or two, it is as little as 20 HU.

does not have PACS, the CT scan station will have the ability to do this.

- **Free fluid**. Free fluid from any source tends to accumulate in the most dependent parts of the peritoneal cavity — Morrison's hepatorenal pouch and the pelvis. When there is a large amount of fluid the bowel loops float to the midline. In addition to identifying the presence of fluid, measurement of the fluid density offers some clues regarding its nature: less than 15 HU for transudative ascites, and more than 30 HU for exudative ascites or blood.
- **Solid organs**. While solid organ pathology is a rare cause of non-traumatic acute abdominal conditions, CT is the modality of choice in the investigation of the hemodynamically stable victim of blunt abdominal trauma. *Lacerations* of the solid organs appear as linear or branching low-attenuation areas. *Subcapsular hematomas* appear as crescentic low-attenuation areas at the periphery. *Intraparenchymal hematomas* appear as round or oval collections of blood within the parenchyma.
- **Hollow organs**. The entire gastrointestinal tract from the stomach to rectum can be traced in serial sections and abnormalities should be sought. In the case of small bowel obstruction, the cause (e.g. intussusception, tumor or inflammatory mass) and the site of obstruction (the *transition point*) can be identified. The presence of *pneumatosis* can be identified more readily with CT than a plain film and, if present, suggests intestinal ischemia. (Remember, however,

that there are benign causes of pneumatosis and, as always, correlation with the clinical picture is essential.) CT is also sensitive for identifying inflammation, which is suggested by the appearance of tissue infiltration or *stranding*. If i.v. contrast has been administered, then reduced enhancement of loops of bowel may signal ischemia. Similarly, the origins of the *mesenteric vessels* may be inspected — best seen in the sagittal axis slices at the abdominal aortic plane — to get some idea about patency. Clots within the portal and/or mesenteric veins would provide evidence for the diagnosis of venous mesenteric ischemia.

- **Acute appendicitis** (➲ Chapter 21). The various CT scan findings that are associated with **acute appendicitis** are:
  - **appendiceal signs**:
    - appendix >6mm in diameter;
    - failure of the appendix to fill with oral contrast or gas to its tip;
    - enhancement of the appendix with i.v. contrast;
    - appendicolith.
  - **peri-appendiceal signs**:
    - increased fat attenuation (stranding) in the right lower quadrant;
    - cecal wall thickening;
    - phlegmon in the right lower quadrant;
    - abscess or extraluminal gas;
    - fluid in the right lower quadrant or pelvis.

Remember: when the appendix is not visualized on the CT, and no secondary local inflammatory changes are seen, the diagnosis of acute appendicitis becomes extremely unlikely!

- **Colon**. The presence of diverticula plus stranding in the left lower quadrant, plus thickening of the sigmoid colon suggests *acute diverticulitis* (➲ Chapter 26). Diffuse thickening of the colon suggests an inflammatory process like *colitis* whether infective or ischemic.
- The **retroperitoneum** including the *pancreas* should be looked at; the presence of stranding and fluid collections around the pancreas suggests *acute pancreatitis* (➲ Chapter 17). Retroperitoneal hematoma next to an abdominal aortic aneurysm suggests that the aneurysm is leaking.
- **Pelvic organs**. It is also important to look at the pelvic organs in female patients. Particular attention should be paid to any large cystic masses in the adnexa, which may suggest a complicated cyst, ovarian torsion or a tubo-ovarian abscess.

Your patient doesn't require a CT ticket to enter the OR (■ Figure 5.3), but often CT will change your operative plans or even cancel the need for the operation.

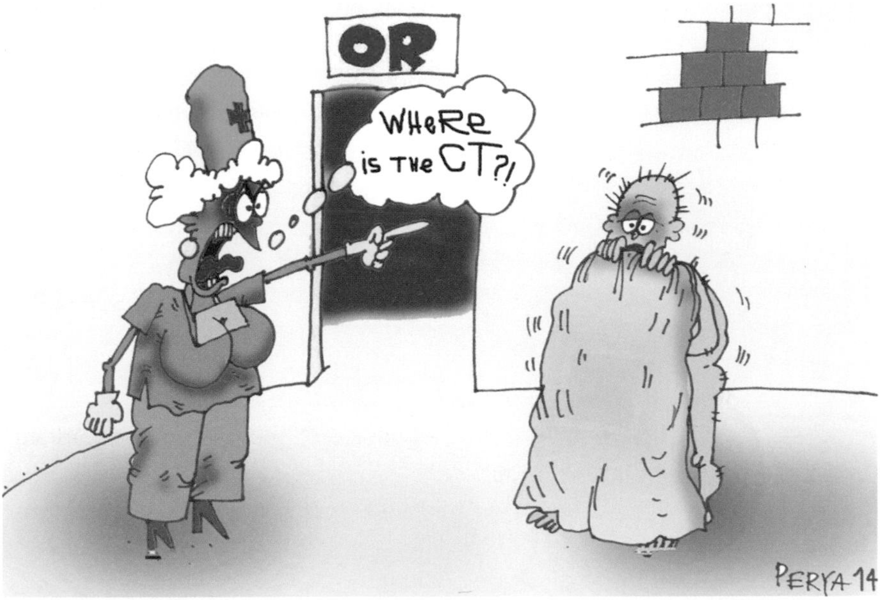

Figure 5.3. You do not need a CT ticket to enter the operating room!

Unfortunately or fortunately — depending on one's viewpoint — in the USA where I practice, the decision about whom and when to scan is no longer in our surgical hands. Aren't we losing control? **The fact of the matter is that most (if not all) patients have already undergone a CT scan before we surgeons are called upon to assess them.** Typically, emergency room physicians or other specialists order such scans before consulting the surgeon. In most hospitals in the USA, even the tiny rural ones, high-tech CT images are much easier to obtain than a gourmet meal or even a cup of *real* coffee. Moreover, radiologists are always readily available to interpret the images in-house or online. No wonder then that physicians and allied providers confronted with what they perceive to be an acute abdomen feel compelled to get a CT. **Is this practice of (almost) routine CT scanning, imposed on us by others, and impossible for us to modify or reverse, 'good' or 'bad' for our patients?** It is very difficult, if not impossible, to prove scientifically that this increased use of CT scanning is beneficial overall. **But what about the individual patient?**

Luckily, gone are the days when the acute abdomen represented a totally black box — days I remember well from my training — when peritoneal signs on examination mandated a laparotomy — which often proved to be 'negative' or 'non-therapeutic', and therefore unnecessary. The gradual introduction of CT imaging (and ultrasound) has made that abdominal black box much more penetrable and less mysterious. **In the individual patient it helps us to be more selective and more conservative; helps us to decide when *not* to operate, when to choose alternative modalities (e.g. percutaneous drainage) and guides us to the choice of incision**. Equally important — for those of us who take emergency calls, those who do not yet work in shifts in the medical factories imposed on us — CT lets us sleep better at night.

So from the individual patient's and surgeon's perspective, I believe that the liberal use of abdominal CT in the setting of the acute abdomen signals a positive trend. There are two caveats: first, we have to try and prevent repeated exposures to CT radiation — particularly in younger patients; second, and most importantly, an experienced abdominal surgeon must be the one interpreting the CT images (together with the radiologist) and deciding how to proceed. **An abdominal image without an abdominal surgeon is only an image — but together, the surgeon and the CT represent the best modern surgical judgment — the human one supplemented and made more accurate.**
Moshe

"Do not treat the image but the patient. A cliché? Yes. But an important one."

Chapter 6

Optimizing the patient

James Rucinski and the Editors

When physiology is disrupted, attempts at restoring anatomy are futile.

The preparation of the patient for surgery may be as crucial as the operation itself.

It's 4 a.m. and you assess your patient as having an 'acute abdomen' — probably due to a perforated viscus. **Clearly your patient needs an emergency laparotomy or laparoscopy. What is left to decide is: what efforts and how much time should be invested in his optimization before the operation?**

Optimization is a double-edged sword: wasting time trying to 'stabilize' an exsanguinating patient is an exercise in futility, for he will die. Conversely, rushing to surgery with a hypovolemic patient suffering from intestinal obstruction is a recipe for disaster.

The issues to be discussed are highlighted below.

- Why pre-operative optimization at all?
- What are the goals of optimization?
- Who needs optimization?
- How to do it?

Why is pre-operative optimization necessary?

Simply, because volume-depleted patients do not tolerate anesthesia and an operation. The induction of general anesthesia and muscle relaxation causes systemic vasodilatation, depressing the compensatory anti-shock physiologic mechanisms. On opening the abdomen, intraperitoneal pressure suddenly declines, allowing pooling of blood in the venous system that, in turn, decreases venous return and thus reduces cardiac output. (Even if you decide to start with laparoscopy, things could turn sour as hypovolemic patients can't tolerate the increased intra-abdominal pressure [IAP] generated by the pneumoperitoneum. Even with an IAP as low as 12-15mmHg, their hearts may fail.)

Thus, an emergency laparotomy/laparoscopy in an under-resuscitated patient may result in cardiac arrest even before the operation is started. In addition, the intra-operative fluid losses are unpredictable: do you want to start with a volume-depleted patient, having to chase your tail?

> **Remember:** Operating on a poorly resuscitated patient is like driving (under the influence of alcohol) a snow mobile on thin ice!

What are the goals of optimization?

Patients awaiting an emergency abdominal procedure need optimization for two main reasons: *hypovolemia* or *sepsis*. Both conditions cause under-perfusion of the tissues and both are treated initially by volume expansion, assisted by vasopressors, as needed. **The chief goal of pre-operative optimization is to improve the delivery of oxygen to the cells**. There is a direct relationship between cellular hypoxia and subsequent cellular dysfunction, organ failure and adverse outcome.

Who needs optimization?

Surgical patients often look 'sick'. The appearance of the patient usually gives an important first impression even before factoring in tachycardia, tachypnea, hypotension, mental confusion, and poor peripheral perfusion. **So look at your patient — not only at his serum lactate level!**

Only basic laboratory studies are necessary. *Hemoconcentration*, reflected in an abnormally high hemoglobin and hematocrit, implies either severe dehydration or extracellular 'third space' fluid sequestration. *Urine analysis* showing a high specific gravity (>1.039) provides similar information. *Electrolyte imbalance* and associated *prerenal azotemia* (with a **blood urea nitrogen** [BUN]-to-creatinine ratio of >20:1) again imply volume depletion. *Arterial blood gas* measurement gives critical information regarding respiratory function and tissue perfusion. **Note that in the emergency surgical patient, metabolic acidosis usually means lactic acidosis — associated with inadequate tissue oxygenation and anaerobic metabolism at the cellular level**. Other causes of metabolic acidosis such as renal failure, diabetic ketoacidosis or toxic poisoning are possible but extremely unlikely. A base deficit of more than 6 (BE less than -6) is a marker of significant metabolic acidosis and adverse prognosis and indicates a need for aggressive resuscitation. Of course, the ER doc or the nurse-hospitalist has already measured the serum lactate.

All patients with any degree of the above physiological abnormalities need optimization. Naturally, the magnitude of your efforts should correlate with the severity of the disturbances.

Measurement of the severity of illness

An experienced surgeon can 'eye-ball' his or her patient and estimate how sick they are by assessing the "gleam in his eye and the strength of the grip...". But terms such as 'very sick', 'critically ill', 'muy enfermo' or 'sehr krank' mean different things to different people. We recommend therefore that you become familiar with a universal physiological scoring system that gives an objective measure of 'sickness'. One scoring system, which has been validated in most emergency surgical situations, is the APACHE II (Acute Physiological And Chronic Health Evaluation) — use one of the online calculators, e.g.: http://clincalc.com/icumortality/apacheii.aspx#Mortality. It measures the physiological consequences of acute disease while taking into consideration the patient's pre-morbid state and age. The scores are easily measured from readily available basic clinical and laboratory variables and correlate with a prediction of morbidity and mortality.

An adjunctive method of assessing pre-operative risk is now available through the American College of Surgeons NSQIP (National Surgical Quality Improvement Program) Risk Calculator. The calculator is an online tool that can be used to determine an individualized risk profile for your specific patient. The calculator utilizes outcome data from all the hospitals that participate in the Program in order to allow a statistical prediction of various outcomes (such as surgical site infection, ileus, respiratory infection, hospital stay or death) associated with the characteristics of your patient. **The tool is**

available at: www.riskcalculator.facs.org. Add the link to the screen of your phone — now calculate the number with the patient at his bedside…

How do I do it? (■ Figure 6.1)

Principles of optimization: air goes in and out; blood goes 'round and 'round; oxygen is good.

Despite the high-tech intensive care unit (ICU) environment, which may or may not be available to you, optimization of the surgical patient is simple. It can be accomplished anywhere and requires minimal facilities. **All you want is better oxygen delivery, i.e. increased oxygenation of arterial blood and enhanced tissue perfusion**. You do not need a five-star ICU but you do have to stick around with the patient! Writing orders and going to bed (until the operation) will unnecessarily prolong the optimization and delay the operation. (Relying on 'hospitalists' to prepare the patient for your operation is like relying on your kids to clean the house when the adults are away.)

So stay with the patient, monitor his progress and be there to decide when enough is enough.

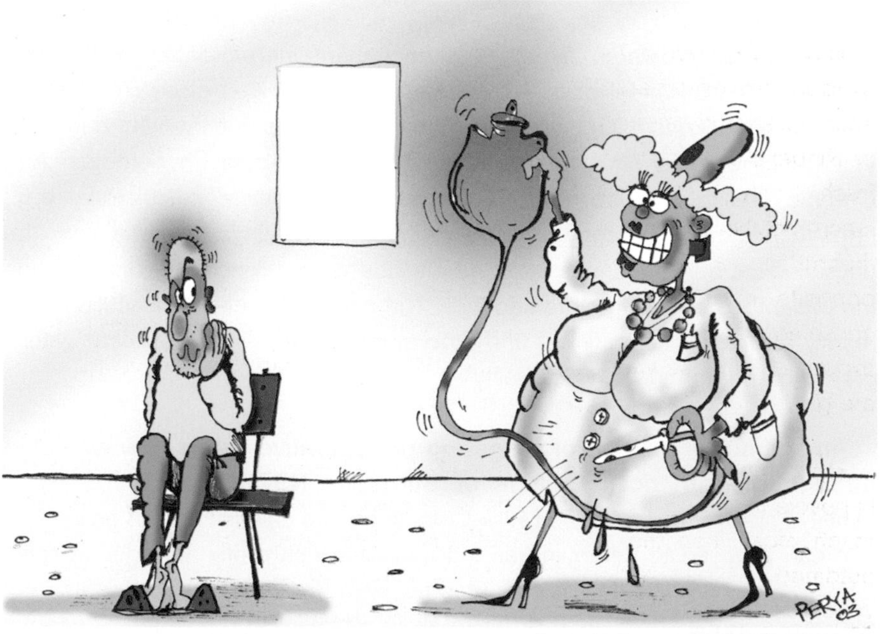

Figure 6.1. "Let me optimize you..."

Oxygenation

Hypoxia not only stops the motor, it wrecks the engine!

Any patient who requires optimization should at least receive oxygen by mask. Look at the patient and his pulse oximetry or arterial blood gases; evidence of severe hypoventilation or poor oxygenation may be an indication for endotracheal intubation and mechanical ventilation. **Do not temporize, the patient will need intubation anyway, so why not now?** Remember, pain and distension associated with any abdominal catastrophe impede ventilation. Effective analgesia impairs ventilation still further. If a nasogastric tube is not already *in situ* this may be the time to insert one. The advantages of NG insertion before intubation are to decompress the distended stomach and reduce the risk of aspiration during the procedure. The disadvantage is that the presence of a tube through the cricopharyngeus may allow regurgitation during rapid sequence induction of anesthesia.

Restoration of volume

The major cause of shock is decreased circulatory volume.
Replace body fluids by the best means at hand.

Alfred Blalock

Now after your patient is well oxygenated you must see to it that the oxygen arrives where it is needed, by restoring blood volume. This is accomplished by an intravenous infusion of crystalloids such as normal saline or Ringer's lactate. Forget about the much more expensive colloids such as fresh frozen plasma, albumin or solutions containing synthetic organic macromolecules such as hetastarch or low-molecular-weight dextran; their theoretical advantages have never been translated into better results — the opposite is true! Hypertonic saline resuscitation may theoretically be advantageous but it remains an investigational therapy at present. (It has been experimental since we entered medical school...). Blood and blood products are given if necessary as discussed below.

How much crystalloid to infuse? An old rule of thumb was that the hypovolemic surgical patient needs more volume than you think they need, and much more than the nursing staff think they need. But this rule is now outdated... **While restoring blood volume is a crucial step before any emergency operation we have to avoid drowning the patients in too much fluid**.

Equipped with huge-bore IV lines and fancy monitoring devices, enthusiastic surgeons and anesthetists commonly flood their patients with too much water and salt. We tend to ignore the 'obligatory' postoperative weight gain caused by too aggressive resuscitation with a shrug: "Well," we say, "the patient is perfusing well and his urine output is excellent — he'll diurese the excess fluids once he's well." But we are wrong!

Accumulating evidence shows that the deleterious effect of excess fluid is not limited to patients who are actively bleeding (by increasing the rate of hemorrhage and the risk of rebleeding) but can, in fact, be demonstrated in all of our patients.

Swollen, edematous cells are bad news in each and every system. Edema contributes to respiratory failure and cardiac dysfunction. It prevents tissue healing — adversely affecting intestinal anastomoses and abdominal closure. It swells abdominal contents producing intra-abdominal hypertension.

This is not a manual on intensive critical care. What we will tell you below applies to your average 'ill' surgical patient lying in the ER or on the floor (on the ward, for non-US surgeons!). Your educated intensivists may be more aggressive… as vasopressors require accurate titration and monitoring.

OK, now we assume that your patient already has a large-bore IV catheter *in situ* — so just hook it up to the solution and open the valve and let it run! You run in a liter and hang up another. **But how much is enough? At this stage you need to assess the effectiveness of what you do.**

Measurement of effectiveness of treatment

Again, the principal goal of non-operative treatment in the emergency surgical patient is the restoration of *adequate tissue oxygenation!* This endpoint is recognized by *physical examination* and measurement of *urinary output*, in conjunction with the information provided by *selective invasive monitoring* and laboratory studies.

With fluid resuscitation one hopes to see improvement of tissue oxygenation by normalization of vital signs and improvement in the visible peripheral circulation. Resolution of hypotension, mental confusion, tachypnea and tachycardia may be seen either partially or fully.

With fluid resuscitation, mottling of the skin and the palpable temperature of the fingers and toes may improve. *Capillary refill* is a clinical test that observes the peripheral circulation in the nail bed. The nail bed blanches when pressed and should return to its normal pink color in less than 2 seconds.

Urine output

Ventilate, perfuse, and piss is all that it is about!

Matt Oliver

A Foley urinary bladder catheter is essential in any patient requiring optimization. It allows an accurate, if indirect, measurement of tissue perfusion and *adequacy of fluid resuscitation*, as reflected in the urine output.

Your aim is at least 0.5 to 1ml urine/kg (patient's weight) per hour. So from the 'average' 70kg or 155lb patient (oh, how rare in our modern practice...), you would want around 50cc of urine per hour. **Adequate urine output is the single best sign of adequate tissue perfusion associated with successful fluid resuscitation**.

Invasive monitoring

The **central venous catheter** and the **Swan-Ganz pulmonary arterial catheter** are tools which permit 'special studies' to be carried out rapidly and repeatedly. The downside of such devices is that they are invasive, expensive, often inaccurate, and associated with potentially life-threatening complications. As technology develops, non-invasive monitoring has also advanced tremendously, allowing the calculation of complex physiological values from 'simple' measurements, such as the wave-form of the pulse oximeter.

These days, we use these modalities very rarely outside a dedicated ICU. Thus we decided not to discuss such tools in this edition. (Consult your ICU text or "Up-To-Date" ☺.)

Laboratory

The information provided by laboratory studies is easy to interpret. Aim for resolution of hemoconcentration, normalization of electrolyte, BUN and creatinine levels, and resolution of metabolic acidosis. As mentioned previously, look at the *base excess* (BE) — if persistently negative, the oxygen deficit at the tissue level has not resolved.

Blood and blood products

Blood products, such as whole blood, packed red blood cells, fresh frozen plasma, cryoprecipitate or platelet concentrate, are indicated selectively to restore oxygen-carrying capacity in actively bleeding or chronically anemic patients, and to correct clotting abnormalities if present. **Do not forget, however, the blood bank blood is a double-edged sword. Beyond the usual and well-known complications of transfusion, blood is immunosuppressive and may be associated with an increased probability of postoperative infections. In addition, the more blood you give the higher the risk of postoperative organ system dysfunction, including the risk of transfusion-related acute lung injury (TRALI) and mortality**.

Do not forget that rehydration with crystalloids may unmask chronic anemia as the hematocrit falls with volume expansion.

Suggested steps in volume optimization

- Institute intravenous fluid therapy and if signs of intestinal dysfunction such as nausea, vomiting or abdominal distension are present then designate nil per mouth (NPO) and, if necessary, nasogastric suction. Intravenous crystalloid may be started at a basic rate of 100 to 200ml per hour with the addition of boluses of 250 to 500ml given over intervals of 15 to 30 minutes. We advise you, however, to sit by your patient…
- Institute procedures for monitoring the effectiveness of treatment including serial physical exams and measurement of vital signs and urine output. **A sick surgical patient needs a Foley catheter. Period**.
- If the main underlying problem is hemorrhage, start a transfusion of packed red blood cells — typed and cross-matched if there is time, type-specific only if there is not. (Add blood components as necessary.)
- Titrate the rate of fluid administration in light of the results of monitoring. Increase or decrease the basic rate of fluid flow and give additional bolus infusions as necessary.
- Pressors should be commenced early in patients with septic shock. But such patients belong to the ICU…

- Wheel the patient directly to the operating room yourself. Do not wait for the porter — aren't they usually late?
- **If the basic problem is continuing hemorrhage then forget this list and go directly to the operating room** (or, if appropriate, to the invasive radiology suite). The best resuscitation in actively bleeding patients is surgical control of the source. In addition, **pre-operative over-resuscitation and transfusion increase the blood loss**.

In the OR...

Give only as much fluid as is necessary and, above all, monitor what the anesthetist is doing on his side of the screen. The old-fashioned formulas used to calculate how much fluid to administer during the operation are exaggerated and outdated. One has to replace blood loss and maintain urine output at 0.5ml/kg per hour, which practically means 30cc per hour — nothing more. **The more unnecessary fluid given before and during the operation — the more problems you'll have with the patient in the ICU and on the floor**.

When is enough, enough?

The above steps in optimization are done with the aim of correcting physiologic derangement as much as possible but without unnecessarily delaying operative intervention. **There is no magic formula for achieving this balance. The disease process itself will determine the duration of pre-operative optimization**. At one end of the spectrum, uncontrolled hemorrhage will require immediate operative intervention after only partial fluid resuscitation or none at all. At the other end of the spectrum, intestinal obstruction that has been developing over several days will require a more complete resuscitation prior to operation. As in life in general, most cases will fall somewhere in between — which means around 3 hours. Stubborn attempts to 'improve' a 'non-responder' beyond 6 hours are usually counter-productive. That you, or your boss, do not feel like leaving your warm beds at 3 a.m. is not an excuse to "continue aggressive resuscitation" until sunrise.

For a 'classification' of the urgency of the case see ■ Table 6.1.

Table 6.1. How urgent is urgent?

Urgency	Example(s)	Meaning
Immediate	Uncontrolled internal hemorrhage, prolapse of cord	Run to the OR
Life-threatening conditions	Leaking abdominal aortic aneurysm	Walk to the OR now
Potentially life-threatening	Perforated viscus Torsion of testis	Take to the OR within 2-3 hours
Should not be delayed	Acute appendicitis, intestinal obstruction	Usually can wait 6 hours until the morning
Can be delayed	Acute cholecystitis	Most cases can wait until the end of the weekend

But stop! Perhaps your patient does not need an operation? One of the cleverest aphorisms in surgery was coined by the late Francis D. Moore: "Never operate on a patient who is getting rapidly better or rapidly worse."

To finally recap...

The key to pre-operative optimization in emergency surgery is oxygenation of the blood and intravenous fluid resuscitation with crystalloid solutions. The only goal of resuscitation is the restoration of adequate tissue perfusion to supply oxygen to the suffocating mitochondria. Accomplish it aggressively to reduce intra-operative and postoperative complications.

These old folks maintain a fragile system quite well... until it gets disturbed — like a house of cards.

Before we forget... resuscitation in the traumatized or bleeding patient

We have to forget what the ATLS courses (and book) previously taught us — to flood the patient with crystalloids. Today we know that overly aggressive fluid resuscitation 'washes' out the clot, disturbs hemostasis, increases bleeding and decreases survival. **Hence, the current paradigm is 'hypotensive resuscitation' — keep the blood pressure just high enough to preserve vital organ perfusion**. In practical terms — do not aim for 'normal' blood pressure but keep systolic at around 90mmHg.

In actively bleeding patients start slowly with Ringer's lactate (do not 'pump' it in) and then switch to blood. Recent studies suggest that whole fresh blood is better than component therapy. **But if you have to transfuse more than a few units of packed red blood cells, growing evidence suggests that mortality and morbidity rates are improved by adding fresh frozen plasma and platelets to the blood given**. (Make yourself familiar with the **massive transfusion protocol** established in your environment.)

This is equally true for the injured patient, the one bleeding from his ulcer and the one with a ruptured aortic aneurysm!

> **"Every operation is an experiment in physiology."**
> **Tid Kommer**

Chapter 7

Pre-operative antibiotics

The Editors

Most men die of their remedies, not of their diseases.

Molière

Curmudgeon is the guy who gets up at the M & M meeting, after you describe your brilliant save with an ER thoracotomy for thoracoabdominal GSW and asks why you did not give prophylactic antibiotics.

Albert I. Alexander

The administration of broad-spectrum antibiotics before a laparotomy for any surgical emergency is an established practice. In this situation, antibiotics are either **therapeutic** or **prophylactic**.

Therapeutic antibiotics: given for an already established, tissue invasive, infection (e.g. perforated appendicitis). They assist the surgeon and the natural peritoneal defenses to eradicate an established infection.

Prophylactic antibiotics: administered in the absence of infection, with the objective of reducing the anticipated incidence of infections due to *existing* (e.g. penetrating injury of the colon) or *potential* (e.g. gastrotomy to suture a bleeding ulcer) contamination during the operative procedure. Be aware that *prophylactic* antibiotics mainly prevent postoperative infection of the laparotomy wound (superficial SSI); they do not prevent intra-abdominal (i.e. deep SSI), pulmonary or urinary infections.

It is very important to distinguish between *contamination* and *infection* (➲ Chapter 13), as only the latter requires postoperative antibiotic administration, a topic to be discussed in the postoperative section (➲ Chapter 40).

The overprescription of antibiotics is a modern curse for which our patients pay the price in terms of morbidity and mortality from antibiotic-associated colitis and the emergence of resistant strains. So use them judiciously and for the shortest duration possible.

When should you start antibiotics?

- If intra-abdominal infection is present or suspected you should administer therapeutic antibiotics immediately — the sooner the better. If there is any delay in proceeding with the operation you may need to repeat administration of antibiotics in the operating room, as adequate levels of the drug should permeate the tissues *at the time of* the incision. This is because immediate vasoconstriction at the incision site would prevent antibiotics — if given later — from reaching the operative wound.
- If you do not suspect any intra-abdominal infection, and so the antibiotics would be purely *prophylactic*, then administer them just prior to the incision — on the way to, or in, the OR.

Remember: The fate of the operative wound is sealed by peri-operative events, including timely administration of antibiotics. Almost nothing done after the operation can change the outcome of the wound (➲ Chapter 46).

So by the way, the nurses may instruct your patient to avoid a shower for 48 hours after the operation, and your ID specialist will cite studies that water increases the SSI rate. But this is BS: a well-sutured wound should be watertight by the next morning (a layer of tissue glue helps…). Let them shower as much as they wish. A public Jacuzzi is another story…

Which antibiotics to use?

Contrary to what is preached by drug companies (■ Figure 7.1) and their various beneficiaries or representatives — including certain clinicians who

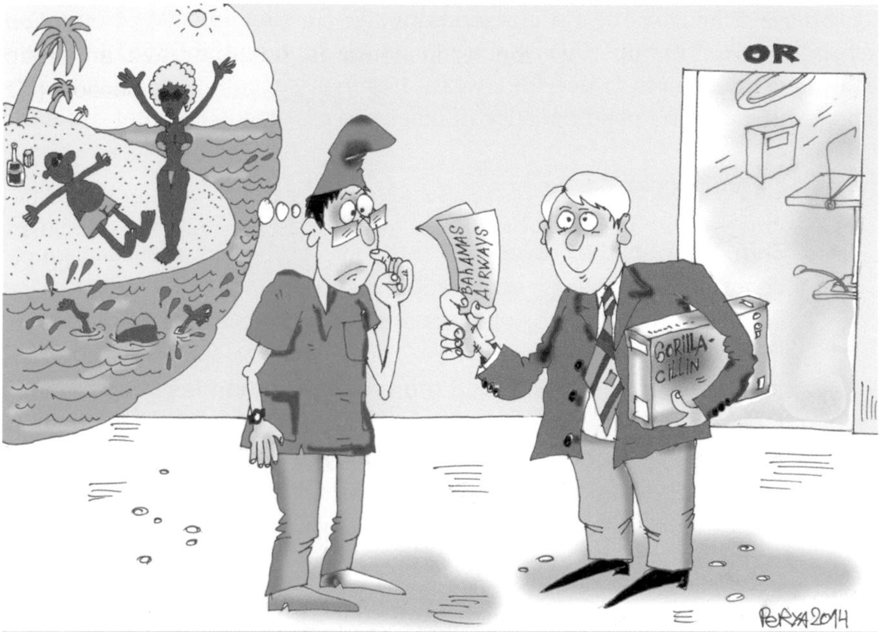

Figure 7.1. "Doctor, try our new Gorillacillin. Here is a recent paper published in the *Zimbabwean Journal of Surgery*... in a study of 75 patients... it proved potent and safe!"

function as 'medical advisers' (we have another name for them...) — the choice of drugs is straightforward. **Many single drug or combination regimens are available and equally effective; the most recent and expensive not necessarily being better**.

The exact regimen of antibiotics to give depends on the pathology you are dealing with. Operating on different organs and disease processes you are likely to encounter a different set of bugs. Therefore, when considering which *empiric* antimicrobial agents to administer you should take into account:

- **The specific pathology** (e.g. perforated colon vs. incarcerated hernia).
- **Severity of disease** (e.g. mild acute cholecystitis vs. emphysematous cholecystitis with severe sepsis).
- **Other factors**: did the pathology develop at home (*community-acquired*) or during hospitalization (*hospital-acquired*)? Was the patient already on antibiotics? Is the patient immunocompromised? Any of these factors could suggest that unusual, opportunistic microorganisms (e.g. fungi) could be involved in the infection.

There are many agents on the market that you can choose from for empiric pre-op administration. For the recommended regimens please consult the

"Executive Summary" of the guidelines by the Surgical Infection Society — available online at: https://www.ncbi.nlm.nih.gov/pubmed/28085573 [1]. It will tell you which agents to use for low- vs. high-risk patients and which agents should no longer be used because of emerging resistance in target bacteria.

A few more general points:

- **Think about the dose**. In the course of fluid resuscitation of hypovolemic patients, antimicrobials may be 'diluted', reducing the availability of antimicrobial drugs at sites of contamination or infection. In these cases, especially in the trauma patient, higher initial doses should be used: "**sooner and more is better than less and longer**." **Don't forget that obese people need higher doses!**
- **One might expect that the bacteriology of postoperative infections at specific sites might be predictable**. Often however this is not so. For example, the biliary system is typically contaminated with *Gram-negative* bacteria but the post-cholecystectomy wound infection is commonly caused by typical skin bacteria — *Staphylococcus aureus* or even methicillin-resistant *Staphylococcus aureus* (MRSA).

But wait a minute, you may be hollering, what about the results of intra-operative cultures? **Well, after finishing this book you will understand that routine microbiological cultures often have no practical clinical value** — in many cases, when the data on the cultured bacteria and the sensitivity to antibiotics are available, the patient is at home and off antibiotics. However, while cultures are useless in 'routine' cases (e.g. acute appendicitis), they should be obtained in **selective situations** as discussed in ➲ Chapter 13.

To summarise...

Remember: Start *empiric* antibiotics prior to any emergency laparotomy/laparoscopy; whether you continue administration after the operation depends on the operative findings (see ➲ Chapter 40). Know the target flora, understand the host, be aware of exceptions, and use the simplest regimen.

"Patients can get well without antibiotics."
Mark M. Ravitch

1 Mazuski JE, *et al.* The Surgical Infection Society Revised Guidelines on the Management of Intra-Abdominal Infection. *Surg Infect* 2017; 18: 1-76.

Chapter 8

Family, ethics, informed consent and medicolegal issues

James C. Rucinski

> *Doctor, my doctor, what do you say…?*
>
> **Philip Roth**
>
> *Stop lying! You know, and I know, that I am dying. So do at least stop lying about it!*
>
> **Lev Tolstoy**
>
> (To understand the 'dying man' you have to read Tolstoy's *The Death of Ivan Ilyich.*)

The wind whistles through the cracks in your call room window when the emergency department (ED) calls and suddenly you find yourself in the maelstrom of that environment, speaking to a small group of extremely anxious strangers — having to explain that an immediate operation will be required to save their beloved one. The operating room is ready.

Obtaining informed consent is a practical combination of salesmanship, ethical problem solving and psychological nurturing. It involves the rapid marketing of one's own skills and plan for treatment. It requires the recruitment of the patient and the family as allies in the decision-making process. More than a legal requirement, however, informed consent requires an ethical commitment to the patient, your peers and to yourself.

Salesmanship

Begin by explaining the problem and your proposed treatment using the same words and language that you might use in speaking to one of your non-medical relatives. **Describe the expected benefits of operation and what the consequences of alternative treatment approaches might be**. (What happens if we do nothing…).

Offer several scenarios; take a case of obstructing carcinoma of the sigmoid colon, for example. At one end of the spectrum is non-operative management, which almost certainly will result in a slow and difficult death. At the other end of the spectrum is rapid recovery from operation with long-term cure of the disease. In between lie the potential difficulties of peri-operative complications or death, recovery with disability or recurrent disease. Another common and 'problematic' scenario is acute cholecystitis. While literature supports early surgery, 'conservative' treatment is also acceptable and widely practiced. When discussing the options you must mention the alternatives, but also be honest about the institution's capabilities as well as your own.

It is crucial that you believe in the plan of treatment that you propose. If this is not the case, and the plan is not acceptable to you but dictated to you from above, then let the responsible surgeon (your boss) conduct his own pre-operative 'negotiations' with the patient and/or his family.

'Sell' yourself to the patient and family as a scientific expert who recognizes the needs of another person, and is participating with them in solving a difficult problem. Include a description, with approximate probabilities, of the most common 'problems' (complications) for the proposed procedure in your particular patient. You will need to make an estimate based on general and specific information. For example, the risk of mortality for elective colon resection may be negligible but in an elderly patient with acute colonic obstruction and hypoalbuminemia the odds of dying may be one in four (➲ Chapter 6). Discuss **general potential postoperative complications** such as infection, hemorrhage (and risk of transfusion), poor healing and death. Then mention the **unique complications specific to the procedure** you are proposing to undertake, such as common bile duct injury or bile leak in laparoscopic cholecystectomy.

The American College of Surgeons online risk calculator (ACS-NSQIP) was already mentioned in Chapter 6 on page 59, and is widely used. It's quick and easy, and can be found at www.riskcalculator.facs.org. Save it on your phone and get into a (good) habit of using it — giving the patient and family a reliable risk estimation as part of the informed consent.

It is crucial that before any major emergency abdominal operation you emphasize that a reoperation may be necessary based on your operative finding or if a problem subsequently develops. This will drastically facilitate the 'confrontation' with the family when a reoperation is indeed indicated; **they will understand that the reoperation represents a 'continued management effort' rather than a 'complication'**. Minor complications, such as phlebitis arising from peri-operative intravenous therapy, may contribute to information overload and probably should be omitted.

Try to conduct the above 'script' in a relatively quiet setting — away from the usual chaos of the ER, SICU or the OR; find a quiet corner and let everyone, including yourself, sit down! Use simple language and **repeat yourself *ad infinitum***, as stressed members of the family may have difficulty in grasping what you say. Offer the opportunity to ask questions and assess whether there is an understanding of your discussion. The more they understand initially, the fewer 'problems' you'll have if complications subsequently develop.

Be 'human', friendly, empathetic but professional. **A good trick is to remind yourself from time to time that the family you are talking to could be yours**. Finally, always leave open the possibility that what you think the problem to be is not correct. Similarly, if you are asked to provide a prognosis always allow for the unexpected, both good and bad, so that if a disaster or a miracle should occur this will not be outside the bounds of the possibilities you outlined earlier. **Never mention *specific* times; for example if you say "3 to 6 months or so" the only thing that will be remembered is that you said "6 months". Then, when the patient dies the following day of an MI… or is still alive a year later…**

Illustrate the problem

When discussing the prospects of an operation with a patient or a family we find that illustrating the problem and the planned procedure on a blank piece of paper greatly enhances the communication. Draw, schematically, the obstructed colon: "here is the colon, this is the obstructing lesion and here is the segment we want to remove; we hope to be able to join this piece of bowel to that one; a colostomy may, however, be needed; this is the place it will be brought out." Below the drawing write the diagnosis and the name of the planned operation. At the end of the consultation you'll be surprised to see how carefully members of the family restudy the piece of paper you left with them, explaining to each other the diagnosis and planned operation. Very often patients and their relatives are very enthusiastic about keeping any drawings you make for them.

The family

When it comes to an operation, you advise the patient and his family and they decide…

The patient's family is your greatest ally in promoting your plan of action. By involving them at an early point in the decision-making process you may be able to make them partners in the relationship that you share with the patient. By avoiding the family you may alienate potential allies or worsen an already 'difficult' group.

The 'difficult' family is not uncommon. Long submerged conflicts and feelings of guilt tend to surface when a member of the group becomes ill. Recruit them as allies by offering them a chance to participate, by 'reading' the nuances of their relationships and by confidently and continuously selling yourself as a knowledgeable and compassionate advisor. Use your first meeting with the family to make a good impression and gain their trust so that you will continue to be trusted when a complication arises or when further therapy becomes necessary. Remember that if things turn out badly it will be the family members that will want to know "what went wrong?"

Ethical problem solving

In order to sell a particular product or idea one must believe in it. In other words, based on your knowledge and experience, the operation you offer should appear ethical to you. **It is ethical if it is expected to save or prolong the patient's life or palliate his symptoms, and can achieve this goal with a reasonable risk-benefit ratio. At the same time you must also be convinced that there are no non-operative treatment modalities that are safer or as effective as your proposed operation. The burden of proof is on you!**

Medicolegal considerations

Surgery is the most dangerous activity of legal society.

P. O. Nyström

The medicolegal dangers associated with emergency abdominal surgery greatly depend on where you practice. In some countries surgeons can get away with almost anything; in other countries emergency surgery is a legal minefield. **There are a few simple but well-proven tactics to prevent lawsuits against you**:

- **Have the patient and family 'on your side'** (as mentioned above) by being empathetic, caring, honest, open, informative, and at the same time professional. Young surgeons tend to be over-optimistic, trying to cheer up the family. A common scenario finds the surgeon emerging from the operating room, assuming a 'tired hero' pose and announcing: "It was smooth and easy, I removed the cancer from the colon, relieving the obstruction. I was able to join the ends of the bowel together, avoiding a colostomy. Yes, your father is stable, he took the operation very well, let's hope he'll be home next week for Easter... (or Passover or Ramadan)." Such a script is somewhat misguided in that it may raise high hopes and expectations, with subsequent anger and resentment if complications should develop. The better script might be: "The operation was difficult, but we managed to achieve our goals. The cancer is out and we avoided a colostomy. Considering your father's age and other illnesses he took it well. Let us hope for the best but you must understand that the road to recovery is long and, as I mentioned before the operation, there are still many potential problems ahead."
- **Detailed informed consent** (■ Figure 8.1). This should be much more than the standard sheet — listing in small print all possible

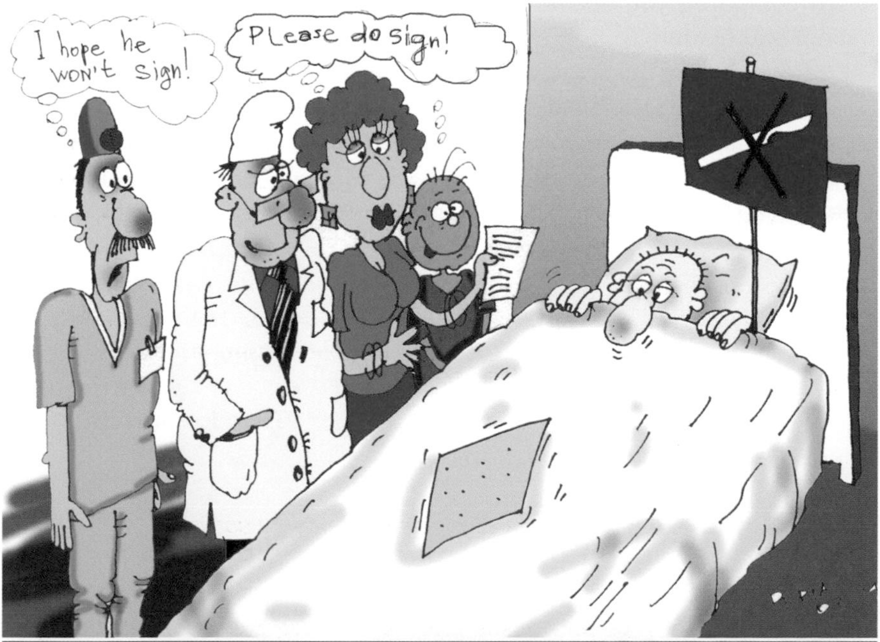

Figure 8.1. "Is he going to sign?"

complications ever described in abdominal surgery. **The chart has to include evidence that you have met with the patient before the operation and discussed the planned procedure and its inherent risks — and alternatives of management.**

- **Documentation**. This is crucial, as what has not been documented in writing did not actually take place. Your notes can be brief but must encompass the essentials. Prior to an emergency laparotomy for colonic obstruction we would write: "78 YO male patient with hypertension, diabetes and COPD. Three days of abdominal pain plus distension. Abdominal X-ray — suggesting a distal large bowel obstruction — confirmed on Gastrografin® study. Therapeutic options, risks and potential complications, including anastomotic leak, wound infection, respiratory failure, explained in detail to the patient and family who accept the need for an emergency laparotomy. They understand that a colostomy may be needed and that further operations may be necessary." **As mentioned above, you may want to include outcome predictions derived from the NSQIP Risk Calculator results for your specific patient. A year or so later, when you have to defend a lawsuit, this short note will prove invaluable!**

Avoid selling autopsies under anesthesia (AUA)

We compared you above to an astute salesman, interacting with the patient and his family. In this capacity, you, a respected clinician, can easily sell anything to the trusting clients. But be honest with yourself and consider as objectively as possible the risk-benefit ratio of the procedure you are trying to 'sell'. It may be easy to convince a worried family that a (futile) operation is indeed necessary, and then at the inevitable M & M (morbidity and mortality) meeting (➲ Chapter 47) to explain that the family forced the AUA on you. Easy and ethical don't always coexist!

> *One should advise surgery only if there is a reasonable chance of success. To operate without having a chance means to prostitute the beautiful art and science of surgery.*
>
> **Theodor Billroth**

Concluding remarks

Not only is what you say important but also how it is said. Introduce yourself and all members of your team who are present. Shake hands with *all* members of the family. Conduct the 'session' in a sitting position — you sitting at eye level, or lower, with the patient and his family. Maintain constant eye contact with each of them — do not ignore the grumpy son hiding in the corner of the room — he may be the one who becomes your nemesis. Be 'nice' but not 'too nice' — this is not the time to smile or joke around. Just play the serious surgeon committed to the well-being of the patient. This surgeon is you, so play yourself!

Nothing is truer than the cliché that should be constantly replayed in your mind — would you recommend the same treatment to your father, mother, wife or son? Studies show that surgeons are much less likely to recommend operations on themselves or their loved ones. **Do unto others as you would have them do unto you — the golden rule. Even if your hands are so keen to operate...**

When the editors asked me to revise/update this chapter for the current edition I looked at it and realized that there is nothing to change: what has been written above was always true and will remain so as long as robots won't totally replace human surgeons. Then I remembered what my late old mentor Dr. Leslie Wise (1932-2016) — he was also Moshe's boss at some stage — would say: "**If you think that you really have to do something, then go out and have a cup of coffee**."

[For much more about "Dealing with patients, families, lawyers and yourself" please consult the so-named Chapter 10 in *Schein's Common Sense Prevention and Management of Surgical Complications*. Shrewsbury, UK: tfm publishing, 2013.]

"The patient's family will never forgive a guarantee of cure that failed and the patient will not let the physician forget a pronouncement of incurability if he is so fortunate as to survive."

George T. Pack

Chapter 9

Before the flight: pre-op checklist

The Editors

> *The pilot is by circumstances allowed only one serious mistake, while the surgeon may commit many and not even recognize his own errors as such.*
>
> **John S. Lockwood**

Aren't we all fed up of being compared to pilots? Richard C. Karl, a surgeon and pilot, has pointed out that the two professions are not exactly the same:

> *Pilots don't fill out a form documenting that they put the landing gear down. This is another fundamental difference in the two professions. We (surgeons) obsess about documentation; aviation worries about getting the wheels down.*
>
> *I do know that it is harder to control bleeding from the back side of the portal vein than it is to land a 737 with an engine on fire.*

Nevertheless, like any military or commercial pilot, prior to any flight, you have to go over a 'checklist' (■ Figure 9.1). In fact, the need to check everything obsessively is more crucial to you than to the pilot. For while a team of dedicated and well-trained maintenance professionals surround the pilot — you are sometimes surrounded only by jerks. We do not want to be abusive or rude or politically incorrect but let's be realistic: at 2 a.m. your intern or junior

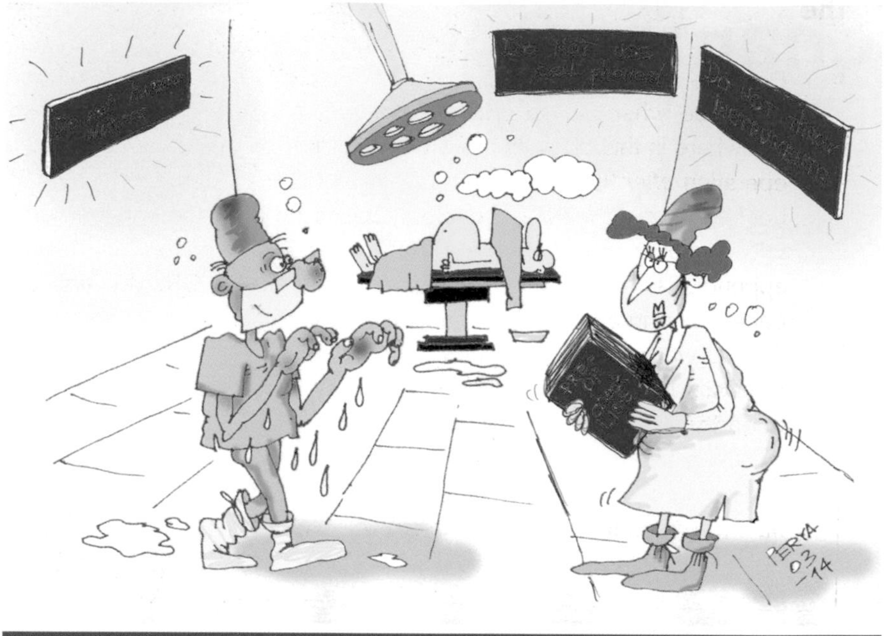

Figure 9.1. "Doctor, show me your pilot's license and CME certificates!"

resident is much more interested in his lost sleep than your prospective operation. And the anesthetist? Your emergency case is just a pain in his ass. The sooner he or she can administer the gases, the sooner they can dump your 'case' in the recovery room, or intensive care unit, the sooner they can crawl under the comfort of their warm duvet. And the nursing staff? Not in vain today are they called OR *technicians*. (Lest we be accused of painting with too broad a brush, there are always the wonderful exceptions — some assist us better than any resident... in this scenario, let them know they are appreciated!)

So face it — assume you are alone; often it is a solo flight and you can count only on yourself. You are responsible for the success, failure, morbidity, mortality, and potential lawsuit. His or her fate is in your hands. This patient, regardless of how many people are buzzing around, is yours. So wake up and go over the checklist.

The formal 'OR time out', dictated by 'big brother' — that mandated final review by the nursing team of the side, site and nature of the procedure — cannot, and should not, come instead of your own checklist.

The surgeon's checklist

- **Does he *really* need the operation?** The cliché that it is more difficult to decide when *not* to operate than when to operate is mentioned elsewhere in this book. But even more difficult is to decide against the operation *after* the operation has been scheduled. So you decided to book the patient for appendectomy based on what the chief resident told you over the phone — that "the CT is compatible with acute appendicitis" — and now, when you arrive in the OR, you find the patient smiling and sitting in bed with a soft and non-tender abdomen. Do you want to operate on the CT or the patient? **You do not need big balls (or ovaries) to book a patient for the operation but you need them to *cancel* the operation.**
- **Examine the patient before he is put to sleep. Never ever — we repeat — never, never, never ever operate on a patient without having examined him yourself; if you do then you are a frickin' butcher!** That the endoscopist visualized a 'bleeding ulcer' and the patient continues to vomit blood may be an indication for operation, but this is your chance to diagnose the large spleen and ascites, which were hitherto overlooked by the others. You do not want to operate on a Child's C portal hypertension patient, or do you? (See ➲ Chapter 23.)
- **Look at the X-rays and imaging studies.** Review all X-rays and imaging studies by yourself. Do not rely only on what the radiologist said or wrote. You may pick up findings, which may move you to cancel the operation or to decide on a different incision. Fine details on the CT may help you to plan the operation. It can show, for example, the safest place to enter the abdomen and avoid bowel loops adherent to the anterior abdominal wall.
- **Position the patient.** Already before you start you have to have a general idea what you are going to do or what you may have to do. This has an impact on your patient's position. For example — does he need a Lloyd-Davies position, offering access to the anus and rectum? This may be needed during colorectal procedures — to insert a scope, to decompress the colon or to insert a stapler. You do not want to have to stop the operation and place the patient in the correct position or to send the intern crawling under soggy drapes playing peek a boo with the anus. Regardless of position, check that all limbs are protected and well padded at potential pressure sites. **Poor positioning on the OR table may result in damage to nerves, skin ulceration and compartment syndrome of the extremities — and a lawsuit.**

- **Warm your patient**. See that the patient is well covered and warmed. **Hypothermia** increases the likelihood of postoperative infections and contributes to intra-operative coagulopathy.
- **Think about preventing deep vein thrombosis (DVT)**. Prevention of DVT should be initiated before the patient is put to sleep — not after the operation. Any abdominal procedure lasting longer than 30 minutes is associated with a moderate risk of DVT; you can add to this specific risk factors such as smoking, the use of oral contraceptives, a previous history of DVT, age, obesity, a cancer and so forth. **But instead of pondering too much — why don't you provide all your patients undergoing an emergency abdominal operation with DVT prophylaxis?** Whether it is in the form of subcutaneous heparin or pneumatic calf compression depends on what your OR can offer. Bear in mind that anticoagulation is not good for an exsanguinating patient! We have seen young patients dropping dead from pulmonary embolism a few days after appendectomy and young women developing intractable post-phlebitic syndromes following appendectomy performed for pelvic inflammatory disease. Always think about this.
- **Is the bladder empty?** Many patients undergoing major emergency operations arrive at the OR with a urinary catheter in place; in the rest you will insert the catheter on the OR table. But if contemplating a lower abdominal procedure (or insertion of lower abdominal trocars) on a non-catheterized patient you have to check that the bladder is empty. When the bladder is full it may look to you like the peritoneum — we have seen residents opening the bladder in search of the appendix ☹. Bladder distension may also mimic a surgical abdominal condition, not rare in a mentally challenged patient. It is your job to see that the nurses insert the Foley properly. Even a senior RN is capable of inflating the balloon in the urethra, causing massive hematuria. We have seen it all.
- **Think antibiotic prophylaxis** (see ➲ Chapter 7).
- **Document everything** (see ➲ Chapter 8).

Now you can go and scrub. While doing so, continue to think and contemplate what you are going to do. Go through the anticipated phases of the operation, refresh the different strategies and options available, think about additional equipment you might be needing, and finally, look in the mirror and give yourself an encouraging nod — what a great profession this is! Don't I look great with that mask covering my face?!

But do not behave like Tolstoy's surgeon in *War and Peace*: "He… joked… and chatted carelessly, as a famous surgeon confident that he knows his job, will often chat while he tucks up his sleeves and puts on his apron, and the patient is being strapped to the operating table. 'I have the whole business at my finger-tips, and it's all clear and definite in my head. When the time comes to set to work I shall do it as no one else could, but now I can jest, and the more I jest and the cooler I am the more hopeful and reassured you ought to feel, and the more you may wonder at my genius.'"

> **Remember:** ***Many lives have been saved by a moment of reflection at the scrub sink.***
>
> **Neal R. Reisman**

You are the captain of the ship — behave like one; the sight of a euphoric surgeon dramatically entering the room with his scrubbed hands held high in the air is pitiful.

> **"Poor judgment is responsible for much bad surgery, including the withholding of operations that are necessary or advisable, the performance of unnecessary and superfluous operations, and the performance of inefficient, imperfect, and wrongly chosen ones."**
>
> **Charles F. M. Saint**
>
> **"The surgeon, like the captain of the ship or a pilot of an aircraft, is responsible for everything that happened. His word is the only one that cannot be gainsaid."**
>
> **Francis D. Moore**

PART III

The operation

Chapter 10

The incision

The Editors [1]

---

*Incisions heal from side to side, not from end to end, but **length** (as you may know) does matter.*

When entering the abdomen, your finger is the best and safest instrument.

Have you ever heard about the novel concept of 'macrolaparotomy' — that it is possible and sometimes advisable to enter the abdominal cavity by cutting into it directly? Yes, with a knife, without inserting scopes or trocars! Did you know that this cutting-edge (yes, we are a little sarcastic) method may be useful — particularly in emergency surgery? This chapter is dedicated to this bold approach to open abdominal entry — read about laparoscopic access in ➲ Chapter 12.

The patient now lies on the table, anesthetized and ready for your knife. Before you scrub, carefully examine the relaxed abdomen. Now you can feel things which were impossible to feel in the tense and tender belly. You may feel a distended gallbladder in a patient diagnosed as an acute appendicitis, or an appendiceal mass in a patient booked for a cholecystectomy. Yes, this can still occur in the era of ultrasound and CT, especially when and where imaging has been skirted or is not available.

Traditionally, abdominal entry in an emergency situation or for exploratory purposes has been through a generous and easily extensible

---

1 Asher Hirshberg, MD, contributed to this chapter in the first edition of this book.

vertical incision, especially a midline one. Generally speaking, the trans *linea alba* midline incision is swiftly effected and relatively bloodless. On the other hand, **transverse incisions are a little more time- and blood-consuming but are associated with a lower incidence of wound dehiscence and incisional hernia formation**. In addition, transverse incisions are known to be less painful and thus 'easier' on the patient and his lung function in the postoperative period. They also provide better exposure when the transverse abdominal axis is longer than the vertical, such as in infants or short obese patients. **Vertical paramedian incisions largely belong to history**.

Keeping this in mind, we should **be pragmatic rather than dogmatic** and tailor the incision to the individual patient and his or her disease process. **We should take into consideration the urgency of the situation, the site and nature of the condition, the confidence in (or uncertainty about) the pre-operative diagnosis, and the build of the patient**.

Common sense dictates that the most direct access to the specific intra-abdominal pathology is preferable. Thus, the biliary system is best approached through a right subcostal ('Kocher') or a transverse incision. Transverse incisions are easily extended to offer additional exposure; a right subcostal incision can be extended into the left side (as a 'chevron'), offering an excellent view of the entire abdomen. When a normal appendix is uncovered through a limited, transverse/oblique, muscle-splitting, right lower quadrant incision, one can extend it by cutting the muscles across the midline to deal with any intestinal or pelvic condition. Alternatively, when an upper abdominal process is found, it is perfectly reasonable to close the small right iliac fossa incision and place a new, more appropriate, one. **Two good incisions are better than one, poorly placed**.

The midline incision is bloodless, rapid, and easily extended affording superior exposure and versatility; it remains the classic '**incision of indecision**' — when the site of the abdominal catastrophe is unknown — and is the safest approach in trauma. Sometimes even a long midline incision is not enough, and you need to make an additional transverse incision to gain exposure to the deep lateral or posterior areas. If needed, don't hesitate to do it. And conversely, a 'chevron' incision can be enlarged by a midline upper extension, creating a 'Mercedes' incision. (Ask your hepatic surgeon about his favourite incision... and vehicle.)

This is the time to mention that an emergency laparotomy without a diagnosis is not a sin! Yes, a patient <u>can</u> enter the operating theater without a ticket from the CT scanner. A clinical acute abdomen — when other diagnoses have been ruled out — remains an indication for laparotomy when the abdominal wall is the only structure separating the surgeon from an accurate diagnosis. Having said this mainly to satisfy and pacify those of you who work under adverse circumstances (e.g. we have visited a city hospital in Eastern Europe where patients had to travel by ambulance for a CT!) — **we have to stress that pre-operative abdominal imaging not only pinpoints the diagnosis but also is of great help in choosing the correct incision**. For example, in a patient needing splenectomy for a delayed rupture of the spleen we could place a left subcostal incision rather than a midline one. The CT has shown us that this is an isolated splenic injury and there is no need to explore the rest of the abdomen.

At what level must the midline incision start and how long should it be? (■ Figure 10.1)

The macho surgeons of previous generations often screamed: "Make it long. It heals from side to side, not from end to end." But today, in the era of minimal access surgery, we are familiar with the advantages of shorter incisions. **In the absence of any obvious urgency, enter the abdomen through a short incision and then extend as necessary; but never accept less than adequate**

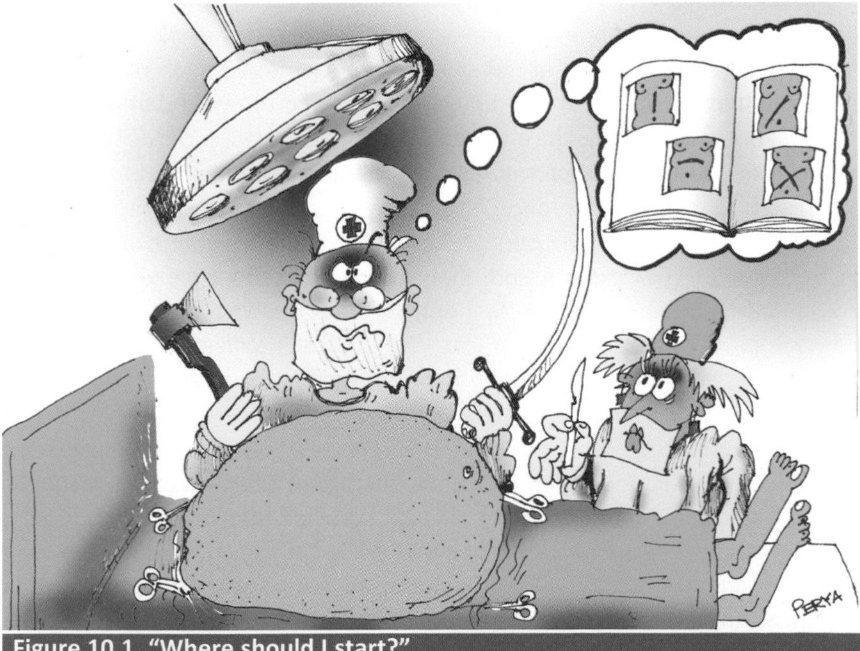

Figure 10.1. "Where should I start?"

exposure — never engage obstinately in keyhole surgery. Begin with an upper or lower midline incision, directed by your clinical/imaging assessment; when in doubt, start near the level of the umbilicus and 'sniff' around from there, then extend towards the pathology. Just remember what the famous Swiss surgeon, Theodor Kocher, said more than 100 years ago: "**The incision must be as long as necessary and as short as possible**." Smart, eh? Before you continue we want you to read a little about Herr Kocher (go to http://www.nobelprize.org/nobel_prizes/medicine/laureates/1909/kocher-bio.html).

When should you extend the incision into the thorax?

Very rarely! In the vast majority of cases, infra-diaphragmatic pathology is approachable through abdominal incisions. The combination of a subcostal and upper midline incision offers an excellent exposure for almost all emergency hepatic procedures, with the exception of retrohepatic venous injuries where insertion of a trans-atrial vena cava shunt necessitates a median sternotomy — usually a futile exercise, anyway. **Thoracoabdominal incisions are mainly reserved for combined thoracoabdominal trauma** (and rarely for tumors at the esophagogastric junction which 'climb' up the esophagus). If not absolutely necessary, avoid extending the laparotomy incision to thoracolaparotomy through the costal cartilage — it heals very poorly! **In most cases, it is sufficient to do a separate anterolateral thoracotomy incision**. This can easily be extended to the other side for a 'clamshell' incision that offers an excellent view to all anterior thoracic structures. **If you need to divide the diaphragm, do it laterally, curve-shaped to avoid damage to the proximal branches of the phrenic nerve**. In some cases, rapid access to the pericardium during laparotomy (for suspected cardiac tamponade for example) is easily done through the central tendon of the diaphragm by grasping the bare area of the pericardium with a Kocher's clamp and opening the pericardium. If blood is found, then extension of the laparotomy incision into a median sternotomy is the best option.

Knife or diathermy?

A few studies suggest that the latter is a few minutes slower while the former sheds a few more drops of blood; otherwise results are comparable. We use either. In extreme urgency, gain immediate entry with a few swift strokes of the knife; otherwise, diathermy is convenient, especially when performing transverse muscle-cutting incisions. **Adequate hemostasis is a crucial surgical principle but do not go overboard chasing individual**

erythrocytes and avoid reducing the subcutaneous fat or skin to charcoal. The hypothesis that "You can tell how bad the surgeon is by the stink of the Bovie (electrocautery) in his OR" has not been proven by a double-blind randomized trial but makes sense nonetheless.

In practice, most incisional 'oozers' stop spontaneously after a few minutes, under the pressure of a moist lap pad or a temporary hemostat. If necessary, use well-directed diathermy to kill the bloody bleeder at the point where is emerges under the skin, and avoid burning blindly in a pool of blood. It is also unnecessary to 'clean' the fascia by sweeping the fat laterally: **the more you dissect and 'burn', the more inflammation and infection-generating dead tissue you create!**

Keep in mind special circumstances:

- If **a stoma is anticipated** then place the incision away from its planned location. You don't want the toilet in the kitchen!
- **Abdominal re-entry into the 'hostile abdomen' of a previously operated patient** can be problematic. You may spend more time, sweat and blood, but the real danger is creating inadvertent enterotomies in intestine adherent to the previous incisional scar. This is a common cause of postoperative external bowel fistula (➲ Chapter 43)! **The prevailing opinion is to use the previous incision for re-entry, *if possible***. When doing so, however, start a few centimeters below or above the old incision and gain entry to the abdomen through virgin territory. Then insert your finger into the peritoneal cavity and navigate your way safely in, taking down adhesions to the abdominal wall. Essentially, you are finished 'getting in' when you are able to place a self-retaining retractor to open the abdomen wide. In a dire emergency or when you expect the abdomen to be exceptionally scarred, it may be prudent to stay away from trouble and create an entirely fresh incision. In this situation beware of <u>parallel incisions</u> in close proximity to one another because the intervening skin may be at risk of necrosis, particularly if the first incision is relatively recent.

Remember: Sometimes, spending an hour to 'get into the abdomen' in order to do a 5-minute procedure (e.g. release of an obstructing adhesion) is not a sign of a timid surgeon but a judicious one! You may want to consider this mnemonic of abdominal entry and exposure: 'the 4 Ps': patience, preservation, persistence, prudence. (Some surgeons may need a fifth p — Prozac®.)

Pitfalls

- When in haste, do not forget that the *liver* lies in the upper extremity of the long midline incision, and the *urinary bladder* at its lowermost. Be careful not to damage either.
- When approaching the upper abdomen divide and ligate the *round* hepatic ligament. Leave it long: it could be used to elevate and retract on the liver or used as a patch for perforated duodenal ulcer if the omentum is not available. Take the opportunity to divide the bloodless *falciform* ligament, which runs from the anterior abdominal wall and the diaphragm to the liver. If left intact it may 'tear' off the liver causing irritating bleeding.
- When performing any transverse incision across the midline, do not forget to ligate or transfix the *epigastric vessels* just behind the rectus abdominis muscles. They may retract, be difficult to control, and cause a delayed abdominal wall hematoma.
- **In the very obese patient**, in the upright position, the umbilicus commonly reaches the level of the pubis. After elevating the fat panniculus you can place a lower midline incision between the pubis and umbilicus, but after the operation it will be macerated by the sweaty (and smelly) panniculus. Thus, in the super-fat, a supra-umbilical midline incision would provide a better access into the lower abdomen. (By the way, be careful with the fatty omentum, it tears easily if pulled too hard, and bleeding from the torn omentum is difficult to control except by resecting that part of the omentum altogether.)

"Pray before surgery, but remember God will not alter a faulty incision."

Arthur H. Keeney

"The key is to make an incision. If it is the wrong incision, then make another incision."

Matthew Reeds

Chapter 11

Abdominal exploration: finding what is wrong

The Editors [1]

In surgery, eyes first and most; fingers next and little; tongue last and least.

Sir George Murray Humphry

Never let the skin stand between you and the diagnosis.

(A little old and outdated aphorism in our modern imaging world — but sometimes still useful in an emergency situation…).

Commonly these days — especially with the prevalent use of diagnostic imaging — when opening the abdomen, the surgeon knows what to expect inside; the clinical picture and/or ancillary tests direct him to the disease process. In some instances, however, he explores the unknown, led on only by the signs of peritoneal irritation, assuming that the peritoneal cavity is flooded by blood or pus. Usually the surgeon speculates about the predicted diagnosis but always remains ready for the unexpected (in some places 'Big Brother' compares our pre-op and post-op diagnoses — we are expected always to be 'correct' whereas they are allowed to screw up the budget…). **This is what makes emergency abdominal surgery so exciting and demanding — the ever looming catastrophe and the anxiety about whether or not you are able to tackle it competently**. Yes, even in the days of CT and MRI the abdomen can be full of surprises! If you don't like surprises then go and be a dermatologist.

---

1 Asher Hirshberg, MD, contributed to this chapter in the first edition of this book.

Abdominal exploration (■ Figure 11.1)

While the specific sequence and extent of abdominal exploration are to be tailored to the clinical circumstances, the two principal stages of any exploration are:

- Identification of the specific pathology which prompted the laparotomy.
- Routine exploration of the peritoneal cavity.

There is a sharp distinction between a laparotomy for non-traumatic conditions such as bowel obstruction, inflammation or peritonitis, and laparotomy for trauma with intra-abdominal hemorrhage.

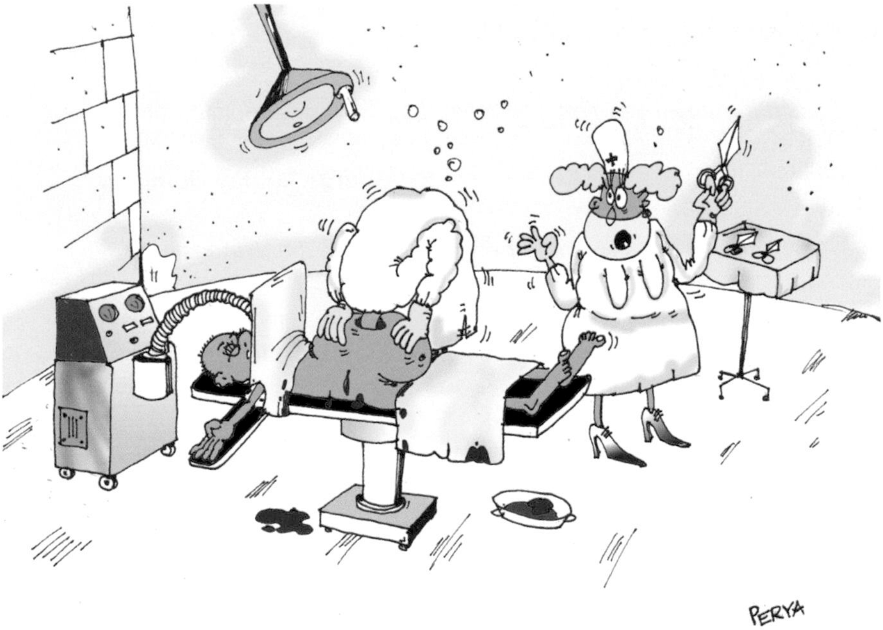

Figure 11.1. "Hey Doc, did you find anything?"

So you incise the peritoneum, what now? Your action depends on the urgency of the situation (condition of the patient), the mechanism of the abdominal pathology (spontaneous versus trauma), and the initial findings (blood, enteric content, bile or pus). Whatever you find, follow the main **priorities**:

- Identify and arrest active bleeding.
- Identify and control continuing contamination.

At the same time — **do not be distracted by trivia**. Do not chase isolated red blood cells or bacteria in a patient who is bleeding to death. For example, do not repair minor mesenteric tears in a patient who is busy exsanguinating from a torn inferior vena cava. This is not a joke — surgeons are easily distracted.

Intraperitoneal blood

The patient may have suffered a blunt or penetrating injury or no injury at all; in the latter case he is suffering from **spontaneous intra-abdominal hemorrhage (abdominal apoplexy)**, an uncommon entity the etiology of which is summarized in ■ Table 11.1.

You may have been expecting the presence of free intraperitoneal blood from the clinical findings of hypovolemic shock, or the results of CT or ultrasound. Your action depends on the magnitude of hemorrhage and the degree of resulting hemodynamic compromise. **When the abdomen is full of blood, and the patient unstable, you should act swiftly.**

Control the situation:

- Enlarge your initial incision generously (avoid the liver and bladder).
- Lift out the small bowel completely (quickly but gently — avoid tearing the mesentery).
- Evacuate the blood as fast as possible — always have two large suckers ready. **However, in massive hemoperitoneum it is better to scoop out the blood with hand/towels/kidney dish, because suckers get easily blocked**.
- Pack the four quadrants tightly with laparotomy pads.

Evacuation of massive hemoperitoneum temporarily aggravates hypovolemia. It releases the tamponade effect and relieves intra-abdominal hypertension (➲ Chapter 31), resulting in sudden pooling of blood in the venous circulation. At this stage, compress the aorta at its diaphragmatic hiatus, or through the lesser omentum, and let the anesthetist catch up with fluid and blood requirements.

Table 11.1. Causes of spontaneous intra-abdominal hemorrhage ('abdominal apoplexy').

Vascular

- ✓ Ruptured abdominal aortic aneurysm
- ✓ Ruptured arterial visceral aneurysm (hepatic, gastroduodenal, splenic, pancreatico-duodenal, renal, gastroepiploic, middle colic, inferior mesenteric, left gastric, ileocolic) — may be associated with Ehlers-Danlos syndrome or other connective tissue disorders
- ✓ Intraperitoneal rupture of varices associated with portal hypertension
- ✓ Spontaneous rupture of the iliac vein

Gynecological

- ✓ Ruptured ectopic pregnancy
- ✓ Spontaneous rupture of the pregnant uterus with placenta percreta
- ✓ Postpartum ovarian artery rupture
- ✓ Spontaneous ovarian hemorrhage (idiopathic, ruptured follicular cyst or *corpus luteum*, ovarian cancer)

Pancreatitis

- ✓ Erosion of adjacent vessels involved in the process of severe acute pancreatitis, chronic pancreatitis or pancreatic pseudocyst

Liver

- ✓ Rupture of benign (typically adenomas) or malignant hepatic tumors

Spleen

- ✓ Spontaneous rupture (infectious mononucleosis)

Adrenal

- ✓ Spontaneous hemorrhage: normal gland (in meningococcemia) or secondary to tumor

Kidney

- ✓ Spontaneous rupture: normal kidney or secondary to tumor (angiomyolipoma)

Anticoagulation

- ✓ Patients on anticoagulation are prone to spontaneous retroperitoneal, intraperitoneal or abdominal wall bleeding (rectus sheath hematoma) — often prompted by unrecognized minor trauma

Unrecognized or denied trauma

- ✓ Patient 'forgot' the kick to the LUQ, which broke his spleen

Miscellaneous

- ✓ Acute ruptured cholecystitis
- ✓ Mediolytic arteritis of an omental artery
- ✓ Polyarteritis nodosa

Be patient, do not rush; with your hand or a Deever retractor (carefully!) on the aorta, the abdomen packed, and the patient's vital organ perfusion improving, you have almost all the time in the world. Do not be tempted at this stage to continue with the operation, which can result in successful hemostasis in a dead patient. Relax and plan the next move, remembering that from now on you can afford to lose only a limited amount of blood before the vicious cycle of hypothermia, acidosis, and coagulopathy — 'the triangle of death' — will further impede your efforts to achieve hemostasis.

Primary survey (see also ➲ Chapter 30)

Now you are ready to identify and treat the life-threatening injuries. The initial direction of your search will be guided by the causative mechanisms. **In penetrating injury the bleeding source should be in the vicinity of the missile or knife track; in blunt trauma, bleeding will probably originate from a ruptured solid organ — the liver or spleen, the pelvic retroperitoneum or a tear in the mesentery**.

Unpack, suck and repack each quadrant consecutively noting where there is blood reaccumulation (active bleeding) or hematoma. Having accurately identified the source (or sources) of bleeding, start definitive hemostasis, the rest of the abdomen being packed away. Simultaneously, if the situation permits, **control contamination** from injured bowel using clamps, staplers or tapes, or repacking in desperate situations.

Stay tuned constantly to events behind the blood-brain barrier (BBB) — which is the screen between you and the anesthetists. Wake them up from time to time and ask how the patient is doing. Take this opportunity also to explain how and what you are doing. Communication among members of the medical team in this situation is vital. **While you are busy repairing the iliac vein the patient may be developing a pericardial tamponade or pneumothorax**. So avoid tunnel vision and keep your antennas up all the time!

Secondary survey

Now the exsanguinating lesion is permanently or temporarily controlled and the patient's hemodynamics have stabilized. With less adrenaline floating around you and the patient, you can divert your attention to all the rest, and look around more precisely. With growing experience your abdominal exploration should become more efficient but never less thorough, **as 'missed' abdominal injuries continue to be a common source of preventable**

morbidity. The practicalities of systematic abdominal exploration are described below.

Intraperitoneal contamination or infection

- First you register the offensive **fecal smell** or **fecal-looking** fluid that denotes the abundance of anaerobic bacteria and usually an infective source in the bowel. Note, however, that neglected infections from any source can be *pseudofeculant* due to the predominance of anaerobes.
- When, on opening the peritoneum, **gas escapes** with a hiss, be aware that a viscus has perforated. In the non-trauma situation this usually implies perforated peptic ulcer or sigmoid diverticulitis.
- **Bile-staining** of the exudate points to pathology in the biliary tract, gastroduodenum or proximal small bowel.
- **Dark stout-beer fluid** and **fat necrosis** hints at pancreatic necrosis or infection in the lesser sac. The great John Hunter (read about him: https://www.rcseng.ac.uk/museums-and-archives/hunterian-museum/about-us/john-hunter/) observed that "the gastric juice is a fluid somewhat transparent, and a little saltish or brackish to the taste" but we do not suggest you go that far! **Whatever the nature of contamination or pus, suck and mop it away as soon as possible**.

Generally, bile directs you proximally and feces distally, but 'simple' pus can come from anywhere. When its source remains elusive, start a systematic search keeping in mind all potential intraperitoneal and retroperitoneal sources 'from the esophagus to the rectum'. Be persistent with your search. We recall a case of spontaneous perforation of the rectum in a young male, twice explored by experienced surgeons who failed to appreciate the minute hole deep in the rectovesical pouch. It was found (by a lowly resident) during a third operation.

Occasionally, however, the origin of contamination or secondary peritonitis is not found. A Gram stain disclosing a *solitary* bacterium — as opposed to a few — suggests the diagnosis of **primary peritonitis**, since *secondary peritonitis* (e.g. secondary to a visceral pathology) is always polymicrobial. More about this in ➲ Chapter 13.

The direction and practicalities of exploration

This depends on the reason for the laparotomy; let's start with a general plan.

The peritoneal cavity comprises **two compartments: the supracolic and the infracolic compartment**. The dividing line is the transverse (meso)colon, which in a xipho-pubic midline incision is located approximately in the center of the incision (a little above the *bauchnabel* or the belly button).

Our preference is to begin with the infracolic compartment: the transverse colon is retracted upwards, the small bowel eviscerated (covered with moist, warm sponges), and the rectosigmoid identified. Exploration begins with the pelvic reproductive organs in the female, and then attention is turned to inspection and palpation of the rectosigmoid, progressing to the left, transverse and then right colon and cecum, including inspection of the mesocolon. The assistant follows the exploration with successive movements of a hand-held retractor to retract the edge of the surgical incision and to enable good visualization of whichever abdominal structure is the focus of attention. Exploration of small bowel then proceeds in a retrograde fashion from the ileocecal valve to the ligament of Treitz, with special care being taken to inspect both 'anterior' and 'posterior' aspects of each loop of bowel as well as its mesentery.

Attention is then turned to the **supracolic compartment**. The transverse colon is pulled down, and the surgeon inspects and palpates the liver, gallbladder, stomach (including the proper placement of a nasogastric tube), and spleen. **Special care should be taken to avoid iatrogenic damage to the spleen caused by pulling hard on the body of the stomach or the greater omentum**.

A complete abdominal exploration also includes entry into the **lesser peritoneal sac**, which is best undertaken through the **gastrocolic omentum**. This omentum is usually only a **thin avascular membrane** on the left side, and this should therefore be the preferred entry route into the lesser sac. Take care to avoid injury to the transverse mesocolon which may be adherent to the gastrocolic omentum. A misdirected surgeon can be convinced that he is entering the lesser sac when in fact he or she is cutting a hole in the transverse mesocolon. If 'vascular', the gastrocolic omentum is divided between ligatures (or one of your modern energy emitting devices) bringing the body and tail of the pancreas into full view. **Should you decide to enter the lesser sac through the lesser omentum (above the stomach) be careful to not divide any pulsatile vessel coursing within the upper lesser sac as it may be an aberrant left hepatic artery originating from the left gastric artery!**

Exploration of retroperitoneal structures involves two key mobilization maneuvers, which should be employed whenever access to the retroperitoneum is deemed necessary:

- **'Kocher's maneuver'** is mobilization of the duodenal C-loop and the head of the pancreas by incising the thin peritoneal membrane (posterior peritoneum) overlying the lateral aspect of the duodenum and gradually lifting the duodenum and pancreatic head medially. This maneuver is also the key to surgical exposure of the right kidney and its hilum and the right adrenal gland. Kocher's maneuver may be extended further lateral and caudad, around the hepatic flexure and along the 'white line' on the lateral aspect of the right colon, all the way down to the cecum. This extension allows **medial rotation of the right colon** and affords good exposure of the right-sided retroperitoneal structures such as the inferior vena cava, iliac vessels and the right ureter. Further extension of this incision angles around the caecum and continues in a superomedial direction along the line of fusion of the small bowel mesentery to the posterior abdominal wall. Thus it is possible to mobilize and reflect the small bowel upwards, the so-called *Cattell-Braasch maneuver*. This affords optimal exposure of the entire inframesocolic retroperitoneum, including the aorta and its infrarenal branches.
- The second key mobilization maneuver is called the '**left-sided Kocher**' or '**medial visceral rotation**' (also called by some the '**Mattox maneuver**') and is used especially to gain access to the entire length of the abdominal aorta and to the left-sided retroperitoneal viscera. Depending on the structures to be exposed this maneuver begins either lateral to the spleen (splenophrenic and splenorenal ligament) working caudally or in the 'white line' of Toldt lateral to the junction of the descending and sigmoid colon, working upwards. The peritoneum is incised and the viscera, including the left colon, spleen and tail of the pancreas are gradually mobilized medially. The left kidney can either be mobilized or left *in situ*, depending on the surgical target of the exploration.

In cases of **spontaneous hemoperitoneum**, you'll have to look for a ruptured aortic, iliac or visceral arterial aneurysm, ectopic pregnancy, bleeding hepatic tumor, spontaneous rupture of an enlarged spleen, or any of the other causes listed in ■ Table 11.1.

In **penetrating trauma** you'll follow the entry-exit track, taking into consideration the missile's energy, velocity and potential to fragment. **Wherever there is an entry wound in a viscus or blood vessel look for the**

exit one! The latter may lie concealed on the lesser sac back-wall of the stomach, the retroperitoneal surface of the duodenum, or the mesenteric edge of the small bowel. **Missing an exit wound is often a death sentence to your patient!**

It is the **blunt abdominal injury**, however, that requires the most extensive and less directed search, from the surface of both hemi-diaphragms to the pelvis, from gutter to gutter, on all solid organs, along the whole length of the gastrointestinal tract, and in the retroperitoneum (the retroperitoneum selectively, as discussed in ➲ Chapter 30). **The exact sequence of exploration is less important than its thoroughness**.

Use your common sense...

Are you already snoring? A little boring, eh? So wake up and listen: because this book is aimed also at trainees we had to be complete and describe the 'classical abdominal exploration'. But frankly, if the patient is bleeding from a ruptured liver we would explore the upper abdomen, but if the infracolic compartment looks pristine and dry we would leave it alone. **So use your common sense**: do not look for ovarian cysts in a patient with a bleeding spleen. Like Dr. Leo Gordon said: "**When common sense interferes with a protocol, follow common sense**."

What about retractors?

Use whatever is available at your institution. In most circumstances we prefer one of the **hand-held retractors** in the hands of the assistant. But not all assistants are as passive or active as you wish them to be. As Arthur E. Hertzler wrote: "If I ever deliberately commit murder I shall select an inattentive and awkward assistant as my victim. I shall select one who has assisted enough to delude himself into thinking he could himself do the work better than the surgeon who is operating. This usually reaches the high point at about the third week of the intern's experiences."

In some situations a 'passive' fixed' retractor (a.k.a. a 'mute intern') should be used — especially when operating in the pelvis or upper abdomen. The good old Balfour retractor is useful when doing a midline laparotomy. Of course, your hospital may have one of those fancy multi-arm retractors (called the Omni-Tract® or whatever) or the ingenious Bookwalter® ring retractor; some surgeons like to use them — particularly those who do not have residents but have to rely on sleepy nurses. We try to use those types of mechanical retractors selectively: often the time needed to place them is longer than the operation and we hate operating with a sharp metal frame piercing our paunch. But when you expect a deep and long dissection — a fixed, smart retractor can change your operation from a struggle to pure fun.

Additional points: grading the severity of injury

Abdominal exploration for trauma ends with a strategic decision about the subsequent steps. Forget at this stage the many available organ injury scales, which are of academic value only; **from the operating surgeon's point of view there are essentially two patterns of visceral damage: 'minor trouble' and 'major trouble'**:

- **'Minor trouble'** involves easily fixable injuries, either because the injured organ is accessible or the surgical solution is straightforward (e.g. splenectomy, suture of mesenteric bleeders, or resection of a colon perforation). There is no immediate danger of exsanguination or loss of surgical control. Under these circumstances you can immediately proceed with definitive repair or source control.
- **'Major trouble'** is when the injury or spontaneous condition is not easily rectified because of complexity or inaccessibility (e.g. a high-grade liver injury, a major retroperitoneal vascular injury in the supracolic compartment, or destruction of the pancreatoduodenal complex). **Here the secret of success is to HOLD the operation** when temporary (usually digital or manual) control of bleeding is achieved. Update all members of the operating and anesthesia teams on the operative plan. Allow your anesthesiologist to use the time needed to stabilize the patient hemodynamically and to obtain more blood products. This is also the appropriate time to seek more competent help, and to plan the operative attack, including additional exposure and mobilization. Such preparation is crucial for the survival of your patient.

Remember: Very often the initial exploration of the abdomen in the trauma patient is incomplete, because the patient's critical condition creates a situation where every minute counts and injuries are simply repaired as they are encountered. **Under these circumstances you must complete the exploration before terminating the procedure**.

Finally, *primum non nocere* (**first do no harm**). This applies everywhere in medicine but is of paramount importance during abdominal exploration. The injured or infected contents of the peritoneal cavity may be inflamed, swollen, adherent, friable and brittle. Careless and sloppy manipulation and separation of viscera during exploration can induce additional bleeding and may produce additional bowel defects, or enlarge the existing ones. And as always, new problems translate into additional therapies and morbidity.

As an emergency abdominal surgeon, you have the chance to be excited and highly satisfied. Try not to screw this up by harming your patients; the fall from the adrenalin-induced 'high' to the failure-induced 'down' can be painful.

> **"When the doctor is in doubt and the patient in danger, make an exploratory incision and deal with what you find as best as you can."**
>
> **Robert Lawson Tait**

Chapter 12

The laparoscopic approach to emergency abdominal surgery

The Editors

> *Laparoscopy shares many similarities with the emperor's new clothes. If you do not join in the choir of praise you are considered either stupid or unfit for the job. But someone has to tell the truth.*
>
> **Roland Andersson**

General principles

Laparoscopy has long ago become part of our daily routine, and even if we still argue about its value in certain procedures, you surely feel familiar and confident, after some training and experience, to enter the abdomen and use the relevant instruments. **So, what is so special and different in emergency laparoscopy, compared to your usual laparoscopic cholecystectomy?**

Well, quite a lot...

- Diagnosis may be elusive.
- The patient's physiology may be deranged.
- Abdominal conditions may be unfavorable.
- Speed may be critical.
- Timing is usually inconvenient: experienced staff may be lacking, available staff may be tired, and you may need to handle unfamiliar situations, with less assistance.

So in general, both decision making and operating technique are more complicated in a surgical emergency. Even procedures you are confident with (laparoscopic cholecystectomy) may become a challenge — for example, in acute gangrenous cholecystitis. But, as you know from elective surgery, reducing surgical trauma to the abdominal wall is beneficial, maybe even more so in a patient with an acute condition who needs his 'healing energy' to overcome the disease itself. The usual potential advantages of laparoscopy — less pain, shorter ileus, and enhanced mobilization — are relevant in the acute setting. On the other hand, the list above makes it obvious that **emergency laparoscopy is not a walk in the park, and the risk of complications is increased**.

But before you decide to use this excellent tool, you must recognize its limitations, and even more important — **you must acknowledge YOUR own limitations. Selectivity, dexterity, and clinical judgment must guide your decisions when and if to use laparoscopy, how to carry it out safely, when to convert, and when to avoid it altogether**.

Potential advantages

- **Diagnosis**. Despite modern imaging, we still operate on patients that may surprise us. The use of CT scans has not eliminated surgery for the non-inflamed appendix. The free air may come from perforation of a viscus we did not suspect. The bowel obstruction in a patient with metastases can be the result of a single adhesive band. **These situations and others can of course be detected and treated by a large, 'formal' laparotomy, but what if we could reduce the cost of exploration by limiting the abdominal wall trauma?** Laparoscopic exploration can establish the diagnosis and direct us to the required intervention. **And even if open surgery is eventually required — it may be done in a more directed way, through a limited incision sited where the pathology lies**.
- **Surgical trauma**. In a patient suffering from an acute abdominal condition, reducing the additional physiologic burden of a large abdominal wound is a highly desired objective. Pain, ileus, immobilization, respiratory dysfunction — are all expected in a patient with an inflammatory or obstructive abdominal condition — why add to that a long incision, which can pour fuel on the inflammatory fire? **Reducing tissue trauma contributes to enhanced recovery**.
- **Wound-related problems**. In acute conditions, the risk of wound infection is increased, and so are the chances of wound healing disorders, wound dehiscence and eventual incisional hernia.

Laparoscopy may prevent these conditions, or at least diminish them by allowing the use of smaller, directed incisions.

Potential flaws

The significant advantages listed above should be balanced against many potential difficulties and risks expected in a patient with an acute abdomen. These relate both to the general condition of the patient, and the specific conditions found inside the abdomen. **The resulting complications, or even mortality, may be fully preventable by an open approach or a timely conversion.**

Here are a few drawbacks of laparoscopy:

- **Hemodynamic stability.** Inflating the abdomen with CO_2 is well tolerated by most patients in elective conditions, despite the known effects on the cardiovascular and respiratory system. This may not be the case in the hypovolemic or septic patient, suffering from a distended abdomen and respiratory insufficiency. **The delicate physiological balance, if still maintained before surgery, may be easily lost by the added insult of increased abdominal pressure and decreased perfusion. In fact, an open abdomen may actually be required as part of the treatment...**
- **Need for speed.** Procrastination is certainly not something a bleeding patient needs. A trauma patient in shock is not the correct patient on whom to practice your hand-eye coordination skills. **Open up and stop the bleeding!**
- **Need for space.** This is a pre-requisite for safe and successful laparoscopy. Colonic obstruction will not leave you enough working space and is almost out of the question for laparoscopy. A thick, edematous abdominal wall (common after aggressive resuscitation) with limited compliance will hardly let you create a working space or will mandate high (and dangerous) insufflation pressures. Obstructed small bowel may still leave you enough working space but will not make your life easy — **extreme care and a high degree of expertise are needed to avoid catastrophic injuries like major spillage of obstructed contents; we have seen mortality from this.**
- **Technical limitations.** The local conditions found in the acute abdomen may limit the ability to handle the situation laparoscopically. Adhesions, tissue edema, bowel distension — **all of these can interfere with the handling, retraction, manipulation and mobilization needed to complete the procedure promptly and safely.**

- **Missed pathology**. The limited palpation, limited access to retroperitoneal structures and sometimes limited visibility may result in missing the actual pathology. **Conversion is a good solution but only if the surgeon realizes that something is missing…**

Remember: I have never seen a patient dying because he was converted to open; I saw them dying because they were not converted in a timely manner. **Moshe**

Setting the scene

Laparoscopy is a team procedure, even more so than open surgery. You rely on equipment and technology that should be familiar to your OR staff, who should help you operate and trouble-shoot them. You also rely on good assistance, for holding the camera and additional instruments.

Achieving smooth laparoscopic procedures out-of-hours, for non-routine cases, performed on patients in non-optimal conditions, is not an easy task. The tired anesthetist and the thirsty scrub nurse may not be eager to join you in what is conceived to be a longer and more difficult procedure. **To become an emergency surgery laparoscopist you should train your OR team to function in these conditions, and it starts by realizing that laparoscopy is possible, and that it's in the patient's best interests to have the procedure done laparoscopically, even at 2 a.m.**

You should start with simple procedures, like appendectomy or maybe cholecystectomy for acute cholecystitis if you feel proficient enough, and make sure the *system* functions well. Only then can you embark on more challenging conditions like duodenal perforation or small bowel obstruction.

And don't buy all that is described in the literature — we will forgive you if you continue to remove the shattered spleen via a midline laparotomy.

You should also make sure you are well equipped for completing the task in front of you. You may know how to suture laparoscopically (you should!) but you need a suture holder. You may need to work in more than one quadrant so better have another monitor ready. You may need to aspirate infected fluid so make sure your suction is connected and functioning. Energy sources, staplers — think about your possible needs in advance, while you think about your impending procedure and plan it, and make sure you have what you need to make the operation safe and successful — **your elegant hands are important but not enough on their own**.

Technique

Planning the procedure

The beauty of emergency surgery is in the surprises it holds for you. And yet, try to minimize surprises and be ready. If you plan to tackle an *incarcerated hernia* laparoscopically — think about the possible scenarios and how you will tackle them: what will you do if you find necrotic bowel? If you go in for *small bowel obstruction*, try to identify the location of the obstruction in the pre-op CT scan: this will help you plan the trocar placement for your scope and instruments, and the location of the monitor at a convenient spot in front of you.

Getting in

We are not here to solve the eternal debate — Veress or Hasson? You may have your own preferences for elective surgery, and it's fine by us. **But we expect you to be familiar with both techniques, because in emergency conditions selectivity is the key, and the closed, blind entry may be more dangerous in certain conditions. For example, with *bowel obstruction* — both the distended bowel and the adhesions from previous operations mandate that you choose the open entry to avoid inadvertent bowel injury**.

Choosing the camera

As you have probably realized by now, a 30° scope will increase your field of view and your overall versatility, and is recommended as a standard. It may be even more valuable in emergency operations, where the need 'to look behind', due to adhesions or bowel distension, is more pronounced. Provided you have a good optical system with a good light source, a 5mm scope may allow you to easily move the camera between different trocars, enabling different viewing angles. A second monitor on the other side of the table may be a good adjunct for this situation. But if you don't have a high- quality 5mm optical system, and especially when you know you are going to work in a single quadrant (*appendectomy, cholecystectomy*), don't compromise, and

get the best viewing conditions you can, using a 10mm scope. This will keep your illumination maximal, even in harsh conditions like blood pooling in your field.

Placing the working trocars

You should have a general working plan, to achieve the surgical task in hand. Some surgical emergencies are 'straightforward', and have a standard scheme: laparoscopic cholecystectomy or appendectomy are usually done the same way (with some minor variations), and are limited to one abdominal quadrant. **Bowel obstruction, on the other hand, can have its 'transition point' in an unexpected abdominal location**. Analyzing the CT scan and understanding where the obstruction point is, even approximately, will help you to plan the trocars' locations in the most effective way (■ Figure 12.1).

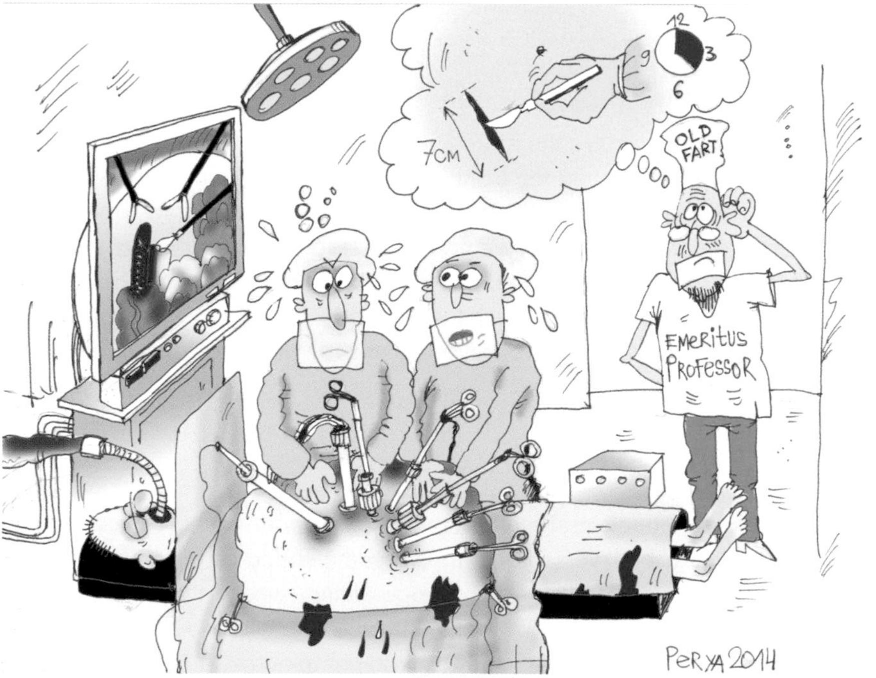

Figure 12.1. Surgeon: "I had to insert a few more trocars for exposure." Assistant: "But Sir, you should have used the robot..."

Tissue handling

Dealing with swollen, edematous and inflamed tissues, or obstructed, distended bowel, is a surgical challenge, requiring both delicacy and firmness in the exact amounts. Holding too delicately or too aggressively — you can rip softened tissue. Manipulating a distended bowel — you can perforate it. Dissecting inflamed tissue too much — you can produce excessive bleeding.

Much experience is needed, but a few rules and tips can help you sail more safely through stormy emergency waters until you gain that experience:

- 'Big bites' are less likely to tear delicate tissues you need to hold.
- Suction tip is a wonderful tool for dissecting inflamed tissues.
- Blunt dissection will help you follow the anatomical planes, especially when separating relatively fresh adhesions.
- Collapsed, post-obstruction bowel loops are the best place to start when you look for the obstruction point.
- When 'running' the bowel, holding the mesentery just below the bowel and not the bowel itself may reduce the risk of inadvertent bowel injury.

Procedures

Choosing which emergency procedure to attempt laparoscopically is not always simple. Some procedures are within the consensus — a 'hot' gallbladder will rarely be approached initially by open surgery. Others will rarely involve a laparoscopic attempt — like abdominal trauma. In most cases the final decision will be a complex outcome of multiple factors, but if the necessary conditions (equipment, experience) are met, we still have to ask ourselves: **is it worthwhile? What do we gain from laparoscopy and what do we risk?**

The best emergency procedures, listed below, to accomplish laparoscopically, are those having a large advantage/disadvantage ratio compared to open surgery.

Here are only a few 'laparoscopic' comments for each of these procedures, as a comprehensive discussion of them is given in the relevant chapters.

Laparoscopic cholecystectomy (see ➲ Chapter 18.1)

Depending on your local practice, acutely inflamed gallbladders may be either operated upon or treated conservatively. **But while open surgery for acute cholecystitis was once the bread and butter of surgical residents, laparoscopic surgery for this condition is quite demanding, requiring the presence of an experienced laparoscopist, and familiarity with several maneuvers that will make safe removal of the gallbladder possible**:

- **Grasping** a distended gallbladder is difficult. Aspirating the bile (you can use the Veress needle for that) will make grasping possible.
- **Blunt dissection**, using the suction tip, is especially rewarding in edematous, inflamed tissues.
- **Anatomy** may be obscured in inflamed conditions — **don't take shortcuts; insist on obtaining the 'critical view of safety'**.
- **If you can't delineate the anatomy — consider alternative approaches, like subtotal cholecystectomy**. Opening the gallbladder just above Hartmann's pouch, carefully evacuating the stones into a pre-placed collection bag and looking down into the gallbladder outlet may assist you in delineation of the anatomy, and understanding where the cystic duct hides. If still unclear — make sure you have cleared the stones and then suture the cystic duct from within, or close Hartmann's pouch with sutures or an Endoloop®. If these maneuvers seem 'impossible', you can simply leave a drain and bail out!
- **Don't forget the option of conversion!** 'Remembering' that option in hindsight *after* the patient has suffered a CBD injury or *after* you have been sued, is not too helpful. Conversion should not be regarded as 'failure'.

Laparoscopic appendectomy (see ➲ Chapter 21)

The advantages of laparoscopy, compared to open appendectomy, are not pronounced, and therefore the debate regarding which approach is preferable is not over. Be that as it may, in practice, we have seen a major increase in the rate of laparoscopic appendectomy, so it's here to stay. **Its advantages are more evident in obese patients, in females and where imaging modalities are less available**.

We will not dwell too much here on the technique (see ➲ Chapter 21.1), and the trocar arrangement is really not that important — use what you were taught to do and what you feel comfortable with. **But if you want to decrease the most quoted disadvantage — postoperative pelvic collection — you**

probably have to be careful while handling the inflamed appendix, and avoid overzealous irrigation.

Perforations and peritonitis (see ➲ Chapters 13 and 16)

You may not want to take an elderly, unstable, septic patient and pump his abdomen with CO_2 (anyway you better resuscitate and stabilize him before he crashes under anesthesia), but in many cases laparoscopy is useful in dealing with peritonitis. **If you already have a diagnosis**, like a *perforated peptic ulcer*, all you need is peritoneal toilet and a few sutures to complete the *Graham patch* (see ➲ Chapter 16.1) and laparoscopy is ideal: it will certainly reduce the wound infection risk and other incision-related problems. Just make sure your laparoscopic suturing skills are well practiced.

If the diagnosis is not known — laparoscopy may be a perfect diagnostic tool, once you decide that the patient needs surgery. Even if conversion is needed — it may be done through a directed, limited incision. The *small bowel perforation*, due to a fish-bone, may be exteriorized and repaired (or resected), without a major midline laparotomy. *Perforated diverticulitis* can also be handled laparoscopically, especially if you like (and trust) the modern 'lavage and drainage' approach for Hinchey 3 cases (non-fecal peritonitis) (see ➲ Chapter 26). If resection is needed, probably with a Hartmann's procedure, and you have laparoscopic colectomy skills, they can be of use now. Otherwise, a conversion through a lower midline laparotomy will usually suffice. **But again — these procedures are for the experts — you need to polish your elective advanced laparoscopic skills before venturing into such potential minefields**.

Small bowel obstruction (see ➲ Chapter 19)

Though probably one of the more challenging emergency procedures for laparoscopy, this may also be one of the most rewarding: cutting a single adhesive band can be a quick procedure that prevents a closed loop obstruction from quickly progressing to bowel necrosis. Indeed, some obstruction cases are the result of multiple adhesions, and extensive adhesiolysis is needed — not a task for a laparoscopic spring-chicken. But, when laparoscopic adhesiolysis is successful, the advantages to the patient are significant: the quick return of bowel function and the reduced risk for new adhesions and wound-associated complications (dehiscence is a real risk after laparotomy for obstruction, due to the distended bowel and increased abdominal pressure).

In order to achieve these advantages, your technique must be flawless. The risk of perforating an obstructed bowel is real, and spillage of the high-pressure, static contents may lead to an uncontrollable and irreversible sepsis. **Going 'in reverse' from the collapsed, distal bowel, avoiding bowel handling as much as possible, and avoiding the use of energy sources will help you avoid disasters**.

Incarcerated hernia (see ➲ Chapter 20)

Commonly an indication for an open procedure, incarcerated hernias, whether incisional or inguinal, can be approached laparoscopically. Indeed, reducing the incarcerated contents by *pulling* (gently!) is usually easier than by *pushing*, assisted of course by the muscle relaxation of the abdominal wall. The hernia defect can also be repaired laparoscopically, but if you find necrotic bowel then conversion, resection and primary hernia repair is your best bet. **Of course, if your open hernia skills are better than the lap ones in the elective situation this is what you should use in the emergency**.

Trauma (see ➲ Chapter 30)

As repeatedly mentioned above, abdominal trauma is not an indication for laparoscopic surgery, but a few specific conditions make laparoscopy more appealing.

Diaphragmatic laceration is sometimes difficult to diagnose, and if highly suspected, and no other indications for abdominal exploration currently exist, laparoscopy, in a stable patient, is a good alternative (especially on the left side). Diagnosis, and non-absorbable suture repair are relatively easy. In a hemodynamically-normal patient it may even be worthwhile to delay surgery until the next morning — make sure the patient really has no other injuries, and have the procedure done by your expert laparoscopist, who doesn't like to be moved out of his bed at night.

> **"Laparoscopy is a path, not a goal.**
> **The goal is a safe outcome!"**
>
> **Vinay Mehendale**

Chapter 13

Peritonitis: classification and principles of treatment

The Editors [1]

> *The mechanical control of the source of infection, while itself nonbiologic, determines the extent of the host biologic response to the disease.*
>
> **Ronald V. Maier**

> *In peritonitis — source control is above all.*

The finding of inflammation, bowel contents or pus, localized or dispersed throughout the peritoneal cavity, is common at emergency laparotomy. How should you best handle this scenario? This chapter will discuss *general aspects* of the surgical treatment. For the management of individual causes of peritonitis look at the specific chapters.

Nomenclature

Inflammation of the peritoneum is termed **peritonitis**. It is generally caused by a bacterial inoculum. This explains why peritonitis and **intra-abdominal infection (IAI)** are used interchangeably. It is important to note though that these two terms are not synonymous, because **peritonitis may also be sterile** as with the chemical peritonitis of early perforation of a peptic ulcer or inadvertent infusion of enteral feeding through a misplaced jejunostomy tube. Here are some definitions to confuse you more:

- **Intra-abdominal infection**. For a condition to be labelled IAI, both the intraperitoneal presence of micro-organisms (or their toxins) and the

1 Roger Saadia, MD FRCS(Ed), contributed to previous versions of this chapter.

inflammatory response of the peritoneum are required. When a purulent exudate is found at laparotomy this is termed by some as 'established peritonitis'.

- **Peritoneal contamination is different.** It consists merely of the soiling of the peritoneal cavity by a fluid rich in micro-organisms, as in the immediate aftermath of a penetrating intestinal injury, before an inflammatory response has taken place.
- **IAI can be diffuse as in generalized peritonitis or localized as in intra-abdominal abscesses.** The latter develop as a result of effective host defenses and represent a relatively successful outcome of peritonitis. **The mainstay of treatment is drainage** (see ➲ Chapter 42).
- **Abdominal sepsis** is still a term used by some but we, semantic *nudniks*, do not like it. **According to modern consensus 'sepsis' means the conjunction of both the host's inflammatory response to infection and a source of infection.** Strictly speaking, **local contamination, infection and sepsis refer to different processes.** Yet, they may coexist in the same patient, developing simultaneously or consecutively — a *continuum*. Abdominal contamination may lead to infection, which is invariably associated with a systemic inflammatory response — sepsis. **Significantly, residual abdominal inflammation or indeed the systemic response (fever, leukocytosis) may even persist after the intraperitoneal infection has been eradicated. Once set in motion, the inflammatory cascade cannot be stopped simply by turning off the trigger.**

Classification of peritonitis

Secondary peritonitis

Ninety-five percent or more of the cases of peritonitis in your practice will be 'secondary'.

This is caused by a breach in the anatomical integrity of a hollow viscus (e.g. perforation or transmural necrosis). It is usually characterized by an aerobic and anaerobic polymicrobial inoculum, reflecting the flora of the gastrointestinal tract. Examples include perforated appendicitis, perforated diverticular disease of the colon, strangulated obstruction of the small bowel and (non-GI) ruptured tubo-ovarian abscess. **It is largely because of secondary peritonitis that you should train yourself to become an expert in surgical infections and the use of antibiotics!** (Try at least to be as knowledgeable as your local infectious disease guru...).

Primary peritonitis

In contrast to secondary peritonitis, this is not caused by a loss of gastrointestinal wall integrity and is not associated with leakage of intestinal contents into the peritoneal cavity. **The responsible micro-organism, typically single (as opposed to the complex flora of secondary peritonitis), originates from a source outside of the abdomen**. In **young girls**, it is usually a *Streptococcus* gaining access via the genital tract. In patients with cirrhosis, *Escherichia coli* is thought to be a blood-borne agent infecting pre-existing ascites — a condition referred to as *spontaneous bacterial peritonitis*. In patients receiving **peritoneal dialysis**, *Staphylococcus* migrates from the skin along the dialysis catheter.

In patients with a known predisposing factor (e.g. ascites associated with chronic liver disease), suspected primary peritonitis can be diagnosed by paracentesis (a polymorphonuclear count in the ascitic fluid greater than 250 cells/mm^3); a positive culture confirms the diagnosis but, even with a negative culture, antibiotic treatment should be instituted. **Whenever possible, a diagnostic exploratory laparoscopy or laparotomy should be avoided because of its prohibitive mortality**. Initial antibiotic treatment is empiric, until results of bacteriological sensitivities become available.

Primary peritonitis in patients without a known predisposing factor is extremely rare. It is usually diagnosed at laparotomy/laparoscopy for an 'acute abdomen' revealing an odorless exudate without an apparent source. The diagnosis is reached by exclusion after a thorough abdominal exploration and is confirmed by a Gram stain and culture that usually isolates a solitary, aerobic organism — **it is a 'single-bug disease'**.

The ever more common use of CT is why we so rarely encounter this entity these days. In primary peritonitis, CT would show free intraperitoneal fluid but no definitive source. Rather than rush to operation, the fluid is sampled percutaneously. The diagnosis is established and managed with antibiotics.

Risk ranking

In order to help select the appropriate management and to estimate prognosis you should rank patients with IAI into two main groups: low risk and high risk.

Low-risk group

Most of your patients will belong to this group:

- They suffer from '**community-acquired IAI**': the patient walks through the ER doors with abdominal pain due to a perforated appendicitis, strangulated bowel or perforated diverticulitis.
- They are not physiologically compromised: stable hemodynamically, no significant organ system failure.
- They are relatively healthy: no advanced comorbidities, no immunosuppression.

High-risk group

- Patients with '**hospital-acquired IAI**' belong to this group. It is a much more morbid event occurring in an already hospitalized patient; for example, ischemic perforation of the colon in a ventilated patient treated for severe pneumonia.
- Obviously, patients with so-called '**postoperative peritonitis**' also belong to this group; for example, a leaking colonic anastomosis on postoperative day 6.
- All critically ill and/or severely immunocompromised patients (steroids, anti-cancer drugs, post-transplant) belong to this category.

These two groups differ significantly:

- The **diagnosis** of peritonitis is much easier to make in the ER than in an ICU patient with multiple comorbidities.
- The **antibiotic** treatment is standard broad-spectrum in community-acquired peritonitis, whereas it needs to be tailored to a hospital-acquired, more pathogenic and often unexpected flora in the patient with nosocomial peritonitis.
- The **source control** of IAI may be more difficult to achieve in the high-risk group (and requires repetitive efforts).
- Finally, the **prognosis** is much less favorable in the high-risk variety.

We have decided to omit from this edition a detailed discussion of **tertiary peritonitis**. This entity has never received widespread recognition and thus has disappeared from the recent literature. **However, we believe it exists. It represents the end-stage of 'high risk IAI'.** Typically, the scenario is like this: the patient lies in the ICU with multi-organ dysfunction; <u>source control has been achieved</u> after multiple operations; the abdomen has been left open; the peritoneal cavity contains a thin, cloudy, poorly walled-off exudate which grows opportunistic micro-organisms (e.g. *Staphylococcus epidermidis*, *Enterococcus* and *Candida albicans*).

This syndrome illustrates the paradox of modern medicine. On the one hand, it is an outcome of unsuccessful treatment of a 'high-risk IAI'. On the other hand, high-tech interventions have permitted the emergence of this category of patients who would have succumbed much earlier to their disease only two or three decades ago (so, yes, a measure of success). **The frequently fatal outcome of tertiary peritonitis indicates that current antibiotic-assisted, aggressive mechanical answers to advanced IAI have about reached their limits.** (Oops, we wanted to omit the topic altogether... as with any book, the decision of what to omit/delete is more difficult than what to write about.)

Management

> The outcome of IAI depends on the patient's premorbid reserves, his current physiological compromise and the virulence of the infection. Your goal is to assist the patient's own local and systemic defenses.

The philosophy of management in a typical case of IAI consists of initial adjunctive measures, source control, followed by peritoneal toilet.

Adjunctive measures

These refer to the stabilization of a sick patient by means of appropriate fluid and electrolyte replenishment. The invasiveness of the monitoring should be tailored to the physiologic status of the patient. **In peritonitis, operating on a poorly resuscitated patient is like throwing both ends of the rope at a drowning man.**

Antibiotics

Empirical, broad antibiotic coverage for aerobic and anaerobic gut flora infection should be started early, as discussed in ➲ Chapter 7. Again, we won't tell you which specific agents to use — your hospital should have its own protocols based on what's available locally and on known patterns of bacterial susceptibility and resistance. In general the 'simpler' regimen should be used in patients with 'low-risk IAI' while the 'big guns' are reserved for the 'high-risk' entities. Read about the *duration* of administration in ➲ Chapter 40.

What about the need for peritoneal cultures?

No, you don't need to obtain cultures of the infected peritoneal fluids in patients with community-acquired, 'low-risk' IAI. The microbiology of this type of IAI is predictable (you don't need to culture s**t!) and it responds readily to an empiric broad-spectrum antibiotic regimen, initiated pre-operatively, that includes anti-anaerobic coverage. In most cases, culture results become available only well after completion of the antibiotic course. Such (costly) cultures won't change your management — but can only confuse some ignorant members of the team.

However, peritoneal cultures are indicated and potentially useful in the following scenarios:

- **Hospital-acquired peritonitis**; the best example being postoperative peritonitis.
- Peritonitis in the **immunocompromised patient** (e.g. AIDS, on chemotherapy).
- Patients who are already on antibiotics, for whatever reason, or have been recently treated with antibiotics.
- Patients with a history of methicillin-resistant *Staphylococcus aureus* (MRSA).
- Patients with suspected **primary peritonitis** where there is no intra-abdominal source of infection.
- **Tertiary peritonitis** which is commonly associated with a peculiar microbiology (see above).

Source control

Source control is the intervention to interrupt the delivery of bacteria and adjuvants of inflammation (bile, blood, fecal matter, barium) into the peritoneal cavity. It is the key to success and survival. **All other measures are futile if the intervention does not successfully eradicate the source and reduce the inoculum to an amount that can be handled effectively by the patient's defenses, supported by antibiotic therapy**.

Source control does not always mean that you must jump immediately on the IAI patient with an operation. Instead, you must be selective, fitting the punishment/treatment to the crime — the individual patient and his disease process. Here are a few nuances to consider:

- **Non-operative management**. In some cases (e.g. acute uncomplicated diverticulitis or acute cholecystitis), i.v. antibiotics alone suffice to effect source control.
- **Invasiveness**. Use the least invasive approach that can accomplish source control (e.g. percutaneous drainage for pericolic abscess).
- **Temporizing measures**. In patients with major physiological compromise, consider temporizing measures to allow optimization before the definitive operative onslaught: *diversion* (e.g. proximal stoma in a patient too unstable to tolerate a colon resection) or *drainage* (e.g. leaking duodenum).
- **Timing**. Source control should be effected as soon as possible after the diagnosis and of course after an appropriate period of physiological optimization. The sicker the patient the more urgent the need for source control. So simple appendicitis can wait until the morning, or the end of the elective list. But perforated appendicitis should be managed ASAP. **Remember: an unintended delay in source control means increased morbidity and mortality**.

In most etiologies of secondary peritonitis, source control involves a simple procedure such as an appendectomy or a patch closure for a perforated ulcer. Occasionally, a major resection to remove the infective focus is indicated, such as a gastrectomy for a perforated gastric carcinoma or a colectomy for perforated diverticulitis.

Generally, the choice of procedure (e.g. stoma versus primary anastomosis), depends on the anatomical source of infection, the degree of peritoneal inflammation, the patient's premorbid reserves and the degree of systemic sepsis, as discussed in the individual chapters.

More aggressive modalities of management?

In doubtful cases do not wait too long
Before exploring, for it is quite wrong
To act upon the slogan Wait and See,
When looking may provide the remedy.

Zachary Cope

Most IAI patients respond to the combination of adequate source control, appropriate antibiotics and competent supportive management. Some patients, however, need more:

- A **planned relaparotomy** would be needed (the next day or day after) if the source could not be controlled at the index operation (because of technical difficulties and/or the patient's critical condition forcing an 'abbreviated laparotomy') or because of the specific pathology (e.g. infected pancreatic necrosis).
- **Leaving the abdomen open (laparostomy)** to prevent and treat the abdominal compartment syndrome. Furthermore, a laparostomy facilitates re-exploration — why close the abdomen if you have to go back! **Thus the two methods are usually combined.**

You will find a detailed discussion on laparostomy and reoperations in ➲ Chapters 31 and 44. Meanwhile, ■ Table 13.1 shows our indications for using these modalities.

Table 13.1. Indications for an 'abbreviated laparotomy'/ laparostomy/planned relaparotomy.*

- ■ **Critical patient condition** (hemodynamic instability) precluding appropriate source control at the first operation, thus calling for an 'abbreviated laparotomy' or 'damage control' strategy.
- ■ **Abdominal compartment syndrome** due to excessive peritoneal (visceral) swelling preventing tension-free abdominal closure.
- ■ **Massive abdominal wall loss** (e.g. post-traumatic, necrotizing fasciitis).
- ■ **Inability to eliminate or to control the source of infection.**
- ■ **Incomplete debridement** of necrotic tissue (e.g. infected pancreatic necrosis).
- ■ **Uncertain viability** of remaining bowel (e.g. acute mesenteric ischemia).
- ■ **Uncontrolled bleeding** (the need for 'packing').

* Remember: there is no need for a planned relaparotomy if the source is well controlled.

Peritoneal toilet ('drain the swamp' ☺)

Once the source of infection is eradicated, cleaning the peritoneal cavity is aimed at minimizing the intraperitoneal bacterial load. Several maneuvers deserve discussion:

- Liquid contaminants and infected exudates should be aspirated and particulate matter removed by swabbing or mopping the peritoneal surfaces with moist laparotomy pads (gently, the peritoneal surface is your friend!).

- **There is no scientific evidence that intra-operative peritoneal lavage, cosmetically appealing and popular with surgeons as it is, reduces mortality or infectious complications in patients receiving adequate systemic antibiotics**. Similarly, *peritoneal irrigation with antibiotics* is not advantageous, and the addition of antiseptics may produce local toxic effects.
- Irrigate (if you wish (■ Figure 13.1) with warm crystalloids but try to confine the irrigation to the contaminated area — to avoid spreading s**t all around — and do remember to suck out all the lavage fluid before you close; there is evidence that leaving irrigation fluids behind interferes with peritoneal defenses by 'diluting the macrophages'. **Perhaps bacteria swim better than macrophages!**

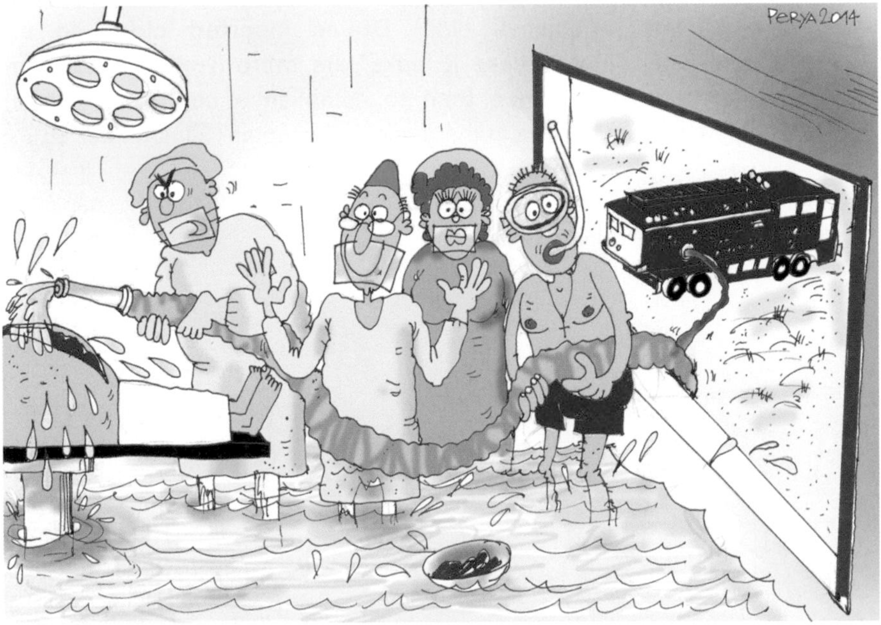

Figure 13.1. "OK guys, now it's enough. I think the abdomen is clean..."

What about drains?

- Despite the dictum **that it is impossible to drain the free peritoneal cavity effectively**, drains are still often misused. They are rarely required. Their aim must be restricted to the evacuation of an 'established' abscess (when the residual cavity would not collapse or cannot be filled with omentum or adjacent structures), to allow escape of potential secretions (e.g. bile, pancreatic juice) or, rarely, to establish a controlled intestinal fistula when resection or exteriorization of the intestinal source is not possible.

- To prevent intestinal erosion, soft drains should be left in place for the shortest duration possible and well away from bowel wall. In general, *active-suction* drainage may be more effective than the *passive* kind, and infectious complications can be reduced by choosing 'closed' systems.
- **Drains often provide a false sense of security and reassurance** (■ Figure 13.2). We have all seen a moribund postoperative patient with an abdomen 'crying' to be re-explored with a surgeon in denial because his tiny four-quadrant drains are dry and non-productive. (By the way, this is particularly true of drains uselessly inserted to deal with postoperative hemorrhage; a tiny trickle of blood from a drain may hide a huge intra-abdominal clot.) **Drains inserted close to an anastomosis "just in case it leaks" are more likely to cause an anastomotic dehiscence than to establish a controlled fistula**. Read more about drains in the dedicated chapter (➲ Chapter 36).

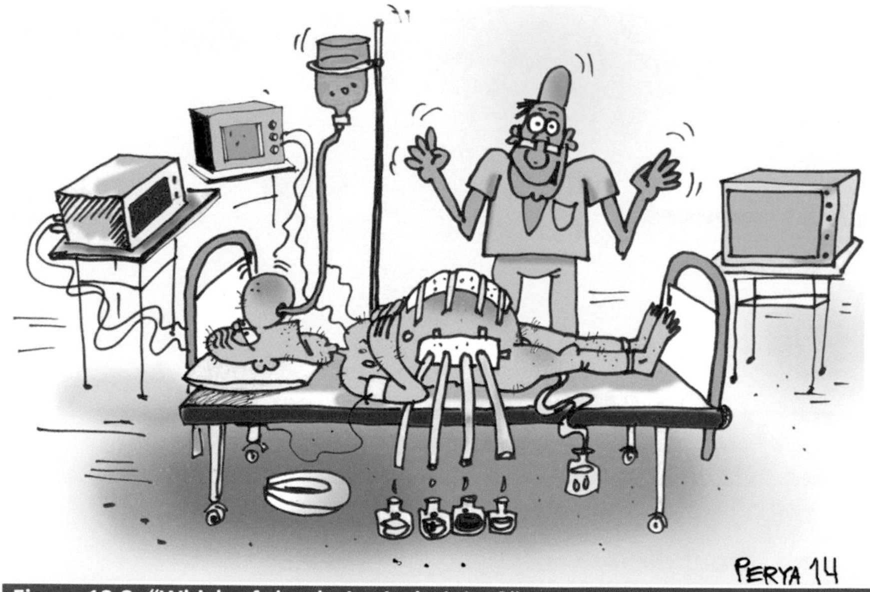

Figure 13.2. "Which of the drains is draining?"

Treatment failure

You have to recognize treatment failures. Ongoing or increasing evidence of systemic sepsis (plus organ system dysfunction) for more than 24-48 hours suggests that your initial source control may not have been adequate — that perhaps more needs to be done.

Repeated imaging combined with clinical judgment (which you will surely master after reading to the end of this book...) will help you to decide how to continue: whether to reoperate?; insert a PC drain?; or 'wait and see'? The initial treatment of a patient with IAI is relatively straightforward. **Trying to rescue a treatment failure is more complex. Thus, the quality of surgeons and hospitals is often best measured using the 'failure to rescue' index.**

Remember: the reason your patient continues to be ill lies at the primary site of operation unless proven otherwise. Do not behave like a 'surgical ostrich' by ignoring the real problem!

> **"Shakiness of the hand may be some bar to the successful performance of an operation, but he of a shaky mind is hopeless."**
>
> **Sir William MacEwen**

Look at the Surgical Infection Society revised Guidelines on the management of intra-abdominal infection. *Surgical Infections* 2017; 18: 1. https://www.ncbi.nlm.nih.gov/pubmed/28085573.

Chapter 14

The intestinal anastomosis (and stomata)

The Editors

This chapter has been subdivided into the following two sections:

1. The intestinal anastomosis.
2. Intestinal stomata.

1 The intestinal anastomosis

Best is the enemy of good: the first layer is the best — why spoil it?

The ideal anastomosis

The ideal intestinal anastomosis is the one which does not leak [1]. Leaks, although relatively rare, are a dreaded and potentially deadly disaster (➲ Chapter 43). In addition, the anastomosis should not obstruct but allow normal function of the gastrointestinal tract within a few days of construction.

Any experienced surgeon thinks that his own anastomotic technique, adopted from his mentors and with a touch of personal virtuosity, is the 'best'.

1 For a comprehensive treatise on anastomotic leaks, look at Chapter 6, *Schein's Common Sense Prevention and Management of Surgical Complications.* Shrewsbury, UK: tfm publishing, 2013.

Many methods are practiced: end-to-end, end-to-side or side-to-side; single- versus double-layered, interrupted versus continuous, using absorbable versus non-absorbable and braided versus monofilament suture materials. We even know some obsessive-compulsive surgeons (do you know any?) who carefully construct a three-layered anastomosis in an interrupted fashion. Now add staplers to the mix. **So where do we stand? What is preferable?** (■ Figure 14.1).

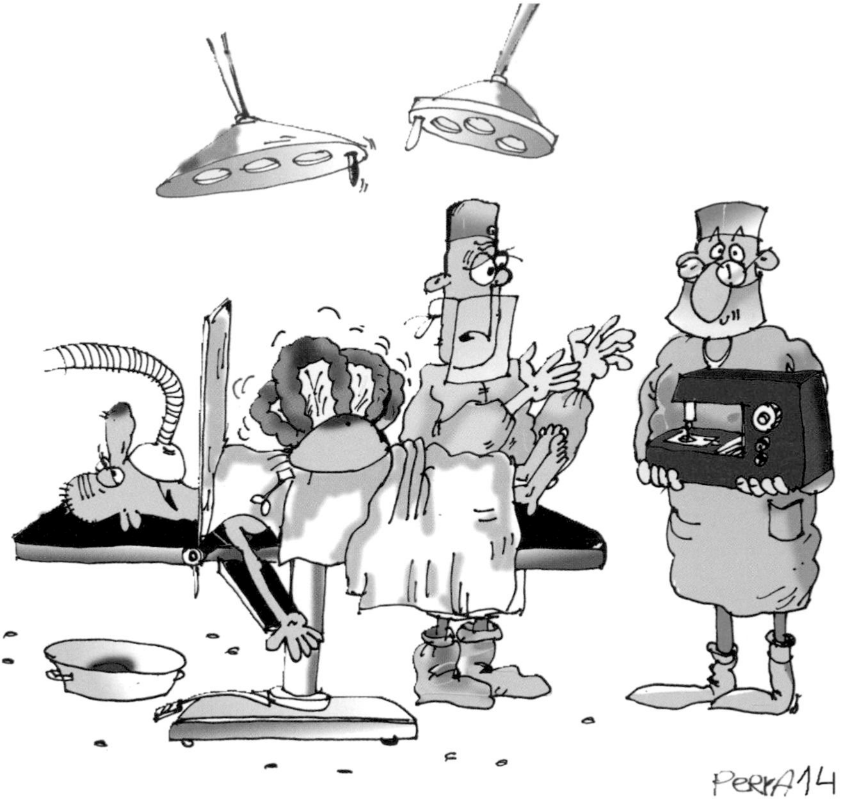

Figure 14.1. "Give it to me, nurse... This will be a perfect anastomosis!"

Pros and cons

Numerous experimental and clinical studies support the following:

- **Leakage**: the incidence of anastomotic dehiscence is not influenced by the method used, **provided the anastomosis is technically sound; constructed with well-perfused bowel without tension, and rendered water and airtight**.

- **Stricture**: the single-layer anastomosis is associated with a lower risk of stricture formation than the multi-layered one. Strictures are also commoner following the end-to-end anastomosis performed with the circular stapler (especially when the smaller sizes are used).
- **Misadventure**: intra-operative technical failures with staplers are more frequent due to 'misfires'. And you know the rule: "**tools in the hands of fools are prone to disasters**."
- **Speed**: stapled anastomoses, on average, are slightly faster than those sutured by hand. The fewer the layers, the faster the anastomosis and the continuous method is swifter than the interrupted one. In practice, the time consumed in placing two hand-fashioned purse-string sutures for a stapled circular anastomosis is not that different from that required to complete a hand-sutured, single-layered, continuous anastomosis.
- **Suture material**: braided sutures (e.g. silk or Vicryl®) 'saw' through tissues and, experimentally at least, are associated with greater inflammation and activation of collagenases than monofilament material (e.g. PDS®, Monocryl®, Prolene®). Monofilament slides better through the tissues and, when used in a continuous fashion, is self-adjustable allowing equal distribution of the tension around the entire circumference of the anastomosis.
- **Cost**: staplers are much more expensive than sutures and, thus, generally not cost-effective. The single-layer continuous technique requires less suture material and is therefore more economical than the interrupted method.

The choice of anastomotic technique: international perspective

To gauge the current 'anastomotic philosophy' around the world we conducted an informal poll among members of the international online surgical forum — SURGINET. And here is a summary of the prevailing trends:

- **Staplers vs. hands**. A minority of surgeons are addicted to 'stapler-only' or 'hand-only' technique. Most use both techniques on a selective basis. **The emphasis is to avoid staplers on 'non-healthy bowel' — e.g. edematous, irradiated — or in what they would consider 'difficult circumstances'**.
- **Location**. Most would use **staplers** when access seems 'difficult' — for example, for **esophageal** and **rectal** anastomoses. Fashioning a new gastric lesser curvature and closure of the duodenal stump during gastrectomy are other popular indications for staplers. **In all other sites, hand-suturing is more popular**.

- **Lap vs. open**. For obvious reasons staplers are used during laparoscopic procedures, unless the anastomosis is performed extracorporeally. The advent of robotic surgery has somewhat revived 'hand'-sewn anastomoses.
- **Suture material**. Absorbable material is used by the vast majority. The braided Vicryl® is popular but those who prefer the continuous-running technique (see below) opt for monofilaments such as PDS®, Maxon™ or Monocryl®.
- **Single vs. two-layered anastomosis/interrupted vs. continuous**. Interestingly, European surgeons tend to practice a continuous single-layer anastomosis using a monofilament. Single-layer interrupted is practiced by many, especially in 'difficult circumstances' or for the sigmoid and rectum. Old school teaching prevails still in some places where two-layered anastomoses are preferred — both continuous, but more commonly the inner layer continuous (absorbable) and the outer interrupted (absorbable or not). Some US surgeons still use silk for the second layer — the power of old dogmas!

Our recommendations

Well, each of us has his own view and we cannot write four different versions of this chapter based on each of our dogmas, can we? (Danny, for example, prefers staplers from the mouth to the anus…).

Using the **WTLS (what the literature says)** test, since all methods, if correctly performed, are safe, nobody can fault you for using the anastomotic method with which you are most familiar and comfortable. However, applying the **IIWM (if it were me) concept** this is our (MS) bias:

We maintain that the one-layer, continuous method, using a monofilament suture material, is the one that a 'modern surgeon' should adopt, because it is fast, cheap and safe. What is good for the high-pressure vascular anastomosis should be just as good for the low-pressure intestinal one. If the first layer suffices why narrow and injure it with inverted and strangulated tissue? Would you put a well-done hamburger back on the grill? **As with any beautiful piece of art, less is more**.

We acknowledge that staplers are elegant, admired by the operating room staff, 'fun' to use and of great financial benefit to the manufacturers. Certainly, staples may be advantageous in inaccessible areas, deep in the pelvis or high under the diaphragm, for rectal or esophageal anastomoses, respectively. **But those types of anastomoses are seldom performed in emergency** situations. **Furthermore, as a surgical trainee you should start using staplers only after achieving maximal proficiency in manual techniques, and in difficult circumstances**. Even the stapler aficionado has to use his hands when the instrument misfires, or cannot be used because of specific anatomic constraints such as the retroperitoneal duodenum. The modern surgeon, and the trainee too, need to be equally proficient in hand-sewn and stapled anastomotic techniques; we suggest, however, that before driving a large truck you should be able to manage a car.

The edematous bowel

There is some evidence (not level I) that, in **trauma patients, stapled intestinal anastomoses are more prone to leak than hand-sewn ones**. This has been attributed to the post-resuscitation bowel edema which develops after severe injury (the staplers cannot 'adjust' to the swelling of the bowel — the surgeon's hands can). It is also our impression that **a continuous, monolayer anastomosis occasionally fails when performed in edematous bowel** (e.g. after massive fluid resuscitation or severe peritonitis). From findings at reoperation we have learned that subsequently, as the bowel edema subsides, the suture becomes loose, leading to anastomotic dehiscence. The same arguments may apply when resection for obstruction has been performed; the proximal dilated and thickened bowel does not conform to the staples in the same way that the distal gut does.

Therefore, when anastomosing swollen, edematous bowel (a common scenario in emergency situations) we prefer not to use staplers or the continuous hand-sutured method. Instead, we use a closely placed single layer of interrupted sutures — individually tied "not too tight, not too loose" — in order to avoid cutting through the bowel edges, but also to obviate the risk of loosening after the edema subsides. We take big bites on the outside and tiny on the inside, inverting the mucosa. All sutures, except the last few at the front, are tied inside the lumen.

And remember: when the bowel edges are not 'perfect' take deeper bites! Incorporate more tissue into the anastomosis! Yes — up to a cm! When assisting younger surgeons we constantly hear ourselves pleading: take a larger bite!

Now raise your right hand and repeat: BIG BITES, BIG BITES, BIG BITES, BIG B...

A few more words on staplers

You will learn the correct use of staplers from your mentors. Despite appearances, we are not rigidly *staplerophobic*. We use staplers generously in emergency situations to *occlude*, rather than *anastomose*; a classic example would be closure of the rectum after a Hartmann's procedure or small bowel transection in an abbreviated laparotomy for trauma or ischemia. Doing a *functional end-to-end* small bowel or ileocolic anastomosis after, respectively, small bowel resection or right hemicolectomy — using a linear cutting (GIA™) and linear occluding (TA) staplers makes sense to us (that is if the bowel appears 'healthy'). But a side-to side gastrojejunostomy, when you insert the GIA™ into the stomach and small bowel through two holes, which you then have to close with sutures, makes no sense, as the combined size of the gastric and jejunal enterotomies is almost that of the gastrojejunostomy which you could have created and sutured by hand. Moreover, these enterotomies which are used to insert the jaws of the linear cutting staplers, and are then closed by hand, seem to be the *Achilles' heel* of the anastomosis — they, rather than the staple line, are often the site of a leak.

As much as we the authors wish to come out with a uniform 'consent' opinion, sometimes our views differ a little.

So here Danny wishes to add: As is true for anything in surgery — it's the final outcome that matters. And what determines the outcome of an anastomosis are mainly the conditions of the bowel, the surroundings and the patient. The technical variant has little effect as long as it is done in an accurate and meticulous way. So for me, all these calculations about size of enterotomies or overall time from start to finish of an anastomosis are meaningless. We have seen laparoscopic hand-sewn anastomoses done quicker than open stapled ones... And we have seen places where the cost of 15 minutes of OR time is greater than the cost of the staplers... So the choice is multifactorial, based on cost, speed, and mainly personal preferences. **If your leak rate is not exceptional, and you are proficient in all the variations — you are free to choose. Danny**

To this Moshe would reply: Danny's view above is from a master advanced laparoscopic surgeon. My view would apply to the average Joe — like me. **Moshe**

When not to perform an anastomosis?

We wish we had an exact answer! In broad terms, whenever the probability of a leak is high, avoid an anastomosis since any anastomotic leak portends disastrous consequences (➲ Chapter 43). **So how do you accurately predict anastomotic failure?**

Traditionally, the avoidance of colonic suture lines during emergency operations for trauma, obstruction, or perforation was the standard practice. But times have changed; during World War II a colostomy was mandatory for any colonic injury, but nowadays we successfully repair most of these wounds (➲ Chapter 30). Furthermore, three- or two-stage procedures for colonic obstruction have been replaced in selected cases by the one-stage resection with anastomosis (➲ Chapter 25). And, as you will read in ➲ Chapters 25 and 28, the issue of whether the large bowel is 'prepared' or not has become a non-issue (at least to most of us). Multiple trials show that safe colorectal suture lines can be effected in unprepared bowel (although, like in many surgical 'pendulums', bowel-prep seems to have gained favor again...).

It is difficult to lay down precise guidelines as to when an intestinal anastomosis is not to be made. You should make a careful decision after considering the condition of the patient, the intestine, and the peritoneal cavity. Generally, we would avoid a colonic anastomosis in the presence of established and diffuse intra-abdominal infection (as opposed to contamination) and under the conditions listed in ■ Table 14.1. Regarding the *small bowel*, anastomosis is indicated in most instances; however, **when more than one of the factors listed in the table are present we tend to err on the conservative side and exteriorize or divert, depending on technical circumstances**.

Table 14.1. Factors that may influence us not to anastomose.

- Diffuse established peritonitis.
- Postoperative peritonitis.
- Leaking anastomosis.
- Mesenteric ischemia.
- Extreme bowel edema/distension.
- Extreme malnutrition with low serum albumin.
- Chronic steroid intake.
- Unstable patient (damage control situation).
- Irradiated bowel.

No formula or algorithm is available, so use your judgment and try not to be too obsessive in always attempting an anastomosis — look at Figure ■ 14.2 — is this your boss? Yes, we know that you wish the patient well by wanting to spare him a stoma, but he will not be impressed if he is dead! You should not be fearful of creating a high small bowel stoma. Previously these were considered to be unmanageable, but with total parenteral nutrition, techniques of distal enteric feeding and reinfusion, somatostatin, and stoma care, these temporary proximal intestinal 'vents' can be life-saving (see also ➲ Chapters 43 and 44). **On the other hand, do not be a *wussy* (look at the Urban Dictionary) by avoiding an anastomosis when it is indicated and possible.**

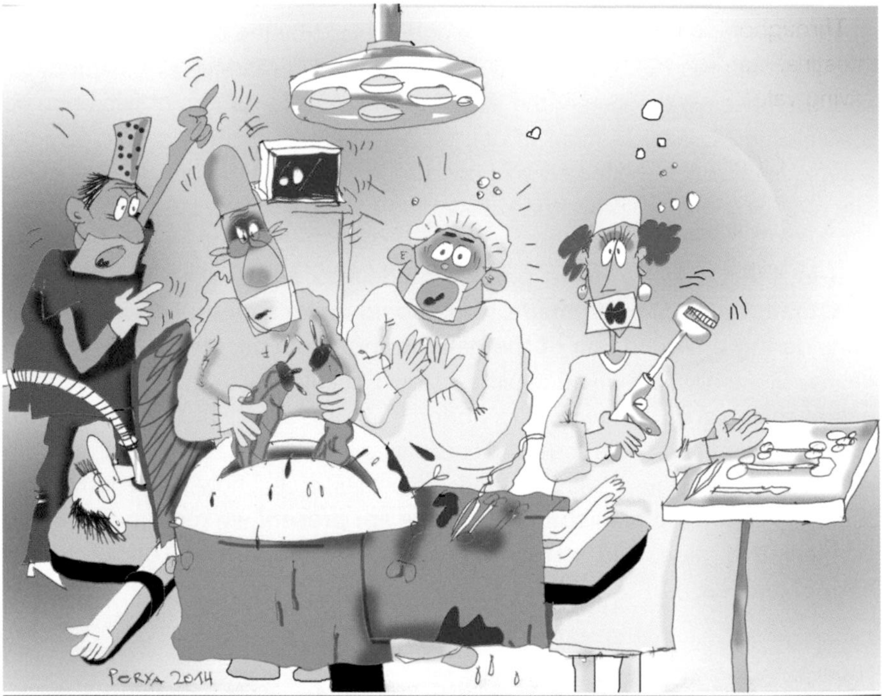

Figure 14.2. Anesthetist: "Systolic blood pressure 60... hemoglobin 5..." Assistant to surgeon: "Boss, pre-op albumin was 1.5..." Surgeon to nurse: "Get me the TA and GIA™. Let me join the ileum with the colon. Will take me 3 minutes..."

Whatever you do, some people will be unhappy. You can't please everybody, can you? **If you do a colostomy there will be always someone to ask you why not primary anastomosis? If you do a primary anastomosis there will be always someone to say why not colostomy? Only being a football coach is worse in this regard.**

So let us leave you with this...

The intestinal anastomosis is the 'elective' part of the emergency operation you are going to perform. Remember — your aim is to save life and minimize morbidity; create an anastomosis when its chances of success are at least reasonable. **There are many ways to skin a cat and to fashion an anastomosis. Master a few methods and use them selectively**.

2 Intestinal stomata [2]

Throughout surgical history, surgeons have viewed the creation of an intestinal stoma with distaste but at the same time understood its potential life-saving value — as reflected by these two quotes from master surgeons:

> *Of all the diseases to which man is liable, there is no one so inconvenient and disgusting as the artificial anus. How wretched is the patient from whom, despite his will, the alimentary, bilious and fecal matter contained in his intestines are constantly escaping.*
>
> **Guillaume Dupuytren**

> *About colostomy: But it is surely far better to part with one of the conveniences of Life, than to part with Life itself. Besides, the excrements that are voided by this passage, are not altogether so offensive, as those that are voided per anum.*
>
> **Lorenz Heister**

This is perhaps the right time and place to discuss general concepts concerning the construction of intestinal stomata. You will read more about specific indications for small or large bowel stomata in the relevant individual chapters.

> *There are only two indications to create a stoma; when you want to and when you need to.*
>
> **R. John Nicholls**

Patients and surgeons have differing views of stomata. For a psychologically unprepared patient who recovers from emergency surgery, a stoma is a devastating insult to their body image and sexuality. To the surgeon, a stoma may be seen as an insult to professional pride; its mere presence implies that he cannot even join a piece of bowel together properly. Go to any

[2] Professor Luis Carriquiry, MD, contributed to this section in the previous edition.

surgical conference and you will see papers on how clever surgeons completely avoid stomata with their robotic/SILS/blah, blah blah...

But common-sense surgeons know that a well-made stoma in the right setting can be life-saving (and also improve the quality of life for some patients — but that's another story). In this chapter we will discuss the whys and wherefores of common stomata and also some tips for more unusual situations.

The emergency stoma: why and when

The most common reason to create a stoma as part of an emergency abdominal operation is that the risk of anastomotic leakage is considered too high. For example, during an operation to correct a left colon anastomotic leak it is wise either to exteriorise the leak or if this is not possible, then completely take down the anastomosis by stapling off the distal limb and creating a proximal end stoma (à la Hartmann).

One could summarize the most common indications for a stoma in emergency surgery as follows:

- Surgery for anastomotic leak.
- Surgery for faecal peritonitis.
- Bowel resection in a patient with major risks for anastomotic failure.
- Surgery for fulminant colitis.
- To allow healing of a perineal wound or sepsis.
- To divert proximal to a fistula (e.g. rectovaginal fistula).

There are a few types of stoma from which to choose for the above indications:

- End colostomy.
- Loop colostomy (sigmoid or transverse).
- Double-barrel colostomy.
- Blow holes.
- Cecostomy.
- End ileostomy.
- Loop ileostomy.
- Jejunostomy.
- Ileocolostomy (double-barrel).

How to make an emergency stoma

Siting a stoma

Patients who have planned surgery involving a stoma typically see a 'bag lady' (a stoma nurse or enterostomal therapist) prior to operation. This consultation helps to prepare the patient psychologically and practically for their surgery. A key part of this process is marking the site for the planned stoma. The patient is usually examined lying and standing, and their clothing preferences are considered. **An emergency abdominal surgeon does not have the luxury of access to a stoma nurse at 2 a.m. when confronted with a sick patient with a perforated colon** (actually, even if you can find one, a stoma nurse will often tell you that they cannot site a stoma in a patient with a tender distended abdomen). So you need to have a reasonable understanding of where to place your stoma.

You should aim to place your stoma through a flat part of the skin away from scars, bony prominences and skin creases. In practice, think of an imaginary triangle with points at the umbilicus, anterior superior iliac spine and the mid-point of the costal margin and then site your stoma through this triangle (on either side) — **the triangle of stomata** (■ Figure 14.3).

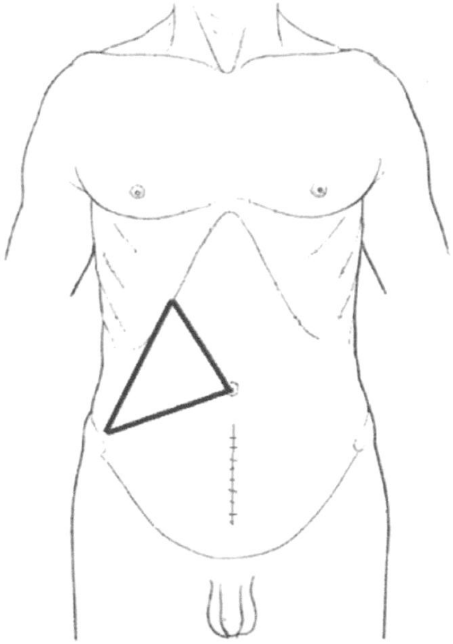

Figure 14.3. The 'triangle of stomata'.

For a more nuanced version of this, you should vary how high or low in the triangle you cut according to the clinical situation. Skinny young girls with Crohn's disease tend to prefer a stoma low down in the abdomen to fit with their wardrobe. This site would, of course, be a disaster in a 250lb beer-swilling man needing a Hartmann's procedure; for him, place the stoma higher, above the beer belly, so he can see to change his stoma pouch. **In practice, with visceral oedema and distended bowel loops you may need to place your stoma wherever it can reach the skin without tension, rather than the optimal site**. Whatever you do, bringing the stoma, or even a mucous fistula out through the surgical wound, is not something that we would advise (see ■ Figure 14.4).

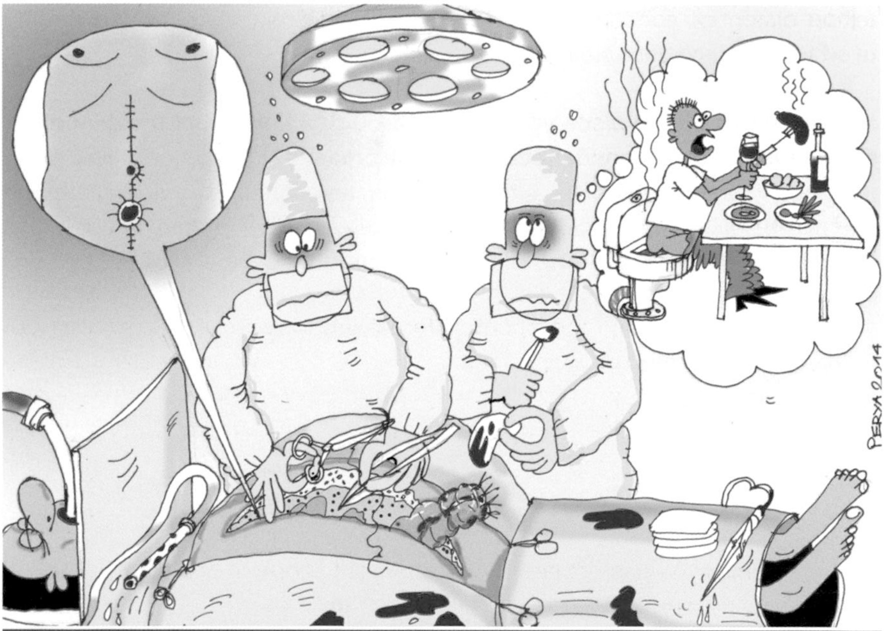

Figure 14.4. Bringing a colostomy out through a laparotomy incision is like putting a toilet in the kitchen.

Making a stoma — general principles

Consider a stoma as an anastomosis between bowel and skin; you should aim to bring together well-vascularized tissues with minimal tension and pay attention to surgical technique.

You should make the stoma *trephine* as small (or large) as possible to allow delivery of the bowel without any vascular compromise. The trephine may be made by elevating the skin with tissue forceps and using a scalpel to excise a disk of skin. For some, this may result in a much too large, ragged skin defect. **So as an alternative, place a cruciate incision at the site of the stoma, excising the corners to make a circular trephine**. Conventionally, the external oblique aponeurosis is incised in a cruciform manner, and the underlying rectus abdominis is split in the line of its fibers. The posterior rectus sheath and peritoneum are elevated between two clamps and incised to enter the abdominal cavity. **Be careful not to injure the inferior epigastric artery at this point** — it's a real pain in the arse to have to fuddle in the depths of a small stoma incision to stop bleeding at the end of a long laparotomy.

The bowel to be used for the stoma is grasped with an atraumatic clamp inserted through the stoma trephine and delivered outside. If you are making a loop stoma, a nylon tape can be looped through a hole in the mesentery and used to guide out the bowel.

Maturation of the stoma is performed (after any other wounds have been closed and dressed) as follows:

- **An ileostomy should be spouted** (known as the 'Brooke's ileostomy') to facilitate collection of liquid effluent. The spout is created by inserting a Babcock clamp into the lumen, grasping the mucosa, and pulling to create the spout. Alternatively, three everting sutures are placed though the serosa about 4-5cm from the opened bowel. These sutures are held in clamps until all are placed and then tightened to spout the ileostomy. Be careful with these everting sutures; if placed too deeply they can cause a difficult fistula at the mucocutaneous junction. By varying the height of these everting sutures, it is possible to create a slight downward tilt to the ileostomy spout which will make stoma management easier. **If the patient is obese or the small bowel mesentery is short, it may be extremely difficult to form a spouted ileostomy without any tension**. **In these circumstances, it IS useful to close the end of the ileum with a linear cutting stapler and form a loop ileostomy just proximal to this (an end-loop ileostomy)**. A loop ileostomy is formed in a similar manner with the proximal end everted to form a spout. It is crucial that the correct (i.e. proximal) limb of the ileostomy is everted; as an alternative both proximal and distal limbs can be spouted. A rod is usually unnecessary when creating a loop ileostomy.
- **A colostomy, in contrast, does not need a spout**. Although traditionally a colostomy was formed flush with the skin, there are some advantages to creating a 'minimally-raised' colostomy which reduces leaking and pancaking (pooling of semi-solid stool under the

stoma appliance). Again, fine absorbable sutures should be used to stitch the full thickness of the bowel, including the mucosa, to the skin, following wound closure.

End colostomy

In the setting of emergency surgery, an end colostomy is usually performed during a Hartmann's procedure to resect the sigmoid colon for perforation or (perhaps less commonly nowadays) for large bowel obstruction. The stoma is usually sited in the left iliac fossa. The challenge here is to deliver a sufficient length of healthy colon to create a tension-free colostomy. **It may be necessary to formally mobilize the splenic flexure and pedicle the colon based on the middle colic vessels to achieve this**. Ensure that the end of the bowel to be matured as the colostomy sits 'comfortably' on the surface of the skin before closing the abdomen. **If you are worried that it is too tight, then it probably is; under these circumstances further mobilize the colon now before closing**.

Loop colostomy

Two types of loop colostomy are useful in the emergency setting — a transverse loop colostomy or a sigmoid loop colostomy:

- **A transverse loop colostomy** is useful to relieve obstruction in a patient who is unfit for a major resection or more rarely as part of a staged procedure (you will then later proceed with a planned resection). It is possible to perform a loop transverse colostomy without a laparotomy by making a trephine incision in the right upper quadrant; indeed on rare occasions, we have even performed this under sedation and local anaesthetic (although this wasn't much fun for surgeon or patient!). Distal limb prolapse is a fairly frequent problem with a loop transverse colostomy, but this can be dealt with later.
- **A sigmoid loop colostomy** is easier for a patient to care for; certainly, there are fewer problems with colostomy prolapse with this stoma. It is useful for 'defunctioning' in a patient with a major perineal wound (an emergency setting of Fournier's gangrene or an open fractured pelvis would be typical examples of this).

End ileostomy

In the setting of emergency surgery, an end ileostomy is usually performed as part of a subtotal colectomy for colitis. Typically, it is sited in the right iliac fossa, although the mobility of the small bowel mesentery means that it can be sited almost anywhere if necessary. The small bowel mesentery should be trimmed back carefully to pedicle the bowel leading up to the stoma. Do this carefully or you risk completely devitalising the stoma. Also be careful when delivering the stoma through your trephine incision; if the incision is too small or you are rough with the tissues, you may strip back the mesentery during delivery (another way of devitalising the stoma). One more important issue is to preserve the vasculature for a future ileal pouch — that will be both viable and able to reach the pelvic floor.

Loop ileostomy

A loop ileostomy has a limited use in emergency surgery. **One example where it may be used is in a morbidly obese patient with acute perforated diverticulitis**. An emergency sigmoid resection in this setting is a formidable challenge; occasionally it may be better to make a proximal stoma and then later perform an elective resection. **When operating on a morbidly obese patient with a thick abdominal wall and a short mesocolon, a loop ileostomy may be the only feasible stoma**.

Another role for diverting ileostomy would be proximal to a 'high-risk' colorectal anastomosis or in the treatment of a 'minor' left colonic anastomotic leak which is left *in situ* rather than dismantled.

Mucous fistula

A mucous fistula is a stoma created from the proximal end of a distal, diverted part of the bowel. The classic example would be following an emergency colectomy for colitis, when the end of the rectal stump would be brought to the surface and matured as a second stoma. Patients and their stoma nurses on the whole hate mucous fistulae; they smell and result in a second stoma appliance. There is good evidence that in most cases of ulcerative colitis, it is safe to close the rectal stump and leave it intraperitoneally. Very rarely the colon is so friable that it is not possible to close the stump safely either with sutures or staples. In these circumstances, we have left a long stump and exteriorised it through the left iliac fossa. As the colon is friable it will not hold sutures well and we have used a neonatal umbilical clamp to hold the colon above the skin level (this sloughs off in a few weeks, leaving a neat and secure mucous fistula).

Ileocolostomy (double-barrel)

If you have resected the right colon, but maintain that it is unsafe to perform an ileocolic anastomosis, it is worth considering creating a double-barrel ileocolostomy. Here, both ends of the bowel (terminal ileum and colon) are brought out through the same trephine — you can suture the back walls of the two segments together if you wish. The advantages of this approach are that for the patient there is only one stoma appliance needed and for the surgeon it is then possible to close this later without a formal laparotomy. **An ileocolostomy is useful in two situations: following a reoperation for a leaking ileocolic anastomosis or at the primary procedure when the risk of a leak is high** (classic examples of this are an emaciated, steroid-dependent patient with Crohn's disease or a patient with faecal peritonitis from a perforated caecum).

Jejunostomy

Rarely will you need to create a jejunostomy. There is often a reluctance to create a proximal stoma due to the perceived risks of a high-output stoma; however, in some situations you will need to balance this risk against that of an anastomotic leak or uncontrolled abdominal sepsis. You may need to make a jejunostomy when there is an unrecognised enterotomy in the proximal bowel or to divert the intestinal contents from a complex enterocutaneous fistula. **This is the ultimate bailout stoma and usually indicates that the patient has had an abdominal catastrophe or that the surgeon has cocked up**. Because you will rarely need to do this it will be an unfamiliar procedure to you. Here are some tips:

- Make your stoma trephine where the relevant piece of jejunum will reach (this is usually in the left upper quadrant).
- Pull the end or loop of jejunum through the trephine as normal.
- You will find that it is much harder to spout a jejunostomy than an ileostomy due to the thickness of the bowel wall and the length of the mesentery; don't worry too much about that, remember this is a bailout stoma!

- The vascular pattern of the jejunum does not allow you to pedicle the bowel as you would do for an end ileostomy, so don't bother trying; you are likely to devascularize a section of jejunum if you do.
- Open and mature the stoma as usual with interrupted fine absorbable sutures
- It is likely to look awful compared to your usual stomata, *c'est la vie!*

'Blow-hole' colostomy and cecostomy

Some surgeons think of blow-hole stomata as obsolete, and others don't even know what they are. **But we think this deserves a brief mention, for the rare case when it may be the best solution available.**

A blow-hole stoma is constructed using only the anterior bowel wall, which is opened and sutured to the skin, without mobilizing or exteriorizing the bowel above the skin level. The sole purpose of this stoma is decompression, as it does not completely divert the fecal stream, so it may be useful to alleviate colonic obstruction when more complicated solutions are not appropriate due to the patient's general condition. **Naturally, it is reserved for old, debilitated, high-risk patients, and its main advantage is the simplicity that makes it possible to construct under local anesthesia.**

The classic blow-hole stoma is a surgical cecostomy — as opposed to tube-cecostomy, that rarely functions as expected due to blockage of the tube and leakage around it. Take for example a 90-year-old patient with severe heart failure and an obstructing tumor at the splenic flexure: his best chance to leave the hospital would be by performing the minimal procedure to decompress the bowel before it perforates, without trying to 'cure' him by a heroic colectomy. Even a transverse loop colostomy, which mandates general anesthesia, may be too much for him. **So through a McBurney incision (as for appendectomy) you eviscerate the cecum and fix the eviscerated segment to the abdominal wall defect all around.** Then you open the cecum, suck the crap out, and you mature the opening to the skin. The skin level stoma is not bulky, and usually easy to manage (■ Figure 14.5).

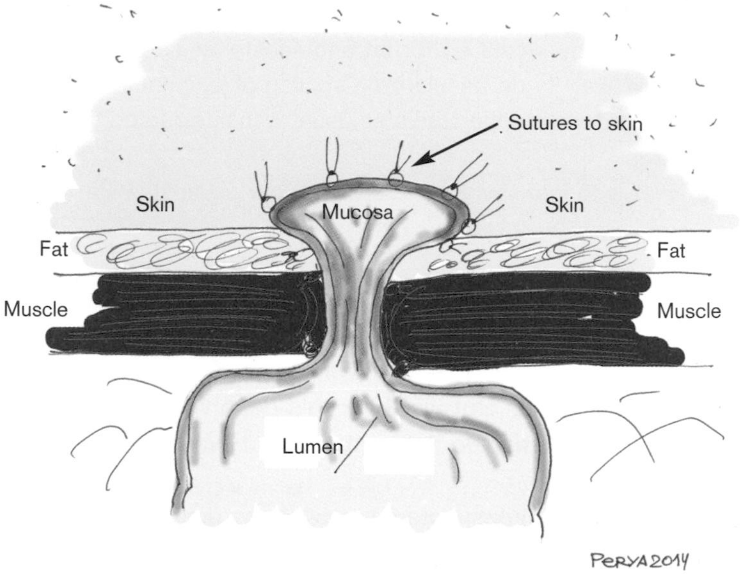

Figure 14.5. Blow-hole stoma.

Making a stoma in a fat person

The challenge of making a stoma in the ever too frequent morbidly obese patient cannot be underestimated. Here are some tips for when you find yourself in this sorry (reflected by the number of times the F word is uttered during the operation) situation:

- Site the stoma higher than you would normally do (it will not be visible to the patient if it is under the fat apron).
- Make the stoma trephine larger (the mesocolon will be thick and friable and will not come through a conventional-sized hole).
- Make sure that you fully mobilize the colon before making a colostomy (the panniculus and its attached colostomy descends several inches on standing).
- **Consider an end-loop stoma if you are still struggling for length** (to do this staple off the end of the bowel and then make a loop stoma just proximal to this).
- Go back to your room and open the well-earned bottle of *Glensomething*.

A tip for the wound

After an operation to create a stoma, we usually seal the laparotomy wound with a liberal application of skin glue, the theory being that if there is an early leak from the stoma appliance it will not contaminate and infect the wound. Anecdotally this does seem to work, although if the wound is grossly contaminated at the time of an emergency operation (e.g. faecal peritonitis), this is probably pointless (under these circumstances, we either leave the skin open or gently approximate it with a few interrupted nylon sutures).

Postoperative care of a stoma

Although not quite a window into the soul, a stoma does allow you direct access to visualize the visceral circulation. **You should therefore look at the stoma directly on the first postoperative day**. A transparent stoma pouch usually allows a good view of a stoma, but if you can't see it properly don't be lazy; remove the stoma pouch and make sure that you have a good view; if the light on the ward is poor then use a torch (Americanos would call it a flashlight).

Stoma ischemia

Stoma ischemia is usually evident early in the postoperative period. This is caused by either a generalized state of hypotension or, more commonly, a technical problem during the construction of the stoma. The severity of ischemia may vary from minor mucosal hypoperfusion to a black, completely necrotic stoma. **Again, all newly formed stomata should be inspected the day following surgery to assess their viability**. If a colostomy looks ischemic, it can be useful to use either a proctoscope or a test tube inserted into the stoma to assess the viability of the bowel under the fascia. Use a pen torch to assess the viability of the mucosa.

Urgent surgery to resect and refashion the stoma is needed if the bowel leading up to the colostomy is necrotic. Conversely, if the bowel immediately under the stoma is pink, then you can afford to wait. It is likely that the mucosa will slough off the stoma and that the late result will be a stenosed stoma. This can be dealt with on its own merits later, but this is preferable to a difficult relaparotomy in the early postoperative period. **A black ileostomy in contrast should usually be revised urgently** (here length is usually less of an issue, and it is often possible to revise an end ileostomy locally without a laparotomy).

If the colostomy appears black, then it is black — do not succumb to that stupid little voice in your brain telling you that it isn't black!

High-output stoma

A fully adapted end ileostomy has a daily output of approximately 500ml. In the initial postoperative period, ileostomy output is often much greater than this (1000-1800ml). A high-output state occurs in about 15% of patients having an ileostomy. This high volume of stoma output usually reduces in the first few postoperative days. **The factors causing a high-output stoma (greater than 2L/day) are all more common in patients having emergency surgery**:

- Proximal stomata (i.e. jejunostomy).
- Intra-abdominal sepsis.
- Following resolution of postoperative ileus or small bowel obstruction.

If a stoma is producing more than 1000ml/day, then intravenous fluid replacement with Hartmann's solution (Ringer's) or normal saline is needed. Restriction of oral hypotonic fluids will help reduce stoma output. Close monitoring of electrolytes is important as deficiencies of sodium, magnesium, and potassium are common. Other adjuncts to reduce a high-output stoma include:

- Low-fiber diet.
- Proton pump inhibitors.
- Antimotility agents such as loperamide (in this circumstance, a high dose of up to 8mg four times a day may be needed) or codeine phosphate (60mg four times a day).

Mucocutaneous separation

Mucocutaneous separation is relatively common after an emergency operation to form a stoma. The degree of separation is usually minor and with careful stoma management most will heal on their own. Attempts at resuturing are usually not helpful; resist the urge to revise the stoma early on as this will be difficult and potentially hazardous.

Other stoma complications

As a surgeon practicing emergency abdominal surgery, you will be well aware of the many other later complications which can occur after creating a stoma. Further discussion of the management of these complications is beyond the scope of this book. The interested reader is advised to consult Chapter #14 in *Schein's Common Sense Prevention and Management of Surgical Complications* for a more in-depth discussion.

Final remarks

A well-constructed stoma can make all the difference between success and failure of an emergency abdominal operation. Consider the stoma to be an anastomosis between skin and bowel and you won't go far wrong. Don't close the abdomen and go for a coffee, leaving the resident to mature the stoma unsupervised; a tiny error here can make a huge difference.

This book is about *emergency* treatment so we won't bore you with late complications or the 'take down' of the stoma. But we'll end with a comment by a wise man.

"There is no law that says that a colostomy must be closed."

Leo A. Gordon

Chapter 15

Diaphragmatic emergencies

Danny Rosin

The diaphragm is a muscular partition that separates disorders of the chest from disorders of the bowels.

Ambrose Bierce

The diaphragm normally separates the abdomen from the chest. The surgeon is interested when it fails in this function. When its integrity is disturbed, either acutely (trauma), chronically (herniation) or congenitally, the pressure difference between the two cavities causes the abdominal organs to shift upwards. The diaphragm is also a powerful muscle that allows us to breathe — but this is not so interesting to us right now.

Most diaphragmatic operations are elective, so when discussing emergency abdominal operations we are limited to only two situations:

- **Diaphragmatic laceration**, which results from either penetrating trauma (knife, bullet) or blunt trauma (rupture).
- **Acute presentation of chronic or congenital diaphragmatic hernia**, due to incarceration or twisting of the herniated contents.

Although this chapter is short and simple we still need some background knowledge in order to understand the treatment options when faced with a diaphragmatic emergency. Our aim is to treat the contents, preferably by just putting the organs back where they belong (but resection is sometimes necessary), and restore diaphragmatic integrity, hopefully by a lasting repair.

So let's start with some definitions, to get familiar with the common pathologies.

Diaphragmatic hernia

This can be congenital or acquired. Being a defect in the integrity of the diaphragm, the congenital hernias result from 'non-closure', while the acquired arise from widening of an existing opening — the hiatus.

There are two types of congenital hernias:

- **Bochdalek hernia** is the more common, representing a congenital *posterolateral* defect — usually on the left side. Its main effect is respiratory, as the protrusion of the abdominal organs into the chest cavity leads to pulmonary hypoplasia; **the life-threatening respiratory distress after birth makes it a neonatal emergency**, which is beyond the scope of this book.
- **Morgagni hernia** is a much less frequent form of congenital hernia, defined by an *anterior, retrosternal defect*.

Rarely, congenital hernias are small and can go unnoticed, only to be diagnosed later in life, presenting similarly to acquired hernias.

Hiatal hernia

Sliding hiatal hernia is an upward shift of the stomach (the gastroesophageal junction migrates proximal to the hiatus) and, therefore, anatomically it is a 'sliding' hernia, without a hernia sac. Hence, **there is no risk of acute surgical complications (e.g. incarceration, strangulation, obstruction) related to such herniation**.

Paraesophageal hernia, on the other hand, is more relevant to our topic. The defect in the diaphragm is actually the hiatus itself, which widens and allows the passage of the stomach (and other organs, if big enough) alongside the esophagus. This hernia is potentially the most problematic, as its symptoms are related to changes in the stomach position, and it has the potential to incarcerate.

Much mental effort is sometimes expended in an attempt to accurately classify different types of hernia on an anatomical basis: true sliding, true paraesophageal and mixed types. In practice, as you will read later, this does not help in surgical decision-making.

Diaphragmatic trauma (see also ➲ Chapter 30)

Diaphragmatic rupture or **laceration** is the result of trauma, the former usually the result of blunt trauma and the latter associated with a penetrating one. **In diaphragmatic trauma the tear includes the peritoneum, so there's no hernia sac but direct shift of abdominal organs into the pleural space.** As in congenital and acquired hernias, the liver protects the right diaphragm, so problems are more common on the left — but it doesn't mean that the right diaphragm is immune to injury, and we have seen herniation of the liver itself into the chest.

Diaphragmatic rupture is usually associated with other injuries and is treated at the same time (primary repair by non-absorbable sutures). While it may be obvious (you see the NG tube curling inside the left chest and you know the stomach is up there), it can sometimes be missed, even by a CT scan. When suspected, and there is no other indication for laparotomy, it is one of the few conditions in abdominal trauma where laparoscopy may have a role (at least in penetrating left thoracoabdominal wounds): explore the diaphragm, and repair if necessary.

When not suspected, and consequently missed, a diaphragmatic laceration can slowly enlarge and present, even years later, as a diaphragmatic hernia, possibly with incarceration. The lack of a hernia sac, and the resultant adhesions to the thoracic organs, may make surgery difficult, and for this reason some surgeons prefer to approach these cases by thoracotomy.

And now we come to the main item of this chapter… gastric volvulus!

Gastric volvulus in a paraesophageal hernia

Gastric volvulus, abnormal rotation of the stomach, is usually associated with a paraesophageal hernia, although it can rarely be seen without any herniation — caused by what I call 'general floppiness' of the stomach.

The stomach can twist along two different (and perpendicular) axes. In **organoaxial volvulus** — which is the more common variant — the stomach rotates around the axis that connects the gastroesophageal junction and the pylorus. The less common variant, **mesenteroaxial volvulus**, occurs around the more horizontal axis that runs from the center of the greater curvature of the stomach to the lesser curvature, twisting around the 'mesentery' where the left gastric artery can be found. (Online you'll find lots of images to help you understand…).

This classification is nice for the radiologists who interpret the CT scan (or the good old barium swallow), **but to you what matters is whether the stomach is obstructed, and if there is any possibility of gastric ischemia and necrosis, regardless of the exact axis.**

Clinical presentation

Many years ago Moritz Borchardt (1868-1948, a surgeon from Berlin who was later forced to emigrate to Argentina, where he died) described the diagnostic triad of gastric volvulus:

- **Epigastric/substernal pain.**
- **Retching without vomiting.**
- **Inability to pass a nasogastric tube.**

You will not be wakened at night by uncomplicated hiatal hernias, and even those with complex reflux problems will be managed by the gastroenterologists and their medications. **The trouble lies with the paraesophageal hernia and its 'relatives' — the missed diaphragmatic injury and the late-presenting congenital hernia — that act like real hernias and may lead to incarceration and even strangulation.** Interestingly, until relatively recently every diagnosed paraesophageal hernia was a clear indication for surgery, even the asymptomatic ones, because of the perceived risk of strangulation and the associated morbidity and mortality. **Some surgeons stick to this approach even today... But as the typical patient is usually old and frail we are more selective in offering surgery — to symptomatic patients only.**

Presenting symptoms relate to a difficulty or pain with swallowing, as the herniated part of the stomach presses upon the esophagus which can be partially obstructed at the hernia neck. **Acute obstruction** will be associated with retrosternal pain (the abdomen is usually soft and non-tender), and retching — as the incarcerated part of the stomach cannot empty, even with forceful attempts to vomit (■ Figure 15.1). A nasogastric tube may be difficult to pass, or fails to decompress the incarcerated stomach.

Since the ascent of the stomach into the chest is rarely straight, some element of torsion is almost always present, but true acute gastric volvulus may quite rapidly lead to gastric necrosis. As these patients

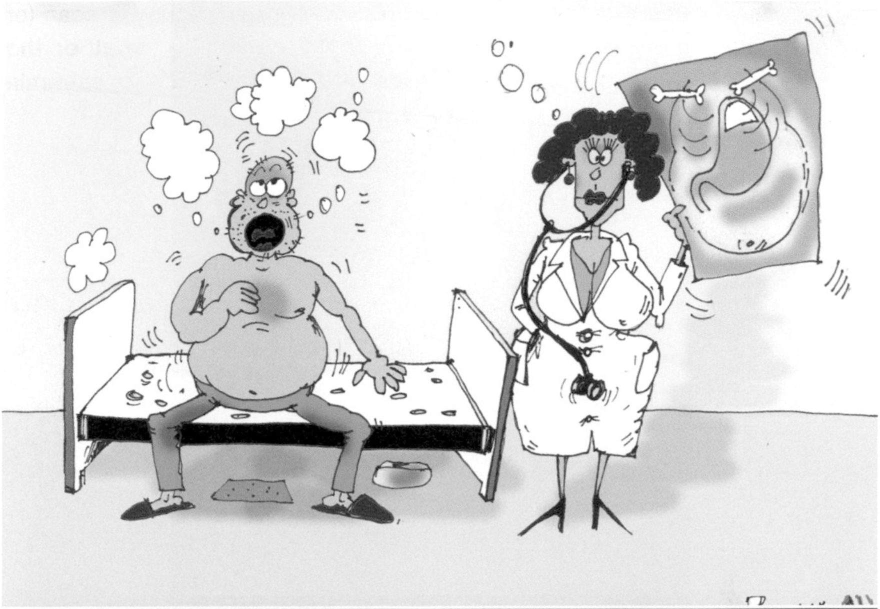

Figure 15.1. Patient: "Please help me to vomit." Doctor: "Your stomach is in the chest. I am afraid of aspiration..."

complain of retrosternal pain, and are usually in some respiratory distress, you can be sure that a chest X-ray will already be available when you are called by the ER doc; but the gastric air bubble up in the mediastinum may have been missed — have a look yourself (■ Figure 15.2).

Of course, nowadays a CT scan is an integral part of the diagnosis and decision-making in the ER (■ Figures 15.3 and 15.4). It will also show you other structures that may be involved: the transverse colon may be stuck up there too, and you really don't want to procrastinate when the colon is at risk of ischemia and perforation high up in the chest.

Although CT is diagnostic, these patients commonly land in the hands of internists/gastroenterologists who feel obliged to insert an endoscope. **The typical endoscopic features of gastric volvulus** (organoaxial) are: a tortuous stomach, paraesophageal hernia (viewed by retroflexing the scope) and an inability to locate, and pass through, the pylorus; evidence of gastric ischemia may be observed. There are reports of successful endoscopic-guided insertion of a nasogastric tube and detorsion — allowing a subsequent elective operation.

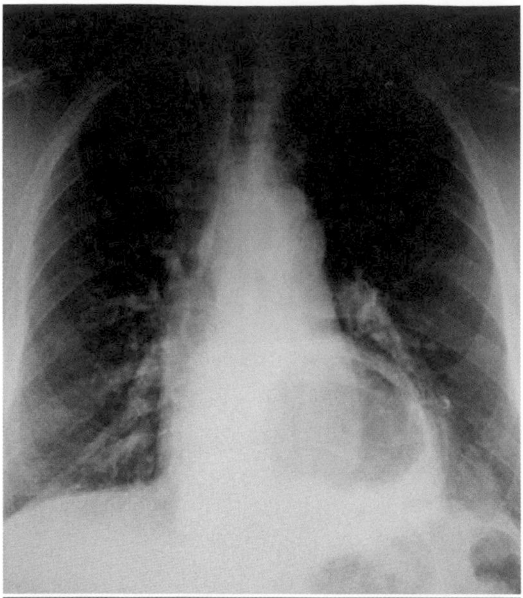

Figure 15.2. Chest X-ray of an incarcerated paraesophageal hernia with a gastric bubble in the mediastinum.

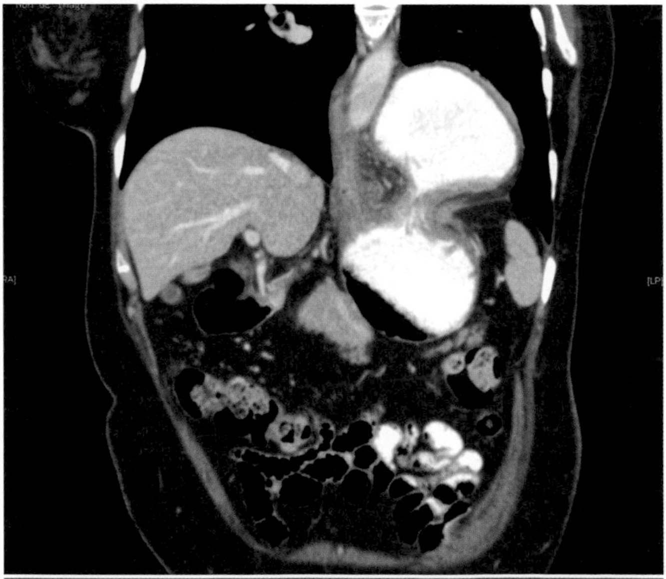

Figure 15.3. CT of gastric volvulus. In this mesoaxial rotation, the lower part of the stomach is found high in the chest — after herniating through a paraesophageal defect. The incarcerated part of the stomach still has a narrow connection with the intra-abdominal part, allowing contrast to enter — but it is distended and compressing the lung upward and the esophagus medially.

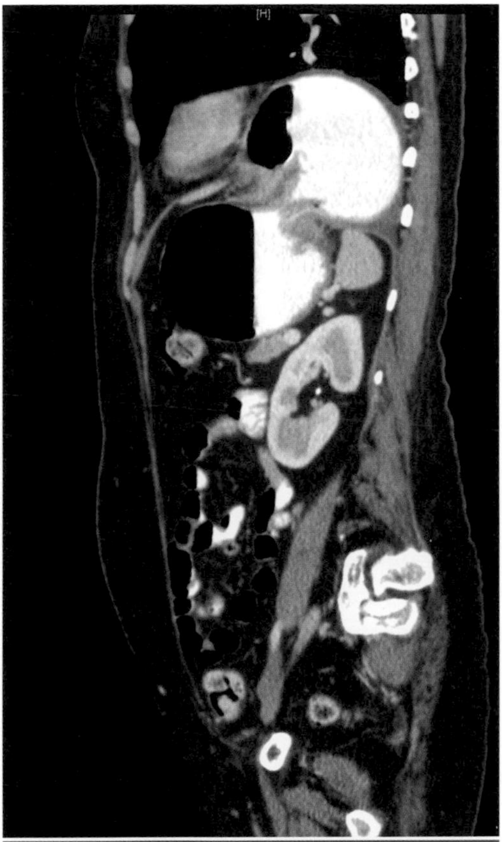

Figure 15.4. CT of gastric volvulus — lateral view, which better delineates the posterior pressure on the heart.

Management

Inserting a nasogastric tube may change an emergency into an elective problem, because if you succeed in decompressing the stomach, and the stomach has not yet necrosed, you will be able to operate in better conditions: these patients are commonly elderly and debilitated, and the added respiratory distress, together with the local conditions of the edematous, incarcerated stomach, make an emergency repair less favorable. **Unfortunately, in true and complete gastric volvulus, you will not be able to place a tube and decompress**.

When surgery is unavoidable, with the imminent risk of gastric necrosis, you'd better act fast (obviously after having optimized the patient and given broad-spectrum antibiotics). Access is through the abdomen — to reduce the contents and, if needed, resect if it is too late. Upper midline **laparotomy** is the classic approach, but **laparoscopy** may allow you to achieve what you need to do — if you are familiar enough with this approach for this pathology.

Reduction of the herniated viscera may be difficult, and sometimes adding a thoracotomy is inevitable. **Reduction may be aided by two maneuvers**: inserting a wide tube through the diaphragmatic defect abolishes the negative, 'sucking', thoracic pressure and then a nasogastric tube may be manipulated into the distended stomach to reduce its size. If still unsuccessful you can try and directly aspirate air and fluid via a needle puncture, or even through a small gastrotomy — but be careful to avoid spillage and protect your patient from empyema.

After a successful reduction of a viable stomach you should continue with your diaphragmatic repair, completing all the familiar components you know from elective surgery: excise the hernia sac, close the defect by suturing the diaphragmatic crura, and complete a fundoplication, or not, based on your beliefs (I do). Some surgeons will recommend gastropexy to prevent a recurrent volvulus, or even a tube gastrostomy for both fixation and drainage, but these are rarely necessary if you complete the repair. **If, however, the patient is not in 'great shape', and you need to get out of there quickly — forget the diaphragmatic repair and the fundoplication. Under unfavorable conditions just fixing the reduced stomach to the abdominal wall (with a few sutures — some would add a tube gastrostomy) is a good idea**.

If the patient, the ER doc or you have waited too long — which in real life is not a rare scenario — and you find a necrotic stomach, your options are more limited. **In such dire circumstances the patient will also limit your options by his/her grave condition, and the eventual mortality is high**. **Do only what you really have to do**: resect the gangrenous portion of the stomach, clean the mediastinum of spilled contents if perforation has already occurred, and close the stomach if you can. If total gastrectomy and reconstruction are needed — make sure the patient is in a condition to withstand such a long and difficult procedure. **If not — consider staging**: insert a tube to drain the distal esophagus, close the duodenal stump and place a tube jejunostomy. Roux-en-Y jejunoesophagostomy will be performed once the patient is stabilized and ready for a major reintervention.

We recall some cases presented in the M & M meeting with a storyline like this: an old thin lady with vague chest pain, hours in the ER 'ruling out heart attack', admission to medicine for dyspepsia, interns or even nurses failing to insert a nasogastric tube, gastroenterologists scoping the patient and failing to realize what they see. At operation the next day, or even later, the whole stomach is dead. Very few survive! We hope you will do better. **The Editors**

Remember: **Presentation may be vague and a delay in treatment is disastrous. Think about it — suspect — proceed rapidly with diagnostic steps and treat accordingly.**

"The diaphragm — the most important and underappreciated muscle in your body." *

* The second part of the aphorism has been censored by the Editors — for details email mosheschein@gmail.com.

Chapter 16

Upper gastrointestinal emergencies

The Editors

This chapter has been subdivided into the following two sections:

1. Perforated peptic ulcer.
2. Upper gastrointestinal bleeding.

For the times they are a-changin'.

Bob Dylan

Let's face it. Upper GI emergencies in need of surgical intervention have become rarities; at least in the developed world. Thanks to modern anti-ulcer drug management peptic ulcers are being prevented or easily healed. Thus, they tend not to perforate and if they bleed, in most instances bleeding can be controlled endoscopically by us or our gastroenterologist buddies. **Furthermore, if surgical treatment is necessary it has become simpler, much less aggressive — dealing with the complication and leaving the healing of the ulcer to medicine.**

For these reasons we decided to combine the two topics of 'perforation' and 'bleeding' into a single shorter chapter.

1 Perforated peptic ulcer

Every doctor, faced with a perforated ulcer of the stomach or intestine, must consider opening the abdomen, sewing up the hole, and averting a possible or actual inflammation by careful cleansing of the abdominal cavity.

Johan Mikulicz-Radecki [1]

Although seldom seen in our own practice, perforated ulcers are still common in socioeconomically disadvantaged or stressed populations worldwide. Usually perforations develop against a background of chronic symptomatic ulceration but patients can present with a perforation 'out of the blue', without any previous history of peptic ulcer disease whatsoever. In the Western World, perforated duodenal ulcers (DUs) are much more common than perforated gastric ulcers (GUs), which are seen more in lower socioeconomic groups — associated with the 'holy' combination of stress, drugs, booze and smoke.

Keep in mind the fact that not all perforations arise in peptic ulcers: **rarely, a gastric adenocarcinoma or lymphoma can perforate as well**.

Natural history

John Blair Deaver of Pennsylvania (1855-1931) — yes, the guy who invented the retractor — wrote: "[in perforated peptic ulcers] it must be remembered that the exudate in the early cases is sterile or nearly so, and the peritoneal reaction is a response to chemical irritation by the gastric and duodenal contents rather than the result of bacterial invasion."

Classically, the abdominal pain caused by a peptic perforation develops very suddenly in the upper abdomen. Most patients can accurately time the dramatic onset of symptoms. The natural history of such an episode can be divided into three phases:

- **Chemical peritonitis/contamination**. Initially, the perforation leads to chemical peritonitis, with or without contamination with micro-organisms (note that the presence of acid sterilizes gastroduodenal contents; it is when gastric acid is reduced by acid-reducing treatment or disease, e.g. *achlorhydria* of gastric cancer, that bacteria and fungi are present in the stomach and duodenum). Spillage of

[1] Read about this Polish surgeon (the Germans claim him to be German...): https://en.wikipedia.org/wiki/Jan_Mikulicz-Radecki.

gastroduodenal contents is usually diffuse but may be localized in the upper abdomen by adhesions or the omentum. Spillage along the right gutter into the right lower quadrant, mimicking acute appendicitis, is mentioned in every textbook but is almost never seen in clinical practice (see ➲ Chapter 21 about the 'Valentino appendix').

- **Intermediate stage**. After 6 to 12 hours, many patients obtain some spontaneous relief from the pain. This is probably due to dilution of the irritating gastroduodenal contents by the ensuing peritoneal exudate.
- **Intra-abdominal infection**. If the patient initially escapes the scalpel, then intra-abdominal infection supervenes 12 to 24 hours later. The exact point in time in the individual patient when contaminating micro-organisms become invasive/infective is unknown. **Therefore, you should consider any perforation operated upon with a delay of more than 12 hours as infection rather than contamination**. This bears on your postoperative antibiotic therapy as discussed below. Neglected patients may present a few days after the perforation in septic shock. Shock in the earlier stages is very rare, although quoted commonly by medical students, **but when confronted with a combination of *shock* and *abdominal pain* think about ruptured aortic aneurysm, mesenteric ischemia or severe acute pancreatitis**. Untreated perforation can lead eventually to an early 'septic' death from peritonitis or the development of an intra-abdominal abscess.

Diagnosis

Most patients present with signs of diffuse or localized peritoneal irritation; they lie still, groaning, and have a board-like abdomen as described in textbooks (some call it 'textbook peritonitis'). Spontaneous 'sealing off' of the perforation, or localization of the spill or leakage into the lesser sac, causes an atypical and delayed presentation. We had a patient who perforated his ulcer into the retroperitoneum — behind the pancreas, the left colon and into the scrotum — he was in septic shock while the abdomen remained soft.

There is free gas under the diaphragm in about two-thirds of patients with perforation. That free air in the peritoneal cavity is the hallmark of perforated ulcer is known even to medical students. However, remember that free gas is visualized better on an upright chest X-ray than on plain abdominal radiographs (➲ Chapters 4 and 5). If your patient can't stand, or sit up, order a left lateral decubitus abdominal film. **Be aware also that free gas without clinical peritonitis is NOT an indication for an emergency laparotomy**. As mentioned in ➲ Chapter 4, there is a long list of 'non-operative' conditions that may produce free intraperitoneal gas. **Free gas in a 'soft' abdomen may also mean that the perforation has sealed spontaneously and is thus amenable to non-operative therapy as discussed below.**

Faced with such a patient today we would advise you to obtain a CT scan of the abdomen, looking for free gas, extraluminal oral contrast and free peritoneal fluid. CT is excellent at picking up minute amounts of free intraperitoneal gas and helping to suggest its source; it is thus a valuable tool in clarifying the diagnosis in patients with an ambiguous clinical picture — **is it acute diverticulitis to be managed non-operatively or a perforated ulcer to operate upon?** Those of you who are lucky to practice in the United States know that in most such patients a CT is available even before you have had a chance to see them. From a self-interested point of view, this is not such a bad idea. Imagine the 13th edition of this book (2049?) — this whole chapter will consist of one sentence: "Obtain a CT; seal perforation with CT-guided injection of glue." But perhaps, before then, perforated peptic ulcers will disappear completely?

Don't forget that in the absence of free air, acute pancreatitis — the 'great simulator' — should be considered and excluded (➲ Chapter 17). Again: elevated pancreatic enzymes and imaging will establish the correct diagnosis.

Philosophy of treatment

The primary goal of treatment is to save the patient's life by eliminating the source of infection and cleaning the abdominal cavity. The secondary goal is to cure, if possible, the ulcer diathesis. The former goal is achieved by simple closure of the ulcer. The latter goal — the permanent cure of the ulcer — is accomplished in most patients by modern anti-acid drugs and the eradication of the causative *Helicobacter pylori* bacteria. Consequently, emergency definitive ulcer surgery should be reserved to rare situations when the perforations are too 'complex' to be simply closed (see below).

A few years ago we asked the international membership of SURGINET (an online general surgical discussion group) about their experience with perforated ulcer disease. And here is what we found:

- **How common is the problem?** It is very rare in developed countries. Surgeons in the US, UK or Australia do not deal with more than one or two cases per year. When western lifestyle and availability of medications reaches a previously developing region, perforated ulcers become rare. **On the other hand, perforated ulcers are still common in indigent populations, as in South Africa, India or even Russia**, where some surgeons report as many as 25 cases per month!

- **What is the site of perforated ulcers? The vast majority are situated in the duodenum**. A few are pre-pyloric or gastric (associated with NSAID use). Because gastric resections for benign disease are so rarely performed, perforated *anastomotic ulcers* have almost disappeared, although they are resurfacing following **bariatric gastric operations**. In this latter group, perforations of the excluded gastric remnants are also being reported.
- **Which operation?** All responders would use *simple closure* as the preferred operative treatment. Some would add, very rarely, and in special circumstances — only if 'forced to do' — a definitive anti-ulcer procedure, as described below.

Management

There is no need to repeat how important it is to optimize these patients along the lines discussed in ➲ Chapter 6.

Antibiotics

As soon as the diagnosis of perforation is made, and the patient is booked in for an operation, administer a dose of broad-spectrum antibiotics. **Most patients present for treatment within 12 hours of perforation and therefore suffer from peritoneal contamination rather than infection**. In many of them, in fact, the peritonitis is purely chemical and does not exhibit any micro-organisms. Antibiotics in this group will serve for prophylaxis. Prolonged postoperative therapeutic antibiotics are not needed. Those who present later than 12 hours may suffer from an established intra-abdominal infection; here antibiotics should be continued in the postoperative phase (➲ Chapter 40). The antibiotics given, either in the form of monotherapy or combination therapy, should 'cover', empirically, Gram-negatives and anaerobes. Routine culturing of the peritoneal fluid in perforated patients is not indicated (➲ Chapter 13). (But you may be crucified by the infectious disease specialist and probably by your boss if you fail to comply with their guidelines.) **Candida, often cultured from the peritoneum in these cases, is a *contaminant* and does not need specific therapy**.

Operative treatment

Open surgery versus laparoscopy?

Omentopexy and peritoneal toilet can be executed laparoscopically. **We suggest that a laparoscopic procedure is a reasonable option in stable and well-resuscitated patients and when the perforation can be promptly and securely closed**. Conversely, a prolonged pneumoperitoneum will be poorly tolerated in the high-risk or severely septic patients. And, of course, you must be a skilled laparoscopist (do you know any surgeon who does not consider himself 'skilled in everything'?) to be able to perform a safe, watertight laparoscopic omentopexy.

By the way, the laparotomy for omentopexy need not always be a *macrolaparotomy*. Instead, with accurate pre-operative diagnosis on CT, you can repair the perforation and suck out the free peritoneal fluid through a limited transverse right subcostal incision or a short midline epigastric incision both of which are easier on the patient than the traditional long midline approach (➲ Chapter 10).

Some surgeons would opt for a **'lap-assisted' procedure**: the diagnosis is confirmed at laparoscopy, the peritoneal cavity is cleansed, a small incision is then placed just on top of the perforation and the hole is fixed.

In sum, do what is safe in your hands — even if open surgery seems to you not so 'sexy' it is still considered 'OK'.

Simple closure of the perforation (■ Figure 16.1)

The key word is OMENTOPEXY! Classically, simple closure of the ulcer is best achieved by an **omental patch** (termed **Graham's patch**, although described earlier in 1929 by Cellan-Jones — well, the Russians claim that it was V. A. Oppel who first described the operation in 1925), also called *omentopexy*. Place a few 'through-all-layers' interrupted sutures (we use 2-0 Vicryl®, but monofilament is OK) through both edges of the perforation (creating transverse closure in order not to narrow the lumen). Leave the sutures untied. Fashion a fat pedicle of the greater omentum and flip it up and over the perforation; then *gently* tie the sutures over the omentum in order *not to strangulate* it (■ Figure 16.2). At this stage ask the anesthetist to inject saline, with or without dye, through the nasogastric tube to ascertain that the patch is waterproof. **If it is not then do it again!** If the omentum is flimsy or absent for some reason, you can do the same with a mobilized **falciform ligament**, flipping it down over the perforation.

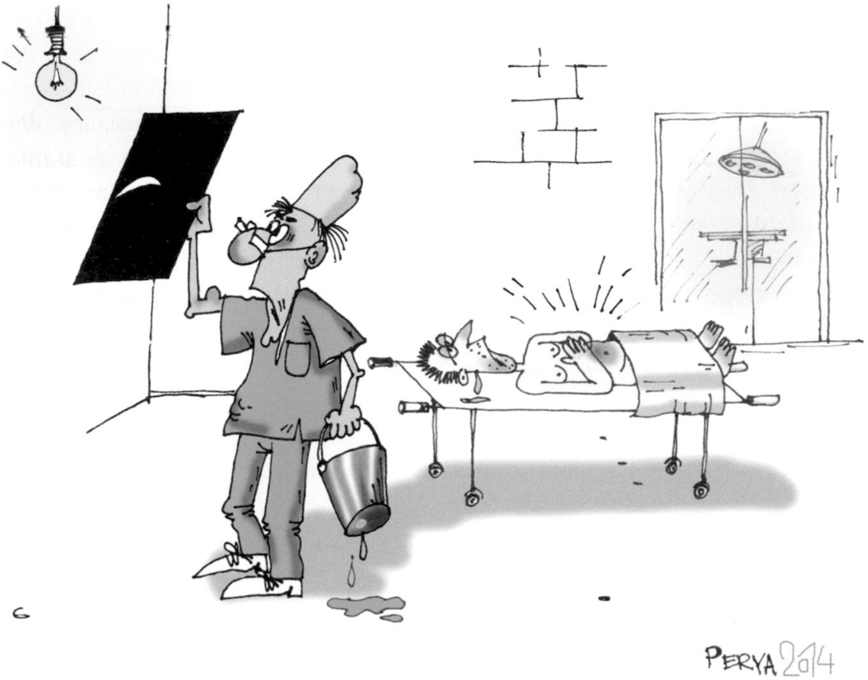

Figure 16.1. "How should we mend it?"

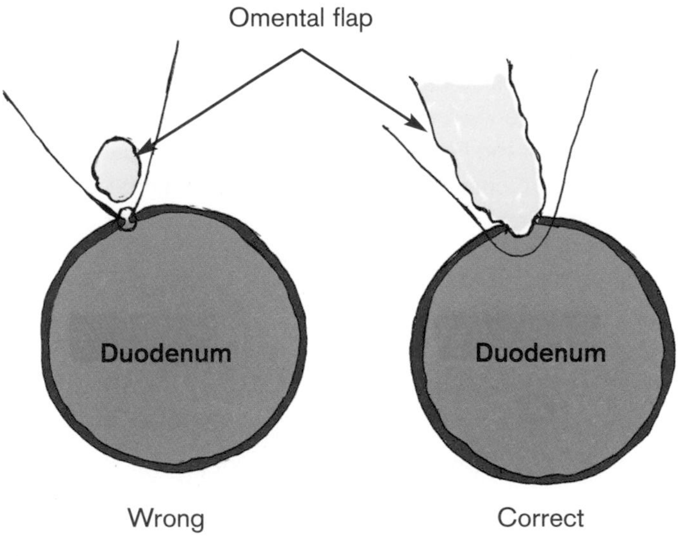

Figure 16.2. Simple closure. Note: the omental patch should 'plug' the hole with the sutures tied over it. Suturing the hole first and then sticking omentum over the repair is wrong.

More than a few surgeons misunderstand this operation; they initially suture-close the perforation and only then cover the suture line with the omentum. Some, mainly inexperienced laparoscopic surgeons, 'cut corners' and avoid the patch altogether — it is easier in their hands to suture-close the perforation. Often they get away with this but not always. **This is a recipe for disaster! This is how postoperative leaks occur!** Approximation of the edematous, friable edges of the perforation can be troublesome. It may be successful in small perforations when the edges of the defect are fresh, but in all cases of **postoperative duodenal fistula** witnessed by us, simple suture-closure of a perforated DU was the causative mechanism. **Be smarter, do not stitch the perforation but plug it with viable omentum**.

Should you leave a drain behind? Some surgeons do (Danny). Some not (Moshe, Paul). Do what makes you feel safe and happy. It appears that drains are left more often after laparoscopic repairs — this makes sense: the lap surgeons suspect that their repair is not always fantastic... but it may also be that solo surgeons are more confident than those who assist residents...

Simple surgical drainage (in 'difficult' circumstances)

In the absence of basic anesthetic facilities (e.g. somewhere in the bush or remote India) and when confronted with a patient who clearly needs an operation, there is a viable (and well-described) option. Under local anesthesia the upper abdomen may be entered through a limited incision and, after aspiration of as much muck and pus as possible, a large drain can be left under the liver in the region of the duodenum. If the perforation seals spontaneously the drain helps to control the associated abscess; if not, then it forms a lifesaving controlled duodenal fistula, to be dealt with — conservatively or operatively — later and elsewhere (not in the bush!). Our friend, Dr. Kuldip Pandey, a surgeon in rural India told us: "In moribund patients, if conditions don't permit for laparotomy, I generally put in a drain under vision (under local anesthesia). Quite often I do it bedside or in the minor OR cum dressing room attached to my ward. In quite a number of cases only this much has led to great improvement in the general condition of the patient who was later operated [upon] and discharged successfully."

Operative treatment: definitive surgery and which definitive procedure?

Surely, you do not want to embark on a lengthy definitive procedure in a critically ill and septic patient. But in what type of patient should you consider doing it?

It is, according to Dr. Alex Berzoy of Odessa, Ukraine: "The patient who would buy vodka instead of a proton pump inhibitor." And he is right! The very patients who are susceptible to perforation also suffer from substandard access to medical care and reduced compliance, both adversely affecting successful medical anti-ulcer therapies. This is obviously much more common in the developing world. Consequently, if the operation for a perforated ulcer can kill two birds with one stone (especially if the environment around you cannot ensure optimal medical management and follow-up of your patient), why not add a definitive procedure? That is, if you know how to do it. **While *intractability* as a real issue seems to be limited to the developing world, other special problems that could indicate a definitive procedure may exist anywhere.**

Ideally, in an emergency you should choose the anti-ulcer procedure with which you are most familiar in the elective situation. **Whatever you do please remember that if your patient is sick and you are not a skilled gastroduodenal surgeon — forget about the definitive procedure. Just patch the hole and get out!**

Special problems

These are the situations which may require more than simple closure:

- **'Kissing' ulcers: coexisting active UGI bleeding suggests the possibility of 'kissing' ulcers — the anterior perforated, the posterior bleeding.** Simple closure of the former, without hemostasis for the latter, could lead to a severe postoperative hemorrhage. In such circumstances enlarge the duodenal perforation into a duodenotomy and explore the inside of the duodenum. If a bleeding posterior ulcer is found, suture-transfix its base as described in the next section of this chapter.
- **Perforated giant ulcers**: while omentopexy should be used to repair most perforated DUs, a giant perforated DU (>2cm) may create a huge anterior bulbar-pyloric defect, which is not amenable to safe closure and thus **mandates partial gastrectomy**. In our hands, in order to avoid a 'difficult' duodenal stump, this would be a Billroth I gastroduodenostomy as depicted in ■ Figure 16.4 in the next section.
- **Perforated gastric ulcers**: these are usually larger than the duodenal ones. For those positioned on the greater curvature of the stomach, a wedge resection of the ulcer, hand sutured or stapled, may be easier and safer than omentopexy. For chronic and large lesser curvature ulcers, omentopexy is notoriously difficult and unsafe; partial gastrectomy may serve the patient better. Perforations of **malignant gastric ulcers** are very rare in the West (but in India, for example, many gastric perforations are malignant). Be that as it may, if we decide to patch a gastric perforation we would take a few biopsies

from its edges before closing it. If positive for cancer, an elective reoperation for 'oncological' gastrectomy may be necessary.

- **Pyloric obstruction**: perforated DUs are rarely associated with chronic narrowing of the gastric outlet. But if the patient gives a history of prolonged postprandial vomiting and/or at operation his stomach appears dilated and thickened, consider that possibility. Insert your index finger through the duodenal perforation and up the pylorus, or feed in a Foley catheter and check whether the inflated balloon (5cc) passes easily through the pylorus. **Documented pyloric stenosis would demand the addition of some form of drainage procedure** (pyloroplasty or gastrojejunostomy). Whether you wish to add a truncal vagotomy is up to you.
- **Intractable cases**: selected patients with a clear history of chronicity or intractability (e.g. a recurrent perforation), with no easy access to healthcare and medications may benefit from a definitive anti-ulcer procedure. That surgeons in London or Houston no longer find indications for acid-reducing procedures does not mean that there are no patients in Tbilisi who would benefit from it.

Non-operative management of perforated ulcers

A non-operative approach consisting of nil per mouth, nasogastric suction, systemic antibiotics, and acid secretion inhibitors, has been proven effective by a few enthusiastic groups. The *sine qua non* for success is the spontaneous sealing of the perforation by the omentum or other adjacent structures; if this occurs, a non-operative approach would be successful.

Non-operative treatment may be of particular value for two types of patients: the 'late presenter' and the 'extremely sick'.

- The '**late presenter**' comes to you a day or more after the perforation occurred, with an already improving clinical picture and minimal abdominal findings. This, together with radiographic evidence of free air, hints at a localized and spontaneously sealed perforation. Non-operative treatment, following a Gastrografin® UGI study, or contrast CT, to document that the perforation is sealed, should be successful in most instances.
- The '**extremely sick**' are the other candidates for conservative therapy: those in whom the risk of any operation could be prohibitive, such as the early post-massive myocardial infarct patient or the one with severe COPD (chronic obstructive pulmonary disease). Also in this group, however, conservative treatment may be successful only if

the perforation is sealed and radiographically proven to be so. Of course, localized collections or abscesses developing at the site of the sealed perforation can be drained percutaneously under CT guidance (➲ Chapter 42).

Leaks after the operation?

If you have performed a proper omentopexy you do not need to bother reading about how to deal with leaks. However, series of patients developing leaks from the perforation repair sites are being reported — reflecting, as mentioned above, a faulty operative technique. Details on how to manage such leaks you will find in ➲ Chapter 43.

Let us not forget:

...a course of anti-*Helicobacter* antibiotics after the operation, combined with appropriate acid-reducing agents. Patients with patched gastric ulcers would need endoscopic follow-up to document the healing of the ulcers. High-risk elderly patients may need acid suppression for the rest of their lives. The duration of such management in younger patients, and whether they will be reinfected with the ulcerogenic bacteria, is controversial.

To summarize...

Patch a perforated ulcer if you can. In almost all patients this is possible, but if not then you must resect. Consider adding a definitive anti-ulcer procedure on an extremely selective basis (almost never), and do not forget that a non-operative approach is possible, beneficial and indicated in selected patients. Whatever you do, large studies show that one-third of these patients will be dead within 5 years — the same factors which led to the perforation shorten their lives.

> *We have no responsibility to such patients but to save their lives. Any procedure, which aims to do more than this, can quite significantly be considered meddlesome surgery. We have no responsibility during the surgery to carry out any procedure to cure the patient of his duodenal ulcer.*
>
> **Roscoe R. Graham**

2 Upper gastrointestinal bleeding

Why are gastroenterologists more imaginative and courageous than we surgeons in employing new and bizarre invasive therapeutic modalities? Because they have somebody (us) to bail them out!

Eli Mavor

The problem

Upper gastrointestinal bleeding (UGIB) implies a source of bleeding proximal to the ligament of Treitz. What is the etiology of bleeding which could need your surgical attention?

- **Chronic *duodenal* (DU) or *gastric* ulcers (GU)**, while much less prevalent than before, are still predominant among the cases you are called upon to operate for bleeding. You will see more DUs than GUs.
- **Bleeding gastrointestinal stromal tumors (GISTs)**.
- **Dieulafoy's lesion**, a manifestation of a gastric submucosal vascular abnormality, has emerged as a relatively frequent indication for an emergency operation.
- **Rare causes** are seen from time to time, e.g. necrotic gastric cancer after chemotherapy or aorto-enteric fistula.
- **Acute gastric mucosal lesions** (e.g. stress ulcers, erosive gastritis and other terms that mean more or less the same) are usually due to ingestion of analgesics and/or alcohol (aspirin for the hangover). With the routine use of anti-ulcer prophylaxis in hospitalized 'stressed' patients, significant UGIB from mucosal lesions is now extremely rare — luckily, you will never be called upon to operate on such cases. In practice nowadays, hemorrhage in stressed patients often originates from reactivated chronic peptic ulcers.

So the pattern of etiology of the bleeding has shifted and, in addition, **failed, repeated attempts at non-operative management leave us with sicker patients who then present with more complex surgical anatomy** (e.g. the duodenum repeatedly tortured by the endoscopist is pristine no more). As a result, the cases you are called to save, after the others have failed, are becoming more demanding, while you, in all likelihood, are less and less familiar and skilled in the operative management of UGIB. (Confess — on how many cases of bleeding duodenal ulcer did you operate during your residency? How many partial gastrectomies have you done?). Therefore, you need to listen to us...

What about bleeding esophageal varices?

We do not know of a surgeon anywhere around the world who still operates on acute variceal bleeding in patients with portal hypertension. Anybody who remembers the bloody-morbid emergency devascularization procedures, or the no less exasperating portocaval shunts, must be relieved that modern endoscopic and radiological approaches have replaced the old butchery. Hence, we have moved the section on bleeding varices from this chapter to ➲ Chapter 23.

Approach

As introduced above, in many parts of the world, patients presenting with UGIB are initially seen by internists and/or gastroenterologists. We surgeons are usually called to take part in the management only when these specialists believe that they cannot stop the bleeding without our help — and this may be too late — which means that they may call you 'to operate' when the patient is already unsalvageable. **Oh yes, even in today's era of fancy endoscopic hemostasis and intensive care units, patients can die from bleeding ulcers** — Moshe recalls a young man admitted to a New York teaching hospital and undergoing two attempts at endoscopic control of his bleeding DU. He continued rebleeding in the ICU; by the time Moshe was called the patient had bled out. Moshe operated but too late — **the patient's life was lost because a simple hemostatic stitch to block the pumping gastroduodenal artery was not inserted in time. We have to know better how to manage these patients and encourage the early involvement of surgeons in their management**.

What to do if you are taking care of the bleeding patient?

- **Check vital signs. Aggressive management of hypovolemic shock is the first priority**. <u>Do not over-transfuse (!)</u> as there is evidence that excessive blood product administration exacerbates bleeding and results in a higher incidence of rebleeding.
- **With resuscitation underway, take a history**. Previous *peptic ulceration*? Dyspepsia? Anti-ulcer medications? (Remember, bleeding patients do not have pain because blood is alkaline and serves as an anti-acid.) Recent consumption of analgesics or alcohol? Severe vomiting or retching (*Mallory-Weiss*)? Chronic liver disease and/or *varices*? Nose bleed (swallowed blood)? Coagulopathy? Amount of blood vomited or passed per rectum (extremely inaccurate)? Full medical history (operative risk factors)?

- **Pass a large-bore nasogastric tube**, flush the stomach with 50ml of water, and aspirate: fresh blood indicates active or a very recent hemorrhage; coffee ground denotes recent bleeding which has stopped; clean aspirate or bile means no recent hemorrhage. **Note**: very rarely, a bleeding DU is associated with pyloric spasm with no blood refluxing into the stomach; a bile-stained aspirate excludes this possibility.
- **Perform a rectal examination**: fresh blood or juicy soft melena indicates active or very recent bleeding, while dry and solid melena signifies a non-recent UGIB (■ Figure 16.3).

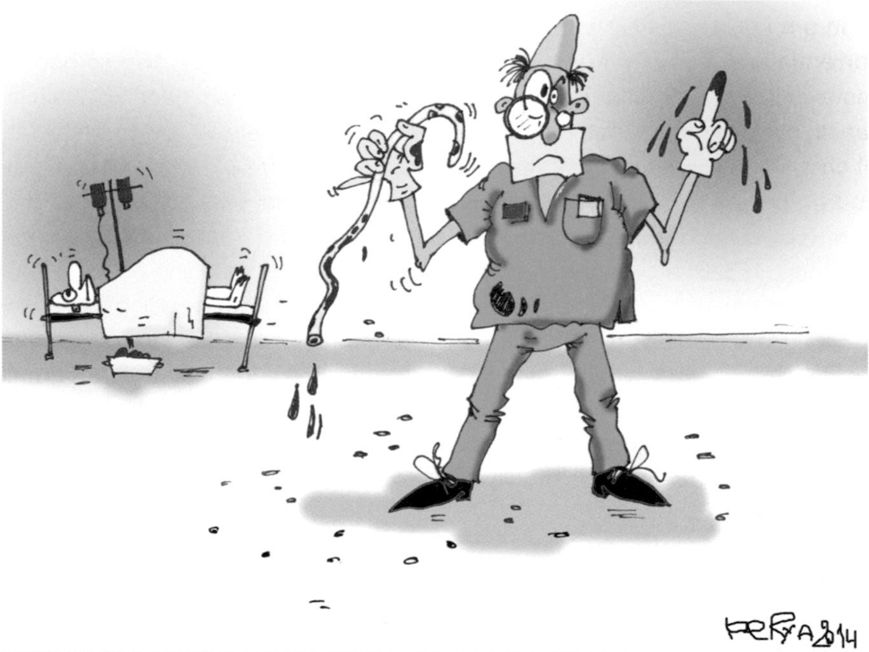

Figure 16.3. "This is a 'serious' UGI hemorrhage."

How to proceed?

Look at ■ Table 16.1. With all the basic information in mind you can classify the patients into one of the three groups.

The 'non-serious bleeders'

These patients have suffered a minor hemorrhage, which has stopped. **Do not rush to endoscopy in the middle of the night**. Semi-elective investigation suffices, and is more accurate and safe. **Note that a very low hematocrit/hemoglobin in patients belonging to this group results from a chronic or intermittent ooze**. The very anemic patient will tolerate endoscopy better after his general condition is improved. These patients do not require an emergency operation and therefore they won't be discussed further.

The 'serious bleeders'

In a minority of patients belonging to this group, fresh blood is pouring torrentially from the stomach; they are virtually exsanguinating! One has to move fast. Esophageal or gastric varices often bleed this way — like an *open tap*. In such cases a previous history of portal hypertension or clinical stigmata of chronic liver disease often coexist, suggesting the diagnosis. Remember — **you do not want to operate on varices** (see ➲ Chapter 23).

Table 16.1. Stratification and management of patients with upper gastrointestinal hemorrhage.

	Serious	Potentially serious	Not serious
Vomiting or nasogastric tube	Fresh blood	Coffee ground/fresh	Nothing/coffee ground
Per rectum	Fresh melena/blood	Fresh melena	Old melena
Hemodynamically	Compromised	Responded to resuscitation/stable	Stable
Hemoglobin/ hematocrit	<9/27	Use your common sense ☺	>9/27
Approach	Endoscopy now	Endoscopy soon	Endoscopy tomorrow
Prognosis	Requires hemostasis	Variable	Self-limiting

In any event, you should transfer the exsanguinating patient to a critical care facility or the operating room. **Intubate and sedate him/her to facilitate gastric lavage and subsequent endoscopy, and, most importantly, to reduce the risk of aspiration of gastric contents in the shocked, obtunded, bleeding patient**. You should attempt endoscopy (use a large-lumen irrigation endoscope that is capable of suctioning a clot rapidly and irrigating with high force) because, even if gastroduodenal visualization is totally obscured by blood, fresh bleeding from esophageal varices (usually at 40cm from the teeth, at the gastroesophageal junction) can always be detected, mandating a subsequent non-operative approach. **In the absence of varices you should MYA [2] rapidly: to surgery or angiography**.

The 'potentially serious bleeders'

They should undergo an emergency endoscopy as should the 'serious' ones who are not exsanguinating.

Emergency endoscopy for UGIB

This should be done only after you have resuscitated the patient and are in a controlled environment. Endoscopy induces hypoxemia and vagal stimulation; we have seen it cause cardiac arrest in unstable and poorly oxygenated patients (in addition, closed cardiac massage on a patient with a stomach ballooned with blood may lead to gastric rupture).

To improve the diagnostic yield the stomach should be prepared for endoscopy. Pass the largest nasogastric tube you can find and flush the stomach rapidly and repeatedly (tap water would do), aspirating as many clots as possible.

At endoscopy in addition to visualizing the potential sources of bleeding mentioned above, look also for the following **prognostic stigmata**:

- Active bleeding from a lesion.
- A 'visible vessel' in the ulcer's base, indicating that the bleeding originated from a large vessel and that there is a high chance of further hemorrhage.
- A clot adherent to the ulcer's base, signifying a recent hemorrhage.

---

2 Move your ass.

Endoscopic management

Having visualized the lesion you should now treat it endoscopically in order to achieve hemostasis and to reduce the risk of further hemorrhage. In broad terms, endoscopic therapy has a better chance of success in shallow lesions, which contain small vessels. However, you should also attempt endoscopic hemostasis in deeper, large vessel-containing lesions, with the aim of achieving at least temporary cessation of bleeding. This will permit a safer, semi-elective, definitive operation to be performed in a better-prepared patient. The specific method of endoscopic hemostasis, be it a 'hot' probe, clips, rubber bands, injection with adrenaline or a sclerosant, or even glue (frankly, it may be that even injection of *Coca Cola* may be effective in stopping bleeding, which in the old days would stop spontaneously...), depends on local skills and facilities. In fact, some experts claim that single-mode endoscopic treatment has no role and advocate 'triple endoRx'. Since it will be performed in most places by the gastroenterologists we will not concern ourselves here with technique.

Post-endoscopy decision-making

At the end of endoscopy you, or the 'other endoscopist', are left with the following categories of patients:

- **Actively bleeding**: **failed endoscopic hemostasis!** The source is usually a chronic ulcer and emergency operation is indicated. But if you have a readily available and skilled invasive radiologist, you may wish to consult him...
- **Bleeding (apparently) stopped**: e.g. chronic ulcer with a 'visible vessel' or adherent clot visualized. **The chances of further hemorrhage, usually within 48-72 hours, are substantial**. Treat conservatively but *observe closely* — you may want to rescope the next day as you may be sitting on a time bomb!
- **Bleeding stopped**: e.g. acute shallow lesion or chronic ulcer without the aforementioned stigmata. In these patients further hemorrhage is unlikely; treat conservatively and *relax*.

Conservative treatment

The mainstay of conservative treatment comprises completion and maintenance of resuscitative measures, and observation for further hemorrhage. There is now good evidence that the administration of high-dose

PPIs in patients with peptic ulceration reduces the incidence of rebleeding and the need for surgery following endoscopic hemostasis. Obviously, you should correct any coagulopathies. **All you need to do is to sustain the patient's organ systems, and watch for rebleeding, which usually occurs within 48-72 hours and can be massive and lethal. Careful monitoring of vital signs, observation of the number and character of melena stools and serial hematocrit measurements will detect episodes of further hemorrhage.** A nasogastric tube on suction is often advocated to provide early warning. In our experience, however, it is often blocked by clots, is of great discomfort to the patient and is therefore worse than useless. If, nonetheless, you choose to use it, flush it frequently.

The management of rebleeding

The patient has bled again! What now? Re-endoscopic treatment? Rush to the operating room? Transfer to the arteriography suite? Well, it all depends...

We do not suggest that you use cookbook recipes or formulas, as they are of little help in the individual patient. Instead, use clinical judgment. That the exsanguinating patient, and the one who continues to bleed after endoscopic hemostasis fails, need an emergency operation is clear and has been discussed above. But what to do with *recurrent hemorrhage*?

Factors that may or may not modify your decision to operate include the magnitude of recurrent hemorrhage, its source, and the age and general condition of the patient.

In general terms, **recurrent hemorrhage is an ominous sign**, meaning that bleeding will continue or, if stopped again, may well recur!

So our advice is:

- **If hemodynamically significant you have to operate!**
- **If rebleeding seems of mild or moderate magnitude** you may elect to continue conservative treatment or retreat endoscopically.
- The **source of the bleeding** may influence your decisions: e.g. a chronic, large ulcer may tilt the scale towards surgery; a superficial, acute source may guide you to avoid an operation.

Gastroenterologists are nowadays very keen to repeat endoscopic therapy in rebleeding patients — all of them, even those who squirt it out in a pulsatile stream — and even to do so a few times. Commonly, those patients 'belong' to them and you cannot interfere, but you should watch them 'from the side' and be ready to act. (After repeated endoscopic maneuvers sometimes not much will be left of the first part of the duodenum when you eventually operate.)

But, whatever you do, remember that old and chronically ill patients poorly tolerate repeated episodes of bleeding; do not mess around with them. As a rough guide, when the transfusion requirement exceeds 4 units of blood in a patient over 65 years of age, consider surgery (or angiography). Yes, we know it is a rough guide but surgical decisions are rough.

Angiographic transarterial management?

As mentioned above, in some centers therapeutic arteriography is the next stop for patients failing endoscopic hemostasis. Not surprisingly, assessing and comparing the results of various management options in such patients is difficult as so many factors are involved. Of course, as everything in life, it depends — in this case on your local expertise. We would consider this option as an alternative to an operation in special circumstances — for example, a bleeding DU when the risk of operative intervention would be prohibitive (e.g. after myocardial infarction) or UGIB from a pseudoaneurysm of the splenic artery associated with chronic or acute pancreatitis. But again, in many 'high-tech' centers, angioembolization has become the default — not the alternative treatment.

Operative management

What is true in acute surgery in general is true for UGIB: the volume of bleeding, the degree of physiological compromise, the number of units transfused — all correlate with morbidity, the risk of rebleeding, the need for surgery and mortality rates.

So finally, you decided to take the (optimally resuscitated, we hope) patient to the OR.

Exploration

Through a midline upper abdominal incision! No laparoscopy is advised in such patients, except in special circumstances (e.g. bleeding gastric GIST). A paraxyphoid extension and forceful upward sternal retraction lets you deal with anything in the foregut. In obese patients with a wide costal angle, however, a transverse chevron-type incision may take a few more minutes but affords a more comfortable exposure. In addition, **a generous reverse-Trendelenburg tilt of the patient will bring the upper stomach almost into your nose**.

Start by searching for external visual or palpable features of chronic ulceration. The latter are invariably associated with serosal inflammatory changes. Look for evidence of chronic ulcers from the duodenum to the gastric cardia. Duodenal *'Kocherization'* (Theodor Kocher is perhaps the only surgeon in history to have his name used as a verb) will be necessary to reveal the now almost extinct **post-bulbar ulcer** in the second portion of the duodenum. Occasionally, a **posterior or lesser curvature gastric ulcer** will become palpable only through the lesser sac. **Acute superficial mucosal lesions** are unfortunately not identifiable from the outside, although a **Mallory-Weiss** lesion may be *tattooed* by bluish serosal staining at the gastroesophageal junction.

The finding of a chronic ulcer in accordance with the pre-operative endoscopic finding tells you where the trouble is; **but what is to be done in the absence of any external evidence of pathology?** Yes, a rare situation but plausible. You have a few options:

- Proceed according to the endoscopist's findings — if you trust them... but they will not always be correct.
- Surgical exploration (gastrotomy, duodenotomy...).
- Intra-operative endoscopy.

Intra-operative endoscopy

Having endoscopically visualized, with your own eyes, an actively bleeding DU, you should not have any doubts. A doubtful endoscopic report, however, may promote a negative duodenotomy, extending it — piecemeal — proximally, until the high gastric lesion is found. **All that was needed was a small gastrotomy and suture ligation of the lesion; instead you are left with a very long, messy and unnecessary duodenogastrotomy to repair**. **To obviate such a mini-disaster we would unscrub for a moment and shove in an endoscope**.

Specific sources of bleeding

Duodenal ulcer (DU)

If anyone should consider removing half of my good stomach to cure a small ulcer in my duodenum, I would run faster than he.
Charles H. Mayo

About gastrectomy for duodenal ulcer: in this operation... a segment of an essentially normal stomach is removed to treat the disease next door in the duodenum. It is like taking out the engine to decrease noise in the gear box.
Francis D. Moore

The source of bleeding is always the *gastroduodenal artery* at the base of a posterior ulcer. Hemostasis is accomplished through an anterior, *longitudinal* duodenotomy, underrunning the base (and bleeding vessel) with two or three (2-0 or 0, a *monofilament* or *Vicryl®*) deeply placed sutures — each placed on a different axis. When bleeding is active, successful ligation of the vessel will be evident; in its absence you may want to abrade the ulcer's base, dislodging the clot and inducing bleeding. Otherwise, just underrun the base, deeply, and in a few directions. **The theoretical danger of underrunning a nearby common bile duct has been mentioned but we are unaware of even a single report of such a case** — however, never say never; s**t can happen! Others have described ligating the gastroduodenal artery from the outside, above and behind the duodenum. We have no experience with this and would be anxious fishing for the artery at the base of the gastrohepatic omentum which would be inflamed by the adjacent ulcerating process. Now carefully close the duodenotomy without constricting the lumen, and get out. Local hemostasis can be achieved even in the base of large ulcers or when the duodenum is extremely inflamed or scarred. **When simple closure of the duodenotomy appears to compromise the lumen just close the duodenum and do a posterior gastroenterostomy (GE)**. Of course, this is an 'ulcerogenic anastomosis'! But such patients will receive proton pump inhibitors for life. **The eventual cure of the ulcer is left to acid-reducing and anti-*Helicobacter* drugs**.

Which definitive procedure should you select in the rare patient? Obviously, only in a patient who is stable hemodynamically and otherwise in reasonable shape! Our choice would be adding a **truncal vagotomy (TV), extending the duodenotomy across the pylorus, and closing it to form a Heineke-Mikulicz pyloroplasty**. When and if the duodenum is extremely scarred and friable we would do a **gastroenterostomy** rather than pyloroplasty — just patch the duodenotomy the best you can and hook a proximal loop of jejunum, side to side, to the antrum.

Is there any indication for an antrectomy? The proponents of antrectomy plus vagotomy for bleeding DUs claim an increased incidence of rehemorrhage when gastric resection is avoided. In numerous emergency operations for bleeding DUs, this has not been our experience and we believe that there is no sense in removing a healthy stomach, producing a gastric cripple, for benign duodenal disease — which in any case can be subsequently cured with medications. When, however, the duodenum is virtually replaced by a huge ulcer involving the anterior and posterior wall of the duodenal cap-bulb, **one essentially is forced to perform an antrectomy** (with or without a truncal vagotomy) — this is similar to the scenario posed by a perforation of a giant duodenal ulcer (see above). In this situation, to avoid creating a duodenal stump which can be difficult to close and can leak, we prefer a Billroth I gastroduodenostomy as depicted in ■ Figure 16.4. This, we believe, is a

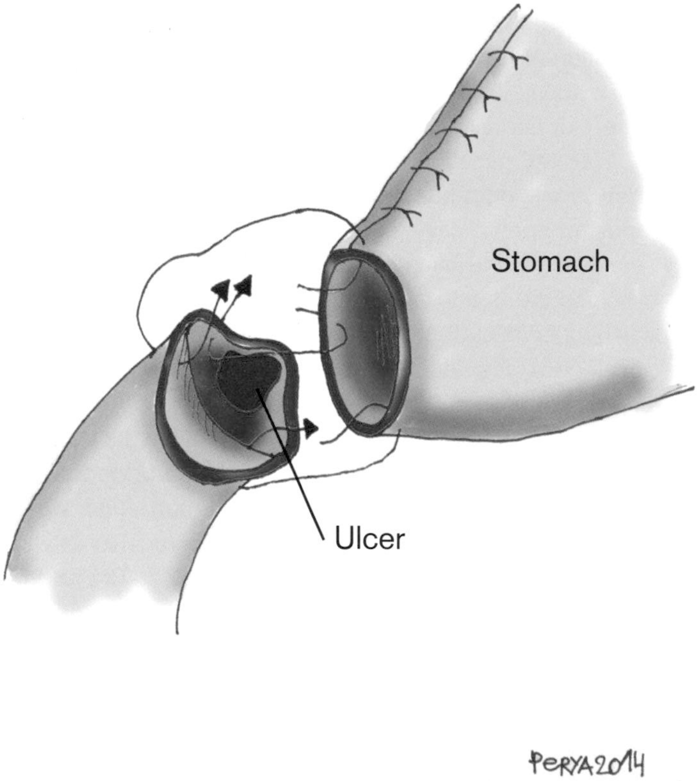

Figure 16.4. Gastroduodenostomy: note that the posterior aspect of the anastomosis is performed with 'heavy' (e.g. Vicryl® 2-0) interrupted sutures, taking 'big bites' in the posterior 'lip' of the duodenum (which is adherent to the pancreas) — well into the scar tissue at the base of the (now excluded) ulcer.

'healthier' solution than other methods, like Billroth II gastrojejunostomy and the insertion of a duodenostomy tube.

Gastric ulcer (GU)

In the previous editions we bored the hell out of our readers with a complex classification of gastric ulcers, recommending different definitive anti-ulcer procedures, based on the specific type of the GU. **This has become irrelevant as, irrespective of the location and type of the ulcer, your aim is to achieve hemostasis by the simplest possible maneuver. In most cases all that is required is simple underrunning of the lesion through a small gastrotomy**. In large chronic gastric ulcers we first underrun the bleeding point with an absorbable suture; with a heavy absorbable suture we then obliterate the ulcer's base. UGIB from a malignant ulcer very rarely requires an emergency operation. We would, however, take tissue from the ulcer's edges for histology. For bleeding ulcers situated at the greater curvature, **wedge resection** of the bleeding ulcer may appear more practical. **Partial gastrectomy** becomes necessary only in cases of a giant GU on the lesser curvature with direct involvement of the left gastric or splenic arteries.

Juxtacardial lesser curvature GUs and the so called 'riding GU'

A riding GU, also called a 'Cameron ulcer', is a variant of a high GU associated with a sliding hiatal hernia, produced by injury to the herniated stomach, 'riding' against the diaphragm. Typically, such ulcers are multiple and shallow, and present clinically with chronic UGIB and associated iron deficiency anemia. However, solitary, deeper ones can present as life-threatening UGIB. Rarely, when conservative/endoscopic therapy fails, an operation may be indicated: it comprises reduction of the stomach by pinching the ulcer away from the adherent diaphragm, local hemostasis, and crural repair. This may be easier said than done since occasionally the huge riding ulcer adheres to mediastinal structures and may require major resective surgery.

In conclusion, the generation of surgeons raised on the dogma that a complicated GU has to be resected is busy retiring or dying off (this includes us...). The modern surgeon should attack the bleeding GU with the simplest procedure possible, as dictated by the specific anatomy encountered.

Anastomotic (stomal) ulcer

This ulcer develops on the jejunal side of the gastrojejunal anastomosis following a previous vagotomy (or when vagotomy was omitted or is 'incomplete') and GE or Billroth II gastrectomy. **Because stomal ulcers almost never involve a large blood vessel, hemorrhage is usually self-limiting or amenable to endoscopic therapy**. Remember also that all stomal ulcers will heal on modern acid-suppressing medications. Persisting or recurrent hemorrhage, however, will force you, rarely, to operate. In the high-risk patient do the minimum: through a small gastrotomy, perpendicular to the anastomosis, examine the stoma and ulcer; underrun the latter with a few deeply placed absorbable sutures; close the gastrotomy and put the patient on H_2 antagonists or PPIs for life.

The role of a definitive procedure is limited, following the above stated philosophy. If the previous operation was a vagotomy plus GE, look for a missed vagal nerve or add an antrectomy. In the case of a previous Billroth II gastrectomy, add TV or consider a higher gastrectomy (do not forget to rule out Zollinger-Ellison syndrome later on). **Remember — hemorrhage from a stomal ulcer can be arrested with a simple surgical maneuver (underrunning); try to stay out of trouble by not escalating the emergency procedure into complicated reconstructive gastric surgery, which may kill your bleeding patient**.

UGIB after gastric bypass procedures for morbid obesity

This not uncommon entity should be addressed as any stomal ulcer. If endoscopic hemostasis fails, just overrun the bleeding ulcer through an incision in the 'gastric pouch' immediately above the anastomosis.

However, bleeding ulcers may develop in the distal, excluded stomach or the duodenum — locations which are not accessible to conventional endoscopy. Angiography (diagnostic/therapeutic) is a reasonable option; percutaneous, lap-assisted endoscopy has been described as well. **If forced to operate you may want to resect the excluded, ulcerated stomach**.

Dieulafoy's lesion

This small, solitary and difficult to diagnose gastric vascular malformation typically causes a recurrent 'obscure' massive UGIB. If not controlled by endoscopic maneuvers (or angio), they have become these days not an uncommon indication for UGIB surgery. Surgeons continue to debate what to do after the lesion has been exposed through an anterior gastrotomy: local excision?; underrunning?; do it through a laparoscope? Well, just stop dithering and deal with the bleeding the best you can!

Acute superficial mucosal lesions

Due to effective anti-ulcer prophylaxis in critically ill patients, you may never be called upon to operate on such lesions. In the remote past we had to intervene in a few such cases whose diffuse bleeding from 'stress gastritis' persisted despite management with PPIs and vasopressin. **Of course, endoscopic treatments are useless in this situation as the involved gastric mucosa looks and behaves like a blood-soaked and dripping sponge**. Surgical options mentioned by the standard textbooks include TV and drainage or total gastrectomy. The former is associated with a very high rate of rebleeding and the latter with a prohibitive mortality rate. **In this situation we have carried out gastric devascularization by ligating the two gastroepiploic, and left and right gastric arteries near the stomach's wall. In our experience, this relatively simple and well-tolerated procedure results in an immediate drying of the gastric sponge**.

To recap...

Admit patients with significant UGIB to your surgical service, to avoid treatment delays. After resuscitation diagnose the source of hemorrhage and stage it. Give endoscopic treatment a chance but do not delay an indicated operation. **At surgery the goal is to stop the bleeding — remembering that most ulcers can be cured later on by medication. Life comes first**.

Perhaps this rhyme will help you to remember...

> **"When the blood is fresh and pink and the patient is old**
> **It is time to be active and bold.**
> **When the patient is young and the blood is dark and old**
> **You can relax and put your knife on hold."**

Chapter 17

Acute pancreatitis

Ari Leppäniemi

During millions of years of evolution the pancreas wandered to the retroperitoneum for a reason; surgeons should think twice before messing with it!

In this chapter I will deal with acute pancreatitis, using alcoholic pancreatitis as the main example. For additional emphasis on gallstone-biliary pancreatitis read ➲ Chapter 18. Abbreviations are listed in ■ Table 17.1.

Table 17.1. Abbreviations.

ACS	Abdominal compartment syndrome
ANC	Acute necrotic collection
APACHE II	Acute Physiological and Chronic Health Evaluation (score)
APP	Abdominal perfusion pressure (APP = MAP - IAP)
CRP	C-reactive protein
ERCP	Endoscopic retrograde cholangiopancreatography
FNA	Fine needle aspiration
IAH	Intra-abdominal hypertension
IAP	Intra-abdominal pressure
MAP	Mean arterial pressure
MODS	Multiple organ dysfunction syndrome
MOF	Multiple organ failure
MRCP	Magnetic resonance cholangiopancreatography
SIRS	Systemic inflammatory response syndrome
SOFA	Sequential Organ Failure Assessment (score)
SvO_2	Mixed venous oxygen saturation
WON	Walled-off necrosis

Now that you have memorized by heart all the abbreviations, you are allowed to continue. **The Editors**

The incidence of acute pancreatitis varies significantly and can be as high as 102/100,000 population in countries such as Finland where alcohol is the most common etiological factor (and source of fun, except sauna and fishing); gallstones are the next most common etiology. Following these two causes (accounting for 70-80% of cases) there are many others: metabolic (hypercalcemia, hypertriglyceridemia), external or iatrogenic (ERCP) trauma, many drugs (look at Google — you will be surprised to see how many drugs have been implicated in the etiology of acute pancreatitis), infections, postoperative conditions (cardiac surgery), anomalies (pancreas divisum), tumors, hereditary and autoimmune diseases. Oh yes, don't forget snake bites!

In daily practice, out of those rare etiologies, post-ERCP pancreatitis seems the most common. In all other cases ask again about alcohol use…☺, and only then classify it as 'idiopathic', meaning that you are an 'idiot' — you have no idea what caused this attack of acute pancreatitis. However, in older patients it is important to rule out an underlying pancreatic neoplasm with a follow-up CT when the inflammation has subsided.

In a normal (Finnish) general hospital ED, about 3-4% of patients with an acute abdomen have acute pancreatitis. **For a differential diagnosis, round up the usual suspects**, such as perforated peptic ulcer, gastritis, reflux esophagitis, biliary colic, acute cholecystitis, acute mesenteric ischemia, intestinal obstruction, acute hepatitis, ruptured abdominal aortic aneurysm, inferior myocardial infarct, basal pneumonia, etc., **and remember that the clinical picture of severe acute pancreatitis resembles peritonitis**. Often a CT (we do not use i.v. contrast in this situation, but contrast is used at a later stage to look for pancreatic necrosis) is needed to exclude pancreatitis (and pinpoint another diagnosis) before operating on a patient with clinical peritonitis. But we'll get to the diagnostics later on…

Natural history

Following the initial triggering factor causing acinar cell injury and intrapancreatic activation of the pancreatic proenzymes, a local inflammation of the pancreas activates inflammatory cells and the release of inflammatory mediators. If this process is not localized, a systemic inflammation develops. This is when patients arrive at your emergency room. **In most cases, the disease is self-limiting, requiring only supportive and symptomatic treatment, but in about 15-20% a more severe form of pancreatitis develops leading to MODS** characterized by dysfunction of the pulmonary, cardiovascular, renal and other organ systems. In the severe forms the peripancreatic fat tissue and sometimes the pancreas itself undergoes necrosis — **necrotizing pancreatitis**; and if the necrotic tissue is invaded by microbes (believed to migrate transmurally from the adjacent colon), causing **infected pancreatic necrosis**, the prognosis gets instantly much worse, and the patient often requires surgical intervention.

Clinical presentation and diagnosis

Clinical features

A history is important. **A typical patient with acute pancreatitis in Finland presents with a history of drinking a bottle of vodka** (have you heard about the vodka called *Finlandia* which in Finland costs more than double what it costs in the USA?) a day for the last 3 weeks, and then he got so much pain that he could drink no more. Most such patients have so called 'darts-habitus' — you know the big guys in the pub throwing darts with their jeans lying low and showing the hairy lower back... Of course, there are also guys who "only had a couple of beers", so ask again.

The other typical patient is a dame (as Humphrey Bogart would say...) with intolerance to certain foodstuffs (greasy food, apples, etc.) causing colicky upper abdominal pain but this time it is different, and feels like a belt around the epigastrium. The problem: a tiny gallstone migrates to the common bile duct causing at least temporary outflow obstruction of bile (and pancreatic juice); the stone itself usually passes spontaneously through the papilla to the duodenum and signs of biliary stasis are minimal and transient (mild elevation of liver enzymes, no dilated bile ducts on ultrasound).

In addition to epigastric pain, patients often suffer nausea and vomiting; fever is uncommon unless there is accompanying cholangitis. Alcohol-induced pancreatitis is often associated with mental restlessness and sometimes even delirium.

Besides assessing the vital signs and reacting to severe physiological derangement (as in all severely ill patients), physical examination typically reveals a distended abdomen, epigastric or generalized tenderness and absent bowel sounds indicating paralytic ileus. In more severe cases, the abdomen might be filled with pancreatic ascites, and in patients with a delayed presentation the typical signs of necrotizing pancreatitis with discoloration around the umbilicus (*Cullen's sign*) or at the loins (*Grey-Turner's sign*) can be seen.

Lab work

Elevated plasma *amylase* levels (pancreas-specific, three times upper normal limit) confirms the diagnosis but be aware that the amylase levels may have returned to normal if the symptoms have been present for several days. Therefore, some also measure serum *lipase* levels that stay elevated for a longer time. **Other abdominal catastrophes can cause mild elevation of the amylase levels, so when in doubt, request a CT!** ***CRP*** is usually significantly elevated in severe acute pancreatitis but it takes 24-48 hours before that happens. Other lab tests such as blood count, liver tests, electrolytes, glucose and renal function (creatinine) are important to complement the overall picture and are helpful when planning treatment. If you suspect **hyperlipidemia** as the cause, check triglycerides. In really sick patients with suspected cellular hypoperfusion, lactate levels and arterial blood gases are needed.

Imaging

If CT is available in your hospital, forget plain abdominal X-rays; they are not helpful except in some cases to rule out mechanical bowel obstruction or perforation of a hollow viscus (if you believe the absence of free air is enough to rule out perforation — I don't...). **Chest X-rays** are helpful in a later phase to assess pulmonary congestion and possible pleural effusion.

Abdominal CT is the best diagnostic tool available. It detects even mild acute pancreatitis (edema around the pancreas, sometimes confined to the head or tail). We have stopped using oral contrast and use mostly tap water as a contrast medium. As I mention above, we do not use intravenous contrast in the initial phase to avoid damage to the already stressed kidneys. If severe (necrotizing) pancreatitis is suspected, a later CT scan with i.v. contrast to assess pancreatic enhancement and vitality can be used after volume restoration and assessment of renal function. And to be honest, it seems that the risk of contrast-induced kidney injury is not so big after all, so we have become more liberal in its use. Of course, there must be a good reason to use contrast...

Ultrasonography is used early as a complementary study to identify or rule out cholelithiasis (CT is not reliable in detecting gallbladder stones) and a dilated common bile duct, but it is not helpful in diagnosing pancreatitis. **If the liver enzymes are elevated and ultrasound shows the presence of gallbladder stones and/or a dilated common bile duct, we usually perform MRCP to see if the stone is still present or has passed through spontaneously**. In cases when a persistent stone causes biliary stasis, especially when associated with a high fever (cholangitis), **ERCP** and sphincterotomy are indicated to clear the common bile duct. This is unusual, though, in most cases of biliary pancreatitis.

Estimation of severity and classification

Although a *continuum* — ranging from edematous acute pancreatitis, with mild symptoms lasting a couple of days, to a critical, severe form of necrotizing pancreatitis, with MODS — for everyday clinical purposes acute pancreatitis can be divided into mild, intermediate, severe and critical forms.

It is not always clear in the early stages (when you are in the emergency room) to which category the patient belongs, i.e. what natural course the disease will take.

So how do we assess the severity of the disease?

- The initial level or progression of amylase levels does not correlate with severity; CRP is better (150mg/L is some kind of threshold for severe acute pancreatitis), but manifests a couple of days too late; *procalcitonin* is increasingly used as a marker of severe disease and sepsis (even though we in poor Finland don't use it routinely...).
- Clinical **scoring systems** such as those described by the late Ranson, USA, or Imrie, Scotland (you probably do not remember the time when medical students, like us, knew all Ranson's criteria by heart), are inaccurate and not used anymore. The **APACHE II** score measures nicely the severity of the disease — a score higher than 8 indicates significant physiological derangement. In our hospital we use the **SOFA**[1] score routinely (remember what it means?) to monitor the degree of organ dysfunction; we rely especially on the cardiovascular, pulmonary and renal components of the SOFA score (and also measurement of the intra-abdominal pressure [IAP] — see ➲ Chapter 31) to determine if the patient should go to the ICU directly from the emergency room.

1 http://clincalc.com/IcuMortality/SOFA.aspx.

- **At the end of the day we classify the severity of acute pancreatitis by combining the local and systemic determinants of severity**. The **local determinants** are related to the presence or absence of peripancreatic and pancreatic necrosis and whether it is sterile or infected. The **systemic determinant** is related to whether there is organ failure or not and, if present, whether it is transient (resolves within 48 hours) or persistent. These factors are connected, and the relationship between necrosis, be it infected or not, and the development of organ dysfunction has been established in multiple studies. The key is the development of persistent organ failure. The mortality in acute pancreatitis is mainly associated with MOF whereas the risk of dying is minimal in patients with no or transient organ dysfunction.

In this day and age patients rarely die from the early-acute manifestation of acute pancreatitis (e.g. hypovolemia); they die from its late sequelae (e.g. SIRS, sepsis, MOF). But beware of the patient coming in with early ACS-induced renal and respiratory failure after undergoing massive fluid resuscitation. Measure the IAP; the patient might need early decompressive surgery!

The 4-week approach to the management of acute pancreatitis (■ Figure 17.1)

1st week: inflammation

About 85% of patients with acute pancreatitis have the mild form of the disease. In the past we used to admit these patients to the ward, keeping them starved and inserting a nasogastric tube, and treating the pain, nausea and delirium with medications. In most cases, the patient recovered within a few days and was discharged. These days we treat the symptoms with medications, start oral feeding as soon as the patient tolerates it, and look for signs of severe acute pancreatitis hoping to recognize it early. If all is going well, the patient has mild acute pancreatitis (a '1-week disease'), where the inflammation resolves without major systemic or local complications.

Any signs of continuous severe pain, restlessness, respiratory distress, decreasing urine output, greatly distended abdomen, increasing CRP levels, or increasing IAP could indicate that the inflammatory process continues and the patient will progress to the second stage: necrosis (see below '2nd

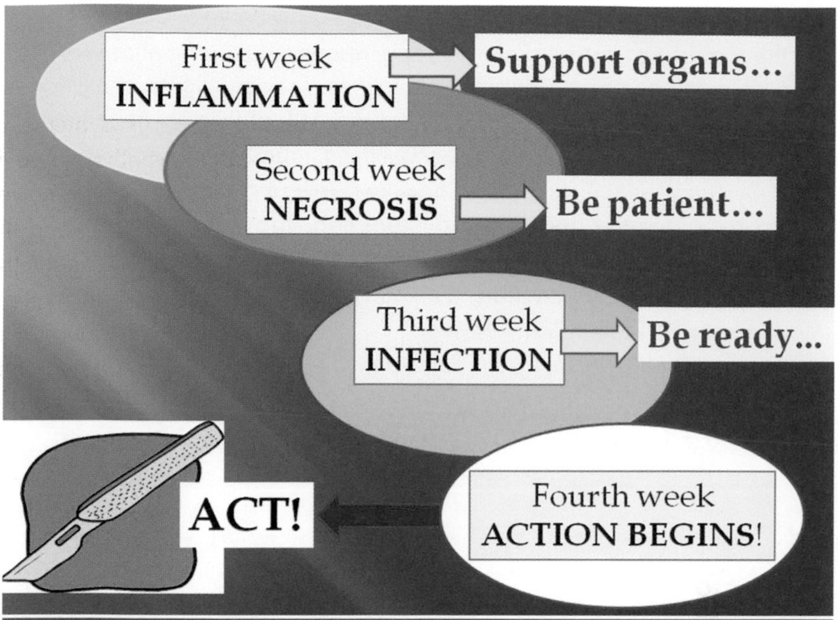

Figure 17.1. Severe acute pancreatitis: week by week.

week'). **Remember: mild acute pancreatitis is maximally a 7-day disease. Anything that lasts longer is not so mild...**

OK, time for a little theory: MOF is a consequence of excessive activation of a systemic inflammatory response cascade, where inflammatory mediators induce end-organ endothelial cell activation leading to increased permeability. Leaking microvessels cause a loss of intravascular fluid and in conjunction with vasodilatation lead to hypotension and shock. Accumulation of inflammatory cells in tissues, increased interstitial fluid and activation of coagulation with microvascular thrombosis further impair oxygen supply of tissues (OK, now you can wake up!).

The clinical manifestation of all this is MODS that develops early during the course of acute pancreatitis. Over half of patients with severe acute pancreatitis have signs of organ dysfunction on admission and most organ dysfunction develops within the first 4 days. So, when that happens, get your patient to the ICU!

Besides monitoring and supporting organ dysfunction as in all ICU patients, below are some specific comments about patients with severe acute pancreatitis in the ICU.

Fluid resuscitation

In the past, aggressive fluid therapy during the early phase of acute pancreatitis was one of the dogmas we followed religiously (God have mercy on the resident who had not ordered at least 5-10L of fluid for the patient). Of course the rationale behind fluid resuscitation is sound: to correct hypovolemia caused by 'third space' fluid loss; however, to put it simply: **too little fluid leads to hypovolemia and organ dysfunction, too much fluid can cause tissue edema, intra-abdominal hypertension (IAH) which — if untreated — can lead to organ dysfunction**. Our current fluid resuscitation goals are summarized in ■ Table 17.2.

Table 17.2. Summary of early treatment of severe acute pancreatitis.

- ■ Early admission to the ICU or high dependency unit.
- ■ Goals for fluid resuscitation with crystalloids:
  - MAP >65mmHg;
  - SvO_2 >65% (requires pulmonary artery catheter);
  - normal lactate;
  - urine output >1ml/kg/hr (about 50-100ml/hr);
  - routine measurement of IAP (goal <25mmHg);
  - norepinephrine and/or dobutamine in cardiovascular failure;
  - APP (MAP-IAP) >60mmHg.
- ■ Analgesia, sedation, lung-protective ventilation.
- ■ Normoglycemia.
- ■ Thrombosis prophylaxis.
- ■ Early enteral feeding, prophylactic antibiotics.
- ■ Early biliary decompression, if obstruction.

Enteral nutrition

Fasting does not help, and it does not alleviate the inflammatory response or 'rest the pancreas'. **Enteral feeding (a product of millions of years of evolution) is superior to parenteral feeding, prevents bacterial overgrowth in the intestine and reduces bacterial translocation, reducing the risk of systemic infections, organ dysfunction and mortality**. **The only contraindication is the inability to eat because of the associated ileus or gastric outlet obstruction**. So, offer tasty hospital food (e.g. Finnish smoked salmon) to a conscious patient if it is tolerated without vomiting or aggravating pain.

In a ventilated and sedated patient this is what we do:

- Try a nasogastric tube first and start feeding.
- If gastric residual is >250ml/6hr, insert a self-advancing nasojejunal tube or ask your endoscopy friend to insert one.
- Then start with 10ml/hr and increase gradually until caloric needs are met.
- Avoid exceeding 40ml/hr (we have had some intestinal catastrophes with high-volume enteral feeding...).

Enteral feeding is probably more beneficial in reducing the risk of infectious complications than prophylactic antibiotics, so use it!

Prophylactic antibiotics

There are many randomized controlled trials and probably even more meta-analyses (BTW — "Meta-analysis is to analysis as metaphysics is to physics," said H. Harlan Stone) and systematic reviews, that try to convince us that prophylactic antibiotics do not benefit patients with acute pancreatitis. **Acknowledging the limitations of the trials and that patients with organ failure are susceptible to infections, we believe (not evidence but maybe error-based medicine) that the use of prophylactic antibiotics in patients with severe pancreatitis is justified — the balance of risk is in favor of administration**. We just wait for the scientific pendulum to swing again to our side... We base our indication for starting antibiotics on clinical judgment taking into account the presence of SIRS, IAH, hyperglycemia, low plasma calcium, high creatinine or other signs of organ dysfunction. If it turns out that the patient has mild acute pancreatitis, it is quite OK to terminate the antibiotics. We start with cefuroxime unless contraindicated (allergy). You can use your local *soup du jour*. **But remember to stop the prophylaxis after 5 days, even if the patient ends up in the ICU!**

Who needs surgery on week 1?

Apart from surgical or endoscopic interventions required for gallstone-associated pancreatitis (see ➲ Chapter 18.3), **there are very few reasons to operate on patients with severe acute pancreatitis in the early stage**:

- **Abdominal compartment syndrome (ACS)**. The combination of excessive fluid resuscitation and capillary leakage leads to tissue edema of the abdominal and retroperitoneal organs, and ascites formation. Intestinal paralysis (ileus) usually adds to the increase in intra-abdominal volume leading to intra-abdominal hypertension (IAH) — see ➲ Chapter 31. When IAH (defined as IAP ≥12mmHg) develops, non-operative methods to decrease IAP should be tried first to prevent progression to a full-blown ACS. **If non-operative management, including percutaneous drainage of pancreatic ascites, fails to reduce the IAP (goal APP >60mmHg), surgical decompression is indicated**. Over the years, our non-operative management has improved, which means that fewer abdomens are opened for ACS. **Another observation**: if the radiologist tells you that "there is only a small amount of ascites", ask for US-guided drainage anyway; often you can drain 2-3L and that helps a lot to decrease IAP.

- Unlike some other indications for an open abdomen (trauma, peritonitis, bowel ischemia), in acute pancreatitis surgical decompression usually leads to an open abdomen of several weeks' duration, **which markedly increases the risk for complications including infected necrosis**. On the other hand, with the new methods of open abdomen management, such as the vacuum-assisted closure (VAC) with mesh-mediated fascial traction, the delayed fascial closure rates approach 90%, with a very low enteric fistula rate.
- **Hemorrhage**. Bleeding — usually arising from the necrotic process around the pancreas eroding an artery — is a rare complication in severe acute pancreatitis, but when it occurs, **it requires prompt management, preferably by angiographic embolization**. Sometimes, however, you are forced to go in and pack the bleeding, leaving the abdomen open, and then do a reoperation 2 days later to remove the packs. Obviously, hemorrhage in need of hemostasis may develop during the subsequent weeks.
- **Colon necrosis** (actually, this complication is more common later on…). Necrosis of a part of the transverse colon in acute pancreatitis is associated with high mortality and is difficult to diagnose until perforation occurs. Gas bubbles in the colonic wall seen on CT can be a useful hint. Colon necrosis is probably caused by retroperitoneal spread of the necrotizing process to the colon with fat necrosis and pericolitis. Usually, the inner layers of the colon remain viable longer. The commonest site of colon necrosis is the adjacent transverse colon — caused by thrombosis of the middle colic artery branches involved in the peripancreatic necrosis. We have also seen cecal perforations — probably aggravated by colonic dilatation. **Try to identify any necrosis (gas bubbles and other signs of necrosis in the colon wall on CT) before it progresses to frank perforation and contamination of the peritoneal cavity**. At surgery, removal of the affected segment is performed. Primary colonic anastomosis under these circumstances is risky, and **a colostomy is a better option**.

2nd week: necrosis

The necrotic process in and around the pancreas starts to manifest by the end of the first week, and the severity (and the prognosis) depends on the quantity and extent of the necrotic tissue. **A CT scan (with i.v. contrast now unless the kidneys are really at risk) can show the extent of the necrosis**. There are classification systems based on the CT evaluation (the first one developed in Finland by the radiologist Leena Kivisaari), such as the Balthazar classification (look it up), **but the physiological state and organ function are better determinants of severity**. Fluid collections around the pancreas and in the lesser sac are common. **We used to call them pseudocysts, but acute peripancreatic fluid collection is a more accurate term. They may resolve spontaneously and as such require no treatment. If the necrotic collections remain sterile, there is no reason to operate at this early stage. So, be patient even if the intensivists give you the typical look (while thinking): "Why is he not going to operate, we are tired and bored of this..."** (see ■ Figure 17.2).

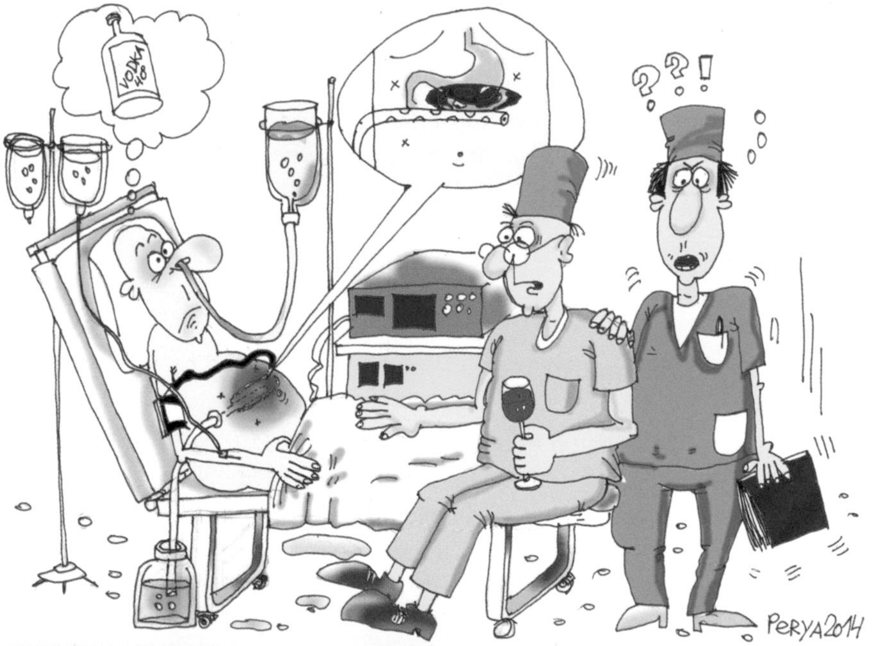

Figure 17.2. Assistant: "Prof, let's operate for God's sake! His pancreas is dead!" Professor: "Are you an imbecile or what? Be patient! We'll operate perhaps next month. Now get me some more vino!"

3rd week: infection

The diagnosis of infected necrosis is difficult. Even US or CT-guided fine-needle aspiration (FNA) of the necrosis has a false-negative rate of 20-25%.

Clinical signs of sepsis are too non-specific for definitive diagnosis, although a new increase in the CRP value without any other good explanation might alert you to look for infected necrosis. **Get a new CT!** If you are lucky, gas bubbles in the CT scan means infection but unfortunately, they are present in less than 10% of cases. What you most commonly see is an **acute necrotic collection (ANC)**, containing variable amounts of fluid and necrotic tissue involving the pancreatic parenchyma and/or peripancreatic tissues; here the possible presence of infection must be based on clinical assessment of progress and organ dysfunction.

What we do at this stage is what the Dutch (who have this remarkable way of doing multicenter randomized studies) invented — **a step-up strategy** (see below): have a US-guided drain inserted into the ANC and take a bacterial sample of the fluid. **If it is positive**, you know there is infected necrosis (still wait up to 4 weeks from the onset of symptoms to see if surgery is needed unless the patient gets really sick). Often removing some of the infected fluid buys you time, so don't hurry! **If the sample is sterile**, remove the drain (within about a week) when the amount of drained fluid has decreased.

4th week: the (surgical) action really starts now

What do you see on CT?

According to the updated **Atlanta classification 2012**, **walled-off necrosis (WON)** is a mature, encapsulated collection of pancreatic and/or peripancreatic necrosis with a well-defined, enhancing inflammatory wall (■ Figure 17.3). **The maturation takes usually 4 weeks** or more after the onset of acute pancreatitis.

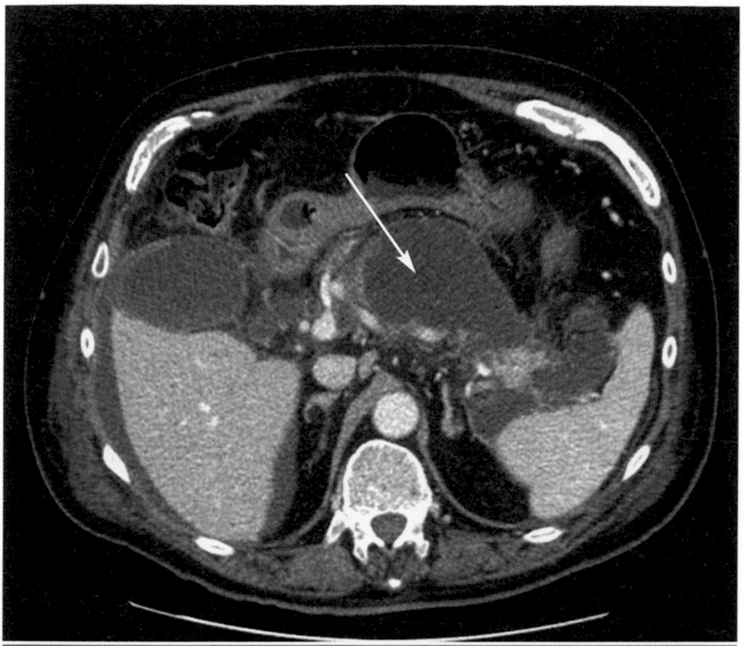

Figure 17.3. Abdominal CT showing walled-off necrosis (WON). Note the encapsulated collection of pancreatic and/or peripancreatic necrosis with a well-defined, enhancing inflammatory wall.

Indications and timing for interventions

According to the International Association of Pancreatology and the American Pancreatic Association evidence-based guidelines for the management of acute pancreatitis [2], **the indications for intervention (surgical, radiological or endoscopic) in necrotizing pancreatitis are**:

- **Clinically suspected or documented infected necrosis with clinical deterioration, or ongoing organ failure for several weeks**.
- Ongoing gastric outlet, intestinal, or biliary obstruction due to mass effect of WON.
- Patient not getting better with WON but no infection (after 8 weeks).
- Disconnected duct syndrome (full transection of the pancreatic duct) with persisting symptomatic collection with necrosis without signs of infection (>8 weeks).

2 IAP/APA evidence-based guidelines for the management of acute pancreatitis. *Pancreatology* 2013; 13(4 Suppl 2): 1-15.

So you see that the timing of intervention is usually postponed until at least 4 weeks after the initial presentation to allow the WON to be formed. As listed above, recommendation for some of the other indications is more than 8 weeks. This requires lots of patience!

Treatment

In patients with suspected or confirmed infected, necrotic pancreatic tissue, the Dutch [3] have shown that by using the so-called **'step-up' strategy consisting of initial percutaneous drainage followed, if necessary, by minimally invasive retroperitoneal necrosectomy, open surgical procedures can be avoided in about one-third of patients**.

So, this is what we do: if the step-up strategy works, fine, don't do anything else; if it doesn't (you put the drain in but the patient does not get any better in a week or so) and at least 4 weeks have passed from the onset of symptoms, think necrosectomy. Depending on your expertise, resources and some clinical features (see below), you have several options on how to do this.

How to do a necrosectomy

There are several ways of doing a necrosectomy ranging from minimally invasive to 'maximally invasive' techniques. The choice depends on the size and location of the WON: whether it is located only in the lesser sac and stays in close contact with the posterior wall of the stomach, or has multiple locations including retroduodenal and/or bilateral retrocolic collections, for example.

The other thing that needs to be considered, is the presence or absence of a disconnected duct, meaning that the necrosis has eroded the body of the pancreas and the main pancreatic duct has been divided leaving a distant isolated pancreatic tail remnant secreting pancreatic juice into the collection. This can easily be seen with an i.v. contrast CT scan, so always have a fresh one before deciding to operate!

You may ask: open or minimal access (including endoscopic) pancreatic necrosectomy? Transperitoneal or retroperitoneal? Close the

[3] van Santvoort HC, Besselink MG, Bakker OJ, *et al.* A step-up approach or open necrosectomy for necrotizing pancreatitis. *N Engl J Med* 2010; 362: 1491-502.

abdomen or leave it open? In reality, you do what you know best but, if possible, tailor the procedure to that which benefits the patient most. It is always useful to have more than one option.

Minimally invasive variations for the management of peripancreatic necrotic collections are routinely used in some centers and include endoscopic retroperitoneal drainage or lumboscopic necrosectomy, and percutaneous necrosectomy and sinus tract endoscopy. The value of these techniques is still controversial, but many centers use them as a primary option. We have sporadically tried some of them, but found them to be cumbersome and, to our minds at least, inadequate. So we aborted the experiment...

A more promising approach in selected patients is the surgical (open or laparoscopic) transgastric necrosectomy of which the Canadians have published a large series with excellent results [4].

The open surgical version starts with a small upper midline laparotomy and anterior gastrotomy. Then, a needle is inserted through the posterior stomach wall to the WON collection (need the pre-op CT!), and the posterior gastric wall is opened through which a careful (avoiding injury to blood vessels and penetration of the WON capsule) necrosectomy is performed. The common ostomy between the posterior gastric wall and fibrous WON capsule is reinforced around its edges with a running locked 3-0 suture on a large needle, and the anterior gastric wall is closed following confirmation of nasogastric tube placement within the WON cavity.

This approach is feasible in selected patients where the WON collection is located and limited to the lesser sac. It is especially useful for patients with a pancreatic leak or disconnected pancreatic duct, where the pancreatic fluid drains into the stomach instead of spreading all over the place. If this single-stage procedure is anticipated or planned, then one should avoid the pre-operative placement of percutaneous drains to avoid losing the containment of the WON collection and risking postoperative external pancreatic fistula.

When the WON collections are multiple and located in areas not feasible for the transgastric approach, open necrosectomy is still a valid alternative. We prefer an old-fashioned anterior abdominal approach where you can actually see what you are doing... ☺.

---

4 Driedger M, Zyromski NJ, Visser BC, *et al.* Surgical transgastric necrosectomy for necrotizing pancreatitis. A single-stage procedure for walled-off pancreatic necrosis. *Ann Surg* 2018; Sep 13. doi: 10.1097/SLA.0000000000003048.

Open necrosectomy

When you do open necrosectomy for the right indications at the right time, removing the black clay-like stuff by scooping with your fingers is easy. Getting through the gastrocolic ligament (yes, I prefer not to go through the transverse mesocolon), opening the correct tissue planes with blunt dissection and utilizing the Harmonic Scalpel® or old-fashioned ligatures gives good exposure.

Usually the necrosis is mostly found around the pancreas while the pancreas itself is firm and protrudes like a transverse ridge. Leave it alone! If on the other hand (and pre-operative CT helps) the necrotizing process has destroyed the middle part of the pancreas leaving the tail without connection to the remaining part of the pancreas (the **disconnected duct syndrome**, or **disconnected left pancreatic remnant**), you can squeeze the separated tail out with gentle finger dissection, but be careful with the splenic vessels and leave the spleen alone. Once you have removed the dead distal pancreas (■ Figure 17.4) (sometimes only a small proximal remnant is left), you can try to find the divided pancreatic duct and ligate it. Usually you don't see it, and a pancreatic fistula occurs, but you can deal with that later on. Pack the area for a few minutes and check hemostasis. Deal with clear bleeders, don't worry about minor oozing. Draining the peripancreatic area with a couple of well-placed drains (one coming behind the left hemicolon into the pancreatic area if the necrosis is mainly on the left side) completes the procedure. **Usually, in 80-90% of cases, we close the abdomen after necrosectomy unless the IAP was clearly elevated prior to surgery or if there is considerable intestinal oedema**. Obviously, in a patient already with an 'open abdomen' (for ACS for example), and who, later on, needs necrosectomy, we almost always leave the abdomen open and continue with the mesh-mediated VAC system.

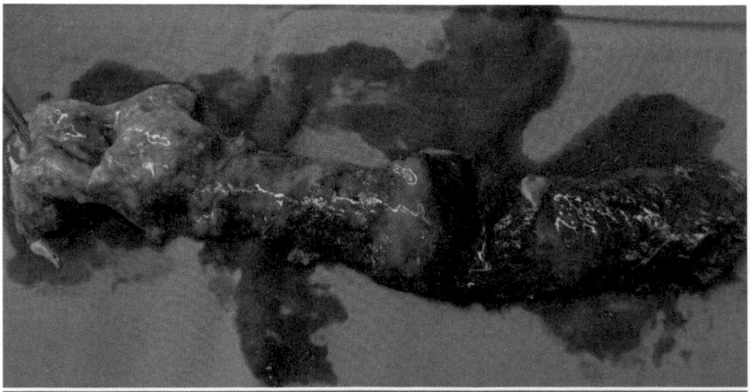

Figure 17.4. Removed dead pancreas.

The vacuum and mesh-mediated fascial traction is a temporary abdominal closure (TAC) method described by our Swedish colleagues [5]. It combines the vacuum effect with mechanical traction induced by a mesh. The intra-abdominal contents are first covered by a polyethylene sheet followed by suturing of an oval-shaped polypropylene mesh to the fascial edges. A polyurethane sponge is then placed on the mesh and covered with an airtight occlusive plastic sheet. A vacuum is introduced by connecting the dressing to a suction apparatus creating continuous topical negative pressure (usually minus 125mmHg). **TAC changes are performed every 2-3 days in the operating theatre or at the bedside in the ICU**. The mesh is divided at the midline during the first change to allow the changing of the underlying plastic sheet. **During the TAC changes, fascial edges are approximated by tightening the mesh and resuturing it in the midline. When the gap between the fascial edges has been reduced to about 5cm, the mesh is removed, and the fascia and skin are closed with sutures.** Using this method the delayed fascial closure rate is about 80-90%, higher than with any other TAC method published. Furthermore, the enteric fistula rate is also the lowest among TAC methods.

About two out of three cases need only a single necrosectomy (probably because we do it late enough and can do a fairly complete necrosectomy). These days reoperations are not 'planned' but performed 'on demand' for complications.

Complications after necrosectomy

After necrosectomy, don't expect everything to go smoothly...

Postoperative **bleeding** is common so don't panic! The drainage fluid tends to be bloody in the first couple of days; it then turns brown and ugly, and finally grey-brown or pus-like. But if the blood in the drainage bag is 'pure' or the patient becomes hemodynamically unstable and requires multiple blood transfusions, don't hesitate to go in, evacuate the blood and clots, stop any bleeding from visible sources or just pack the area and leave the abdomen open. **Angioembolization is an alternative to reoperation — and is probably a better choice if it is readily available**.

Residual necrosis after 'incomplete' necrosectomy is more common if you do the initial necrosectomy too early. Completing the necrosectomy in a second (or more) operation is acceptable, so don't try to remove every tiny bit of necrosis at the first operation if it causes more harm (usually bleeding).

5 Peterson U, Acosta S, Björck M. Vacuum-assisted wound closure and mesh-mediated fascial traction — a novel technique for late closure of the open abdomen. *World J Surg* 2007; 31: 2133-7.

Pancreatic fistula is common especially after necrosectomy that involves distal pancreatectomy. You cannot measure amylase levels from the drains if the secretion is thick but eventually you will find out that there is a fistula. Keep the drains and, when feasible, ask your endoscopist friends to insert a stent into the pancreatic duct. If the drain amylase levels stay high (tens of thousands or more) for more than a few days, stenting is useful as soon as the patient is able to tolerate duodenoscopy. Some use octreotide; we routinely do not.

Bile-stained secretion from the drains is a bad sign. Accidental injury to the duodenum during necrosectomy sometimes happens. If the duodenal fistula is controlled (bile not floating all over the place) and the patient is not septic, have patience. Closing the duodenum at this stage is virtually impossible; it is better to have a controlled fistula and deal with the duodenum later (if necessary). If it is not controlled then you have a big problem — read ➲ Chapter 43.

Colon necrosis and/or perforation is seen not so uncommonly after necrosectomy. It happens also in conservatively managed patients, probably because we wait longer to operate and the necrotic process has more time to affect the adjacent tissues (see above). We seem to see it more today, maybe because we wait TOO long... **Discovering stool-like material in the drain after necrosectomy really ruins your day**. You can of course pretend that it is just necrotic material that looks like stool, but if it looks like s*** and smells like s***, that's what it is. Now, have a CT scan anyway to see where the problem is, have a double dose of cereals for breakfast and get on with it. Use the same incision if possible, but don't hesitate to change from a transverse to midline if needed. Remove bad colon (no mercy), avoid primary anastomosis, and clean and drain the abdominal cavity.

Please note:

- In managing patients with severe acute pancreatitis, the emphasis is on EARLY and AGGRESSIVE supportive management, and LATE and MEASURED surgical treatment.
- These patients are best treated in centers that can provide long-term ICU support, combined with radiological, endoscopic and surgical expertise — by people who remember and understand all the acronyms used in this chapter (!) — not in the small 'high-care unit' in your little community hospital. So ship them out to the experts...

Let me conclude with some Finnish wisdom...

Remember — we Finns drink a lot so we see tons of these cases.

When our hospital (the Meilahti hospital) in Helsinki was built (about 1965), the mortality rate for severe acute pancreatitis was over 90%. When I started my surgical residency (early 1980s), it was still around 50%. **Gradually it came down to 20% with greatly improved intensive care and early surgical conservatism**. The last 10-15 years have seen tremendous progress in our understanding of this very complex disease. Recognizing, preventing and treating the ACS associated with aggressive fluid resuscitation and tissue edema has further improved the prognosis, and we have further improved the non-operative management of ACS, avoiding open abdomens. Even if we have to open the abdomen and leave it open, we are able to manage the open abdomen much safer than in the past. We see about 40 patients with open abdomens (not just pancreatitis) every year, and with modern temporary abdominal closure methods, such as the mesh-mediated vacuum-assisted closure technique, we can close the fascia (and skin) in about 90% of patients. Only a small proportion end up with skin grafting and subsequent abdominal wall reconstruction.

The biggest improvements in recent years have been associated with better defining the indications for surgical interventions, improved surgical techniques and appropriate timing of necrosectomy (not too early, not too late). In our most recent analysis of 435 patients with severe acute pancreatitis treated over a 17-year period, the overall 90-day mortality rate was 18% [6]. During the last 11 years, the mortality rate for 109 consecutive patients undergoing necrosectomy was 23%. However, in the absence of multiple risk factors including age over 60, comorbidities, early (<28 days) necrosectomy, MOF at the time of necrosectomy and a couple of other factors (about half of the patients), the mortality rate for open necrosectomy was zero.

So, until a 'magic pill' is invented that stops the inflammatory cascade at its beginning (or a safer brand of booze is developed), we still need — with the help of our intensivists — to treat these patients as 'surgical' patients.

The proper management of severe acute pancreatitis requires that you understand its natural history and be armed with lots of patience. During the early phases of the disease "our patience will achieve more than our force" (Edmund Burke); later on, when called to operate on necrotic and infected complications, remember that "patience and diligence, like faith, remove mountains" (William Penn).

6 Husu H, Leppäniemi A, Lehtonen T, *et al*. Short- and long-term survival after severe acute pancreatitis: a retrospective 17 years' cohort study from a single center. *J Crit Care* 2019; 53: 81-6.

I wish to conclude with some wise words from the famous pancreatic surgeon Kenneth W. Warren (1911-2001).

"The most common errors in the surgical treatment of acute pancreatitis are to operate too early in the course of the disease and to do too much, or in the secondary or septic phase of the disease to operate too late and to do too little."

Kenneth W. Warren

Chapter 18

Gallbladder and biliary emergency surgery

The Editors

This chapter has been subdivided into the following three sections:

1. The acute gallbladder.
2. Bile duct emergencies.
3. Biliary pancreatitis.

1 The acute gallbladder

In dropsy of the gallbladder... and in gallstones we should not wait 'til the patient's strength is exhausted, or 'til the blood becomes poisoned with bile, producing hemorrhage; we should make an early abdominal incision, ascertain the true nature of the disease, and then carry out the surgical treatment that necessities of the case demand.

James Marion Sims

Biliary surgery, and especially gallbladder surgery, is considered as one of the pillars of 'general surgery'. Yet you will find a great diversity of clinical presentations, treatment options and local customs and dogmas — that will all affect the selected approach. **In acute biliary surgery the disagreements are even greater, and the debate between non-operative treatment and**

endoscopic, radiologic and surgical interventions is more heated. Therefore, in this chapter we will try to simplify this maze for you, and lead you through a common-sense approach, focusing on problem areas. As always, you will be able to find in the literature a large spectrum of views and approaches which contradicts ours — but by now you know who is right... We trust you to know the basics (and more) from your medical school, surgical training and practice.

For the sake of simplicity we will divide the chapter between **gallbladder emergencies** and **bile duct emergencies** — but you should remember that the clinical picture may be 'mixed' — **it's the patient with acute cholecystitis and simultaneous elevation of bilirubin and amylase that will force you to think hard about the next step**.

Acute cholecystitis

Acute cholecystitis (AC) is either *calculous* or, much less commonly, *acalculous*. Since the clinical picture of these two entities differs, they are discussed separately. We will start with the calculous one.

Obstruction of the gallbladder outlet by a stone is by far the most common etiology for acute cholecystitis (AC). It is a spectrum:

- **Short-lived obstruction** with spontaneous dislodgment of the obstructing stone causes **biliary colic**.
- **Impaction of the stone at the neck** of the gallbladder will lead to distension, pressure elevation, ischemic changes and, if left to progress, secondary bacterial infection — AC. **Untreated, it may progress to complicated conditions such as necrosis, perforation, empyema, liver abscess, peritonitis and systemic sepsis**.

How do you know where the patient is along this spectrum? You use all the information you can gather from the history, physical examination, laboratory results and imaging studies. **Biliary colic is self-limiting and of short duration**: the pain — typically in the epigastrium, but maybe the right upper quadrant, radiating to the right loin, back and/or shoulder and associated with nausea/vomiting — lasts no more than a few hours, and there are no clinical/laboratory markers of inflammation. In contrast, in **AC the pain will last longer**, as a persisting pain, and will be associated with local tenderness (usually), peritoneal signs (sometimes) and (rarely) a mass — denoting a palpable gallbladder — as well as systemic inflammatory signs (fever, leukocytosis, elevated CRP). **Remember: inflammation alone cannot**

always differentiate between the 'early', mechanical/chemical acute cholecystitis and the 'late', bacterial phase.

Often at surgery, we are surprised by how advanced the AC is, which clinically had been assessed as 'mild'. More advanced forms, such as gangrenous cholecystitis or gallbladder empyema, will be associated with higher levels of inflammation, greater leucocytosis, and more systemic manifestations of sepsis.

Diagnosis

Diagnosis is not considered complete without supporting imaging.

Ultrasound

Ultrasound is your best friend: available, cheap, simple, radiation free, and usually accurate. It will demonstrate the stones, the distended gallbladder with its thickened walls, and provide information about associated findings such as pericholecystic fluid collection, bile duct dilatation and the nearby structures — liver, kidney, and pancreas. **Note, however, that often, ultrasonographic features of AC lag behind the clinical picture** — a patient can have an advanced AC even if the wall of the gallbladder is not thickened and/or the gallbladder is not surrounded with fluid. **Remember also that an almost constant feature of AC is gallbladder distension (a feature which is sometimes not mentioned by the radiologist) — so: a non-distended gallbladder on imaging is usually not AC!**

CT

Many patients will already have had a **CT scan** of the abdomen when you are called for a consult, and a distended, thick-walled gallbladder with surrounding fat stranding will support the diagnosis, even when the US is 'not diagnostic'. However, the US is more accurate in this situation and will show stones missed by the CT. Often we ask for an US to confirm the CT diagnosis. You may be correct if you call this a 'defensive approach'...

HIDA scan

In **doubtful situations** you can still use the old and trusted HIDA (hepatic imino-diacetic acid) radionuclide scan. It is highly sensitive for non-visualization of the gallbladder in cases of cystic duct obstruction, although specificity is affected by impaired hepatic bile secretion with hyperbilirubinemia. **A negative scan (i.e. visualization of the gallbladder) will exclude the diagnosis of AC and make you think again.** Be aware however that the cystic duct could be *chronically obstructed*, leading to the development of a **hydrops** (mucocele) of the gallbladder without any acute manifestations.

Again, remember that some findings may be lacking, without excluding the diagnosis. We have seen AC without distension (due to chronic changes), with a thin wall (about to burst) or with stones so small that are easily missed by imaging. Don't rush to label the condition as 'acalculous cholecystitis', as this rare diagnosis is usually limited to sick, ICU patients — but to make our life complex, seen occasionally in otherwise perfectly healthy patients.

You may also get confused by some abnormal associated parameters. For example, **mild jaundice (bilirubin levels of up to 5mg/dL [85μmol/L]) and minimal elevation of liver enzymes can accompany AC, even without *choledocholithiasis* and *cholangitis*.** Whether this is caused by pressure on the bile ducts, reactive inflammation around the gallbladder or absorption of bile from the gallbladder through its pressurized, ischemic wall, does not really matter. **What matters is that you know to differentiate this condition from ascending cholangitis (see below) that merits a different plan of action.**

The trick is not to jump to conclusions but hold to your guns and **remeasure liver functions a day later**: if improving, go ahead with your operation; if deteriorating, you must image the duct — preferably with magnetic resonance cholangiopancreatography (MRCP) as discussed below.

Management

Have you ever popped a potato out of the oven in your mouth? What happens? And what if you let it cool and then enjoy it!

Amjad Siraj Memon

Here lies the main dissociation between what's recommended in the literature and what is practiced in many places around the globe. **The simple, 'correct' management of acute cholecystitis is surgery, and nowadays it means laparoscopic cholecystectomy. So why isn't it always practiced?**

Non-operative management

Conservative management will be successful in most cases to relieve the acute episode. Antibiotics, to cover Gram-negative enteric bacteria (adding anti-anaerobe agents in sicker patients), along with i.v. fluids, analgesics and anti-emetics, will make more than 90% of your patients better within a few days. The price for this approach is prolonged hospital stay, a defined risk of failure — which in turn may necessitate a more invasive approach in worse conditions — and a risk of recurrent episodes during the waiting period of 6-8 weeks for the 'interval' cholecystectomy that is necessary anyway.

So why not 'just take it out'? The reasons vary, but the most common around the world is the lack of an immediate OR/surgeon availability. **If you are lucky to work in a system where early cholecystectomy is feasible (next day is OK, even the day after tomorrow is fine) — then go for it! You will find the operation easier, with the gallbladder wall edema allowing you a relatively easy dissection, before fibrosis ensues making anatomy unclear and surgery more difficult and dangerous. Other reasons for delaying include evidence that bile duct injury is more likely in the acute phase and the observation from large studies that around half of proposed 'interval' cholecystectomies are never actually carried out (see below).**

Delaying cholecystectomy may be justified also in other specific situations. If the patient presents late, after a few days of disease, the operation may prove difficult, with a higher rate of conversion and higher risk of complications. You are probably familiar with the '**golden 72 hours**', although you should not take it too literally — some patients have an 'easy gallbladder' even later, while others will have a horrendous, gangrenous one after 24 hours. **Medically unfit patients** may also benefit from delayed surgery, after optimization, proper evaluation (reversing any anticoagulation drugs) and preparation. **However, this is a double-edged sword, as these frail patients can also succumb more easily to an untreated septic source.** So use your judgment — good judgment comes from experience; experience comes from bad judgment. And so it goes.

Gallbladder drainage

Gallbladder drainage is another option to temporize the acute condition, by relieving the intra-gallbladder pressure and draining the infected bile. It is an effective solution for the high-risk patient (e.g. acute cholecystitis a few days after an acute MI), and for failed 'conservative' treatment a few more days into the disease process.

Performed percutaneously, transhepatically, under imaging (US or CT) by the interventional radiologist, or rarely — if the latter option is not available — under local anesthesia as an open procedure by you, it will usually bring the condition under control, with rapid clinical improvement. In many cases it will also lead to dislodgment of the obstructing stone, and if bile starts to flow down the tube, and a *tube cholecystogram* a few days later shows free flow of contrast to the common bile duct (CBD) and duodenum, you can safely cork the tube until interval cholecystectomy, 6-8 weeks later. Don't expect it to be an easy case!

As a 'footnote' one has to mention here that it is not written in the 'Bible of Surgery' that all patients treated conservatively, or after successful percutaneous drainage, must undergo an interval LC. **Be selective: you can leave the old, frail, high risk and asymptomatic alone!** Longitudinal studies and audits reveal that many patients allowed to 'cool down' never come to surgery, for a variety of reasons. Recurrent problems are not inevitable.

Operative management

Emergency cholecystectomy is not a true emergency, requiring you to rush to the OR, unless you are dealing with the rare **free perforation with bile peritonitis**, or with *Clostridium*-induced, *emphysematous cholecystitis*. **Remember that even with these conditions, a brief resuscitation is a must**.

Early cholecystectomy, as mentioned above, is the preferred approach for most cases of acute cholecystitis. The definition of 'early' may differ between surgeons and systems, but operating in the next available OR list, or after hours in the 'emergency' list, is acceptable as long as it is done within a day or two. **Operating after 72 hours is not recommended — but still possible**. Some patients will improve quickly after the initial non-operative therapy; this may mean that they had a 'protracted biliary colic' and not a true inflammation, but nevertheless — if you can get rid of the source and send them home without a gallbladder, they may benefit.

The algorithm on the facing page summarizes our recommended approach (■ Figure 18.1).

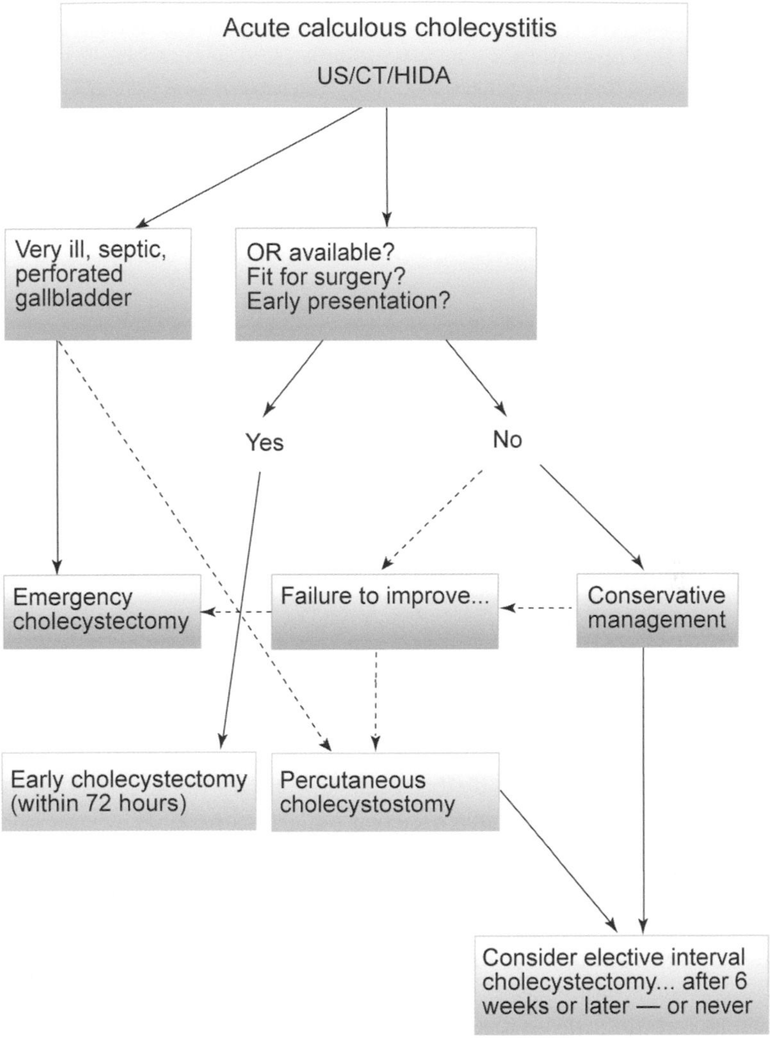

Figure 18.1. Algorithm for the treatment of acute calculous cholecystitis.

The operation

Laparoscopic cholecystectomy (LC) is the standard approach. It is rare nowadays to start with open surgery, unless the patient is very unwell and you do not think it a great idea to pump his tummy with gas; but then think again if surgery is what he needs now. **The need to convert a lap approach to an**

open procedure is related to local inflammatory conditions and inversely related to your own expertise, but what should really guide you is the progress of the operation.

Struggling without making progress (45-60 minutes of no real progress is an acceptable rule of thumb) means that your chance of harming the patient increases, and you should change strategy — calling for help is one such possible change.

With the decreasing exposure of young surgeons to open cholecystectomy, converting to open is not always a safe option (what we call the 'unlearning curve'), and finding a grey-haired surgeon to assist you is not a bad idea. Yes, sometimes one of those 'old farts' may prove useful!

There are some technical 'tricks' that you may use to improve your chances of successfully and safely completing a difficult LC:

- **Decompress the distended gallbladder** (you may use the Veress needle inserted through the abdominal wall or a special 'needle-trocar' connected to suction). After aspiration of the contents, grasping the 'eggplant' becomes easier...
- **Add a fifth or even sixth trocar** to improve retraction of structures that obliterate your view, especially in obese patients.
- **Use gravity**: make sure, before the operation, the patient is well secured to the OR table, and make your anesthetist give you a steep anti-Trendelenburg and left-tilt position.
- **Use the suction tip liberally**; it is a good dissection tool, especially for the 'wet', edematous gallbladder.
- **In a difficult-to-grasp lower segment of the gallbladder** try to milk the stone back up from Hartmann's pouch into the fundus, or just push the gallbladder up with an open instrument.
- **Adhering to the principles of a 'critical view of safety' is even more important in acute conditions, when anatomy tends to be distorted**. If it's not easy — go higher and find the plane between the liver and the gallbladder, and try to come back down from there. This is the equivalent of the open 'fundus-down' technique, which is less suitable for laparoscopic performance.
- While **uncontrolled bleeding should make you convert quickly**, remember that you don't have to panic, as hemorrhage can usually be controlled, at least partially, by pressure. Instead of frantic and dangerous hemostatic attempts, insert a gauze and apply pressure, wait a few minutes and reassess.

We hope that there is no need to explain the 'critical view of safety' (CVS). But if you are not familiar with this term please do read Chapter 16 in *Schein's Common Sense Prevention and Management of Surgical Complications,* for an in-depth discussion on how to avoid problems (and manage them) in gallbladder and biliary surgery.

The crocodiles hiding under the gallbladder fossa

So you have achieved a perfect CVS, and clipped/divided the cystic duct and artery. And now, it's time to fire the diathermy, shave the gallbladder off the liver and relax? Not so fast.

Don't forget that a few millimeters (sometimes 1mm) under the surface of the fossa there may loom crocodiles which can suddenly strike you. The **middle hepatic vein** (or its large tributary) can be easily breached if you dig a little too deep with your diathermy hook. Bleeding will be venous but massive and pulsatile (with respiration). In your chaotic and hasty attempts to control the bleeding you could easily damage or occlude the **nearby right hepatic duct and/or a branch of the right hepatic artery**.

To control the bleeding: increase the insufflation pressure (say to 25mmHg) and ask the anesthetist to temporarily stop ventilation: now bleeding is minimal and you can close the hole with a fine suture. If you can't — convert immediately.

In conclusion: be gentle when removing the gallbladder from its liver bed, Don't dig too deep. You may damage a bile duct, an artery or a major vein. When the gallbladder is grossly glued to the liver think about subtotal cholecystectomy (see below).

Conversion, and open cholecystectomy

Apart from non-progression (■ Figure 18.2), and difficulty in defining anatomy, you may need to convert for bleeding, or — and this means you did not convert early enough — for bile duct injury (clear bile is suddenly accumulating in your surgical field? Something is wrong!).

Don't expect the conversion to easily solve your problems, and continue to be alert, suspicious and careful. You need the best possible working conditions — exposure and lighting, so make sure you have good assistance, proper retraction, and accessories such as a head-light, if needed.

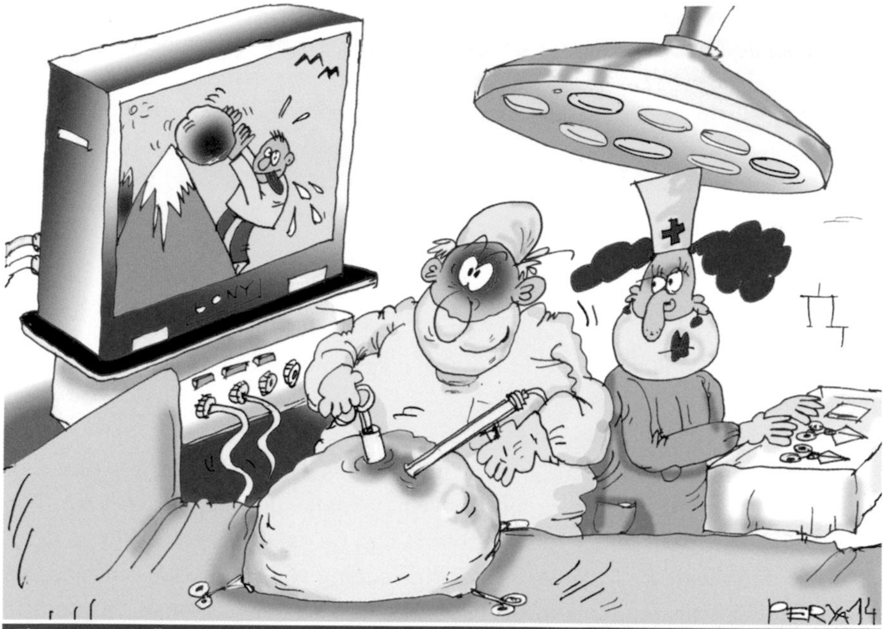

Figure 18.2. "I never convert..."

The most important thing is changing your mindset: this is no longer minimal access, so act accordingly. Forget about 'connecting the dots' (if they do not fit) between your trocars, resulting in a strange and inconvenient incision — make a proper subcostal incision that will allow you to work comfortably. Forget about 'mini-cholecystectomy' unless you have your own experience with this procedure — this is not the time to save a few centimeters but to make sure you complete the procedure quickly and safely. Unlike at laparoscopy, after you have converted, the retrograde 'dome-down' cholecystectomy is the one we recommend — staying near the gallbladder wall and progressing toward the cystic duct and artery, to be disconnected last. What about a drain? Probably not if you feel the cystic duct was well secured, but leaving one is not a sin.

> It may seem paradoxical to your modern surgical psych, but the truth is that patients do not die because they were converted to open. However they may die because they were not converted.

Alternative approaches to avoid *tzures*[1]

In some cases you need to act differently in order to save you (and the patient...) from big troubles. This is commonly the situation in 'neglected'

[1] *Troubles* in Yiddish.

cases, operated late in the disease process, with *a lot of pathology and little normal anatomy*. Sometimes even 'cooled down' cases, operated weeks after the acute infection, may be surprisingly challenging — with a chronically contracted, thick-walled gallbladder, sometimes described by the pathologist as 'xanthogranulomatous'. **Your initial surprise should be quickly transformed into a decision about how to progress safely with a low risk of complications**.

Subtotal (partial) cholecystectomy

Our old friend, Asher Hirshberg, summarized it aptly: "**It is better to remove 95% of the gallbladder (i.e. subtotal cholecystectomy) than 101% (i.e. together with a piece of the bile duct)**."

And yes, yes, yes — **any weathered surgeon will tell you that this is the procedure to use, in order to avoid misery in problematic situations such as a scarred, 'impossible' triangle of Calot — when inflammatory changes obscure the anatomy in such a way that the risk of bile duct injury is significant**. It is also useful in cases where the risk of bleeding from the liver is significant, as in cirrhosis or coagulopathy.

Partial or subtotal cholecystectomy was popularized in the United States by Max Thorek (1880-1960) and some call it the Thorek procedure. Thorek, by the way, was a keen aphorist and said: "**...how old is our newest knowledge, how painfully and proudly we struggle to discoveries, which, instead of being new truth, are only rediscoveries of lost knowledge**."

How should you perform a partial or subtotal cholecystectomy? It seems to us that this most valuable technique, which has saved our butt numerous times, is not well known to the new generation of surgeons. So here are some details...

During open cholecystectomy

Open the gallbladder at the fundus, empty it from all contents. Now start carving out the gallbladder (we do it with the diathermy) leaving its posterior wall attached to the liver. Hemostasis of the rim of the remnant is achieved with the diathermy and clips or Vicryl® 3-0 sutures. When you reach the level of Hartmann's pouch, make sure that all impacted stones have been evacuated — now you can insert your index finger, or instrument tip, all the way down to the internal opening of the cystic duct, which can often be visualized from within. The accurate placement of a purse-string suture around this opening, as depicted by artists' drawings, is not satisfactory, because the suture tends to tear out of the inflamed and friable tissues.

A better option is to leave a 1cm rim of Hartmann's pouch tissue and suture-buttress it over the opening of the cystic duct (we use 2-0 Vicryl®). The exposed mucosa of the posterior gallbladder wall is fried with diathermy (some say until you smell fried liver... but beware crocodiles) and the omentum is brought into the area. Finally, leave a drain below the gallbladder remnant; usually you won't see even a drop of bile in the drain because in such cases the cystic duct is obstructed due to the inflammatory process. However, in the rare case when a bile leak develops, the drain will solve the problem.

What to do if you find that it is impossible to close the cystic duct/gallbladder remnant? Don't panic: it is absolutely safe just to leave a suction drain and bail out. The drain will be producing bile for a few days, up to 2 weeks, but eventually it will dry out!

During laparoscopic cholecystectomy

The gallbladder is opened at a 'safe and comfortable' location, at Hartmann's pouch or above, and the contents evacuated. **Have your suction ready and place a specimen collection bag inside — through an added port if needed — to collect the stones before they spill.** At this point you

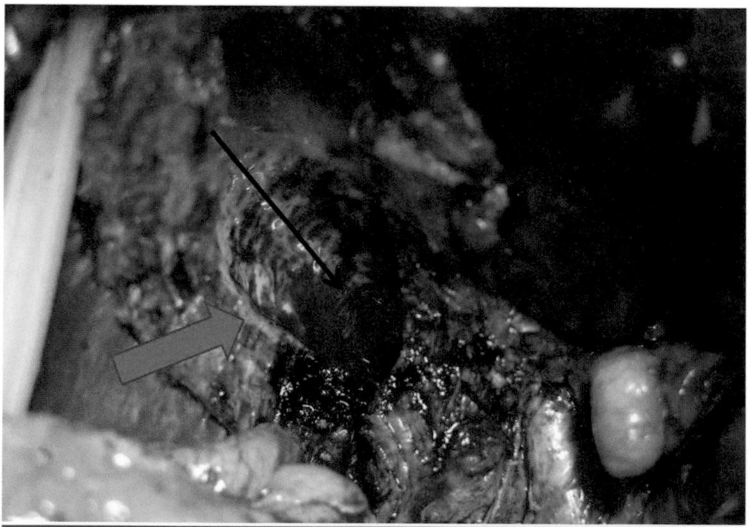

Figure 18.3. Subtotal cholecystectomy. The end result of subtotal cholecystectomy, be it laparoscopic or open. The <u>blue arrow</u> points to the 'rim' of the gallbladder remnant. The <u>black arrow</u> points to the inside of the remnant and down to the Hartmann's pouch, which is now clear of stones and towards the inner opening of the cystic duct. If you can close the remnant with sutures then do it; but sometimes, as in this case, it is impossible... so just leave a drain. Do not worry — everything will be alright!
Image courtesy of Dr. Kristoffer Lassen, Oslo, Norway.

can easily look inside towards the gallbladder outlet and make sure you clear all stones obstructing the cystic duct. Complete the transection of Hartmann's pouch, and close the remnant (you can suture the cystic duct from within, or suture-close the remnant from outside, or simply place an Endoloop® around it). **As with the open technique, if you cannot close the cystic duct or the remnant — just leave a drain and bail out**. Now complete the removal of the body and fundus — you can leave the posterior wall on the liver and fulgurate the mucosa if the risk of bleeding is high. Leave a drain. The end result is depicted in ■ Figure 18.3.

'Fenestrating' versus 'reconstituting' subtotal cholecystectomy

Some surgeons like to invent new terms and then to demand that you adopt such terms. So they decided to divide subtotal cholecystectomy into two types — each associated with specific potential complications:

- '**Fenestrating**': **when you leave the cystic duct and the remnant open**. As expected, this procedure is associated with an increased risk of bile leak through the drain. But if you are patient enough most such leaks will dry out within a few days up to 2 weeks. If you are impatient then ERCP (plus sphincterotomy and stent) will do the job.
- '**Reconstituting**': when you suture the gallbladder remnant. This procedure lowers the risk of bile leak but predisposes the patient to the risk of a **symptomatic gallbladder remnant**.

Symptomatic gallbladder remnant

These patients can present with biliary symptoms (acute or chronic) months or years after their subtotal cholecystectomy. Many of them will tell you about their past 'difficult' cholecystectomy but only a few will know that it was subtotal. When you review the old operative notes you will realize that in some cases even the surgeon did not recognize that he was leaving behind a piece of the gallbladder — most probably having divided and occluded Hartmann's pouch instead of the cystic duct.

Imaging in these patients will show a gallbladder remnant with stones and/or sludge. Differential diagnoses include late enlargement of the cystic duct remnant and a duplication of the gallbladder (one of which was missed during the initial operation), but in the majority of patients the problem is the remnant. The treatment is a 'recholecystectomy' (laparoscopic is possible but not easy) with pre-operative bile duct imaging providing a road map for the biliary anatomy.

Obviously, an empty gallbladder remnant will scar down and won't become symptomatic. **This is why you should do everything you can to clean the**

remnant before 'reconstituting' it. (Even we have started to like the neologism ☺.)

Finally, when doing a subtotal cholecystectomy always write a detailed operative report justifying what was done and why, and explain it to the patient — thus pre-emptively suppressing any future law suit. ("He did not tell me that part of my gallbladder is still inside...").

In conclusion: in this operation, the structures in Calot's triangle are not dissected out and bleeding from the hepatic bed is avoided; it is a fast and safe procedure having the advantages of both cholecystectomy and cholecystostomy.

Surgical cholecystostomy

Another option to bail out in difficult situations is to do a cholecystostomy. This procedure is rarely performed nowadays, as percutaneous techniques prevail, but occasionally you may find yourself alone with a patient in such an extreme condition, that he will be best served by a short procedure under local anesthesia. Another plausible situation can arise during a planned LC when the gallbladder appears 'impossible' — say, an obliterated gallbladder in a morbidly obese patient: **you do not want to convert, and you are not comfortable with laparoscopic subtotal cholecystectomy...**

Whatever the situation, expose the fundus of the gallbladder, place a purse-string suture, and incise it. Suck out the contents; evacuate stones if you can but your purpose is drainage, not a complete surgical solution. Then insert a Foley catheter into the gallbladder, inflate the balloon and tie the purse-string, which is easier done during an open procedure.

You may want to know how to insert the Foley catheter into the gallbladder during a laparoscopic procedure. Well, insert a 5mm grasper through the epigastric port and bring it to lie within the tip of the lateral subcostal trocar. Now remove the latter while 'pushing' the grasper to follow the retracting trocar, through the skin incision. Lubricate a Foley catheter (16Fr will do), grasp it with the grasper and pull it into the abdomen.

With regard to the **management of the cholecystostomy tube**, a tube cholangiogram performed a week later will tell you whether the cystic duct is patent; and if so whether the bile duct is free of stones. The tube can be safely plugged if all is well, and then left as a safety valve until elective surgery; another attack is simply treated by opening the tube. Whether an interval cholecystectomy is subsequently indicated is controversial, but is usually performed (see above). Cystic duct obstruction usually mandates interval cholecystectomy.

Other considerations

Intra-operative cholangiogram (IOC)

Without jumping into this neverending discussion again, an IOC has been mentioned as a way to delineate unclear anatomy in cases of acute cholecystitis. **It may be enough to say that "the authors have not found the need for this measure in their experience"...** We also find it difficult to perform in acute disease, where the cystic duct is obstructed and the tissues are edematous and friable. Transcholecystic needle cholangiography has been described, but it is rarely used. It is best to define the surgical anatomy by proper dissection, using the above-mentioned principles, and if you can't — then avoid this area and resort to subtotal cholecystectomy. **Again: in emergency surgery, simple is beautiful. Why complicate your life?!**

[An] intra-operative cholangiogram is a religion — not science.
Nathaniel J. Soper

Antibiotic treatment

The role of antibiotics in treating acute cholecystitis appears to be trivial, but it is not. It seems that over-treatment is the rule, by type as well as by dosage. The common pathogens are enteric Gram-negative bacteria, secondarily infecting an obstructed gallbladder. So, as mentioned above, the early phase of acute cholecystitis is probably sterile. Not every case of 12-hour RUQ pain with some ultrasonographic signs of distension and wall-thickening mandates antibiotics. And if they are prescribed, the coverage should not automatically include anaerobes, which are not common pathogens. If surgery is carried out, the peri-operative antibiotic coverage for acute cholecystitis should be short (➲ Chapters 7 and 40), and extended only for complicated cases of empyema, gangrene or perforation.

Acalculous cholecystitis

We briefly mentioned this condition above as it is relatively rare, and often mistakenly diagnosed when small stones are simply missed. This entity is a manifestation of disturbed gallbladder circulation in a critically ill patient, usually the outcome of multiple etiologic factors: gallbladder distension due to fasting, a low-flow state, and vasospasm due to the use of amine vasopressors. **The result is a distended gallbladder, with an ischemic wall and secondary infection that risks the patient's life**. (Having said this, apparently there has been a growing number of cases developing 'out of the blue' in otherwise healthy individuals, even young patients, without any of the known predisposing factors.)

The diagnosis may be obscured by the patient's general condition and underlying critical disease, and clinical signs may not be obvious in the sedated patient (e.g. after undergoing an unrelated surgery). But bedside US (or a trip to the CT) will quickly reveal the distended gallbladder, surrounded by fluid, that will explain the septic deterioration and the elevated liver enzymes — if you were suspicious enough to order the study. Questionable cases and unclear studies may require the definitive HIDA scan — but this is difficult to perform in the typical ICU patient, so you may need to act empirically if suspicion is high enough.

Although this condition may lead to necrosis and perforation, most cases, despite old beliefs, will respond to percutaneous drainage. If the patient does not improve, though, cholecystectomy may be required. **In non-critically ill patients diagnosed with acalculous cholecystitis, we would proceed with LC, along the lines discussed above.**

For an in-depth discussion on the complications of cholecystectomy read the relevant chapter in our book on surgical complications [2].

Beware of the easy-looking gallbladder and the overconfident surgeon. Think like this: during cholecystectomy removing the gallbladder is not your main goal. Your main goal is not to damage the main bile ducts!

2 Bile duct emergencies

A stone has passed into the CBD — how does this change your approach?

As in cholecystitis, the same mechanism is responsible for most of the problems — obstruction and build-up of pressure. Obstruction is caused by a stone in most cases, but a stricture or external compression can result in a similar outcome — which can be one of three:

- Non-infected: obstructive jaundice.

2 *Schein's Common Sense Prevention and Management of Surgical Complications.* Shrewsbury, UK: tfm publishing, 2013; Chapter 16: 315.

- Infected: acute ('ascending') cholangitis.
- Acute pancreatitis.

While separated for didactic reasons, 'mixed' presentations do occur commonly in real life. **The common denominator for all these emergencies, though, is that only rarely do they require emergency surgery**. Your goal, and responsibility, is to solve the acute problem, navigating between different imaging modalities and interventional procedures, and lead the patient safely to the eventual elective cholecystectomy.

Obstructive jaundice

If the gallstones are small enough, and the cystic duct wide enough, stones can migrate into the CBD. The sphincter of Oddi is the reason why even small stones may get stuck, at least temporarily, but it is surprising to find even larger stones in the CBD, which make us wonder how the hell did they pass through the cystic duct... but the fact is they did, sometimes after being stuck in the gallbladder outlet for a few days. Of course, small stones that pass to the CBD and stay there can grow over time, but this is a slow process.

Primary CBD stones are much less frequent, and are usually the result of longstanding bile stasis, which may be related to a stricture, or the elusive/alleged 'sphincter of Oddi dysfunction'. We don't have a good explanation why such a slow and quiet process suddenly leads to acute obstruction of the CBD, but the outcome is the same, like that of a passing stone: mechanical blockage of the flow.

The presentation may be different though, as acute obstruction of a narrow duct by a small passing stone is usually painful ('choledochal colic'), while with obstructing stones in a chronically dilated and hypokinetic CBD, symptoms tend to be 'gradual' or 'minimal' — almost like the 'silent jaundice' of malignant obstruction.

The patient will tell you about his dark urine, and his loving wife about his yellow eyes, but obvious jaundice requires a bilirubin of 3mg% (50μmol/L) or more. The liver function tests are both informative and helpful, with direct hyperbilirubinemia, moderately elevated transaminases, and the more specific elevated alkaline phosphatase and gamma-glutamyl transferase. Don't be surprised to see some amylase/lipase elevation as well — the 'common channel' brings along many variants of combined pathology of the biliary and pancreatic systems.

Management

As opposed to cholangitis (see next), obstructive jaundice is not a life-threatening emergency; but the patient is stressed, because of the pain, if present, and the altered appearance — with its frightening associations ("yellow patients have cancer"). **The mandatory ultrasound will confirm your diagnosis (gallstones? dilated CBD? intrahepatic dilatation? pancreatic mass?), although the sensitivity for CBD stones is not more than 50%. If no gallstones are visible in the gallbladder you must look for peri-ampullary malignancy — and CT is your next step.**

Benign obstructive jaundice is a fluctuating condition, and spontaneous resolution is common. It usually means that the stone has passed, but not necessarily so — stones may act like a ball-valve with intermittent obstruction. In these cases you are likely to see that normalization of the hepatic enzymes is not complete. **But even if all laboratory features normalize, you should still consider specific CBD imaging to rule out a CBD stone before deciding to remove the gallbladder**. MRCP availability has significantly increased in recent years and is our preferred study, but endoscopic ultrasound (EUS) is also accurate, albeit more invasive. **Endoscopic retrograde cholangiopancreatography (ERCP) as a <u>diagnostic</u> modality is no longer justified in these cases.**

When the jaundice fails to resolve, or if your investigation proved the presence of a CBD stone — pre-operative ERCP with sphincterotomy (ERCP+S) is the favored approach in most places.

After the CBD has been cleared, in the absence of infection, surgery (laparoscopic cholecystectomy) should not be delayed too much. There are some claims that pre-operative ERCP does induce some inflammatory changes, which can make surgery more difficult, but we have no evidence that delayed surgery has real advantage over early.

We will not conclude without mentioning **cholecystectomy with intra-operative cholangiography, bile-duct exploration (transcystic if possible) and stone removal**. The proponents of this approach (laparoscopic, of course), claim that this is the simplest, one-stage solution, but the fact is that the equipment and expertise required are beyond what's commonly available, so this perfect solution is not so perfect... and thus not widely practiced.

Open CBD exploration is still a valid option but is usually saved for failed endoscopic attempts — we hope that you, or your mentors, remember how to do it and are familiar with the management of T-tubes...

Acute ('ascending') cholangitis

What is the source of infection in patients with choledocholithiasis? Is it really 'ascending' from the duodenum (which is not so heavily colonized anyway)? Is it an infected stone that starts the process? God knows... but complete obstruction, like a malignant one, is probably 'protective' against secondary infection until late into the disease process. **In complete obstruction, invasive biliary intervention is probably the most common cause of cholangitis, and once bacteria are introduced into the system, the risk of recurrent infection is high until the whole problem is solved.**

The most important underlying factor is bile stasis, and the most important element of treatment is restoring the bile flow. Without it — ductal pressure will rise, and the risk of bacterial translocation from the bile to the blood increases, resulting in bacteremia and sepsis.

You are probably familiar with *Charcot's triad* (Jean Martin Charcot of Paris, 1825-1893 — ■ Figure 18.4):

- Right upper quadrant (RUQ) pain.
- Fever (and chills).
- Jaundice.

Add to that the two other elements — confusion and septic shock — and you get Reynold's pentad, which is associated with markedly increased mortality, and should make you move faster. Significant leukocytosis (or even worse — leukopenia), and evidence of organ failure (lungs, kidneys, liver) indicate rapid deterioration and mandate aggressive treatment.

Management

You already know how to diagnose jaundice in the laboratory, but please don't forget to obtain blood cultures as well.

The treatment comprises:

- Fluid resuscitation and hemodynamic monitoring (and support, if needed).
- Antibiotic treatment.
- Unplugging the duct.

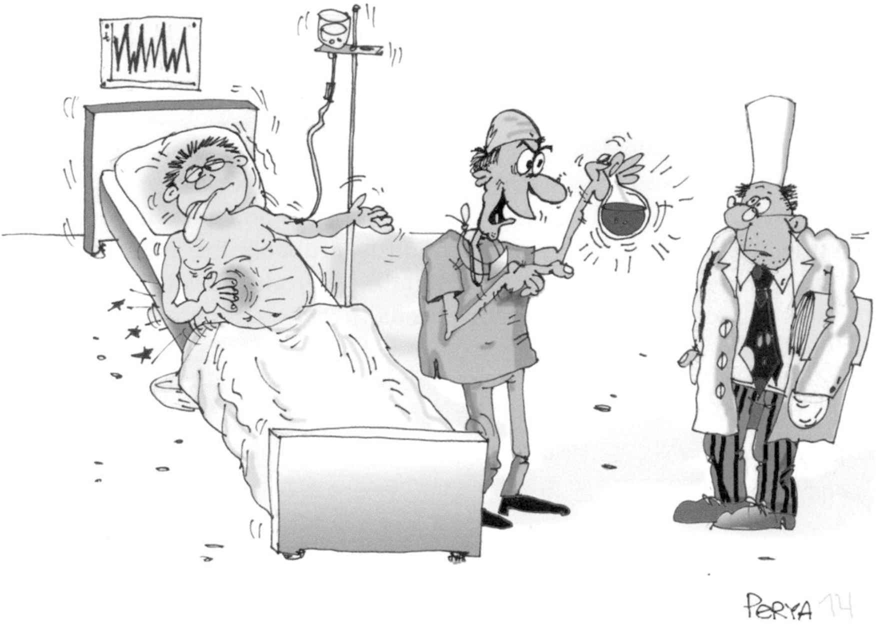

Figure 18.4. "Oh the urine is dark... what do you call that triad? Charcoal triad?"

The antibiotic treatment, started empirically, should cover enteric Gram-negative bacteria (typically *E. coli* and *Klebsiella*), and probably, especially in elderly patients, also anaerobes, which will grow in up to 20% of the cultures.

In most cases of acute cholangitis there will be a relatively prompt response, with defervescence within 24 hours. Therefore, interventional therapies should be used selectively, and saved for patients with persistent septic signs, deterioration of lab results (increasing bilirubin), and diagnosis of non-resolving biliary obstruction. **Only in a handful of patients, presenting in septic shock as a result of pyogenic bile, is emergency ERCP+S at presentation justified**. Make sure that the extreme condition is not the result of an associated condition, like gangrenous cholecystitis.

ERCP+S is the modality of choice for biliary drainage. If possible the obstructing stone should be removed after sphincterotomy, but in a septic patient a shorter drainage procedure may suffice, by inserting a plastic stent.

Failed or impossible ERCP (a gastric bypass patient, for example), will mandate an alternative procedure, like percutaneous transhepatic drainage. If the gallbladder is distended, a percutaneous cholecystostomy may drain the CBD as well.

Surgical solutions, as in obstructive jaundice, should be on an elective basis, after solving the acute condition, except in rare conditions that mandate emergency surgery, like gallbladder perforation. Taking a septic patient for an emergency exploration of the CBD is a rare event nowadays, but if deemed necessary (e.g. failed ERCP+S to remove large CBD stones or an impacted 'basket') — it should be kept to the minimum possible — like a choledochotomy and T-tube insertion. **Forget about complex biliary anastomoses in a septic patient**.

3 Biliary pancreatitis [3]

Please read about acute pancreatitis in general in ➲ Chapter 17. **Here we'll focus on the approach to patients with gallstone pancreatitis**.

You should suspect **gallstone** pancreatitis in patients who present with acute pancreatitis and are found (on US/CT) to harbor stones in the gallbladder. Suspect it also in non-alcoholic patients even if stones are not visualized as occasionally 'idiopathic acute pancreatitis' is caused by tiny gallbladder stones or sludge (*microlithiasis*).

Commonly, in addition to the elevated pancreatic enzymes, there is some degree of chemical liver dysfunction (like that described above in patients with ascending cholangitis). **It is believed that biliary pancreatitis is caused by small stones dropping into the CBD from the gallbladder, and migrating distally through the papilla**. More than 30 years ago Dr. John Acosta established his name in the Hall of Fame of surgery by sifting through the feces of patients with suspected **gallstone** pancreatitis, finding small stones in their feces within 10 days of their admission (■ Figure 18.5). In those patients who underwent a laparotomy, within 48 hours impacted stones in the papilla were found in more than two-thirds of individuals (and the morbidity/mortality was high); in those who underwent a *delayed* operation no impacted stones were found and the M&M was minimal. From John Acosta (and the other stool strainers who duplicated his findings and added more information) we learned:

- Most CBD stones responsible for pancreatitis pass spontaneously.
- Most of the so-called 'impacted stones' will pass into the duodenum if you wait long enough.
- In most such patients pre-operative ERCP is negative for bile duct stones.

[3] B. Ramana, MS DNB FRCS, contributed to the previous versions of this section.

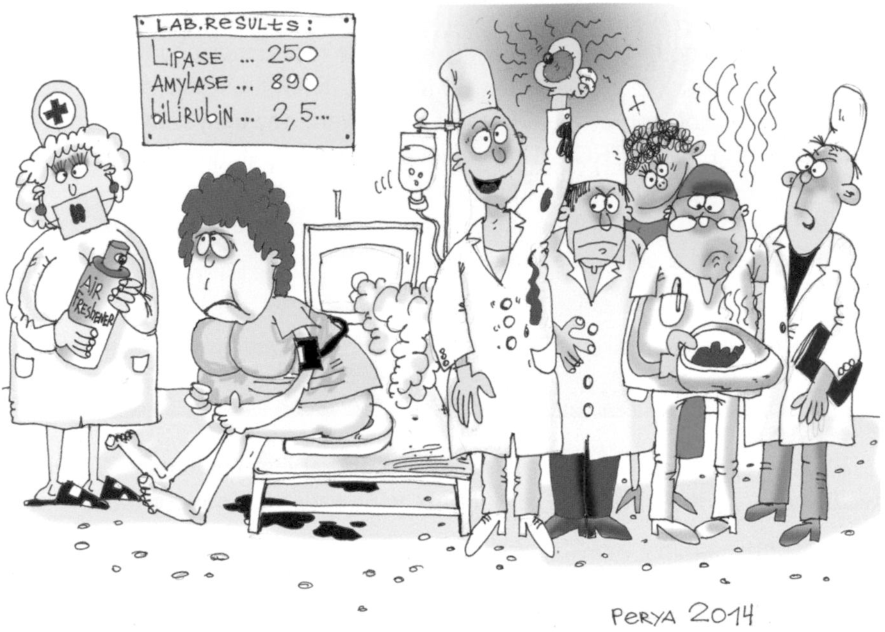
LAB.RESULTS:
LIPASE ... 250
AMYLASE ... 890
biLiRUbiN ... 2,5...
AiR FRESHENER
PERYA 2014

Figure 18.5. "Eureka, we found it!"

- In most such patients (intra-operative) cholangiography during LC is normal.
- Sifting through patients' feces may change your life and make you famous!

This has taught us how to manage these patients...

Start conservative treatment as described in ➲ Chapter 17. In most patients, resolution of the clinical features of pancreatitis occurs within a few days and is marked by normalization of white cell count and pancreatic and liver enzymes. It is then — within a week or so — that you want to go ahead with laparoscopic cholecystectomy — preventing recurrent biliary pancreatitis by removing the source of the problem. There is no need to wait longer — once signs of pancreatic inflammation have subsided and chemical cholestasis is improving you can safely go ahead with surgery. **The aim should be to perform cholecystectomy during the same hospital admission as the episode of pancreatitis.**

What about 'suspected' CBD stones? How can you be sure that they have indeed migrated into the duodenum?

- **If the CBD is not dilated on US and liver enzymes are back to normal** there is no need for any pre-operative imaging of the CBD. Adding a routine intra-operative cholangiogram in this situation is controversial. Cholangiography may indeed demonstrate small stones, but stones which would pass spontaneously in most instances.
- **If the CBD is dilated and/or liver function is deteriorating** you have to suspect impacted CBD stones (often associated with cholangitis). An urgent therapeutic ERCP may be needed and, if successful, followed a day or so later by LC. Whether an early endoscopic sphincterotomy to remove an impacted stone is beneficial in aborting the episode of acute pancreatitis is controversial. Some claim it is — if performed early enough (within a few hours...) — but try and find a center where patients undergo ERCP within a few hours after their pains have started!
- **Nowadays, MRCP is a good option**, selecting which patients need to undergo invasive ERCP before cholecystectomy. If normal you can proceed with LC.

What to do with patients with complicated acute pancreatitis? You surely do not want to operate on them. Treat conservatively as described in ➲ Chapter 17. Delay the cholecystectomy until pancreatitis and its complications are resolved.

What to do with patients who are not fit for LC? Clearly, you do not have to rush with LC in medically unfit patients. Let them recuperate from the acute disease and try to improve their general condition before proceeding with cholecystectomy. Do note, however, that some patients may suffer recurrent acute pancreatitis during the waiting period. **Another option (as in high-risk patients with cholangitis) is ERCP+S — leaving the gallbladder *in situ*.** Now the stones can enter the CBD and rapidly fall into the duodenum without producing pancreatitis. This is a viable option in the very old, frail and medically unfit and it has been shown to reduce the risk of recurrent AP.

> **In short:** in most patients let the pancreatic inflammation subside, wait for the CBD stones to pass spontaneously and then remove the gallbladder. Some patients need bile duct imaging and possibly ERCP and sphincterotomy. In a few patients you will have to wait longer for the acute pancreatitis to resolve.

So this is the end of the long *spiel*. You surely understand that there are many ways to catch the fish and one has to find the best option for the specific case scenario. By now you surely know what that option is…

> **"The most important aim in this operation is to not injure the CBD, the second most important aim is to relieve any sepsis. The third — if it can be done safely — is to remove the gallbladder."**
>
> **Kristoffer Lassen**

Chapter 19

Small bowel obstruction

The Editors

It is less dangerous to leap from the Clifton Suspension Bridge than to suffer from acute intestinal obstruction and decline operation.

Fredrick Treves

By far, the most common causes of small bowel obstruction (SBO) are adhesions (usually as a consequence of prior operations) and hernias. The list of other, less common etiologies of mechanical obstruction is long, and includes bolus obstruction (e.g. bezoar), malignant (e.g. primary small bowel tumors or metastases), inflammatory (e.g. Crohn's disease), volvulus (primary or around a fixed point like Meckel's diverticulum) or intussusception. Hernias causing SBO are discussed in the next chapter (➲ Chapter 20), while early postoperative small bowel obstruction (EPSBO) and paralytic ileus are discussed in ➲ Chapter 41). For SBO developing in the aftermath of bariatric abdominal surgery please consult Chapter 23 in our book on surgical complications [1]. Mention will be made below of SBO in the 'virgin' abdomen, intussusception, the cancer patient, radiation enteritis and gallstone ileus. **The bulk of this chapter is, however, devoted to the most common type of SBO — adhesive SBO.**

Sir William Osler used to say that "intestinal adhesions are the refuge of the diagnostically destitute" as an explanation for abdominal pain. This remains true except when the adhesions produce obstruction. Iatrogenic surgeon-made adhesions are responsible for more than two-thirds of episodes of obstruction, but in the absence of obstruction they are NOT a cause of

1 *Schein's Common Sense Prevention and Management of Surgical Complications.* Shrewsbury, UK: tfm publishing, 2013: Chapter 23.

abdominal pain. **Remember that upper abdominal, supracolic procedures (e.g. cholecystectomy) are much less likely to be associated with small bowel adhesions than infracolic ones**. Finally, as you are not an internist, we scarcely need remind you that adhesions almost never (never say never in surgery) cause colonic obstruction.

Please note that in this **era of laparoscopic surgery** some patients may not volunteer a history of previous surgery and the abdominal scars may be almost invisible when the previous operation has been, say, something as banal as laparoscopic tubal ligation. Banal — yes; but it could have created a single 'band' adhesion causing complete SBO. On the other hand the risk of adhesive obstruction is lower after laparoscopic compared to open surgery, so assuming 'adhesion' (and treating conservatively) may lead to missed pathology. **This is why we prefer to consider SBO in patients with a history of laparoscopic surgery more like a 'virgin abdomen' and look for a diagnosis by CT scan** — as discussed below.

The dilemma

The majority of adhesive SBO patients (at least half of them, perhaps many more) respond to conservative (non-operative) treatment. But persevering with conservative management in SBO may delay the recognition of compromised (strangulated) bowel, leading to a poor outcome. Faced with this dilemma, your task is to resolve the following issues.

- Which patients need an urgent laparotomy for impending or established bowel strangulation? And when is initial, conservative treatment appropriate and safe?
- Once instituted, how long should conservative treatment be continued before an operation is deemed necessary? In other words, **how do you avoid an operation without risking intestinal compromise?**

All surgeons acknowledge that symptoms and signs suggesting that the bowel may be compromised call for an immediate operation. You know the signs — severe constant pain, peritoneal signs (but remember that any distended loops of small bowel can be tender — even when the distension is caused by paralytic ileus or gastroenteritis), clinical and laboratory features of systemic inflammation, elevated lactic acid, and so forth. However, surgeons across the world tend to offer a wide range of opinions as to the duration of non-operative therapy before declaring that it has failed. Some still preach the outdated dictum "never let the sun set or rise over intestinal obstruction", while others persist in avoiding an operation seemingly until the next Ramadan season or Christmas (to be politically correct we have to mention Hanukah).

Here we aim to provide you with guidelines to answer these questions and help you develop a common sense approach. But first we need to clarify some terminology.

Definitions

- **Simple obstruction**: the bowel is blocked, compressed or kinked, but its vascular supply is not threatened.
- **Strangulation obstruction**: the vascular supply to the segment of obstructed bowel is compromised.
- **Closed-loop obstruction**: a segment of bowel is obstructed at both a proximal and distal point — typical examples would be a volvulus or a loop of bowel incarcerated within a tight hernial defect. **Commonly, the involved loop of bowel is strangulated**.

Understanding the terms '**partial**' versus '**complete**' obstruction is crucial to the planning of treatment. Some surgeons offer definitions based on symptoms (mild vs. severe) which are notoriously inaccurate. Others consider patients who pass flatus as having partial obstruction, whereas to us the sound of farting is a happy indication that the obstruction has resolved or is resolving. We believe that the best way to distinguish between partial and complete SBO is radiology, starting with the humble *plain abdominal X-ray* (but CT is better..):

- **Partial obstruction**: there is gas seen in the colon, in addition to small bowel distension with fluid levels.
- **Complete obstruction**: no gas is seen in the colon.

Most episodes of partial SBO will resolve without an operation, while most patients presenting with a complete obstruction will require one.

Clinical features (Figure ■ 19.1)

The three important clinical manifestations of SBO are colicky central abdominal pain, vomiting and abdominal distension. Constipation and absence of flatus are relatively late symptoms of SBO but essential for the

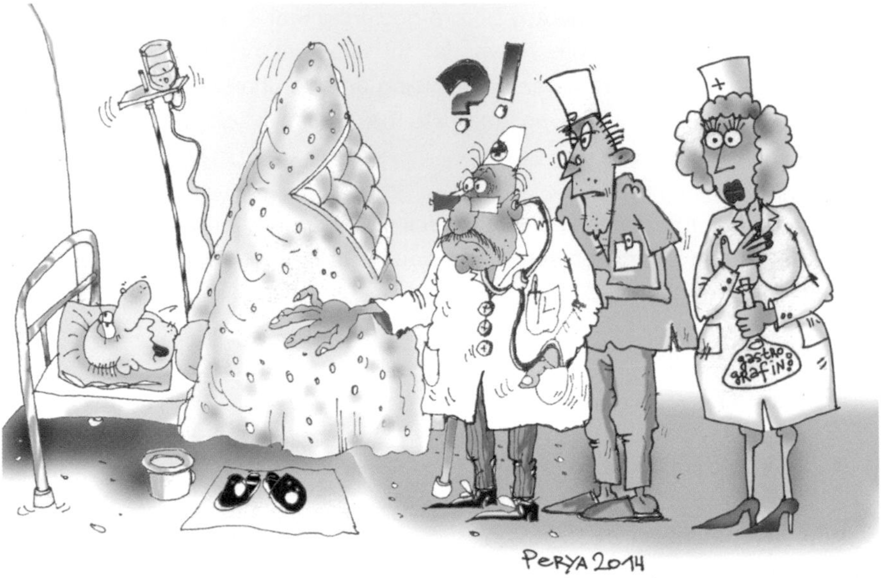

Figure 19.1. "I suspect this is intestinal obstruction. Should we try Gastrografin®?"

diagnosis. We are always surprised how often non-surgeons fail to ask the patient "when was the last time your bowels moved and you passed wind?" — calling you to "assess SBO" in patients with *diarrhea*, because a few loops of small bowel were seen on the abdominal X-ray... **Remember: a patient who continues to pass gas and/or move his bowel is not suffering from a mechanical SBO!**

The pattern of these features depends on the site, cause and duration of the obstruction. For example, in proximal obstruction, vomiting is prominent while pain and distension are absent or mild; as the level of obstruction descends, the crampy pain becomes more marked. In distal SBO, distension is a significant symptom with vomiting appearing later. **Feculent vomiting** is the hallmark of longstanding, distal, complete SBO and is characteristic of massive bacterial overgrowth proximal to the obstruction (*remember* — the main bulk of feces is made of bacteria). **It is a poor prognostic sign — the more thick and smelly the nasogastric aspirate, the less chance there is that the obstruction will resolve spontaneously. When we see s***, sorry, feces coming from the nasogastric (NG) tube we start preparing the patient for surgery!**

Is there strangulation?

This is a crucial question. If it is "yes", not only is an operation compulsory, but it also needs to be performed promptly. **The most important clinical feature of strangulation is continuous pain**. Signs of peritoneal irritation (guarding, rebound tenderness) may be present but remember that:

- Dead bowel can be present in a relatively 'innocent' abdomen.
- Signs of peritoneal irritation are rarely useful in differentiating 'simple' obstruction from strangulation because they may also be found in 'simple' SBO when the distension is severe. As we mentioned above, dilated loops of intestine are tender — you must surely have seen internists poking aggressively into distended abdomens and diagnosing 'peritonitis' in patients suffering from gastroenteritis. Eh?

What about lab tests? Obviously, features of an inflammatory response (leukocytosis, raised CRP) or indicators of tissue ischemia (elevated lactate, negative base excess or metabolic acidosis) point to the existence of compromised bowel. **But never use any such tests in isolation. Look at the whole clinical picture** — the leukocytosis and acidosis may improve after the hypovolemic patient has received a few liters of fluids. And the lactate levels may not rise at all if any ischemic segment is short.

Closed loop obstruction always equals strangulation! Here a loop of bowel is twisted (like in volvulus) and its blood supply is compromised. Plain abdominal X-ray is commonly misleading in this situation. The intestine above the twisted loop may be full of liquid and thus appears opaque — all one sees is a single dilated loop of bowel (but CT would be diagnostic!). **Patients with this type of obstruction tend to cry out in pain — like a siren! Agonizing, steady abdominal pain may be the single most important clue you have**.

Having diagnosed strangulation, you will be congratulated for having expeditiously resuscitated and wheeled your patient to the operating room. However, save yourself the embarrassment of explaining, the next day, the presence of the long midline incision to deal with a knuckle of ischemic gut trapped in the groin! **Never forget that a common cause of strangulated bowel is an external hernia.** The suspicion of strangulation must make you examine, or rather re-examine more carefully, the five external hernial orifices: two inguinal, two femoral and one umbilical (➲ Chapter 20). Oh yes, do pull off those tight jeans — see that the patient is undressed before examining him.

Remember: No isolated clinical feature or laboratory finding can tell you if the intestine is strangulated or dead. Only fools wait for elevated lactic acid levels. Do not wait for fever, leukocytosis or acidosis to diagnose ischemic bowel, because when all these systemic signs are present, the intestine is already dead!

By now you understand that nothing, nothing in isolation can accurately distinguish between 'simple' and 'strangulating' SBO. One must assess the whole clinical picture. So how do you play it safe? Let's take a step back and discuss imaging…

Imaging

Plain abdominal X-rays

The essential **radiographic features** seen on supine and erect abdominal X-rays are: gaseous distension of the bowel proximal to the obstruction, the presence of air-fluid levels (seen with the patient in the upright position) and, in complete SBO, the absence of gas distal to the obstruction. The presence of *parallel striations* (caused by the valvulae conniventes) running transversely, right across the lumen, are characteristic of distended small bowel. Colonic gas shadows lack this pattern (see ■ Figure 5.1 in ➲ Chapter 5).

CT

We reluctantly admit — wherever CT is readily available, it has replaced abdominal X- rays as the primary method of imaging of the abdomen. Many of us are called to see patients suspected of having SBO only after a CT has been obtained. **But even if you are not the one to order the CT, try to educate those who do, to see to it that the 'oral'** (per NG tube) **contrast used is water-soluble** — the water-soluble contrast will act like a '**Gastrografin® challenge**' (to be discussed below).

However, if you need a 'quick CT' and do not have time to decompress the stomach (the usual scenario in the emergency room, where CTs are often obtained before the patients are thoroughly examined), the oral contrast can be omitted. The fluid inside the bowel lumen acts like 'contrast' and the i.v. contrast (given only if renal function is OK) delineates the bowel wall.

What you should look for on the CT is listed in Table ■ 19.1.

Table 19.1. What should you look for on the CT?

✓	Dilated loops with air-fluid levels (present in any SBO)
✓	**Oral contrast 'stacked' in the stomach** — suggesting advanced, complete SBO
✓	A **transition point** — decompressed small bowel distal to dilated small bowel (it is not an indication that conservative treatment will fail)
✓	Thickened bowel wall
✓	Findings suggestive of a **closed loop obstruction** — single, isolated segment of dilated small intestine (usually calls for an operation)
✓	**Small bowel feces sign** — gas bubbles and debris within the obstructed small bowel lumen — *fecalization* (indicates fixed prolonged obstruction)
✓	**Pneumatosis intestinalis** (the bubbles of air within the bowel wall suggest compromised bowel but not always — we saw cases of pneumatosis in obstructed bowel which at operation was found to be viable and didn't require resection)
✓	**Mesenteric edema** as defined by hazy fluid attenuation in the mesentery of the involved intestinal segment and/or vascular engorgement or vascular 'swirling' (suggests compromised intestine)
✓	The presence of **free intraperitoneal fluid** usually indicates advanced SBO — suspect compromised bowel!
✓	**Free intraperitoneal air** or **portal venous gas** — you know what it means... no need to explain
✓	**Surprise findings suggesting that it is not adhesive SBO** — the list is long, just to mention a few examples: obstructing cecal carcinoma (causing distal SBO), diverticular mass adherent to the small bowel, small bowel neoplasms, intussusception...

While CT has been shown accurately to define the level of obstruction (the 'transition point') and identify strangulated bowel segments, **it does not mean that it is indicated in all cases of SBO**. Take, for instance, the 'frequent traveler' who presents to the ER every other month with adhesive SBO, responding to a day of NG decompression — CT-induced 'radiotherapy' has not been proven to be a valuable mode of treatment in such a patient!

CT, however, is a 'must' in the following circumstances:

- History of **abdominal malignancy**. A CT finding of diffuse carcinomatosis indicates that symptomatic management is the correct option.

- The **'virgin' abdomen** (see below).
- **Clinical picture not consistent with the usual partial adhesive SBO**. Paralytic ileus may be easily confused with a partial SBO (➲ Chapter 41): there is air in the large bowel, the contrast may go through but the patient remains symptomatic; fever and/or leukocytosis may be present. CT will document the underlying cause responsible for the paralytic ileus, such as acute appendicitis.
- **Early postoperative SBO** (➲ Chapter 41).
- **SBO following laparoscopic procedures** (➲ Chapter 41).

Management

The timeline matters: a patient who has been puking for 3 days at home is different from the one rushed to the ER after the first spasms of mid-abdominal colic! Intuitively, the former will require a more vigorous resuscitation but a shorter spell of non-operative management.

Fluid and electrolytes

There is hardly a need to remind you that SBO results in significant losses, or sequestration, of extracellular fluid and electrolytes (into the lumen of the bowel, within its edematous wall, and — as the obstruction progresses — into the peritoneal cavity), which have to be replaced intravenously. The aggressiveness of fluid management and hemodynamic monitoring depends on the condition of the individual patient. The fluid of choice is Ringer's lactate. **The charting of urine output — in a catheterized patient if indicated — is the minimal monitoring necessary**. Oh, how often we find such patients on the 'medical floors' without a Foley catheter — nobody knowing the volume of urine they passed (sometimes even without a nasogastric tube). It seems that this will never change...

Even patients scheduled for urgent laparotomy for strangulation require adequate pre-operative resuscitation (➲ Chapter 6). Patients with SBO sometimes have intra-abdominal hypertension (we have seen patients with distal SBO presenting with a full-blown abdominal compartment syndrome), which may falsely raise their cardiac filling pressures (CVP, wedge). These patients require even more aggressive fluid administration to maintain an adequate cardiac output.

Nasogastric (NG) aspiration

"My work essentially has been that of plumber of the alimentary canal. I have worked on both ends, but largely in between," wrote the late Owen H. Wangensteen, of Minneapolis. And indeed, by the 1930s he had introduced the NG tube as a crucial and indispensable aid in the management of SBO. So how sad and pathetic it is to find — 90 years later — patients admitted from the ER with the diagnosis of SBO, with their abdomens distended, their pyjamas stained in green, and no tube sticking from their nose!

A large NG tube (at least 18Fr in diameter) is needed. **The NG tube has both therapeutic and diagnostic functions. It controls vomiting (and reduces the risk of aspiration), but its main aim is to decompress the dilated stomach and gut proximal to the obstruction**. In a simple obstruction, decompression of the bowel results in rapid pain relief and alleviates the distension. **Essentially, the segment of intestine *proximal* to the obstruction and *distal* to the gastroesophageal junction behaves like a 'closed loop' — decompression of the stomach with a nasogastric tube converts it to a simple obstruction; pain, nausea and vomiting are relieved. Note that in strangulating or closed-loop obstruction, the pain persists despite nasogastric aspiration**.

Insertion of an NG tube is extremely unpleasant. Many patients remember it as the most horrendous experience of their hospital stay (and would certainly resist fiercely any attempt at reinsertion). The procedure can however be made much 'kinder' — soften the rigid tube by immersion for a minute or two in very hot water, spray the nostril of the patient with a local anesthetic, and lubricate the tube. There is no advantage in connecting the NG tube to a suction apparatus; drainage by gravity is as effective. (Long naso-intestinal tubes [Cantor, Linton, Moss, Andersen — you may have heard some of the names] are a gimmick with unproven benefits — requiring cumbersome manipulation and causing delay when operation is necessary. Those who still mention them in your departmental meetings tend to be senile.)

Of course, it is you who has always to ascertain in person that the tip of the NG tube sits in the stomach. (You know how to do it with a large bulb syringe. Our nurses tend now to be more sophisticated — ordering a chest X-ray after each and every insertion of the NG tube to "check the position".) But still, how often we arrive in the morning to find the NG tube inserted in the ER with the tip curled up in the distal esophagus. No wonder the nurses tell you that it had "drained nothing" — that is if anyone bothered to chart the NG output in the EMR...

When to operate?

An hour or two of fluid replenishment is compulsory in the management of every patient. Reassess your resuscitated and NG decompressed patient. What is the pattern of pain now? Is there improvement on abdominal re-examination?

Immediate operation is required in a minority of patients in whom the probability of strangulation or bowel compromise is high: those who do not improve, those who experience continuous pain, or those with significant abdominal tenderness combined with the features stated above (e.g. fecal NG aspirate, systemic signs, abnormal labs). Of course, radiological features should also be considered.

An initial non-operative approach is often possible because most patients improve at first on the 'drip-and-suck' regimen. It would be safe to bet, at this stage, that patients with radiological partial obstruction will eventually escape surgery, whereas those with complete obstruction will eventually visit the operating room. **But how long is it safe to continue with conservative management?**

Some surgeons would abort the conservative trial at 24 hours if the patient fails to 'open up', because of the nagging concern about strangulation even in a benign-looking abdomen. Many surgeons would limit the conservative trial to 48 hours. A few others are prepared to persevere, up to 5 days in a carefully monitored patient — especially in patients who give a history of repeated episodes of adhesive SBO.

In the absence of an immediate indication for operation, **we favor the use of an oral water-soluble contrast medium (e.g. Gastrografin®) as soon as the diagnosis of SBO is made.** Gastrografin®, a hyperosmolar agent that promotes intestinal 'hurry', plays, we believe, two roles: *diagnostic-prognostic* and *therapeutic*.

The 'Gastrografin® (or other water-soluble contrast agents) challenge'

After the initial gastric decompression (an hour or two), instil 100ml Gastrografin® (make sure that your patient does not get barium — ➲ Chapter 4) via the NG tube which is then clamped. **After 4-6 hours, a simple plain abdominal X-ray is obtained.** This is not a formal radiological study under fluoroscopy.

So how exactly does this study help us?

- The presence of contrast in the large bowel proves that the obstruction is partial. In most of these instances, the Gastrografin® is very soon passed per rectum as well — many times the patient has to sit on the commode even before going for the X rays... In partial SBO, Gastrografin® is often therapeutic as it expedites the resolution of the obstructing episode. **On the other hand, failure of Gastrografin® to reach the colon within 6 hours (some surgeons would wait a little longer...) indicates a complete obstruction**. The probability of spontaneous resolution after a failed Gastrografin® challenge is very low; **most of these patients will require surgery anyway so why not operate on them now?**
- **Another sign of a failed Gastrografin® challenge is the failure of the contrast to evacuate from the stomach and enter the small bowel** — it signifies significant back pressure in the obstructed bowel. Thus, if you see the stomach full of Gastrografin®, you know that further delay is futile — you need to operate!

These days a CT Gastrografin® challenge works the same way and provides more information. So if we admit a patient during the evening hours with a suspected adhesive SBO, and without features mandating an immediate operation, we perform the Gastrografin® challenge, **and if by the morning the contrast has not reached the colon we would operate**. If you see the contrast in the colon, expect the patient to defecate very soon. If CT without Gastrografin® has been obtained (which is usually the case in the ER), we would order the challenge in the morning and plan to operate early afternoon, if the obstruction is not relieved.

Of course, the results of the Gastrografin® challenge test should be correlated with the whole clinical picture. Note that Gastrografin® may pass across a chronic small bowel narrowing. **Thus, for the obstructive episode to be considered 'resolved', the abdominal symptoms and signs should disappear as well**.

This approach has led us to modify that old aphorism; the new version should read: "**Never let a patient with a complete intestinal obstruction escape an operation for more than 24 hours**."

The Gastrografin® challenge is safe. The most feared potential complication is aspiration of the hyperosmolar Gastrografin® into the lungs, causing edema and pneumonitis. However, if your patient can protect his airways (he is not obtunded and the stomach has been decompressed beforehand), this should not happen — it has never occurred in any of our patients.

Remember: ongoing pain, be it colicky or steady, continuing for hours after the placement of an NG tube, is a bad sign. It means that you have to operate!

Antibiotics

In animal models of SBO, systemic antibiotics delay intestinal compromise and decrease mortality. In clinical practice, there is no need for antibiotics in patients treated conservatively, and we operate whenever the suspicion of intestinal compromise is entertained. A pre-operative dose of antibiotics is administered prophylactically; beyond this there is no need for postoperative antibiotics even if bowel resection has been performed. **The only indication for postoperative antibiotic administration would be bowel gangrene with established intra-abdominal infection**.

The conduct of the operation

Most surgeons still prefer the open approach. The **laparoscopic one** — is discussed later.

Here is our advice for the conduct of the operation:

- The incision for abdominal re-entry has been discussed in ➲ Chapter 10 but we need to remind you to be careful in avoiding iatrogenic enterotomies with their associated postoperative morbidity. **Finding your way into the peritoneal cavity may take time, but be patient, for this may be the longest part of the procedure**. The rest is usually simpler. In this scenario the gentle hand of the 'slow' surgeon is much preferred over that of the macho cowboy — haste may open the gate to a nightmare.
- **Find a loop of collapsed small bowel and follow it proximally**. It will lead you to the point of obstruction just distal to the dilated obstructed intestine. Now deal with the cause of obstruction, be it a simple band or a bowel kink. Mobilize the involved bowel segment using sharp and blunt dissection with traction applied on the two structures to be separated.
- **Resect only when bowel is non-viable or it is impossible to free the obstructed segment**. Frequently, an ischemic-looking loop of bowel is dusky after being released. Do not rush to resect; cover the bowel with a warm, wet laparotomy pad and wait patiently; it will usually pink up within 10 minutes. If not, it requires resection.

- Concentrate on the loop which is responsible for the obstruction; **there is no need to free the whole intestine by dividing all the remaining innocent adhesions**. This maneuver may be cosmetically appealing, but adhesions lysed today will reform tomorrow. As aptly stated by Timothy Fabian: "**Lysis of all small bowel adhesions is not required because I believe that the bowel is 'locked in the open position' by these chronic adhesions.**"
- However, **following bowel resection** it would be prudent to free all the adhesions distal to the anastomosis to prevent a second narrow part causing back pressure on the anastomosis and then perhaps leading to a leak.
- Occasionally, **multiple points of obstruction** appear to be present with no clear area of demarcation between dilated and collapsed bowel. This is more common in patients after multiple operations for SBO or those with early postoperative SBO. In this situation the whole length of the 'frozen' gut must be unravelled — again, very carefully and patiently in order not to damage the bowel. This is tedious surgery indeed!
- Nowadays, **with so many patients having mesh implanted in their abdomen you will occasionally have to deal with it**. An existing mesh, with the viscera adherent to it, could make any abdominal re-entry dreadful, even if it is not the direct cause of the obstruction. When opening a 'meshed abdomen', try to gain access to the peritoneal cavity above or below the mesh, and work your way from there. Sometimes, however, you will need to cut the mesh at its center. **When separating the intestine from the mesh remember that it is preferable to leave a tiny bit of mesh adherent to the bowel than to leave a piece of bowel on the mesh**. Remove the segment of mesh which caused the obstruction but there is no need for a 'total meshectomy' — any *incorporated* (non-infected) mesh away from the problem zone should be left undisturbed. When closing the abdomen you can include the mesh in the suture line.
- What to do with a **ventral hernia associated with the SBO** will be discussed in the next chapter. Remember, your main aim is to relieve the SBO — don't be obsessed with fancy hernia repairs at this stage. **Only immature surgeons convert an emergency procedure to an elective one...**

How to manage an iatrogenic intestinal injury during adhesiolysis

Transmural enterotomies should be repaired transversely. Use your best suture technique but be careful — **leaking enterotomies result in**

nightmares! Superficial serosal tears should be left alone. Areas where the mucosa pouts through the defect should be repaired with a seromuscular suture.

Decompress or not?

Ah yes, the proverbial double-edged sword. **On the one hand, excessive bowel distension impedes abdominal closure and contributes to postoperative intra-abdominal hypertension with its well-known deleterious physiological consequences**. On the other hand, bowel decompression may contribute to postoperative ileus and even cause peritoneal contamination.

We, like most others, would decompress the distended bowel if abdominal closure seems to need excessive tension. Gently milk the intestinal content towards the stomach, from where it is sucked through the NG tube by the unhappy anesthetist. Milk the bowel very gently by successively squeezing the loops between your fingers in a sequential manner, as the obstructed bowel is thin-walled and very easily injured. Do not pull too hard on the mesentery — it may tear (remember that injury to the peritoneal surfaces promotes formation of adhesions). Palpate the stomach from time to time — if full, gently squeeze and shake it to restore patency of the NG tube. For a distal SBO, you may also milk the small bowel contents towards the collapsed cecum.

Open decompression through an enterotomy is unwise (nay, it is stupid), given the risk of gross bacterial contamination. Needle decompression is not effective with the thick small bowel contents. **Obviously, open decompression should be performed if bowel is being resected** — insert a *Poole* sucker (BTW, people tend to call it a 'pool sucker' but it is named after Dr. Eugene Poole of the Mt. Sinai Hospital in New York, who invented it in 1918) or a large sump drain connected to the suction through the proximal line of bowel transection and gently 'accordion' the bowel onto your suction device. Try to avoid contamination of the surrounding area! Watch with satisfaction how the suction bottle is being filled with fluidy s**t — one senses a great accomplishment.

Before closing, run the bowel again for missed enterotomies. **(Remember: the five minutes invested for this task may save you weeks or months of treating an abdominal catastrophe or sitting in court...)**. Check for hemostasis, as extensive adhesiolysis leaves large oozing raw areas; intraperitoneal blood promotes ileus, infection and more adhesion formation. Close the abdomen safely. **SBO is a set-up for wound dehiscence and a ticket to the M&M conference**.

A word about patience

You will understand by now that in some circumstances a laparotomy for SBO will be a long and difficult operation due to multiple adhesions or radiation enteritis for example. If you begin an operation expecting a quick and easy procedure and are then confronted by a nightmare abdomen the first thing you must do is reset your mental clock. Failure to do this may mean that you will attempt to rush the procedure, and this inevitably leads to disaster with multiple inadvertent enterotomies, peritoneal contamination and ultimately an even longer and more dangerous procedure. When you enter such a disastrous abdomen unexpectedly, tell everyone immediately that the procedure is now going to take a few hours while you unravel all the loops necessary to get at the problem and fix it. And then take your time and fix it carefully and slowly.

Laparoscopic approach (■ Figure 19.2)

Laparoscopic management of small bowel obstruction could be a very attractive option for several reasons:

- **The actual maneuver needed in many cases is one snip of the scissors, and subjecting the patient to a major laparotomy to release a single adhesive band is a pity!**
- Much of the post-laparotomy recovery is related to ileus created by handling the already distended loops of bowel. Saving this manipulation results, in experienced hands, in very swift recovery — almost as if the obstruction was relieved spontaneously. You can actually see the bowel contents propagate after you release the obstruction, and peristalsis resumes under your laparoscopic vision. NG output quickly reduces, allowing early removal, early diet resumption, and early discharge — as early as postoperative day 1 in some satisfying cases.
- As every laparotomy induces new adhesions and adds to the risk of future obstructions, it makes sense to try and avoid such added insult. Laparoscopy induces very few adhesions, although it still needs to be proven whether laparoscopic adhesiolysis indeed reduces the incidence of future obstruction episodes.

These advantages should be carefully weighed against the potential risks. This procedure requires advanced laparoscopic skills! The risk for bowel injury, and uncontrolled spillage of bowel contents from the obstructed bowel, can result in severe, and even lethal sepsis.

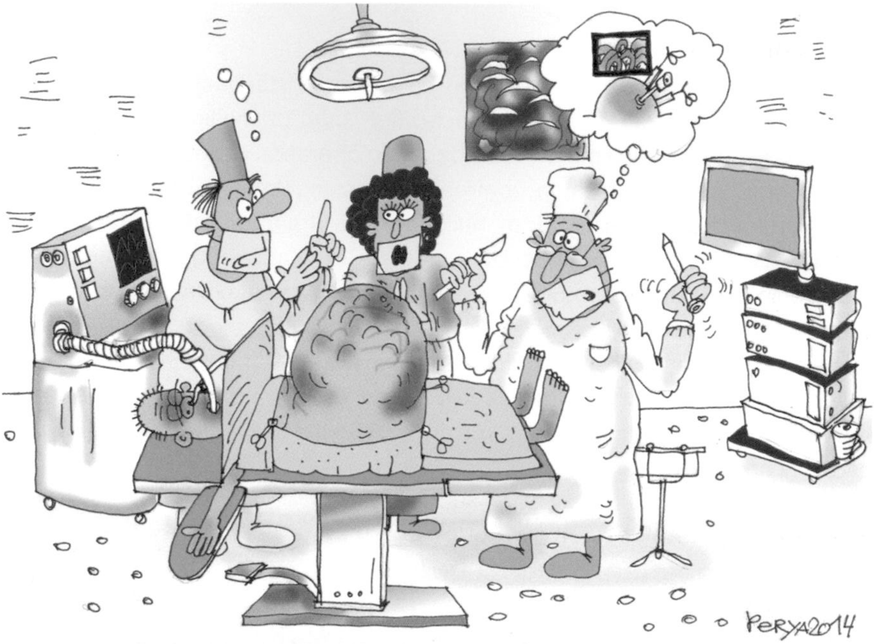

Figure 19.2. Assistant: "Sir, permission to try laparoscopically? Where should I insert the first trocar?" Chief: "Idiot! This is a classical case for the robot. Bring it in!"

Should you wish to attempt a laparoscopic approach do it selectively on the easier cases:

- First episode of SBO.
- Abdomen not excessively distended (e.g. more proximal SBO).
- Patient stable and able to endure a prolonged pneumoperitoneum — superimposed on an already distended abdomen.

A few technical tips:

- The first port should be placed through an *open approach* and away from the old incision.
- Try to work on the collapsed distal bowel, and find your way 'backwards', until you identify the obstruction site.
- Try to handle the mesentery and not the bowel wall itself; a little mesenteric laceration is better than unintended perforation of bowel.
- Move slowly, and use table tilting and gravity to help you with bowel mobilization and retraction — especially of the heavy, fluid-filled obstructed loops.
- Be careful with interloop adhesions!

Most importantly — do not be obstinate; know when to abort — before you create too many holes.

Special circumstances

The virgin abdomen

Patients presenting with SBO, but without a previous history of abdominal surgery need special attention: it is here that you have to suspect non-adhesive causes of SBO, including rare 'zebra-like' conditions, for example, the one and only obstructing *obturator hernia* you are likely to diagnose and treat during your entire glorious surgical career.

So the patient presents with clinical and radiological features of SBO but with no abdominal wall scar of previous surgery. What to do?

> **First, ask again about all past procedures including that laparoscopic ovarian cystectomy and a tiny scar hidden in the umbilicus; and while you're at it, why don't you re-examine the groin for incarcerated hernias!**

Also, ask about a history of cancer (melanoma typically metastasizes to small bowel), a history of abdominal trauma treated conservatively (resulting in adhesions), or about recent ingestion of bezoar-forming food (e.g. persimmon), and so forth...

In the old days a complete SBO in a scarless abdomen was an indication for a laparotomy. **But nowadays, a CT (use water-soluble contrast) is the way to go — mainly to rule out situations when an operation can be avoided**; for example, SBO due to previously undiagnosed but suspected Crohn's disease (➲ Chapter 24) or bolus obstructions (see below).

There is an endless list of potential causes of non-adhesive mechanical SBO, which includes abdominal wall hernias (the ones you have missed on examination), malignancies (e.g. cecal tumors), inflammatory masses (e.g. 'lost' gallstones), internal hernias (e.g. paraduodenal hernia), bolus obstruction (e.g. gallstone ileus) and so forth. There is no point pondering too much; just get the CT and proceed with laparotomy/laparoscopy if indicated. **In the majority of cases there is no place for a trial of non-operative management.**

Intussusception

Although common in pediatric patients (➲ Chapter 34), intussusception is a very rare cause of SBO in adults. In adults, the 'leading point' is usually organic (e.g. neoplasm, inflammatory lesions), and seldom *idiopathic* as in children. Patients with small bowel or ileocolic intussusception present with non-specific features of SBO. A specific pre-operative diagnosis can be obtained with ultrasound or CT, showing the *multiple concentric ring sign* (bowel within bowel), but won't change what you need to do — operate and resect the involved segment of bowel. Although controversial, some would attempt reduction of intussusception when there are no external signs of ischemia or malignancy and if after reduction no leading point is found (i.e. idiopathic intussusception), one could leave the bowel alone. Also, 'partial' reduction, if the intussusception is long, may limit the extent of resection to the bowel in the vicinity of the leading point, saving some length of healthy bowel.

One more thing: you should differentiate between intussusception as a cause for obstruction and that which is an *incidental* finding on a CT scan. The latter is found by CT done for causes other than obstruction, and is probably caused by hyper-peristalsis. **It is harmless, intermittent, physiological, and does not require intervention — despite the pressure to 'fix it'.** Just make sure there is no leading point seen by a good quality 'enterography' CT or MRI. If you succumb to that pressure ("laparoscopy is harmless, just have a look to make sure...") you may find yourself searching in vain, and then open ("just to make sure by palpation..."), and even resect an innocent segment.

The known cancer patient

When a patient is admitted with SBO a year or two following an operation for gastric or colonic or ovarian cancer, you should first attempt to obtain information about the findings at the previous laparotomy. The more advanced the cancer, the higher the probability that the current obstruction is malignant rather than adhesive. Clinically, cachexia, ascites or an abdominal mass suggest diffuse carcinomatosis. **These cases present a medical and ethical dilemma.** On the one hand, one wishes to relieve the obstruction and offer the patient a further spell of quality life. On the other hand, one tries to spare a terminal patient an unnecessary operation. Each case should be assessed on merit. **In the absence of stigmata of advanced disease — precluding any hope of palliation — surgery for complete obstruction is justifiable.** In many instances adhesions may be found; in others, a bowel segment obstructed by local spread or metastases can be resected or even bypassed.

When diffuse carcinomatosis is suspected clinically or on CT scan, a reasonable option would be to insert a palliative, venting percutaneous gastrostomy, allowing the patient to drink, and to die peacefully at home or in a hospice environment. You may consider adding a (prophylactic) gastrostomy even if the malignant obstruction can be relieved. A few months later, when the SBO recurs, the gastrostomy would be of great value. When you open the abdomen to find it 'frozen' with cancer, do not poke around too much. Just insert a G tube (that is if you can easily access the stomach) and get out. **Let the patient die in peace, and not in pieces**, without leaking intestinal contents soaking his abdomen...

A sincere, ongoing discussion with the patient, his family, and his oncologist is crucial to find the optimal balance between 'cure', palliation and futile care. **You may not be aware of some modern 'biological' medications that may significantly extend survival of some cancers, and make 'futile' surgery less futile nowadays (melanoma is a good example)**.

In doubtful cases, it may be better to operate and find end-stage carcinomatosis than to miss an obstruction that can be readily fixed.

Radiation enteritis

SBO following radiation treatment of abdominal or pelvic malignancy usually develops months or even years after irradiation. A relentless course of multiple episodes of partial SBO, initially responding to conservative treatment but eventually culminating in a complete obstruction, is characteristic. There is also the uncertainty about the obstruction being malignant or adhesive in nature. One always hopes that it is adhesive, because SBO due to radiation injury is 'bad news' indeed.

When forced to operate for complete obstruction, one finds irradiated loops of bowel glued or welded together and onto adjacent structures. The paper-thin bowel tears easily. Accidental enterotomies are frequent, difficult to repair, and commonly result in postoperative fistulas. Short involved segments of bowel are best resected, but when longer segments are encountered, usually stuck in the pelvis, it is safest to bail out with an entero-enteric or enterocolic bypass, using non-irradiated bowel for this purpose. Postoperative short-bowel syndrome is common whatever the procedure. **The long-term prognosis is poor — radiation enteritis is almost as bad as the malignancy the radiation had attempted to control**.

Recurrent multiple episodes of SBO

The patient is typically readmitted every second month for SBO and has undergone, in the past, multiple operations for this condition. How should he be managed?

We would treat him as any other patient presenting with adhesive SBO. Fortunately, most such episodes are 'partial', and responsive to conservative treatment. When complete obstruction develops, operative management is obviously necessary. Attempts at preventing subsequent episodes with plication of bowel or mesentery or long tube stenting are recommended by some. The evidence in favor of such maneuvers is anecdotal at best. We do not practice them. Occasionally a patient develops obstruction early in the aftermath of an operation for adhesive SBO: this is a case par excellence for prolonged non-operative management, with the patient maintained on TPN until adhesions mature and the obstruction resolves (see ➲ Chapter 41).

In our experience, most such 'frequent SBO travelers' know how to treat their episodes of obstruction better than the resident (or surgeon) on call. Listen to what they have to say. They know that not every episode requires a CT!

Sometimes one is asked by patients or their physicians to perform an elective adhesiolysis in order to prevent additional episodes of adhesive SBO. This sounds tempting of course. But anyone who has tried doing so knows that even after a complete and most satisfying adhesiolysis these patients can return with the same problem. **Our advice: operate only for non-resolving SBO — prophylactic surgery does not work**.

But of course, never say never...

Gallstone ileus

Gallstone ileus develops typically in elderly patients with longstanding cholelithiasis. It is caused by a large gallstone eroding into an adjacent segment of bowel — usually the duodenum — and then migrating distally until stuck in the narrow ileum. **Presentation is usually vague as initially the stone may disimpact spontaneously — causing intermittent episodes of partial obstruction**.

You will never miss the diagnosis once you habitually and obsessively search for *air in the bile ducts* on any plain abdominal X-ray you order (or

on the CT). The air enters the bile duct via the enterocholecystic fistula created by the eroding gallstone (still remember the differential diagnosis of pneumobilia? If not go back to ➲ Chapter 5).

Treatment is operative and should be tailored to the condition of the patient. In frail and sick patients deal only with the SBO — leave the gallbladder alone. Now, after it has spontaneously drained into the duodenum the likelihood of it generating further problems is very low. So just place an enterotomy *proximal* to the stone and remove it and search for additional stones in the bowel above — you do not want to have to reoperate! In patients who are younger and reasonably fit and well, you may want to also deal with the cause of the problem — the gallbladder. Perform a cholecystectomy and close the duodenal defect: place your suture line transversely to avoid narrowing of the duodenum. **But again: *not* removing the gallbladder after dealing with the obstructing gallstone is a perfectly reasonable option**.

There are those who believe that there is yet a better option: they would remove any large gallstones still in the gallbladder via a cholecystotomy and then simply close the gallbladder again — much easier and safer than cholecystectomy in this situation.

Bezoars

Bezoars are tightly packed collections, or 'balls', of partially digested or undigested material forming in the stomach and then migrating distally, where they may obstruct the terminal ileum. You may encounter one of the following types of bezoars:

- **Phytobezoars**: partially digested agglomerations of vegetables or fruits forming in patients with altered gastric physiology (e.g. following gastric resection, vagotomy or bariatric operation and even in patients with diabetic gastroparesis) or health food aficionados, and elderly 'forget-to-chewers'. Many sorts of fruits and vegetables are implicated, particularly when consumed in large quantities (Moshe once suffered partial SBO after consuming, within an hour, a whole bag of baby carrots; large quantities of popcorn can do the same), but consumption of *persimmons* is especially notorious in this regard — with patients developing multiple episodes of SBO.
- **Trichobezoars**: most commonly occurring in younger patients with psychiatric disturbances who chew and swallow their own hair. Trichobezoars form in the stomach and often reach a huge size; they break into smaller pieces and migrate into the small bowel where they can obstruct at several points.

- **Parasitic bezoars**: consisting of conglomerates of parasites such as *Ascaris lumbricoides* which may obstruct the distal ileum. This is obviously common in endemic areas.

Patients present usually with features of partial or 'smoldering' SBO and a virgin abdomen. History is suggestive, and CT images — showing the actual intraluminal bezoars — are diagnostic. A Gastrografin® challenge can dislodge the obstructing parasites, or other types of bezoars, pushing them into the cecum. But when the obstruction is complete, you have to operate and deal with the obstructing bezoar like you do with the gallstone (see above). **However, some bezoars can sometimes be fragmented, and milked on, without the need for enterotomy**. It is crucial to palpate the entire small bowel, including the duodenum (and also the stomach) for additional bezoars, and remove all of them. **Indeed, intra-operative (or 'next morning') gastroscopy is recommended to remove the 'mother bezoar' before new fragments are passed on**. Pre-operative CT may be helpful in mapping such additional bezoars for you. **You don't want the patient to develop early postoperative SBO — caused by a missed bezoar — needing another laparotomy for removal, do you?**

SBO after gastrectomy

With the disappearance of gastrectomy performed for benign disease, and the declining rate of gastric cancer, there are not too many post-gastrectomy patients to present with SBO, although some do. **However, with the mushrooming of bariatric gastric surgery this entity has become relevant again**.

The potential reasons for SBO in these patients are:

- **Simple adhesive obstruction** — what's common is common! (see above).
- **Recurrent gastric carcinoma**, with loops of bowel 'frozen' by peritoneal carcinomatosis (see above).
- **Bolus obstruction by bezoars**, which tend to form after acid-reducing operations (see above).
- **Internal herniation** of small bowel through defects of the mesocolon or behind the jejunal loop forming the Billroth II (or Roux-en-Y) gastroenterostomy — be it antecolic or retrocolic.
- **Twisting or volvulus** of redundant afferent or efferent jejunal loops.
- Another specific type of obstruction is **jejunogastric intussusception**. Both the afferent or efferent loops can invaginate into the gastric

remnant but the *retrograde* efferent loop intussusception is more common. This can occur from a few days up to many years after the gastrectomy. Sudden onset of epigastric pain, vomiting and hematemesis, and a palpable epigastric mass in a patient with previous gastric surgery are the classic triad.

- **Obstruction of the *afferent* loop** after Billroth II by whichever of the above mentioned mechanisms produces a closed loop obstruction (between the obstructing point and the duodenal stump). High intraluminal pressures are commonly associated with elevation of serum pancreatic enzymes (amylase) and, if the obstruction is not relieved, with necrosis of the involved loop and the attached duodenum. **The clinical picture of epigastric pain, upper abdominal mass and hyperamylasemia may confuse you into thinking that you are dealing with acute pancreatitis.**

Obviously, the more complex the original post-gastrectomy reconstruction, the more potential peritoneal defects created, and the 'looser' the various intestinal loops — the higher the risk for bowel to kink, rotate, herniate and obstruct. (Now you understand why we prefer Billroth I reconstruction after gastrectomy!)

The proximal location of the obstruction is suggested by the frequent vomiting, lack of abdominal distension and paucity of dilated small bowel on plain abdominal X-ray. CT with oral contrast is a superb diagnostic aid showing the exact anatomy of obstruction. Occasionally, endoscopy is needed to clarify the picture. **Do understand that acute *afferent* loop obstruction is a dire emergency — you must operate before the closed loop obstruction results in complete necrosis of the duodenum!**

At operation the anatomy has to be restored and this entails resection of non-viable loops of bowel and reconstruction of the upper gastrointestinal tract, as you would do after partial or total gastrectomy.

Small bowel volvulus

This is also called **'midgut volvulus'** — distinguishing it from '**foregut (gastric) volvulus**' (➲ Chapter 15) and '**hindgut volvulus**' (➲ Chapter 25).

Volvulus — the twisting strangulation of an intestinal segment around an axis formed by a band or an adhesion is a common occurrence in adhesive SBO. A narrow-based loop of small bowel suspended by a Meckel diverticulum can also undergo torsion. **But what about 'spontaneous' volvulus — one that involves the entire, or almost entire, small intestine?**

Spontaneous volvulus of the small bowel, while very rare in the developed world is not uncommon in rural areas of the Indian subcontinent, central Asia and Africa. It seems more common in healthy farmers returning home for a large evening meal or, in Muslim countries, during the fast of Ramadan — when large meals are consumed at night after the day of fasting. The common pathway appears to be a huge load of high-fiber, indigestible food, arriving suddenly in an empty small bowel. The sudden distension creates rotational-kinking forces.

At operation, typically the twisted bowel is loaded with liters of clay-like undigested food and is often suspended on an unusually long mesentery. Occasionally, small bowel volvulus occurs in combination with that of the sigmoid colon, forming the so called **ileosigmoid knot** where the ileum and the sigmoid entangle each other to form a knot and become gangrenous. An arrangement of the small bowel and sigmoid colon on long, narrow mesenteries would appear to be a prerequisite.

As in any other condition resulting in an acute vascular compromise of the bowel, **patients present with severe central abdominal pain that is out of proportion to the abdominal findings**; additionally, systemic signs of hypovolemia and toxemia are dramatic and dominant. An urgent operation is indicated during which the ischemic intestine is managed as discussed above.

Intestinal malrotation

Most cases of **midgut malrotation** present within the first weeks or months of life. The rest can present sporadically throughout childhood and even in adults. The anatomy of malrotation is depicted in ■ Figure 19.3: note how close the D-J flexure (point X) is to the cecum (point Y) and how narrow the base of the mesentery is, and thus prone to torsion.

Strangulating midgut volvulus in these patients can present acutely, but more commonly, especially in older children and adults, volvulus is preceded by **recurring attacks of upper and central abdominal colicky pain**, intermittent vomiting of bile and is often relieved by diarrhea. Once again, patients presenting with acute midgut volvulus are in great pain and appear ill but have minimal abdominal findings on examination!

Classically, the diagnosis was achieved by contrast studies: upper gastrointestinal barium examination showing loss of the duodenal C (corkscrew duodenum) and the D-J flexure to the right of the midline. Barium enema would show the cecum riding high under the liver. **CT however has**

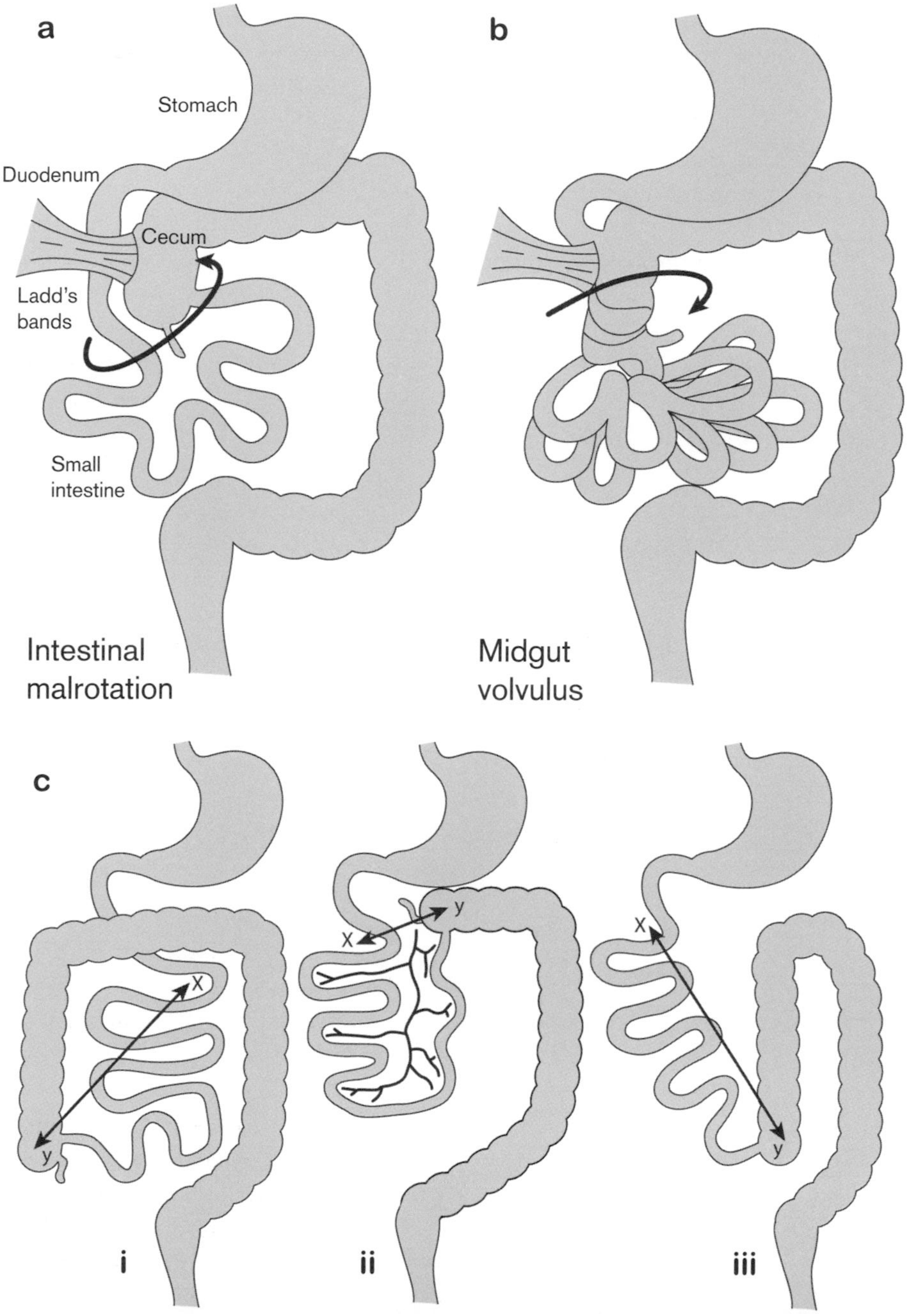

Figure 19.3. a-c) Small bowel malrotation and volvulus; ci) normal; cii) malrotation; and ciii) following Ladd's procedure. X = D-J junction; Y = cecum. *Modified from: Youngson GG. Common Pediatric Disorders. Royal College of Surgeons of Edinburgh, 1998.*

become the optimal diagnostic modality showing the small bowel located entirely within the right hemi-abdomen and the colon situated on the left. Features of the twisted mesentery and intestinal wall ischemia are also seen. Midgut volvulus can also be diagnosed on Doppler ultrasound by demonstrating the 'whirlpool sign' — wrapping of the superior mesenteric vein and the mesentery around the superior mesenteric artery.

Emergency laparotomy is mandated. Remember that these patients are grossly hypovolemic and need aggressive fluid resuscitation. At operation, detort the twisted bowel working in a *counterclockwise* rotation. Ischemic dead bowel needs resection — usually massive resection. For a discussion on whether to anastomose or not and whether a second-look operation is necessary — look at ➲ Chapter 22.

After resecting the dead bowel, or convincing yourself that it is viable, you want to address the anatomical pathology of malrotation by doing what has been described by William E. Ladd below.

- 1. Divide the peritoneal folds (Ladd's bands) that cross from the cecum to the liver, compressing the duodenum.
- 2. Mobilize the right colon.
- 3. Mobilize the D-J flexure, freeing the ligament of Treitz — straightening the duodenal loop.
- 4. Divide any thick peritoneal folds compressing the SMA.
- 5. Place the bowel in a new pattern as depicted in ■ Figure 19.3ciii — note that now point X is far from point Y.
- 6. Remove the appendix to prevent 'atypically situated' appendicitis.

Obviously, after having to resect most of the small bowel you do not need to worry about recurrence of the volvulus and there is no impetus to correct the anatomy, except at points 1, 4, 6.

Prognosis

Overall, about half of the patients presenting with an adhesive SBO can be managed without an operation. About a third of patients operated once for adhesive SBO will have recurrent problems within 30 years. For patients admitted several times for adhesive SBO, the relative risk of recurrence increases each time. More than two-thirds of patients with four or more SBO admissions will reobstruct. The risk of recurrence is a bit lower in patients in whom the previous obstructive episode was treated *surgically* but this does not mean that those patients who were treated conservatively will have an increased need for operation during their future admissions for SBO. **The aim is therefore to operate only when necessary, but not to delay a necessary operation**.

In our minds, anyone who discovers a viable solution to prevent adhesive SBO would deserve a Nobel Prize. So, this is your chance to be famous! However, the guys from Uppsala may think otherwise.

"The only thing predictable about small bowel obstruction is its unpredictability."

Chapter 20

Acute abdominal wall hernias

The Editors

You can judge the worth of a surgeon by the way he does a hernia.

Thomas Fairbank

Acute groin hernia

In most parts of the world, the majority of groin hernias are now repaired electively. Despite this, surgeons are still frequently confronted by acute groin hernias and it is important that you know how to deal with them.

Some words about terminology: groin hernias, inguinal or femoral, may be described as reducible, irreducible, incarcerated, strangulated, or obstructed. This terminology can be confusing and these words, which have come to mean different things to different people, are much less important than the concepts that underlie the recognition and management of acute hernia problems. **The important concept to be grasped is that any hernia that becomes painful, inflamed or tender — and is not readily reducible — should be regarded as a surgical emergency**.

Presentation

Patients may present acutely in one of two ways:

- Symptoms and signs related directly to the hernia itself.

- Abdominal symptoms and signs, which at first may not seem to be related to a hernia.

The **first mode** of presentation usually means pain and tenderness in a tense, irreducible hernia. A previously reducible hernia may suddenly become irreducible. This problem is usually obvious (■ Figure 20.1).

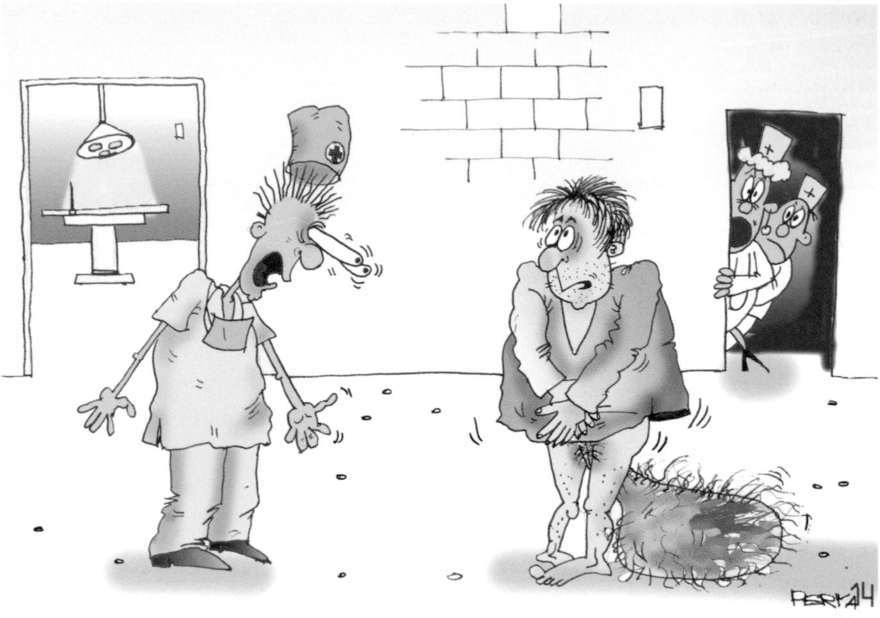

Figure 20.1. "This must be strangulated, eh?"

The **second mode** of presentation may be much more insidious. **Beware the vomiting old lady!** Treated at home for several days by the primary care physician as a case of gastroenteritis, she eventually comes under the care of the surgeons due to intractable emesis. By this stage she is dehydrated and in need of much resuscitation. **It is surprisingly easy in these circumstances to miss the small femoral hernia barely palpable in the groin, trapping just enough small intestine to produce obstruction**. No abdominal symptoms or signs are present and the plain abdominal radiographs may be non-diagnostic. None of these difficulties saves you from the embarrassment of the following morning's round when the hernia is discovered. (Luckily — or sadly, in view of the declining clinical competence — these days such hernias are commonly unearthed in the ubiquitous CT scan.)

Hernias are still one of the commonest causes of small bowel obstruction (➲ Chapter 19). You must look carefully for them in all cases of actual or suspected intestinal obstruction. This may mean meticulous, prolonged and disagreeable palpation of groins that have not seen the light of day, let alone soap and water, for a long time. In most cases, however, the diagnosis is obvious with a classical bowel obstruction and a hernia stuck in the groin or scrotum.

Beware the Richter's hernia — typical of femoral hernias, **where only a portion of the circumference of the bowel is strangulated**. Because the intestinal lumen is not completely blocked, bowel obstruction may not occur and presentation is consequently delayed and non-specific.

A trial of manual reduction

Analgesia is an important part of the management. Opiate analgesia and bed rest with the foot of the bed slightly elevated may successfully manage a painful obstructed hernia of short duration. **Gentle attempts at reduction of such a hernia are justified once the analgesics have taken effect**. A successful reduction of the hernia means that emergency surgery at unsociable hours may be traded for a semi-elective procedure on the next available routine list — a benefit for both patient and surgeon. **Note that manual reduction of an incarcerated hernia should be attempted only in the absence of signs of intestinal strangulation**; it should be gently performed, to avoid *reduction en masse* — when the **herniated bowel and the constricting ring are reduced together**, providing a false sense of achievement and a delay of necessary surgery.

Preparation

Surgery for acute groin hernia problems should be carried out without undue delay, but these patients must not be rushed to surgery without careful assessment and preparation. As we suggested earlier, some patients may need considerable resuscitation on admission to hospital. **Quite often these patients still have a hernia because they have previously been deemed 'unfit' for elective repair; comorbidity in this group of patients may be a significant problem.**

The operation

Inguinal hernia

An inguinal incision is a satisfactory approach. Even if a bowel resection is required it is possible to deliver sufficient length of intestine through the limited incision.

The main difference in dissection in an emergency hernia operation compared to an elective procedure is the moment at which the hernial sac is opened. In the emergency situation the hernia will often reduce spontaneously as soon as the constricting ring is divided. The site of constriction may be the superficial inguinal ring, in which case the hernia reduces when external oblique is opened. **It is recommended, therefore, that the sac be opened and the contents grasped for later inspection *before* the constricting tissues are released**.

What should you do when the hernia's contents have reduced spontaneously before you have opened the sac? There are two main scenarios:

- **You should not worry about missing ischemic bowel**: there were no pre-operative clinical or radiological features of intestinal obstruction; the sac contains clear or serosanguinous fluid. In this situation we would repair the hernia and that's all.
- **You should worry about missing ischemic bowel**: pre-operative features suggested involvement of intestine; the sac contains darker fluid. Now you have to examine the loop of bowel that has popped back into the abdomen. How to do it?

In this era of laparoscopy, it may be possible to inspect the reduced sac contents by insertion of the scope via the hernia sac, or through the abdomen — whatever feels simpler to you. However, if laparoscopy is not available, there is nothing wrong with a limited lower abdominal laparotomy (transverse, muscle splitting in the involved quadrant or a midline) to deliver out the intestine.

When the hernia sac contains only omentum, any tissue that is necrotic, or of doubtful viability, is excised, ensuring meticulous hemostasis in the process — even a tiny bleeder from the stump of the resected omentum may bring you back to the OR! **If, on the other hand, bowel is involved**, then any areas of questionable viability should be wrapped in a warm moist gauze pack and left for a few minutes to recover. Irreversibly ischemic gut should be resected. If there is a limited area of what appears to be traumatised wall of the bowel from the constricting ring of the hernia (looks like a dark ring on the bowel's serosa), then this can be dealt with by invagination rather than by resorting to resection. In this situation the injured bowel wall is invaginated by a seromuscular suture, taking bites on the viable bowel on either side of the defective area of gut. But of course, you may prefer to resect the injured area, rather than invaginate...

Occasionally, particularly if a bowel resection through an inguinal incision has been necessary, edema of the herniated gut makes its replacement in the abdomen difficult. Maneuvers such as putting the patient into a marked Trendelenburg position and gently compressing the eviscerated gut, covered by a large moist gauze swab, will almost invariably allow the bowel to be replaced in the abdomen. It is possible to minimize the chances of this difficulty arising if care is taken during any bowel resection not to have any more gut outside the abdomen than is absolutely necessary. Very rarely, the herniated viscera won't return to the abdomen without pulling on it from *within*; **in such instances La Rocque's maneuver may be useful**: extend the skin incision up and laterally; then extend the split of the external oblique aponeurosis and follow this with a muscle-splitting incision of internal oblique and transverse muscles above the internal ring. Through this incision you enter the peritoneal cavity and reduce the herniated viscera from within (if you think that laparoscopy can help you as well — you may be right, just wait patiently a few more pages). Of course, pulling up the strangulated bowel from inside can be accomplished during a laparotomy performed for one of the indications mentioned above or below.

The question of the type of hernia repair to be employed is a matter for the individual surgeon, with one proviso — in these days of tension-free hernia repair, it seems imprudent to place large amounts of mesh in the groin if necrotic gut has had to be resected. In this situation some other type of non-mesh repair seems advisable to obviate the prolonged misery of infected mesh (but even that is debatable... according to local dogmas and the risks one is ready to take...).

Femoral hernia

You can approach the acute femoral hernia from below the inguinal canal, from above, or through it.

With the **low approach**, you place the incision below the inguinal ligament, directly over the bulge. You find the hernial sac and open it, making sure to grasp its contents for proper inspection. Strangulated omentum may be excised and viable bowel is reduced back into the peritoneal cavity through the femoral ring. When the ring is tight, and usually it is, you can stretch it with your small finger, inserted medially to the femoral vein; occasionally, you'll have to cut the lower fibers of the overlying inguinal ligament to let your finger enter the femoral canal. You can resect non-viable small bowel through this approach and even anastomose its ends, but pushing the sutured or stapled anastomosis back into the abdomen might be impossible. **Therefore, when bowel has to be resected, it is advisable to do it through a small (right or left) lower quadrant muscle-splitting laparotomy; or a short midline laparotomy.**

Some authorities favor an approach **via the inguinal canal** but we see little merit in this approach, which must disrupt the anatomy of the canal and presumably risks a subsequent inguinal hernia.

Yet another approach is **McEvedy's**. This involves entering the extraperitoneal space along the lateral border of the lower part of rectus abdominis. The skin incision is vertical, in line with the border of rectus, or oblique/horizontal. A vertical skin incision has the merit of allowing extension to a point below the inguinal ligament and this may be helpful in reducing stubborn hernias, allowing traction from above and compression from below. Once the space behind the rectus muscle has been accessed, the hernia can be freed from behind the inguinal ligament. The peritoneum can be opened as widely as necessary to permit inspection of the contents of the hernia sac and to carry out intestinal resection if that is required.

All the above approaches are reasonable provided the contents of the hernia sac are examined and dealt with appropriately. As with inguinal hernias, the implantation of large amounts of mesh should be avoided in patients who have contamination of the operative field with intestinal contents. With this caveat the choice of repair is not different from what you would do in the elective situation. **Our choice: in the absence of gross contamination, the femoral canal is obliterated with a mesh plug**. When gross contamination is present, we would 'close' the femoral canal by suturing the inguinal ligament, above, to the pectineal fascia, below. Again, if you wonder about the place of laparoscopy, wait until the end of the chapter. Let's just say that laparoscopy, usually in its transabdominal version, is gaining support for these cases — the reduction of the bowel, if done carefully, is usually easier, and the extraperitoneal mesh placement is safe and less prone to infection.

Incisional/ventral hernias

Incisional hernias are common but are frequently asymptomatic except for the unsightly bulge and discomfort they sometimes produce. **It is the small incisional hernias with the tight neck that become acutely symptomatic — incarcerating omentum or intestine**.

The presentation is well known to you: **an old 'silent' hernia or abdominal scar, which has now become painful**. When bowel is incarcerated there may be associated symptoms of small bowel (or, rarely, colon) obstruction. The hernia itself is tense, tender and non-reducible.

It is important to decide whether the intestinal obstruction is caused by the incisional hernia or simply associated with it (■ Figure 20.2). The latter

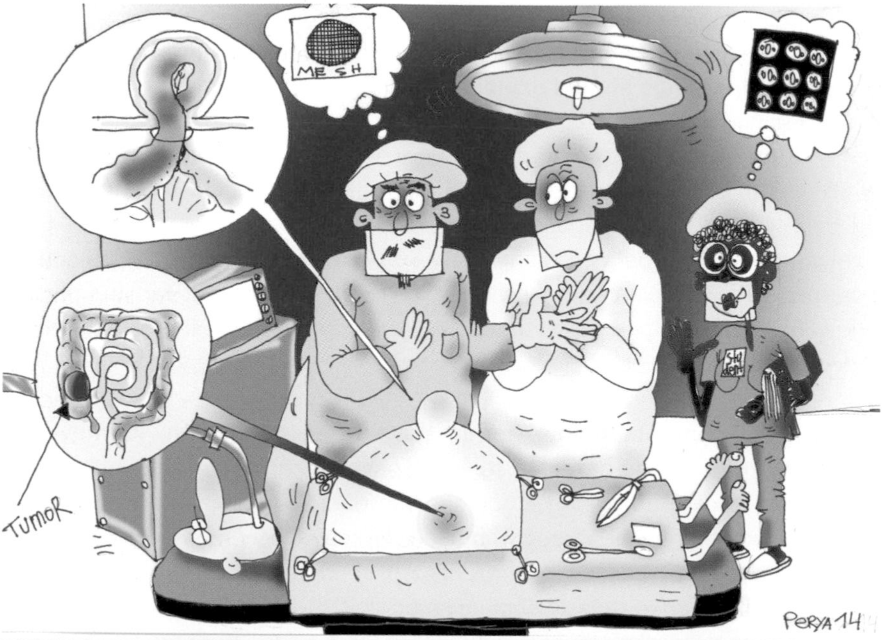

Figure 20.2. Professor of surgery to assistant: "Just reduce the hernia and repair with light mesh..." A medical student: "Excuse me Sir, did you have a chance to look at the pre-op CT?"

situation, which is not uncommon, implies that the patient suffers small bowel obstruction, due to adhesions for example, and the obstructed and distended loops of bowel invade the longstanding incisional hernia as a *secondary phenomenon*. On examination, the bowel-filled tender hernia may mimic incarceration. **It is for this reason that the contents of any hernia associated with obstruction must be examined carefully at operation to ensure that the hernia truly is the cause of the obstruction**.

> **Obviously, with liberal use of pre-operative CT imaging, the site of obstruction and the nature of the contents of the hernia can be accurately delineated, providing a road map for surgery.**

Any 'acute' incisional hernia is a surgical emergency. This is also true with other types of abdominal wall hernias, such as paraumbilical or epigastric ones. It should be noted, however, that epigastric hernias rarely, if ever, cause trouble. They contain only extraperitoneal fat from the falciform ligament, and for this reason need not be repaired routinely in the absence of symptoms. Also, the acutely incarcerated umbilical hernia frequently involves fat only.

At operation, the hernia sac must be entered to evaluate the incarcerated contents that are to be reduced or resected depending on the findings. **And the surgical findings should explain the clinical presentation**. For example, if — operating for what clinically appears as an 'incarcerated hernia' — you do not find strangulated omentum or bowel in the sac, you have to retrieve the whole length of the intestine. If you find pus within the sac you have to look for the source. We have seen patients operated upon for a 'strangulated incisional hernia' when the underlying diagnosis was perforated appendicitis. We have operated for 'strangulated femoral hernia' to find the hernia sac full of pus originating from a tubo-ovarian abscess. (Again, this hints at the usefulness of a pre-operative CT scan!)

After the contents of the hernia have been dealt with, identify the fascial margins of the defect. Use your conventional 'best' repair but do not forget that placing a mesh in a contaminated field is potentially problematic. However, not everybody agrees with such dogma and there are those who do report 'reasonable' results with implantation of non-absorbable mesh in acute situations and even in grossly contaminated fields — after resection of bowel. Note, however, that the risk of infection of mesh inserted during operations for ventral hernia is much higher than after repair of groin hernias.

A few caveats should you plan to use synthetic mesh:

- In contaminated fields use polypropylene, which is relatively resistant to infection rather than polytetrafluoroethylene (PTFE) which is not. Infected polypropylene mesh grafts are occasionally salvageable while infected PTFE patches always have to be removed. **The 'lighter' and more porous the mesh — the less susceptible it is to infection!**
- **Bear in mind also that leaving non-absorbable mesh in contact with the gut could lead to difficulties and disasters later**. Mesh repair of an incisional hernia should always aim to place the prosthetic material outside the peritoneum, ideally in the preperitoneal/ retromuscular position. At the very least omentum should be placed between any unavoidable intraperitoneal mesh and the viscera. Experience with subsequent laparotomies in patients with intraperitoneal mesh shows that adhesions are much denser than with extraperitoneal mesh and as a result small bowel resection is often required simply to access the abdominal cavity. And although uncommon we have all seen spontaneous intestinal fistulas developing at the contact point with the mesh. The manufacturers of the 'dual'-type mesh (smooth or coated on the inside, porous on the outside) claim that their products are safe for intraperitoneal use; however, injury to bowel has also been observed with such types of mesh.

- What about one of the ultra-costly **biomaterials** which are pushed forward by the industry as the ideal 'patches' for abdominal wall hernias in contaminated fields? Well, although somewhat resistant to acute infection, they are prone to late formation of 'weaknesses' and 'bulges' of the abdominal wall, and eventual hernia recurrence. The initial enthusiasm with biomaterials seems to have diminished, as more long-term results are published. 'Slowly absorbable' materials are now being promoted by several companies, but we wait for more results before jumping on this new wagon.

Parastomal hernias are a particular type of incisional hernia with extra problems. The principles of management here are the same as for other ventral hernias. If a 'clean' operation is possible — no necrosis, no bowel resection — then a definitive hernia repair might be attempted. The **Sugarbaker method** currently seems the most favored but it depends whom you are asking...

For a long and detailed assessment of the evidence in emergency hernia repair, see the World Society of Emergency Surgery guidelines here: https://wjes.biomedcentral.com/articles/10.1186/s13017-017-0149-y. It is notable that the recommendations are mostly level 'C', i.e. based on weak (or no) evidence!

Planned hernia

In a critically ill patient, when the repair is deemed complex or is judged to increase the intra-abdominal pressure significantly, we would simply close the subcutaneous layer and then the skin — leaving the patient with a large incisional hernia. We have seen patients dying from respiratory failure prompted by the abdominal compartment syndrome after herniated contents were stuffed back into the abdomen! **Remember — patients do not die from the hernia but from its intestinal complications or a closure that is too tight**.

What about laparoscopy?

The place of laparoscopy in acute hernia surgery is expanding as experience with laparoscopy in the surgical community develops. The same principles apply — treat the contents and then deal with the abdominal wall defect. Laparoscopy has some advantages — sometimes pulling the bowel back into the abdomen (carefully!) is easier than pushing from outside. Also, placing the mesh in an extraperitoneal position, and not underneath a fresh incision, may decrease infection risk. Two factors are important: the skill and experience of the laparoscopist and the condition of the patient. This is not surgery to be attempted by a beginner in laparoscopy. Neither is it suitable for a patient with extensive comorbidity and who might not be able to withstand a prolonged procedure or the additional insult of a pneumoperitoneum. Choose carefully. **Laparoscopy is not widely used in emergency surgery for hernias even by surgeons who do a lot of elective laparoscopic hernia surgery**.

> **"Always explore in cases of persistent vomiting if a lump, however small, is found occupying one of the abdominal rings and its nature is uncertain."**
>
> **Augustus Charles Bernays**

Chapter 21

Acute appendicitis

Roland E. Andersson [1]

This chapter has been subdivided into the following two sections:

1. Acute appendicitis.
2. Laparoscopic appendectomy.

1 Acute appendicitis
Roland E. Andersson

I cannot see what harm has been done if the appendix has been removed. The perfect man is the man without an appendix.
R. H. Harte

We all know: "Whatever the clinical presentation, whatever the abdominal findings, always keep acute appendicitis at the back of your mind."

Acute appendicitis (AA) is among the first diagnoses that a surgeon has to master. You may soon find your way through the complex maze of the patient's history, clinical and laboratory evaluation and diagnostic imaging to get your personal way of handling these patients. Most surgeons soon become 'experts' on AA, or so they think — often with strong opinions based on personal experience. **As a consequence, there are wide variations in how**

[1] The laparoscopic appendectomy section has been written by Danny Rosin, MD FACS.

this group of patients is managed, not only across the world but also between individual surgeons — different cultural and economic situations also play a role. All this impedes establishing generally accepted guidelines on how to manage patients with suspected AA.

> *Why the treatment of obstruction, strangulation, or perforation of the part of the intestine known as the vermiform appendix should have given rise to such a confusion of creeds, such a pandemonium of assertions, doubts, and arguments is not altogether easy to understand.*
>
> **Charles A. Balance**

So what can we tell you that you do not already know? Perhaps nothing. But let us emphasize a few points — trying to wipe out a few dogmas from your head:

- **Untreated appendicitis does not necessarily progress to perforation**. Many cases of mild, simple AA can resolve without treatment. This, often forgotten, natural history of appendicitis has important implications on how we think about and should treat AA.
- **Appendicitis cannot be confirmed or excluded by any single symptom, sign or laboratory finding**. **The opposite is true**: a high diagnostic accuracy can be reached in most cases when the whole clinical picture and the various laboratory parameters of the inflammatory response are considered together.
- **The synthesis of clinical and laboratory findings is easier and more objective with the help of a diagnostic score**. The Alvarado score is the most known but has been outperformed by the **Appendicitis Inflammatory Response (AIR) score** — this is the score that we use (■ Table 21.1). **(But remember: the score should be used as a guide but clinical judgment is still needed in every case!)**
- **Patients with a suspicion of appendicitis are heterogeneous**. We cannot use one single approach for all but need to differentiate the management depending on the clinical presentation and the perceived probability of perforation.
- **If the diagnosis is unclear at presentation it is worthwhile to reassess the patient after a few hours of observation**. This reassessment should include a review of the history, a clinical examination and laboratory workup.
- **Imaging is important in selected cases**, to differentiate between AA and other conditions like ureteral stone, acute sigmoid or cecal diverticulitis, an abdominal cancer, ovarian torsion, torsion of omentum, appendicitis epiploica, Crohn's disease or pelvic inflammatory disease.

Table 21.1. Appendicitis Inflammatory Response (AIR) score. *Andersson M, Andersson RE. The Appendicitis Inflammatory Response score: a tool for the diagnosis of acute appendicitis that outperforms the Alvarado score. World J Surg 2008; 32(8): 1843-9.*

Variable	Level	Score
Pain/tenderness RIF		+1
Vomiting		+1
Defence or rebound (the strongest)	Slight	+1
	Moderate	+2
	Strong	+3
WBC	10-14.9 x 10^9/L	+1
	≥15.0	+2
Proportion neutrophils	70-84%	+1
	≥85	+2
CRP	10-49mg/L	+1
	≥50	+2
Temperature	≥38.5°C	+1

Sum points:

0-4	Low probability of appendicitis
5-8	Indeterminate
9-12	High probability of appendicitis

Will this appendicitis resolve or progress to perforation?

We all fear perforation, with its increased morbidity and mortality. We have been taught that delay is dangerous and that perforations can be prevented by early diagnosis and operation, and that this is worthwhile even at the expense of a high proportion of unnecessary operations (up to 30% of 'white' appendectomies in some series). **This is also what families and lawyers tend to believe**.

But when we compared the number of perforations per 100,000 inhabitants, we found out that this is almost identical at centers that apply 'liberal' or 'restrictive' attitudes to appendectomy [2]. Centers that apply a 'liberal' attitude have of course more negative explorations but the number of perforations is not lower. We also found that they operated on more cases with confirmed appendicitis than centers with a 'restrictive' attitude to appendectomy. **This teaches us that a 'restrictive' attitude allows patients with mild appendicitis to resolve spontaneously — without treatment and without causing more cases to perforate**. However, as fewer cases of mild appendicitis are operated upon, the denominator will be smaller giving a higher proportion of perforation.

A high proportion of perforations may therefore reflect a better management as it is the consequence of allowing mild appendicitis cases to resolve without treatment. *Capisce?* ☺

Charles Mc Burney recognized this more than 100 years ago:

> *But, lest I give a wrong impression, I must distinctly state here, that there are many cases of appendicitis of a mild character which rapidly convalesce under no other treatment than that just referred to, and that not a few severe cases eventually recover without other active aid.*

We know, and you hopefully will know as well, that perforation is a different disease that is essentially unpreventable. Most perforations develop early, before the patient arrives in hospital — they do not perforate while we investigate or observe them. Sure, sometimes a 'masked' perforation is diagnosed after a delay and a perforation may rarely occur in an obstructed appendicitis that arrives very early to hospital but that's another, uncommon story.

Diagnosis

Classification

AA starts as an inflammation. Like most inflammatory conditions, it will, in many cases, resolve without treatment. Sometimes the inflammation may be caused by an obstruction of the outlet of the appendix (by an *appendicolith*

2 Andersson RE. The natural history and traditional management of appendicitis revisited: spontaneous resolution and predominance of prehospital perforations imply that a correct diagnosis is more important than an early diagnosis. *World J Surg* 2007; 31: 86-92.

for example) and **this can progress rapidly to necrosis, perforation and life-threatening free peritonitis**. However, mild attacks of spontaneously resolving **phlegmonous appendicitis** that does not need any treatment are common; if you rush to diagnose it by CT, and then operate upon such early and mild cases, you will never realize how common such self-limited attacks are. **You will continue to believe that you are preventing perforations!** (Isn't that what you tell the family after the operation: "we were lucky to catch it in time!")

Let us bring here a **simple classification of AA** to facilitate the discussion of diagnosis and management. **In essence, AA is either simple or complicated**.

- **'Simple' AA** implies inflammation of the appendix in the absence of appendiceal gangrene, perforation or any associated pus formation.
- **'Complicated' AA** exists whenever any of these features are present.

Some pathologists may report small inflammatory changes as "endoappendicitis", "early appendicitis", "catarrhal appendicitis" or "chronic appendicitis". Such inflammatory changes are commonly seen in asymptomatic patients who have had appendectomy *en passant*. **These entities have no clinical significance**. It is not the beginning of a progressive disease that will end with perforation; it should not be called appendicitis.

Another entity you should be familiar with — because it requires a different approach — is the **appendiceal mass, developing late in the natural history of AA**. The 'mass' is an inflammatory phlegmon made of omentum and/or adjacent viscera, walling off a complicated appendicitis. A 'mass' containing a variable amount of pus is an **appendiceal abscess**. These problems will be discussed below.

"What about '**chronic appendicitis**'?" some of you may ask. While **recurrent attacks** of typical acute appendicitis may occur and require the same approach as 'simple' appendicitis, I do not believe in so-called 'chronic appendicitis'. **Some surgeons label chronic pain and non-specific symptoms as 'chronic' appendicitis and then offer to solve the problems with an appendectomy. In most cases, however, the resulting (short term) 'cure' represents a placebo effect of the operation**.

Clinical features

The *classic* signs and symptoms of AA are well known; **even your dentist can diagnose classic AA** (■ Figure 21.1): a history of 'gastric upset' with

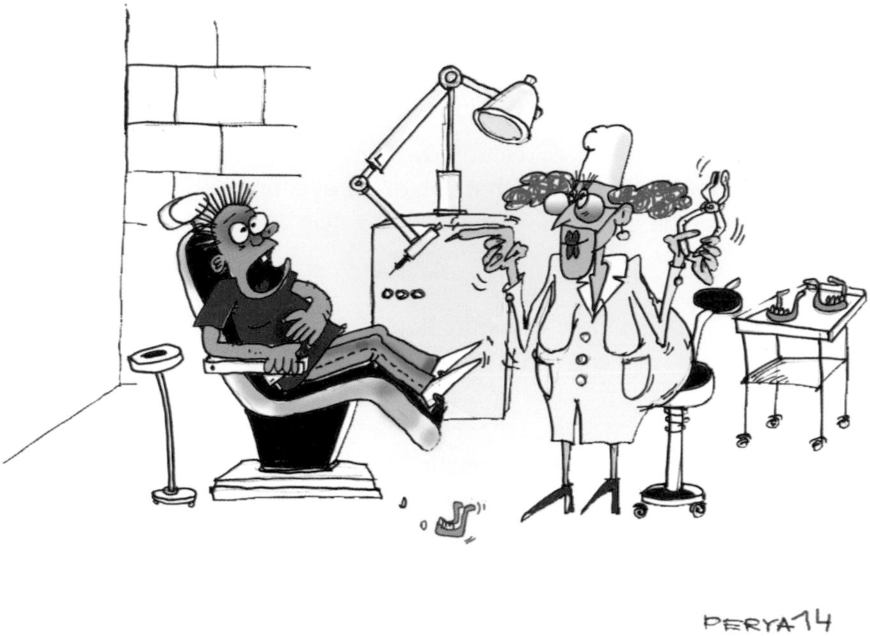

Figure 21.1. "Even dentists can diagnose it!"

vomiting or nausea, associated with mid-abdominal diffuse 'visceral' discomfort, which gradually migrates to the right lower quadrant (RLQ) and becomes 'somatic'. Add to this the physical findings of localized peritoneal irritation and, **most important, laboratory evidence of systemic inflammation. But as you know, several other conditions can have a similar presentation and not all cases of AA follow this classic path.**

In fact, the clinical presentation of AA varies considerably depending on the duration of symptoms, the stage of inflammation, the anatomical position of the appendix (e.g. retrocecal, pelvic). For some patients the diagnosis is evident and for others very vague. Thus, not all patients with suspected AA can be approached the same way. **We need a structured management based on the degree of suspicion.**

An algorithm for a structured approach

Figure ■ 21.2 depicts an algorithm of how we manage these patients. It is based on the AIR score (see ■ Table 21.1), which is a simple tool that can help to determine the probability of appendicitis. **There is nothing magic with it but it can help to put your patient into perspective based on objective findings.**

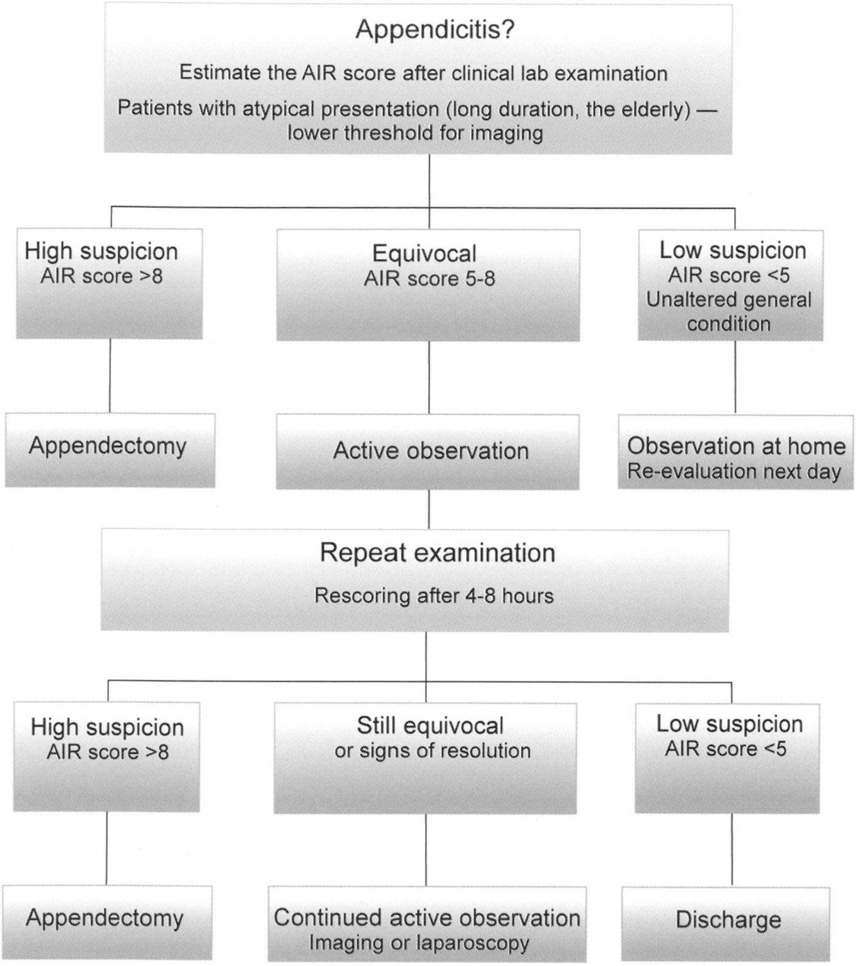

Figure 21.2. An algorithm for a structured approach to suspected AA.

It is based on the variables that are most important for making the diagnosis, and it assigns a proper weight to each of these variables. The cut-off points are chosen based on the outcome of many hundreds of similar patients. **Validation studies on thousands of patients from different hospitals in different countries have shown that the results are valid and can be replicated**. This means that the score has a built in experience of more patients than any surgeon will ever see in his/her career. It can therefore be especially useful for less experienced surgeons at the beginning of their career, let alone for the GP or ER doc who sees these patients initially.

The score divides the patients into three groups according to the probability of them suffering from AA — high, low and intermediate:

- **Patients with a high probability of AA — AIR score >8**. **Such patients, I believe, don't need any further workup unless you want to rule out another cause**. A negative imaging study would not rule out AA in a young man with a classic presentation, the presence of rebound or guarding tenderness and a strong inflammatory response. Before sending such a patient for imaging you may ask yourself what your action would be if it turned out negative. You would probably need to do at least a diagnostic laparoscopy anyway so the imaging will not change your management.
  The situation may be different in older patients or atypical presentation, where diverticulitis or a tumour may cause the same clinical presentation as appendicitis. Diagnostic imaging may be of benefit for a differential diagnosis in such cases. In patients with over 3 days' duration of symptoms, imaging is also indicated to detect an appendiceal phlegmon or abscess. See the section about the atypical patient below.
- **Patients with a low probability of AA — AIR score <5**. Take for example a young patient with abdominal pain but no signs of *peritonism*, no inflammatory response and no other alarming symptoms — **here the probability of complicated AA in need of prompt appendectomy is extremely low!** An imaging study may only lead to a false-positive examination or you may detect a mild appendicitis that may resolve without treatment within a few hours — I hear from my American friends, who almost routinely obtain CTs, about the so-called entity of 'CT appendicitis' (see below). **Most of these patients can be safely observed at home but should be planned for a re-examination after some hours if not improved**.
- **Patients with an intermediate probability of AA — AIR score of 5-8**. ***Periodic re-evaluation* is a time-honored and proven diagnostic modality in the doubtful case**. Unfortunately, the art of active observation and the virtue of patience are disappearing from the scene of modern practice. Instead, the current emphasis is on obsessive activity, where in order to prove oneself one must always 'do something'. **However, in the absence of clear peritonitis and a strong inflammatory response, very rarely are attacks of AA a true emergency requiring an immediate operation**. So if the clinical presentation is indeterminate admit the patient for active observation,

which means planned complete re-examination, including laboratory workup and rescoring after 6-8 hours. **In most instances, AA will declare itself and in non-specific abdominal pain the 'attack' will wane.** A significant decrease in the inflammatory response at the re-evaluation (especially the WBC count and proportion of neutrophils, whereas the CRP can increase as explained below) may indicate a resolving appendicitis. If you give such a patient a second round of a few hours of observation you may often find that he is ready to be discharged home. **Remember: such patients do not perforate under surgical observation!**

Indicators of inflammation

The Editors asked me to explain my views on this topic — here it is: the most important diagnostic information in AA comes from the inflammatory variables — temperature, WBC, proportion of neutrophils and CRP. **Some of these variables are in fact stronger predictors than signs of peritoneal irritation. That is why you should make use of them! But remember that the inflammatory response is dynamic — it takes some time to start up (please do not use the term 'kick-off') and it also decelerates with a delay**. This is especially true for the temperature and CRP which reacts with at least a 12-hour delay while the WBC and proportion of neutrophils can change rapidly within hours. In an AA patient with only a few hours' duration of symptoms you may therefore have (almost) normal laboratory results. **That is why the diagnostic information of the inflammatory variables increases if you repeat them after a few hours of observation**.

Just as an increase in the inflammatory response can suggest the presence of AA, a marked decrease can suggest spontaneous resolution. Here the decrease comes in reverse order. You will first notice it in a decrease in the WBC count and proportion of neutrophils, whereas the slow reacting CRP can still be on the rise. **It may take another 24 hours for the CRP to start the decline**.

What about antibiotics during 'observation'?

If you decide to observe the patient, **do not administer antibiotics** as they may mask the findings or 'partially treat' which may just delay the diagnosis and time until surgery. **Reports and experience that appendicitis may be 'cured' by antibiotics is no proof that the antibiotics were efficient**. The inflammation may have resolved all by itself. Placebo and antibiotics had the same efficiency in a randomized study. **Of course, if you diagnose AA and decide to treat it with antibiotics then this is a different story** (see below).

The atypical patient

The atypical patient is the one where imaging is indicated.

Patients with atypical presentation (>3 days' duration of symptoms, recurrent episodes of abdominal pain, a palpable mass, the elderly or patients where the intensity of pain is out of proportion to the weak clinical or laboratory findings; or when there is a discrepancy between the clinical and laboratory findings) need special considerations. Imaging may be indicated to detect/exclude an appendiceal phlegmon or abscess, Crohn's disease, diverticulitis, tumor, strangulated intestinal obstruction, torsion of the ovary, appendicitis epiploica, torsion of the omentum, ureteral calculi or other differential diagnoses.

Abdominal imaging in acute appendicitis

Imaging has a role, especially in selected patients like the elderly or in those whose presentation is atypical as mentioned above, but its efficiency as a universal tool to detect or exclude appendicitis has been overemphasized. A CT scanner is also not readily available everywhere. CT and ultrasound are two wonderful techniques but "a fool with a tool is still a fool". Indiscriminate and non-selective usage of modern diagnostic technology is not going to help. What is needed is common sense and rational deployment of available investigations. Ultrasound in good hands has been reported to be accurate in the diagnosis of AA and is useful in excluding other diagnoses, which may require a different therapy (e.g. hydronephrosis), or incision (e.g. acute cholecystitis), or indeed no therapy at all (e.g. ovarian cyst — **in women endovaginal US is a great tool to exclude/diagnose pelvic pathology!**). However, most of us do not work in an institution where we can be so confident of the radiologist's diagnosis of appendicitis based on ultrasound. **In most settings CT examination is more reliable than ultrasound**. The diagnostic features of AA on CT and the CT value in diagnosing conditions which mimic AA, but may not need operative treatment (e.g. cecal diverticulitis), are emphasized in ➲ Chapter 5.

I order imaging selectively. **Unfortunately in many places the diagnostic algorithm is increasingly driven by dogmatic emergency room personnel who perform CT scans in lieu of clinical evaluation**. Such indiscriminate use of CT scanning leads to a new syndrome of 'CT appendicitis': you admit for observation a patient with right lower quadrant pain and ambiguous clinical findings. Meanwhile the emergency room doctor orders a CT, which is reported by the radiologist the following morning. At this stage, the patient feels much better, his abdomen is benign, and he wants to go home but the radiologist claims that the appendix is inflamed ("cannot exclude AA..." or "suggestive of AA..."). *But should we treat the CT image or the patient?*

Diagnostic laparoscopy

Diagnostic laparoscopy is a wonderful instrument, but it is invasive and should not replace conventional clinical diagnosis and imaging. It has been recommended to leave a macroscopically uninflamed appendix *in situ*, thus reducing the 'negative appendectomy rate' but this is just a white wash. **(Anyway, most surgeons I know are reluctant to *not* remove the appendix in such circumstances — what about you?)** Negative diagnostic laparoscopy is a non-therapeutic procedure which is associated with unnecessary pain, a risk of complications and increased costs. If your negative laparoscopic exploration rate is higher than 15% you are misusing the procedure.

However, diagnostic laparoscopy is useful for the patient with an equivocal diagnosis of appendicitis that has not improved after observation, imaging has not clarified the situation and the patient's presentation is such that he cannot be discharged.

And this is how I do it in Sweden:

First I gather all the data needed to calculate the AIR score. It helps me put the patient into a wider perspective. I never make any decision until I have all this information. For women of fertile age a gynecological examination including a transvaginal ultrasound is also done, as this can detect ovarian pathology (➲ Chapter 33). The calculated score is my guide:

- **Patients with a low probability of AA — no peritoneal irritation, all inflammatory variables normal (score <5)**. This group represents the majority of all patients with a suspicion of AA. They can safely be observed at home. Plan for a reassessment after 6-12 hours (i.e. the next morning). Imaging is not indicated unless you think the patient may have another disease.
- **Patients with a typical presentation — presence of peritoneal irritation and strong inflammatory response (score >8). These patients need an operation!** A few hours' delay is acceptable, but in

this group of patients there are many with perforation so I would start antibiotic treatment and arrange for an operation without undue delay, especially if the patient is septic (tachycardia, tachypnea or leukopenia). Imaging is not indicated as a negative examination will probably not change this decision. **If I am in doubt about the diagnosis I start the operation laparoscopically** — for many of you this is probably a routine anyway.

- **Patients with an indeterminate presentation (score 5-8) are admitted to hospital and re-examined after 6-8 hours**. The AA patient will by then unfold with a significant increase in clinical symptoms and inflammation. If still atypical you may order a CT or proceed with laparoscopy. If there is a marked decrease in inflammation at the re-examination (especially fever, WBC count, proportion of neutrophils) but the suspicion of AA remains — I plan another re-examination after 6-8 hours. As I will not operate during that time I allow the patient to have a meal and then to fast again. I often find further improvement after a second observation period and sometimes the patient can be sent home. **I have seen this many times also in CT-verified appendicitis patients**.
- **Small children, the fragile elderly and patients with an atypical presentation** (as explained above) need special considerations. **In this situation I have a low threshold for imaging**.

Treatment

Antibiotics

Judicious administration of antibiotics, to cover **Gram-negative and anaerobic bacteria**, will minimize the incidence of postoperative wound (common) and intra-abdominal (rare) infective complications (➲ Chapter 13). In simple AA the antibiotics are considered **prophylactic**, while in complicated AA they are **therapeutic** (➲ Chapter 7). **We encourage you to administer the first dose of antibiotics when you make the diagnosis**.

If at surgery the AA proves to be simple and there is no visible pus, no postoperative administration is necessary. **Should you, on the other hand, discover complicated AA, additional postoperative doses are indicated. We suggest that you tailor the duration of administration to the operative findings**. Gangrenous AA, without any pus formation does not require prolonged postoperative administration. When pus is found or the appendix is perforated you should give 3-5 days of treatment (➲ Chapters 7, 13 and 40).

Non-operative management of acute appendicitis

As already said, simple AA can frequently resolve without treatment. **No wonder that reports have shown that 'assumed' or image-proven simple AA can respond to non-operative management with intravenous broad-spectrum antibiotics. However, I believe that in the majority of patients the symptoms resolve spontaneously and not because of the antibiotics.** This is just a parallel to recent findings that patients with uncomplicated acute diverticulitis have identical healing rates irrespective of whether they receive antibiotics or not. The same efficiency of placebo and antibiotics has also been shown in appendicitis.

I see two problems with giving antibiotics to a patient with 'assumed' AA. The first is that if the patient gets better you do not know if he had AA in the first place and you do not know if the improvement was spontaneous or due to the antibiotics. So you are forced to 'complete' the treatment, which may in fact prolong the hospital stay. The second is that if the patient has complicated AA you may see only a partial response, which will similarly prolong the suffering. Therefore, I do not support non-surgical management with antibiotics for 'assumed uncomplicated appendicitis'.

However, non-operative management of AA with antibiotics can be beneficial and reasonable in the following categories of patients:

- Patients with a **prohibitive surgical-anesthetic risk** (e.g. post-myocardial infarction).
- Patients who **refuse** an operation.
- Patients in the middle of the Pacific Ocean, on a space ship on a trip to Mars, or a nuclear submarine, or in **rural locations where no surgeon is available.**
- **Obviously, patients with an 'appendiceal mass' or phlegmon should be managed non-operatively.** This is accepted by most surgeons and is no longer controversial!

The operation

> *The point of greatest tenderness is, in the average adult, almost exactly 2 inches from the anterior iliac spine, on a line drawn from this process through the umbilicus.*
>
> **Charles McBurney**

> *The appendix is generally attached to the cecum.*
>
> **Mark M. Ravitch**

When to operate?

You don't have to rush to the operating room with each patient diagnosed with AA! Obviously, if your patient is in a septic state with rapid respiration, tachycardia or has impressive abdominal findings (denoting a possible perforation) the patient should receive optimal resuscitation while you start antibiotic treatment, but you should not delay the operation any further. **Otherwise, you can safely defer an operation to daytime**. But of course, local considerations such as workload and OR availability may force you to operate after midnight...

Open versus laparoscopic approach?

As pointed out above, the liberal use of diagnostic laparoscopy for suspected AA leads to a high incidence of unnecessary invasive, non-therapeutic procedures that are not free of complications — which commonly end with an appendectomy even if the appendix is 'normal'. **But what about laparoscopic appendectomy (LA) if the diagnosis has been established?** The voluminous literature on this controversy (most surgeons do not consider this 'controversial' anymore) can be summarized like this: **compared to the open procedure, LA is associated with a better cosmesis, some reduction in postoperative pain, marginally earlier discharge and a lower incidence of wound infection**. However, LA is associated with a higher risk of postoperative intra-abdominal collections/abscesses — rare, but serious complications. Concerning costs, the money saved by an earlier discharge after LA is spent on a more expensive and longer procedure. We can therefore not declare any winner between these methods, so the choice is up to the preferences of the surgeon and the patient and the local situation. **LA may, however, have a clear advantage in the very obese patient** (avoiding a large incision). For details about LA and perhaps another perspective go to the next section of this chapter.

Technical points for open appendectomy

Did anybody ever teach you how to do an open appy? Even if you are a lap-appy aficionado do not deprive yourself of the skills (and pleasures) of being able to remove a diseased appendix through a smallish right lower quadrant incision. **Such skills may come in useful when 'converting' a difficult LA — no, a midline incision is usually not necessary in that situation!**

It is possible that you have done your share of open appendectomies already as an intern. However, having seen many surgeons transform a customary appendectomy to an elaborate operation resembling a Whipple's procedure, we remind you of the KISS principle (keep it simple, stupid!). Here are a few tips:

- **Incision**: you do not need the long unsightly oblique incision — except in the muscular young man whose possible retrocecal appendix may be unreachable through a transverse hole. **Use the *transverse* one!** A common error is to place it too medially over the rectus sheath. If you center the incision slightly lateral to the point of McBurney you will in most cases get it right. Incise the fascia, split the muscles and open the peritoneum. **Start with a small incision about 4-5cm long; it can be always extended to each side by cutting the lateral edge of the rectus fascia and/or muscle.**
- **Appendectomy**: you can remove the appendix in an antegrade or retrograde fashion but there is no need to invert the stump. Just ligate or suture-transfix the appendix at its base and chop off the rest. To control the divided mesoappendix you can use clips, diathermy or ligatures; when the tissue is friable, overrun it with a running suture. The commonly performed fetishes of painting the stump with Betadine® or burning it with diathermy are ridiculous. **If the appendix has perforated just at its base, to secure the stump safely you must include in it some healthy cecal wall — just place a linear stapler across the cecum proximal to the perforation and fire.** If you do not have a stapler then do it by hand — suture the stump together with surrounding cecal wall using your best anastomotic technique!
- **Peritoneal toilet**: just aspirate and mop the fluid (do not forget the pelvis!). **Peritoneal lavage is useless or even harmful — responsible for those fluid collections that you see on post-op imaging.**
- **Hemostasis**: **be meticulous!** The partial evisceration of the cecum places the blood supply on tension and may interrupt the blood flow, thus concealing bleeding. When the cecum is repositioned, its circulation recovers and bleeding from the divided artery or the mesoappendix may declare itself. **Thus, always check the stump of the mesoappendix after returning the cecum to its natural position.** Place some gauze into the depths of the wound: if it comes out pink, you have to recheck the hemostasis.
- **Microbiological culture**: taking it in these cases is unnecessary and wasteful unless the operation is after failed antibiotic treatment (➲ Chapter 13).

- **Drains: are very (very!) seldom necessary after appendectomy** (no, I am not kidding) and have also been shown to be harmful (➲ Chapter 36).
- **Closure**: theoretically, closing the peritoneum is unnecessary because it adds no strength to the repair, and we know that the peritoneum repairs itself within 48 hours. However, this step 'covers' the bulging viscera, facilitating careful closure of the abdominal wall layers and may prevent interstitial hernias. Next the muscles are approximated loosely with a few sutures to obliterate dead space; the fascia is closed with a running suture. The subcutaneous layer, if thick, may be approximated with a few fine sutures. Close the skin in continuous subcuticular fashion, also in complicated cases. Use absorbable sutures and avoid including too much tissue, as this may cause necrosis and infection. Some still advocate **secondary wound closure** in complicated appendicitis. This may prevent a few wound infections at the cost of prolonged suffering from changes of dressings and further manipulations and an ugly scar for all patients. This is not worth the cost as explained in ➲ Chapters 37 and 46.

> *The surgeon who can describe the extent of an appendiceal peritonitis has convicted himself of performing an improper operation.*
>
> **Mark M. Ravitch**

(If you do not understand this aphorism please feel free to email the Editors.)

Special considerations

The 'white' appendix

What should you do when the appendix proves to be pristine? Well, you can rub it to allow the pathologist to diagnose mild acute inflammation (just kidding). The classical dictum is that whenever an abdominal appendectomy incision exists the appendix should be removed in order not to confuse matters in the future. **What about a normal appendix visualized at laparoscopy? Should it also be removed?** The emerging consensus is to leave it alone, informing the patient or the parents that the appendix has been left *in situ*. As we mentioned above, the problem is that most surgeons are reluctant to follow such (alleged) consensus. What about you?

Obviously, when the appendix appears normal (**very unlikely if you had followed our diagnostic approach or obtained a CT scan**) you should search for alternative diagnoses such as Meckel's diverticulitis, adnexal pathology, perforated cecal diverticulitis, or mesenteric lymphadenitis (whatever that is). Extremely rarely, you will encounter pus-looking fluid and no source — primary peritonitis (➲ Chapter 13). In most instances, however, you'll find nothing.

What should you do if foul-smelling, murky, or bile-stained peritoneal fluid is encountered, suggesting a serious alternative pathology elsewhere? If the source of the pathology is not evident you could do a diagnostic laparoscopy through the partly closed gridiron incision. If it is evident then close the incision and place a new one where the action is. Bile should guide you into the upper abdomen. Feces or its odor direct you towards the sigmoid. Do not try to do a colon resection through an extended transverse incision. Think of perforated duodenal ulcer and intestinal perforation. Anyhow, if you follow the diagnostic steps outlined above it is very unlikely that you will find yourself in such an unpleasant situation...

Postoperative appendiceal stump phlegmon/abscess and stump appendicitis

Your patient had an uneventful appendectomy for acute appendicitis following which he happily went home. Seven days later he presents with right lower quadrant pain, a temperature and high white cell count. The wound looks OK. This may be a postoperative abdominal abscess or an appendix stump phlegmon. Nowadays the diagnosis is simple — a CT will demonstrate an abscess or a phlegmon which involves the cecum. **Both are cured by a few days of antibiotic therapy but an abscess may need percutaneous drainage, especially if larger than 5cm**.

With **stump appendicitis** be aware that patients can develop classic acute appendicitis at any time *after appendectomy*. Historically this followed appendectomy for complicated appendicitis, often by a relatively inexperienced family doctor/surgeon. **It is now becoming more common in the era of *laparoscopic appendectomy***, where during the procedure surgeons may misidentify the cecal base of the appendix and consequently leave a long appendiceal stump — prone to stump appendicitis and requiring a re-appendectomy. **Few ER or family practice docs realize that post-appendectomy patients can (rarely) suffer from acute appendicitis — do explain it to them!**

Appendiceal mass (phlegmon)

Typically, patients with an appendiceal mass present late in the course of the disease and this should be suspected when symptoms have persisted for more than 3 days. Occasionally, they report a spontaneous improvement in their symptoms, reflecting localization of the inflammatory process. **On clinical examination you will find a right iliac fossa mass.** Overlying tenderness or obesity may obscure the presence of the mass. Therefore, suspect an appendiceal mass in the 'late presenters' or those with an atypical smoldering picture. When palpation is not rewarding, **obtain a CT scan, which is the best way to document an appendiceal mass**. Another indication for CT is associated evidence of undrained pus such as a spiking fever and toxicity, signifying an **appendiceal abscess**.

Why should you distinguish between AA and appendiceal mass or abscess? **Because the appendiceal mass (and abscess) can (and should) be managed non-operatively**. You could operate on both, as you operate on AA, but removal of the appendix involved in an inflammatory mass may be more hazardous than usual, occasionally necessitating a right hemicolectomy. **On the other hand, conservative treatment with antibiotics leads to resolution of the mass in almost all cases**. Failure of the mass to respond to antibiotics signifies an abscess (rare!). CT or ultrasound-guided percutaneous drainage is then the most rational approach (➲ Chapter 42).

Interval appendectomy?

As no more than one out of ten patients treated conservatively for appendiceal mass will suffer a recurrence of AA (usually within 1 year and not a complicated attack), **the dogma of routine interval appendectomy has become obsolete**. In patients over the age of 40 years we suggest elective colonoscopy/colonic imaging after 1 month to exclude the rare situation in which carcinoma of the appendix or caecum was the cause of the mass. Cancer or inflammatory bowel disease will be detected only in 2 out of 100 such patients. **So apply the "if it were me" test and do not recommend interval appendectomies to your patients!**

Appendicitis epiploica (appendagitis)

We mention this condition here because of its name. You have probably not heard much about it but it is not so rare and often imitates AA. Appendicitis epiploica (some call it '**appendagitis**') follows a spontaneous torsion of an appendix epiploica — the peritoneum-covered tabs of fat attached along the *tenia coli*. It is more common in obese individuals and in the cecum and sigmoid. Since the sigmoid colon often crosses the midline the most common manifestation is localized tenderness and peritoneal signs in the right iliac fossa. Typically, patients do not lose their appetite and do not feel or appear sick despite these findings. Thus, **'AA on examination' in an afebrile and healthy-looking patient should raise your suspicions**. The natural history is spontaneous remission as the appendix epiploica sloughs off, transforming into that loose calcified peritoneal body that you occasionally find during unrelated abdominal procedures. **A CT scan usually identifies the localized area of pericolonic inflammation, excludes AA and thus helps you to avoid the unnecessary surgery or diagnostic laparoscopy** (➲ Chapter 5). **If you are misled into an operation just remove the necrotic piece of fat**. Then look at the mirror and say: "How stupid I was to operate!"

Torsion of omentum

Just to be 'complete' we mention also this relatively rare entity which could impersonate very accurately the clinical features of AA. This is caused by torsion of a pedicle of heavy omentum — causing ischemia and gradual necrosis. If you encounter it during a planned appendectomy for AA, cure is provided by partial omentectomy. CT imaging however can avoid the operation as it would show the inflamed segment of omentum and a normal appendix. **As with appendicitis epiploica, conservative treatment (NSAID, no need for antibiotics) would lead to spontaneous recovery within a week**.

Dr. Andersson of Sweden — whom we consider the ultimate international guru on AA — offers a rational diagnostic approach based on the AIR score and selective imaging. We have no reasons to doubt that this approach must be serving him very well in Sweden. But we wish to present some 'international perspective' reflecting our own environments.

In some countries, like in **the USA, where I (MS) practice, the decision whom and when to CT scan is no longer in our surgical hands**. The fact of the matter is that most patients have already undergone a CT scan, before we, surgeons, are called to assess them. Typically, these scans are ordered by emergency room physicians, or family docs, before consulting the surgeon. In most hospitals in the USA, even the tiny rural ones, high-tech CT images are much easier to obtain than a gourmet meal or even a cup of good coffee. And radiologists are always readily available to interpret the images online. **It's no wonder then that physicians confronted with a potentially acute abdomen feel compelled to get a CT when it is as easily procured as junk food**.

Is such a practice of almost routine CT scanning advantageous over the 'restrictive' imaging policy, combined with the AIR score, advocated by Roland? Well, it is very difficult, if not unfeasible, to prove scientifically that the increased use of CT scanning is beneficial overall. But what about the individual patient?

The advantages of 'liberal scanning' are familiar to those of us who use it (➲ Chapter 5) and include:

- Many patients with '**non-specific abdominal pain' can be discharged safely** after a normal CT scan. Hospital admission for clinical observation (intermediate AIR score) is thus rendered unnecessary.

- **Other pathologies are readily diagnosed and treated correctly**. Dr. Andersson tells us that patients with a 'typical presentation' (score >8) do not need imaging. However, patients with acute diverticulitis of the cecum or sigmoid, gynecological emergencies and other conditions mentioned by Dr. Andersson, may present with typical features of AA. Imaging would save them an unnecessary appendectomy and/or diagnostic laparoscopy.
- **Many small hospitals, especially in rural regions of large countries do not have a general surgeon readily available** to evaluate each and every patient 'à la Dr. Andersson'. Some hospitals do not have a surgeon at all. A negative CT allows the evaluating physician to sleep better at night and avoids unnecessary 'shipping out' (transfer of patients to another institution).
- **Legal considerations**. Juries in the USA have been awarding almost a million dollars for a "failure to obtain imaging" and thus, allegedly, causing a delay in diagnosis of AA — with resulting morbidity. While not advocating 'defensive medicine', it is impossible to ignore such harsh realities.

No, we do not support *routine* CT scanning. But we think that its liberal use makes for swifter and more 'accurate' clinical management. Yes, we understand the issue of 'CT appendicitis' and the dilemma of removing early inflamed appendices which may have settled spontaneously. And anyway, the train has already left the station — we have a useful diagnostic tool, which will improve (become faster and emit smaller doses of radiation) — and there is no way back. **And BTW: in pregnant women — consider MRI**.

A few words about the AIR score. We would like to emphasize what Dr. Andersson said that AA scores should be used only as an adjunct to clinical judgment. While statistically solid they may 'misfire' in the individual patient. Take for example an elderly patient presenting with lower abdominal pain and a minimally elevated WBC count and CRP level. **His AIR score was 5**. He was admitted for observation. Perforated AA was found at laparotomy the next day; he died from overwhelming sepsis. **A CT on admission may have saved him!** Such a patient falls into the 'uncertain category' described by Dr. Andersson. (Oh yes, Dr. Andersson stated that the old and frail patients deserve to be scanned — but this should be emphasized!).

AA is not a single disease that needs one treatment, but has a spectrum of presentations and pathologies that can be treated in different ways — including without an operation. **We wish we knew how to modulate the prevailing educational, cultural, economic and legal components, which still influence most surgeons to believe that any diseased appendix belongs in the formalin jar.**
The Editors

2 Laparoscopic appendectomy [3]
Danny Rosin

Up to the decision to operate, there should be no difference in the decision process between surgeons who prefer laparoscopic appendectomy and the 'open' enthusiasts. They all aim to correctly diagnose, as explained above, and proceed with the treatment. But, as mentioned briefly in ➲ Chapter 4, some perceive laparoscopy as an extension of the diagnostic effort: "We are not sure if the appendix is inflamed or not, let's avoid the CT radiation, let's avoid the annoying observation, let's stick the scope in and know for sure!" And while this approach may make sense, we tend to forget its downsides, the invasiveness and its risks, the anesthesia and its risk (minimal, admittedly, but existent), and the tendency 'to do something', even remove a normal appendix, just a souvenir from a nice trip to the abdomen.

So, while we cannot claim that diagnostic laparoscopy for suspected appendicitis is a gross mistake, or God forbid a crime, we try to minimize its use!

Why laparoscopy?

My first instinctive reply would be: **it's a good procedure**, I do it well, I feel comfortable with it and the patients are happy. After years of almost exclusive appendectomy by laparoscopy I feel it's a good and honest answer, and many young surgeons who trained with lap appendectomy as the routine procedure feel the same, and mainly feel it's easier and 'cleaner' than to struggle through a mini incision. But I realize that some older surgeons will read the above sincere text and say "bulls**t!", and I acknowledge the fact that a serious book like this deserves some more scientific text. And it's not as if we don't have good arguments:

- **Differential diagnosis**. Despite all modern diagnostic modalities, we have not eliminated surgical surprises, and a normal appendix may still wait for us inside, along with some other unexpected pathology. Laparoscopy is a much better diagnostic and therapeutic tool in these cases than a limited RLQ incision. And while 'young fertile women' are nearly in the consensus for lap appendectomy, even Valentino had an unexpected pathology [4].

3 Professor Ahmad Assalia, MD, contributed to this section in the third edition of this book.
4 Remember the case of the famous movie actor and womanizer Rudolph Valentino who underwent an appendectomy for suspected acute appendicitis in New York (1926). He became gravely ill after the operation and died; autopsy revealed a perforated peptic ulcer...

- **Wound infection**. Dealing with an infective process, it's no wonder laparoscopy is associated with fewer incisional problems. Even if a wound infection occurs (surely it's less frequent) — the result is a small annoying wound infection and not an open large one, destined for a long secondary healing and an ugly scar. Although hernia in a McBurney scar is rare, we have seen it following wound infection and impaired wound healing.
- **Pain and recovery**. The problem with 'small' operations, like appendectomy, is that the advantages of laparoscopy are more subtle and more difficult to prove. This does not mean that the advantages are not there, and we (and the patients) witness it daily. McBurney aficionados will wave papers about "no statistical difference" in QOL scores measured by scales we don't really understand, but we **know** our patients do well and, if we didn't f*** up, recover swiftly.
- **Cosmesis**. Yes, this is a minor issue... And yet...

Why not laparoscopy?

- **You don't know how to do it**. This may be the most important contraindication for lap appendectomy. Never attempt a procedure you don't master, just because it's fashionable. No one here claims that open appendectomy is **bad**, only that maybe, under optimal conditions, lap appendectomy may have some advantages. A lack of experience, and lack of proper equipment, are all very good reasons to stick with the safe and proven open approach. **A little more pain is preferable to some horrendous complications we sometimes see after misguided attempts to keep this simple procedure 'minimally invasive'**. (You have to read Chapter 17 in *Schein's Common Sense Prevention and Management of Surgical Complications*, tfm Publishing, 2013.)
- **Intra-abdominal collections**. I'm not sure this issue is solved yet. There have been claims for a higher incidence of post-appendectomy pelvic collections after laparoscopy. While we do see this occasionally, many studies claim that the rate is not different when compared to the open procedure. It may be that excessive irrigation by laparoscopy contributes to spreading the localized infection. We are not sure it's true — **but we don't irrigate, just aspirate the pus, and it seems to work just fine. The other Editors agree with me about this — just suck the crap out!**
- **Relative contraindications**. In situations like pregnancy, or perforated appendicitis with generalized peritonitis, one may argue that laparoscopy is less advisable, or more risky. The level of surgical experience may play a role here, as well as a large dose of common

sense. **Remember that obese patients may actually benefit from laparoscopy, despite the fact that a more difficult operation is expected**.

- **Cost**. No, we will not go into this. Cost is such a complicated topic! Enough to say that if you do have basic laparoscopic equipment, you can remove the appendix quite cheaply, with reusable instruments, a cheap energy source, a few ties and a homemade bag. Leave the Harmonic Scalpel® and the staples to others, use your excellent manual skills, and be thankful you have fewer obese patients to operate on than those poor guys in the USA.

How to do it?

You may have learned your technique from your chief resident and been convinced that this is the 'correct' way to do it. Please remember that surgical variability is good. I will avoid the horrible 'cat skinning' aphorism but just tell you that after almost 20 years of lap appendectomy I still modify the technique from time to time, if only for the fun of it. See ■ Figure 21.3 for some of the **trocar placement options** that are favored by different surgeons. Please note that I skipped the single port and robotic configurations. I advise you to skip them too… But with all the variability, there are several key points you should remember, to make the procedure run smoothly and safely. Here they are:

- **Urine. Let the patient empty the bladder before surgery**. I know that many surgeons prefer a Foley catheter for every lower abdominal laparoscopy, but why give those who oppose laparoscopy another

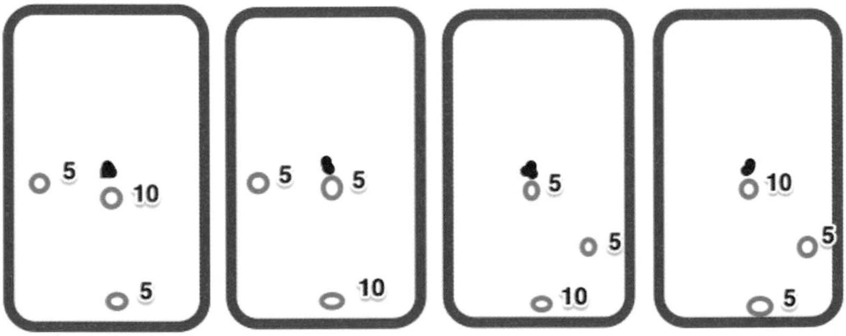

Figure 21.3. Some of the options for trocar placement in laparoscopic appendectomy.

good argument against it? And why give your patient an increased risk for a UTI? An empty bladder will keep the pelvic space free for you, and allow you to safely insert the lower trocar. And no, you don't need urinary monitoring for such a short operation, unless it takes you more than two hours… and then you shouldn't do it…

- **Position**. Make the operation convenient for you. Tuck the arms along the body so you'll be able to stand comfortably, with the assistant standing near you. Secure the patient to the table so the anesthetist will have no excuse against a *steep Trendelenburg and left tilt*. You don't need the small bowel obstructing your surgical field of interest.
- **Equipment**. Use the best equipment you can have. Make your laparoscopic conditions optimal; the less you struggle the better is your operation:
  - **optics and light source** should prevent you from working in the dark. If you have a good 5mm scope (that will allow you to move between the trocars as needed) — fine. If not — use the 10!
  - **energy sources**, depending on availability, can make life easier. The *Harmonic Scalpel®*, *LigaSure®* and other variants from different companies, can all save you time and save the patient his erythrocytes. But remember that a **good laparoscopic surgeon can achieve the same with simple monopolar or bipolar energy, and some pre-tied loops or even simple surgical ties**. We encourage you to master these skills even if you live in Utopia and staplers are for free.
- **Mobilization**. Not every appendix will wait for you in full erection (*oy vey*). The high, low, retrocecal, subhepatic or "WTF — where is it for heaven's sake" appendix may play hide and seek with your nerves and ego. But here comes the real advantage of laparoscopy: you are not limited in the confines of a strange incision in the corner of the abdomen. Look around, explore, follow the tenia, follow the terminal ileum, mobilize the cecum, mobilize the whole right colon — do whatever it takes to find the bastard; you can do it and you have the technology! (I guess most of the readers are too young to remember the citation from my favorite childhood series "The Six Million Dollar Man"... Look it up on YouTube!).
- **Mesenteric transection**. Once you have localized the appendix you have to start working on it. You may need to separate some more adhesions around it, peel the omentum that is already attached to it, or even the bowel around it. You must do it in order to elevate the appendix and expose the mesentery. "**Can I grab it?!**" you ask, sheepishly, and the presidential answer would be, surprisingly, "Yes you can…!" But that is only because you are a common sense surgeon, **you know how to gently manipulate it, or grab the mesentery just underneath, and avoid crushing, perforating,**

ripping and spreading the infection. The mesenteric transection can be accomplished by any means you prefer (and afford) — ties, clips, bipolar, any modern energy source or even a vascular stapler, but please remember, for God's sake, **this is not cancer surgery**: you don't have to cut too proximal if the mesentery is thickened and inflamed. It is perfectly safe to transect close to or on the appendix itself, decreasing the risk of bleeding and the bulkiness of the specimen to be removed.

- **Appendiceal transection**. Although, at times, you start with transecting the base (retrograde appendectomy, when the tip is buried somewhere), this is usually the phase when success can be declared, the anesthetist can be woken up, and the nurse can be promised that coffee is really soon. Do you know how to tie, intracorporeally or extracorporeally, and impress the intern? Do you want to use the friendly *Endoloop®*? Do you expect a 'conference' sponsored by one of the stapler companies? All methods are legitimate as long as the base is secured. And if it is all swollen or necrotic down to the base — get a piece of the cecum with a stapler — exactly like you would in an open case.

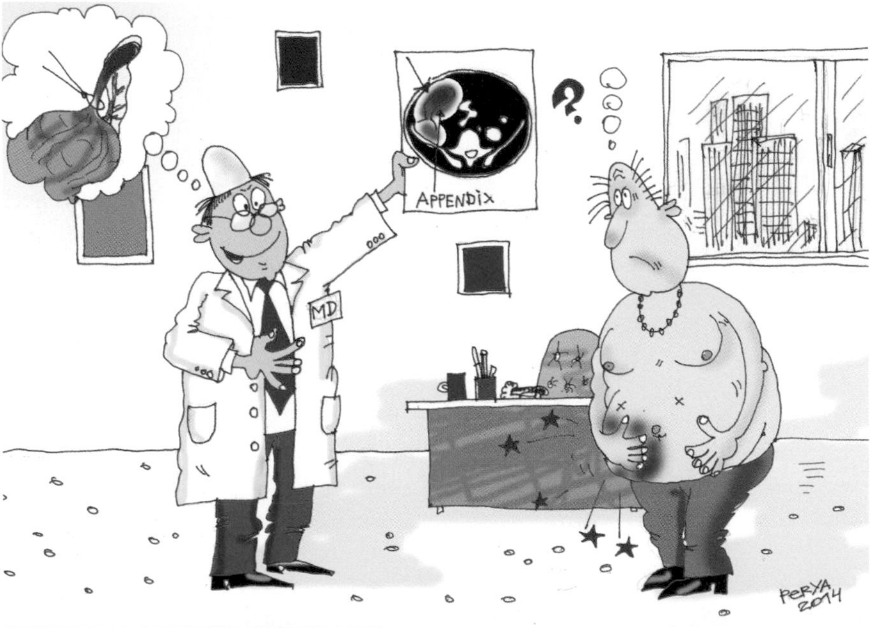

Figure 21.4. Patient: "But Doc, how could it be possible? I had my appendix removed laparoscopically last year at the Mayonnaise Clinic! Could I have two appendixes?"

- **Extraction.** Please don't ruin your beautiful operation with non-elegant extraction of the specimen; this will not only make you look bad in the eyes of the nurses but will also increase the chance of infective complications. Use an extraction bag (unless you remove a slender, white appendix...). Enlarge the incision a bit if the appendix is too bulky. Make it look easy and effortless, and **don't worry about four more millimeters to the incision length. It is better than an infected short incision.**

To conclude, laparoscopic appendectomy is a very good option. It's your responsibility to play it safe, and prove that I am right!

Gosh, I almost forgot, **take care to remove the whole appendix**, not only part of it — not a rare occurrence in laparoscopic hands which are not as skilled as yours... (see ■ Figure 21.4)

Acute appendicitis, like any other surgical condition, has a *spectrum*. To reach the diagnosis, consider historical, physical and laboratory findings together. No isolated variable can confirm or exclude AA. The more typical variables are present, the higher the chance that you are dealing with AA. Whether you operate immediately or tomorrow, whether you observe or obtain additional tests is determined *selectively* based on your individual patient.

It has been said that "The good thing about standards of care is that there are so many to choose from." And this is true of course concerning the choice between open and laparoscopic appendectomies. If you are a well trained laparoscopic surgeon then a laparoscopic approach is almost always preferable. So strive for laparoscopic excellence but be careful. Looking around us — beyond what is published in the literature — we see an epidemic of complications developing after laparoscopic appendectomy which we have (almost) never seen before: intraperitoneal abscesses, intestinal obstruction, cecal fistula, recurrent appendicitis, bowel injury, bladder injury [5]. And yes, hernias can develop also at the trocar site. **So decide for yourself and play it safe!**

Never become blasé about AA; it can kill even today, and may humble even the most experienced surgeon. The Editors

You may ask yourself: why such an extra long chapter, dedicated to such a tiny worm-like organ?

5 For a more detailed discussion of the complications of appendectomy and how to prevent them read Chapter 17 in *Schein's Common Sense Prevention and Management of Surgical Complications*. Shrewsbury, UK: tfm publishing, 2013.

"There are two things in life that we will never understand: women and acute appendicitis."

"There are three types of patients with acute appendicitis: those who do well no matter what we do; those who don't do well no matter what we do; and those in whom our management actually makes a difference. As most fall into the first category ...every surgeon believes that what he/she does is the right thing to do."

Magnus Bergenfeldt

Chapter 22

Acute mesenteric ischemia

Paul N. Rogers and Wesley P. Stuart

Vascular surgery is peculiar because, above all, it is mainly surgery of ruins.

Cid dos Santos

Occlusion of the mesenteric vessels is regarded as one of those conditions of which the diagnosis is impossible, the prognosis hopeless, and the treatment almost useless.

A. Cokkins

Which of you hasn't been called by the internists or ER docs to "rule out mesenteric ischemia" in some elderly patient? As a rule, on such occasions you will find a groaning patient with non-specific abdominal complaints and a hospital chart that outweighs you. **"Rule out mesenteric ischemia" — easier said than done!**

Acute mesenteric ischemia usually involves the region supplied by the superior mesenteric artery (SMA). Thus, the small intestine is predominantly affected but the right colon, which is also supplied by the SMA, can be involved as well. Isolated ischemia of the colon, which is much less common, will be discussed separately under the heading of *Ischemic colitis* in ➲ Chapter 24.

The problem

The problem is a sudden reduction in arterial perfusion of the small bowel, which quickly leads to central abdominal pain. If left untreated, the process progressively involves the muscular layer of the intestines and it is only after some hours, when the serosa is affected, that peritoneal signs appear. To simplify matters, let us divide acute arterial mesenteric ischemia (AMI) into three types:

- **Thrombotic**: due to an acute arterial thrombosis (**of a chronically diseased artery**), which usually occludes the orifice of the SMA, resulting in **massive ischemia of the entire small bowel plus the right colon** — the area supplied by the SMA. This is probably the most frequent form of the disease, and is acute-on-chronic.
- **Embolic**: due to a shower of embolic material originating proximally — from the heart (atrial fibrillation, post-myocardial infarction, diseased valve) or an aneurysmal or atherosclerotic aorta. Emboli usually lodge in the proximal SMA, <u>but beyond the exit of the middle colic artery</u>; therefore, as a rule, the most proximal segment of small bowel is spared, along with the transverse and (probably) the right colon. **While emboli may fragment and re-embolize distally, the patchy ischemia that is sometimes seen is more often due to incomplete arcades and is analogous to the 'patchy' ischemia seen in other situations. Note that while embolism may occur on a background of chronic mesenteric arterial disease, thrombosis *in situ* is much more likely.**
- **Non-occlusive mesenteric ischemia (NOMI)**: due to a 'low-flow state', in the absence of documented arterial thrombosis or embolus. **Note, however, that underlying mesenteric atherosclerosis may be a precipitating/ contributory factor**. The low-flow state is a product of low cardiac output (e.g. cardiogenic shock), reduced mesenteric flow (e.g. intra-abdominal hypertension) or mesenteric vasoconstriction (e.g. administration of vasopressors) — **usually, however, it is due to a combination of these factors, developing in the setting of a pre-existing critical illness**.

Mesenteric <u>venous</u> thrombosis can also produce small bowel ischemia. The features and management of this entity differ drastically from the other three. It will be discussed separately below.

The problem is that in clinical practice, outside the textbook, mesenteric ischemia is usually recognized when it has already led to intestinal gangrene. At that stage the Pandora's box of 'sepsis' has been opened and even removal of the entire gangrenous intestine will not always stop the progression to organ failure and death. Even if such physiological consequences can be overcome, the patient commonly becomes an 'intestinal cripple', suffering from the short bowel syndrome.

Have we depressed you enough yet?

Assessing the problem

Typically, the early clinical picture is non-specific: the patient complains of severe abdominal pain — if he can complain at all — and the doctor finds little on physical examination.

Textbooks will tell you that, early on, **the abdominal pain is out of proportion to the clinical findings** — the patient shouts and groans but his abdomen is innocent! However, we have seen patients with almost a *painless* presentation — the (fully alert) patient presents with what looks like 'ileus', doesn't complain about pain, but at laparotomy a segment of his small bowel is already necrotic.

So the key is always to have the suspicion of AMI in your mind! Remember: what the ER doc or internist admits as a "gastroenteritis", or "partial small bowel obstruction" or "ileus" may prove (often too late) to be AMI. Thus, you must resist the natural temptation to ascribe patients' non-specific symptoms to some other benign condition unless the clinical features, including imaging, for the alternative explanation are fully present. **And by the way — in the elderly — the diagnosis of acute gastroenteritis is rarely the final diagnosis; unless it was the wrong diagnosis!**

There are likely to have been preceding symptoms of a similar sort of pain developing with meals and accompanied by weight loss, suggesting pre-existing *mesenteric angina*. There may also be a history of negative investigation of abdominal pain. A history or evidence of **systemic atherosclerotic vascular disease** is almost the rule in patients with mesenteric thrombosis, while a **source for emboli**, such as **atrial fibrillation**, is usually present in patients with mesenteric embolism. This latter group usually also have arterial disease. Low-flow state patients are commonly moribund due to underlying critical disease and are not infrequently found in the cardiac surgery ICU.

Nausea, vomiting, diarrhea (caused by 'reflex bowel emptying') and hematochezia may come late, if ever, and are, again, non-specific. **Physical examination** in the early stages of the process is treacherously benign; peritoneal irritation appears too late, when the bowel is already dead.

Laboratory tests are not much help here either. Many biomarkers have been recommended to diagnose AMI (e.g. procalcitonin, D-dimer, CRP); the measurement of serum lactate has become an obsession among our young colleagues. When positive they are suggestive but non-specific; when negative they are meaningless. However, **extreme leukocytosis is not uncommon even before the intestine dies.**

Plain abdominal X-rays early in the course of the illness are normal. Later, there may be a pattern of adynamic ileus, with visible loops of small bowel and fluid levels, but with gas and feces seen within the normal colon and rectum.

The bottom line is that initially in acute mesenteric ischemia the physical examination and all commonly available X-rays and blood tests may be *normal.*

At this stage, entertaining the diagnosis of mesenteric ischemia, you have two options:

- The first is to enter in the chart "abdominal examination normal; mesenteric ischemia cannot be ruled out; will reassess later". This, you will do only if you are a lazy moron, which, we trust, you are not.
- **The second option — the right one — is to order a CT scan with intravenous contrast**, which has replaced mesenteric catheter angiography as the initial, screening imaging modality in AMI. Although catheter angiography is more specific and accurate, surgeons have been reluctant to offer such an invasive procedure in patients with a non-specific clinical picture.

Unfortunately, the first option is still common in some places — leading to procrastination, late diagnosis and treatment, and a very high mortality rate.

Computed tomography

To be diagnostic, the examination should include (appropriately timed) intravenous contrast ('CT angio'), with the focus on two areas: the bowel wall and mesenteric vessels. Oral contrast, while making the exam more perfect in the eyes of the radiologist, may lead to more unnecessary and risky delay. Simply ask for an *arterial phase CT.*

The commonest finding is bowel wall thickening, which is, however, non-specific. The bowel wall may appear hypodense due to edema or hyperdense when submucosal haemorrhage is present. Contrast enhancement patterns of the affected bowel loops may improve diagnosis: absence of enhancement may mean no flow (dead bowel) while delayed or persistent enhancement may mean low flow (potentially reversible ischemia). **Pneumatosis** and **portal vein gas** are uncommon but specific, albeit late, signs — due to intraluminal gas dissecting into the friable bowel wall and then into the portal venous tributaries. CT angio can also visualize *acute* changes such as emboli within the SMA and provide a map of the distribution of any thrombotic disease in the same vessel; it can also demonstrate *chronic* changes, such as stenosis or occlusion of the chief collateral sources of mesenteric blood supply — the celiac and/or inferior mesenteric arteries. The CT abnormalities are usually apparent but you (and your radiologist) must be alert to the possible diagnosis and look carefully at the images.

Magnetic resonance angiography (MRA) could be superb in imaging mesenteric vessels (with reduced risk of contrast nephrotoxicity) but, like CT angio, is far inferior to conventional angiography in visualizing distal branches. However, in how many hospitals would MRA be available in the middle of the night?

Mesenteric angiography

This was previously the standard investigation for patients with a suspicion of ischemia but it has been superseded by CT angiography in most instances. Nowadays catheter angiography should normally be undertaken only with an intention to treat suitable lesions already identified by CT angio. **To be beneficial the angiogram should be performed before the bowel has become gangrenous. The clock is ticking; every passing minute reduces the chances of the bowel and the patient surviving. (Note that an acute abdomen with peritoneal signs is a contraindication to angiography.)**

The radiologist should start with biplanar angiography (i.e. including a lateral view to show the origins of the SMA and the celiac axis). An occluded ostium of the SMA denotes *thrombosis* and calls for an immediate revascularization procedure (radiological or surgical) — unless there is evidence of a good collateral inflow — the angiography providing the road map for vascular reconstruction. When the ostium is patent the radiologist advances the catheter into the SMA. Note that ostial disease in these patients is often very severe and not readily amenable to percutaneous angioplasty. Don't waste precious time in futile attempts at endovascular revascularisation when surgery is what is really required. An intra-operative retrograde angio is always possible if necessary. *Emboli* lodge distal to the take-off of the middle colic artery, produce a smooth filling defect on the background of a normal SMA, and can be multiple.

Non-operative treatment

In the absence of peritoneal signs, attempts at non-operative treatment may seem reasonable. Unfortunately, even in the best appointed centers with close cooperation between vascular surgeons and skilled interventional radiologists, these attempts utilising stents, thrombolytics and maybe even papaverine in an attempt to overcome vasospasm, simply amount to further dangerous delay in initiating the required laparotomy.

So you see we are not enthusiastic about the use of non-operative measures in this disorder but if you insist on trying then ensure that the patient is well hydrated before going to the angio suite to oppose the nephrotoxic effects of the contrast media. And in the unlikely event of successful transcather management of embolism consider postoperative systemic anticoagulation.

In the event of non-occlusive mesenteric ischemia, the approach involves attempts at restoring compromised hemodynamics. Again in this situation it has been suggested that a papaverine infusion may be useful. We disagree and have never witnessed successful use of this therapy.

To transfer or not to transfer?

Beyond the usual considerations impacting the decision 'to transfer or not' any acutely ill surgical patient (e.g. local availability of advanced supportive care), a common dilemma arises when confronting an AMI patient: should I deal with him here or should I ship him out to a higher-level center where non-invasive and invasive vascular therapies are available?

Well, the decision should be individualized, asking the following questions:

- Does the patient need arteriography plus/minus a transcatheter therapy rather than rushing to the OR?
- Even if an urgent laparotomy were needed — would it involve a revascularization procedure?
- If embolism is suspected as the cause of AMI — are you confident doing SMA embolectomy?
- Of course you can perform bowel resection in your small hospital, but do you have the supportive infrastructure to allow 'second looks' and intensive care?

So, as you see, in general, patients with suspected AMI could benefit from transferal to a higher-level center. But what you do depends on where you practice. Always remember that the gold standard is treatment in a hybrid OR with the services of both a vascular surgeon and an interventional radiologist.

Operative treatment

As we have already told you — peritoneal signs, considered together with a suggestive clinical (and CT) picture, are an indication *not* to do arteriography but to operate; the same applies to failure of the non-operative regimen discussed above.

Through a midline incision assess the viability of the intestine. **In general there are two main possible scenarios: one is that the bowel is *frankly gangrenous* (dead); the second is when the bowel appears *ischemic* (dusky) and of questionable viability**:

- **Frank gangrene of the *entire small bowel*** is usually combined with the same problem in the right colon and **signifies SMA thrombosis**. Theoretically, a patient could survive resection of the entire small bowel and right colon. He may even tolerate a duodenocolic anastomosis while being nutritionally supported at home with total parenteral nutrition (TPN). But the eventual mortality of such an exercise in the average elderly vasculopath approaches 100% and the cost is immense. **Our recommendation to you when involved in a similar situation is to walk out to talk to the family, and explain that anything done will only increase the suffering of their beloved**. If the family wishes so then return to close the abdomen over the dead bowel. Provide a lot of morphine and comfort. **As with everything in life — there are exceptions**: in a relatively young and active patient, and when local circumstances are favorable (we doubt that there are facilities for home TPN in rural Afghanistan or even Eastern Ukraine), you and the family may want to strive for long-term survival.
- **Frank gangrene of a *shorter segment*, or *multiple segments of small bowel*, usually denotes *embolism***. After excising all dead segments carefully examine the remaining bowel. Measure it: how long is it? **Only about half of patients left with less than 1 meter (3 feet) of small bowel will live without TPN (saving the ileocecal valve improves the prognosis)**. Now, observe the remaining bowel. Is it truly non-compromised? Are the mesenteric arcades pulsating well? Feel the SMA at its root — is it vigorously pulsating?

- **Dusky bowel. When you are not happy with the remaining bowel, or when the bowel is not dead but appears ischemic and of questionable viability from the start, what are you to do?** Many strategies have been suggested to assess the bowel: wrap in warm sponges and wait (drinking coffee in the meantime); assess the circulation with intra-operative Doppler; or fluorescein angiography; or pulse oximetry. But in truth none of these can be completely reliable so the pragmatic solution is always a second-look laparotomy 'tomorrow'. The only reason not to go back and look again is if the patient is dead or dying. This strategy allows the maximum length of ultimately viable bowel to be preserved, and we know that each centimetre may be important in those who have had a massive resection (■ Figure 22.1).

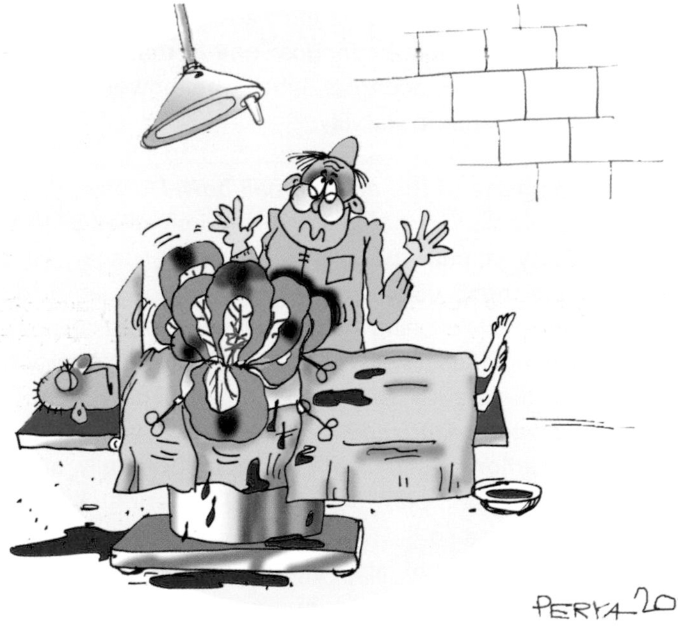

Figure 22.1. "How much should I resect?"

Adjunctive vascular procedures

The ideal setting for surgical improvement of the perfusion of ischemic small bowel is when the operation follows emergency arteriography (plus failed angiographic therapy) and the bowel is viable or doubtful. Obviously, when the bowel is dead it cannot be revived! Arteriography serves as a road map; when the SMA is thrombosed at its origin, a vein or graft bypass, antegrade or retrograde, is indicated to reperfuse it. The two main options here are autogenous vein bypass or externally supported polytetrafluoroethylene (PTFE) inserted in a 'lazy loop' fashion. The origin of these bypass grafts is often determined by the pattern of disease affecting the other intra-abdominal vessels. Usually the iliac vessels are the best source of pulsatile flow but care must be taken when vein is used, to see that it does not kink when the gut is returned to its normal position.

Less commonly you will encounter a picture of SMA embolism. Feel for the SMA just at the base of the mesocolon; if non-pulsatile you'll find it, after incising the peritoneum, to the right (as you look at it from below) of the large, blue superior mesenteric vein. After obtaining control, open the artery transversely and pass up and down a small Fogarty embolectomy balloon catheter. Heparinize the vessels before repairing the arteriotomy.

If you work at an 'ivory tower' the option of **endovascular therapies** may be available as well. Early lysis and stenting of an 'acute on chronic' occlusion of the SMA may obviate the need for laparotomy altogether. **Even if bowel resection is needed, the patient can be transferred directly from the OR to the radiology suite for stenting of the SMA (and/or celiac artery) to improve the blood supply to the remaining, marginally perfused intestine.** (This is why we told you earlier that some patients may do better in an 'ivory tower' than in your little hospital...).

To anastomose or not?

You should be very selective in attempting an anastomosis following any resection of devitalized intestine. The patient must be hemodynamically stable and his nutritional status at least fair. To be hooked-up, the remaining bowel must be unquestionably viable and the peritoneal cavity free of established infection. **Most crucially, the underlying cause of ischemia must have been identified and removed.** The best time to make a decision about an anastomosis is at a 'relook' laparotomy.

Another factor strongly bearing on your decision is the length of the remaining bowel and its predicted postoperative function. When more than half of the small bowel is resected, the resection is considered 'massive'. Restoring intestinal continuity in such cases leads to poorly tolerated and *intractable diarrhea*. And finally, the chief reason not to anastomose the bowel is the possibility that further ischemia may develop.

We recommend, therefore, that whenever the above-mentioned favorable factors are absent, or when resection is massive, the ends of

the remaining bowel should be stapled off and left for a relook laparotomy. Doing this forces you to do a second laparotomy which we believe is required in all but the most exceptional circumstances.

Second-look operations?

A routine planned 'second-look' operation allows direct reassessment of intestinal viability at an early stage, before additional mediators of 'sepsis' have been released, and in a way that aims to preserve the greatest possible length of viable intestine. This concept, which guides our current practice, motivates many surgeons to re-explore their patients routinely after 24 to 48 hours.

This is an ideal situation for an '**abbreviated laparotomy**' at the initial surgery. The sections of bowel that are definitely dead are excised after stapling and dividing the bowel. The stapled ends are simply dropped back into the peritoneal cavity. A delay of 24-48 hours allows the patient's deranged physiology to recover before a second look. At the relaparotomy, originally questionable sections of intestine will have declared themselves viable or not, and the operation can proceed to anastomosis, or resection and anastomosis or, in the case of massive resection, to the formation of a double-barrel stoma to avert the risk of troublesome diarrhea. This last procedure allows eventual anastomosis, when the patient has fully recovered, and the short gut has maximally adapted, to restore intestinal continuity without resort to a major laparotomy.

Obviously, if you plan a second-look operation there is no need to close the abdomen at the end of the first procedure; instead, treat the abdomen as a laparostomy until re-exploration, relieving any intra-abdominal hypertension to improve mesenteric blood flow further. (An alternative would be to close the abdomen and perform a 'second-look' laparoscopy, but we are not persuaded that this is a good idea.)

To sum up — it appears that in most patients a second-look procedure is indicated. In patients whose ischemia is due to embolism, a postoperative search for sources of emboli seems prudent.

Mesenteric venous thrombosis

In this rarer condition, the so called 'DVT of the abdomen', the venous outflow of the bowel is occluded. The clinical presentation is less striking and non-specific. Abdominal pain and varying gastrointestinal symptoms may last a few days until eventually the intestines are compromised, and peritoneal signs develop.

Mesenteric venous thrombosis may be idiopathic (i.e. the doctor is an idiot — ignorant of the underlying reason), but commonly an underlying hypercoagulable state (such as polycythemia rubra vera) or sluggish portal flow due to hepatic cirrhosis, is present. It has also been described in the postoperative phase after upper abdominal procedures such as splenectomy. It can be iatrogenic as well, due to operative injury and ligation of the SMV. Finally, note that it may be the mode of presentation of a previously occult cancer originating in the breast, lung, prostate or elsewhere; look at the chest CT!

Typically, many of these patients are admitted to the medical floor with a surgeon consulted much later — to operate for non-viable bowel. **However, an early trip to a contrast-enhanced CT scan may achieve an earlier diagnosis, helping to avoid an operation altogether and improve survival.**

Characteristic findings on CT consist of a triad:

- A hypodensity in the trunk of the superior mesenteric vein.
- Associated intraperitoneal fluid.
- Thickened segment of small bowel.

Thus, anytime we review a CT in a patient with a non-specific abdominal picture (e.g. alleged ileus), we specifically look at the SMV, and force the radiologist to do likewise. Remember: radiologists read numerous images a day; if you do not ask them specific questions they can miss significant findings...

With the above findings, and in the absence of peritoneal signs, full systemic anticoagulation with heparin may result in a spontaneous resolution of the process. The role of systemic or selective angiographic thrombolysis is not clear. **Failure to improve or the development of peritoneal signs mandates an operation.**

At surgery, you'll find some free serosanguinous peritoneal fluid; the small bowel will be thick, edematous, dark-blue but not frankly dead, with the involved intestinal segment poorly demarcated. **Arterial pulsations will be**

present and thrombosed veins seen. You may need to resect the affected segment, but this decision, to resect bowel, despite its horrible appearance and your surgical temptation, is difficult, unless it's clearly dead. As to whether or not to anastomose and the need for a second look — apply the same judgment as discussed above for arterial insufficiency. Postoperative anticoagulation is mandatory to prevent progression of the thrombotic process. Adding a venous thrombectomy is advocated by some, so is intra-operative thrombolysis; the real benefits of these controversial approaches are unknown.

To sum up...

In most places the mortality rate of acute mesenteric ischemia is still prohibitive. Why? Because surgeons fail to do the following:

- Suspect ischemia before intestinal gangrene develops.
- Proceed with diagnostic/therapeutic angiography.
- Improve intestinal perfusion during laparotomy.
- Exteriorize the bowel or execute a second-look operation.

So here is the 'catch 22': if you wish to see survivors of this horrendous condition you will have to be aggressive. Three misconceptions about AMI exist: it is rare; diagnosis is impossible; and treatment is futile. We hope that by following the advice given here you will be able to see things more clearly.

On the other hand, these patients rarely have simple pathology. They commonly suffer from multisystem disease and even in receipt of optimal care they will have a high mortality. Regrettably, in many patients this condition seems likely to remain an agonal complaint. As our mentors taught us: "you can't save 'em all!"

"The man is as old as his arteries."

Thomas Sydenham

Chapter 23

Hepatic emergencies

Erik Schadde

The liver confounds the surgeon's dependence on anatomy.
J. Foster

When I was an intern I overheard a mid-level resident saying to the chief resident that there is a 'liver patient' in the emergency room. My chief resident appeared gloomy and concerned. I didn't understand what 'liver patient' referred to in this context. Liver trauma? A liver tumor? Soon I learned: 'liver patient' refers to those with chronic liver disease, cirrhosis and portal hypertension or those after a liver transplant. In short, any patient who belongs to the hepatology or liver transplant service.

In this chapter I will address first the acute problems arising in the chronic liver patient. Hepatic trauma will be addressed next. Finally, I will look at some miscellaneous conditions of the liver that may present as an emergency.

The 'liver patient' — chronically diseased hepatic parenchyma

In the emergency room

The patients with chronic liver disease you are called to see in the emergency room usually fall into one of two categories: either they have a problem that the internists can no longer manage or they are in some way involved with liver transplantation — the surgical treatment of end-stage liver disease since the 1980s. It is important that the latter group of patients are seen by their respective transplant physicians. Decompensated patients on the liver transplant list may need to be 'deactivated' (i.e. removed from that holy list) and have their MELD score [1] upgraded. **Decompensated patients with chronic liver disease are generally managed by internists or even better — hepatologists.**

Variceal bleeding

Esophageal varices are the source of upper gastrointestinal (GI) bleeding in about 90% of patients with cirrhosis and portal hypertension. The emergency room usually calls the interventional gastroenterologist, who performs endoscopic variceal rubber band ligation and (rarely) sclerotherapy. If they can't visualize the bleeding and control it, you, the surgeon, may be called and asked whether you can offer a surgical solution — an emergency surgical shunt for example. **Your answer in 2020, however, is almost always "no"!**

The space that surgical shunt procedures still occupy in traditional surgical textbooks is inversely correlated with their use in real life. They are sometimes indicated in *elective* situations where TIPS (transjugular intrahepatic portosystemic shunts) are not possible. However, emergency surgery in this situation is out of the question because you will almost certainly bring the patient to the verge of death.

Your surgical advice however is still needed. **Remember that there is still a minority of chronic liver disease patients in whom the upper GI bleeding is caused by peptic ulcers, Mallory-Weiss tears or Dieulafoy lesions and not variceal disease despite their cirrhosis and portal hypertension.**

Your advice should be to perform another round of gastric irrigation and another endoscopy. You may improve conditions with two simple interventions before the second endoscopy: i.v. administration of somatostatin (or equivalent terlipressin) and forced gastric emptying using erythromycin followed by a 30-minute waiting period. If this fails again — **recommend moving to the interventional radiology (IR) suite to perform an emergency TIPS procedure**. The TIPS creates a connection between the hepatic and portal venous systems to provide central decompression of the hypertensive portal system. It may increase pre-existing encephalopathy or lead to new-onset encephalopathy and therefore the indication must be carefully considered. In Child-Pugh C (see ■ Table 23.1 on page 314) cirrhosis patients with elevated bilirubin >10mg/dL (171μmol/L) undergoing TIPS, there

1 MELD — Model of Endstage Liver Disease based on the patient's age, bilirubin, creatinine and INR levels. To calculate go to: http://www.mdcalc.com/meld-score-model-for-end-stage-liver-disease-12-and-older/.

is a real risk that the liver will decompensate. **But when sclerotherapy and variceal banding fail twice, this is the logical next step in an emergency despite this risk**.

However, you may become a little bit more involved if your interventional radiologist does not routinely do TIPS or (even better... and more common) there is nobody around who has ever heard about it. Your hemorrhaging patient will have to be transferred to a different center (only God can help the patient if such a center does not exist in your country) and a **balloon tamponade will be necessary to temporize the situation** — and it is possible that the emergency room will need your assistance for that. It is rare nowadays to find any surgeon who has placed more than a few, if any, balloon tubes (Sengstaken-Blakemore or Linton-Nachlas) in his life, so below are a few words about the technique.

Advice on the technique of balloon catheter placement:

- **Make sure you insert balloon tubes only after the patient has been intubated and the airway is protected**. (BTW, patients with a massive upper GI hemorrhage should have already been intubated for the endoscopy.)
- Find out what type of balloon tube you have available, take the time to understand the different access channels and the different balloon tubes, and test the integrity of the balloons. **It is useful to keep the balloons in the freezer, as it makes them rigid and easier to insert**.
- Insert the tube with the help of a laryngoscope and *Magill's* forceps, or — even better — side-by-side with endoscopic assistance, because your endoscopist is already there. Test the position of the gastric lumen with a stethoscope, as with an NG tube. If in doubt about the position get an X-ray.
- Inflate the gastric balloon stepwise to a 200-250cc final volume; if necessary, stop and readjust if there is resistance. (I admitted an unstable cirrhotic patient with a balloon tube from an outside hospital. He had a torn gastroesophageal junction and died after salvage surgery.) Adjust the tension to the gastroesophageal junction by fixing the tube to the patient (*not to the bed*), with the split tennis-ball technique — using a 'bite block' to provide counter resistance.
- If the patient stabilizes, don't inflate the esophageal balloon if you are using a Sengstaken-Blakemore tube (the Linton-Nachlas doesn't have an esophageal balloon, which is why I prefer it — ■ Figure 23.1), but leave it alone. In most cases there is no need to inflate the esophageal balloon. But if you get the impression that the esophageal bleeding hasn't stopped, connect the esophageal balloon (with a three-way stopcock) to a manometer and **do not inflate above 35mmHg**.

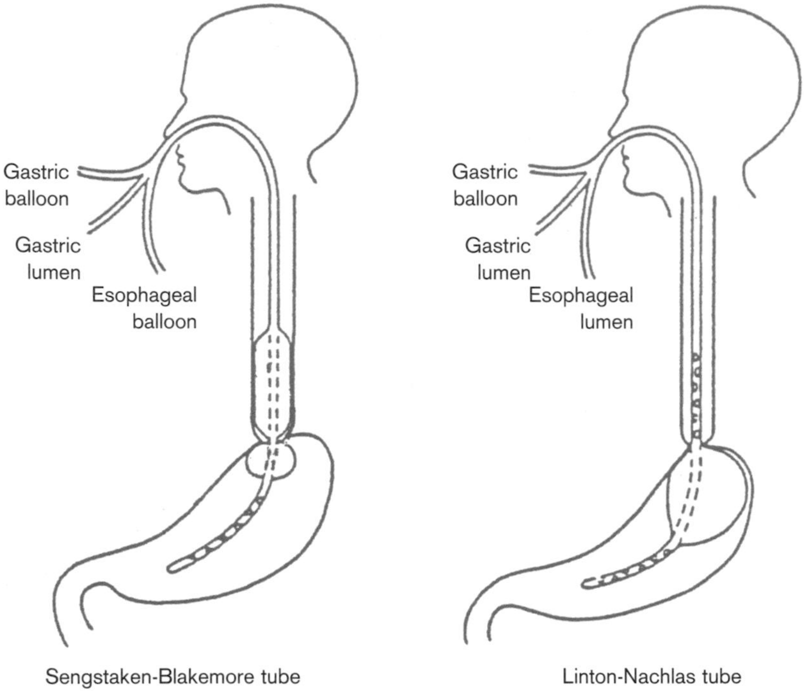

Figure 23.1. Sengstaken-Blakemore vs. Linton-Nachlas tubes.

- If the patient does not stabilize, deflate the balloon, take it out and perform another endoscopy and if visualization is still bad, perform a CT arteriogram or regular arteriogram, because you might be dealing with a bleeding peptic ulcer or a Dieulafoy gastric lesion.

The esophageal 'hemostatic' stent

Patients do not always survive the ordeal. And there remain difficult decisions further down the road from this emergency. For example, **a massive hemorrhage from an ulcer developing at a variceal site banded by gastroenterology**. In this situation we have advocated a newly available **variceal stent**. Originally designed for blind insertion in the ambulance, it was, however, never used in that setting. But in the emergency room after intubation it may be a promising option to stop esophageal bleeding from ulcers or varices in severe reflux esophagitis, where rubber bands are not applicable. The device comes with a temporary Linton balloon to define the esophagogastric junction. The device is introduced over an endoscopically-placed guidewire. Having inflated the gastric balloon, under gentle traction, the large (30 x 135mm) covered self-expanding metal stent is released (■ Figure 23.2). The stent can be left in place

a Introduction of the delivery system over the guidewire. This step follows previous insertion of the guidewire through the working channel of the endoscope.

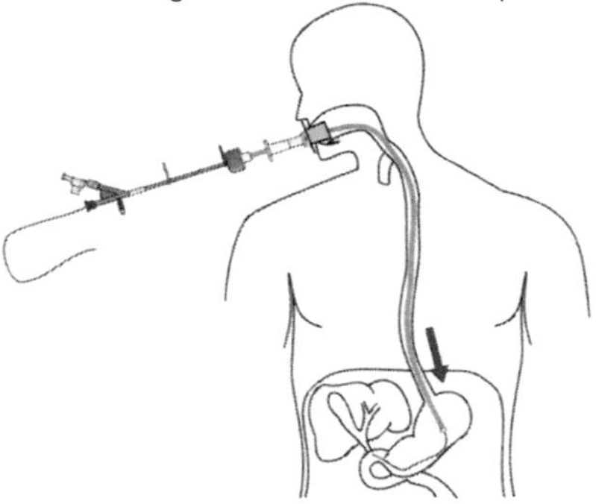

The protecting plate touches the mouthpiece.

b Fixation of the delivery system in the stomach.

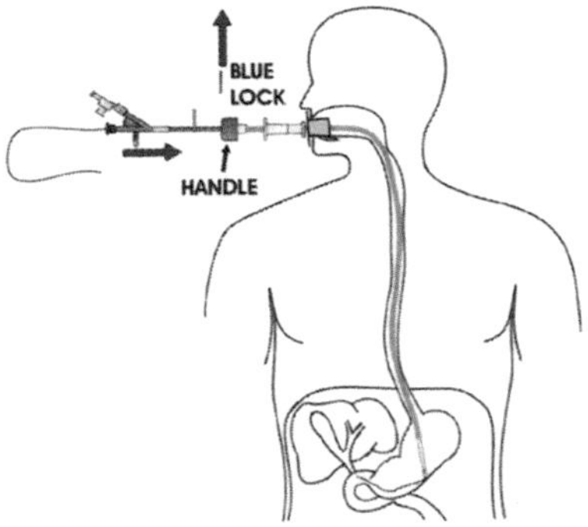

Remove the blue lock. Push the balloon out of the sheath until the white lock touches the sheath handle.

c Fixation of the delivery system in the stomach.

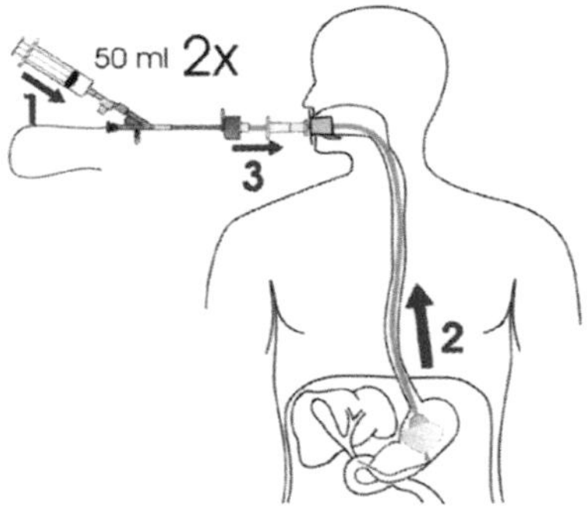

1st step: Inflation of the balloon. 2nd step: Fixation of the ballooon in the cardia by pulling it back. 3rd step: Move the protecting plate to the mouthpiece and lock it.

d Stent deployment.

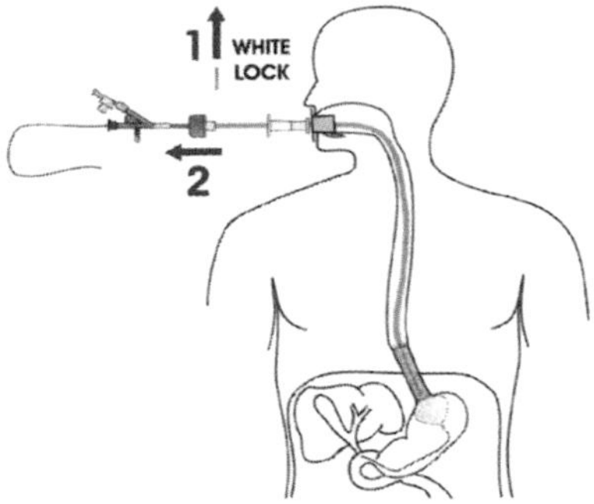

1st step: Remove the white lock. 2nd step: Pull the sheath handle until it reaches the Y-connector.

e Delivery system removal.

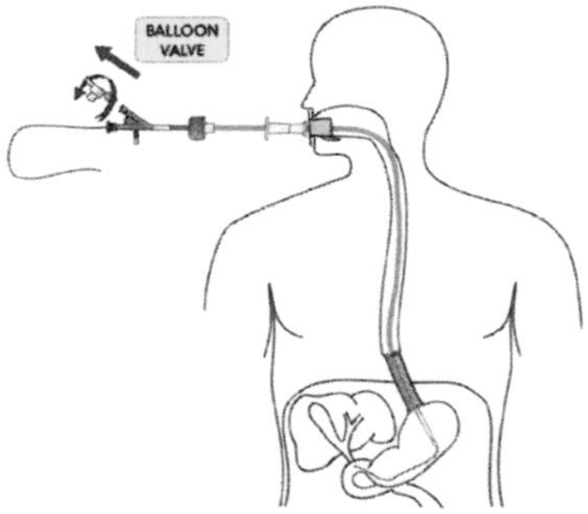

Unscrew the balloon valve and remove it. The balloon gets empty (cca 30 sec).

f Delivery system removal.

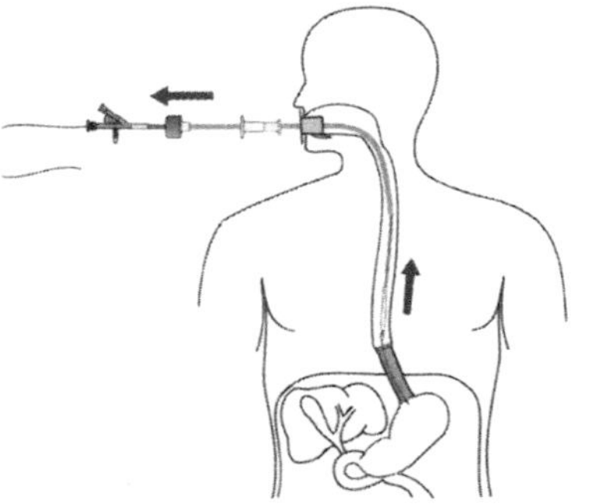

Remove the delivery system. Finally, remove the guidewire.

Figure 23.2. The esophageal hemostatic stent. ***Promoted and introduced to me by Christoph Gubler, MD, at the University Hospital of Zurich.***

for 1 week. Usually this time interval is enough to come up with a better treatment plan...

The patient with cirrhosis and portal hypertension who needs emergency general surgery

The liver patient does not make an attractive surgical candidate — for any surgery except for one operation: **transplantation**. **Therefore, elective surgery should be avoided if possible; even a dental procedure may end up with a blood transfusion due to coagulopathy**. However, liver patients not infrequently present with general surgery emergencies and a general surgeon needs to know what to do about these.

A time-honored and well-validated tool to assess the risk of liver patients is the Child-Pugh score (■ Table 23.1). Although initially developed

Table 23.1. The Child-Pugh classification.*

	Score**		
	1	2	3
Bilirubin (mg%)	<2	2-3	>3
Albumin (g%)	>3.5	2.8-3.5	<2.8
INR	<1.7	1.7-2.3	>2.3
Encephalopathy	None	Mild	Marked
Ascites	None	Mild	Marked

* Charles Gardner Child III (1908-1991) was Professor of Surgery at the University of Michigan. R.N.H. Pugh published his classification in 1973 (Pugh *et al*. Transection of the esophagus for bleeding esophageal varices. *Br J Surg* 1973; 60: 649-90).

** The individual scores are summed and then grouped as:

<7 = Child A
7-9 = Child B
>9 = Child C

(A Child C classification forecasts a survival of less than 12 months) in the context of surgery for portal hypertension, the score has been useful to generations of surgeons to assess the mortality risk of chronic liver patients undergoing anything from a hernia repair to a Whipple procedure.

The score categorizes patients as follows:

- **Child A**: those with an acceptable risk for any general surgery procedure.
- **Child B**: those where the indications must be very selective due to an increased risk of decompensation.
- **Child C**: those who should not undergo any procedure due to very high mortality.

The score is useful, even though some of the parameters assessed depend on the clinician's subjective judgment. Some authors prefer the MELD score — consisting of three laboratory values (International Normalized Ratio [INR], bilirubin and creatinine). MELD reflects 3-month mortality on the liver transplant waiting list. The MELD score (see the link to the calculator on page 310 and ■ Figure 23.3) was introduced to rationalize organ utilization among centers who 'cheated' by transplanting patients who were less sick than others. A score that depends only on laboratory values indeed requires minimal subjective judgment. However, to judge the severity of liver disease for general surgery candidacy, the Child score is perfect and doesn't need any improvement. **There are some tools that can hardly be improved upon, such as hammers — the Child score is such a tool**.

Typically, you are called because a Child B patient has an incarcerated inguinal hernia and his internist wants it fixed. **Make sure you explain that the hernia repair may easily kill him, get an experienced anesthesiologist involved and, if you can, perform the repair under local anesthesia**. Correcting coagulopathy with fresh frozen plasma (FFP) is difficult and frequently does not help; vitamin K should be obligatory but frequently doesn't help either in improving coagulopathy in cirrhotic patients.

By the way, what you learn when you do liver transplants is that a liver patient with an INR of 2.5 is not necessarily coagulopathic like a patient who takes coumadin and has an INR of 2.5. While correcting the INR with FFP in anticoagulated patients may sometimes be indicated and effective, most surgeons dealing with cirrhotic patients do not attempt this before the operation. Giving people 6 units of FFP upfront will volume-overload them, cause ascites and more bleeding from venous congestion. I always avoid

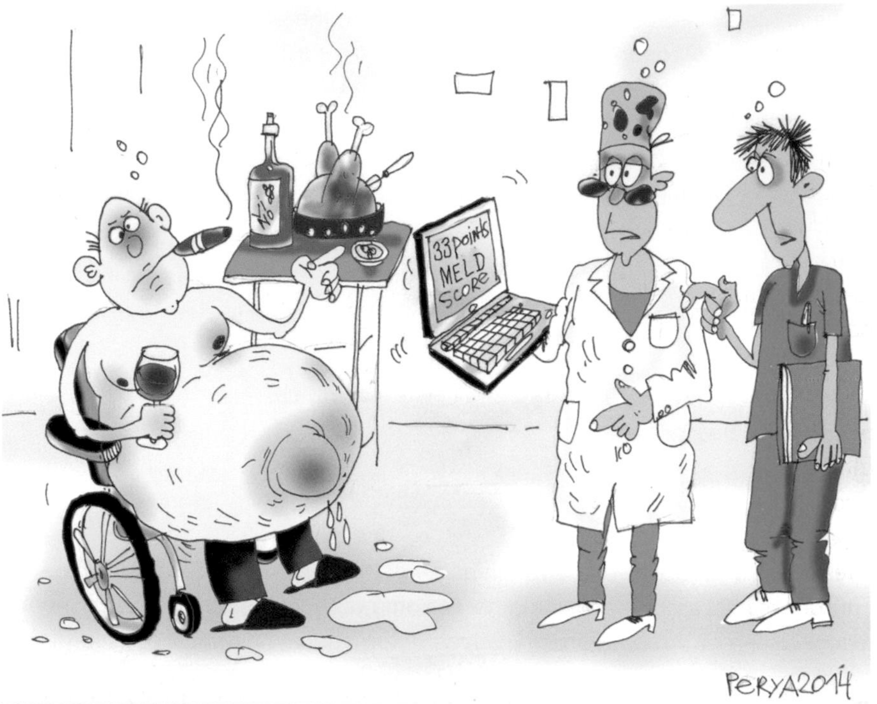

Figure 23.3. "Sir, you have 33 points on the MELD score. We need... to find a new liver for you. Perhaps from China?" Patient: "Actually, I would like another piece of chicken. And get me some better wine. This one sucks!"

giving FFP pre-operatively. Now you will ask me about the evidence... ("**Definition of a modern surgeon: one whose ignorance is due to lack of experience, but evidence-based**"), but it is an area where it is difficult to perform a clinical trial.

Obsessive hemostasis and meticulous respect for peritoneal integrity to avoid postoperative leak of ascites (leading to its infection) are the mainstays of successful surgical management. These patients tend to develop postoperative hematomas, infectious complications, ascites and renal failure. **Fluid management should be restrictive**; low doses of peri-operative diuretics are helpful in correcting the volume retention physiology found in chronic liver disease. Make sure your residents avoid volume overloading at night when called by the nurses about oliguria. **Unlike in the routine postop surgical patient, oliguria here usually means 'Lasix®' rather than 'lactated Ringer's'...**

Child C patients have a short life expectancy (unless transplanted...) **and they should only be operated on if there is no other option and should be clearly informed about their high mortality risk**.

Typically, due to the large-volume ascites, Child C patients have **umbilical hernia emergencies**, that require emergency surgery. I have spent many hours at the bedside of patients high on the transplant list slowly reducing a few loops of bowel that had incarcerated, but were not strangulated, to spare them the umbilical hernia repair that could easily bring them to the ICU with a 20 MELD point gain within 24 hours. At the same time I have seen courageous (reckless? inexperienced?) young transplant surgeons taking Child C patients to the OR arguing that in the event of decompensation "they are already listed for transplantation". It is important to consider here that the outcome for patients who are transplanted after decompensation is dramatically worse.

Another typical emergency for a jaundiced Child C patient with massive ascites is a sprinkling little fountain of ascites at a thinned-out skin ulceration at the base of a large umbilical hernia filled with ascites. I strongly recommend that you do not perform a conventional umbilical hernia repair here, but just suture the folded skin over the ulcer under local anesthesia and put the patient on antibiotics to prevent bacterial peritonitis. The dermis has a lot of mechanical stability and ultimately these lesions can heal.

On occasion, however, you will have no choice but to bite the bullet as in a recent case of colon perforation during elective colonoscopy as part of the work-up for a liver transplant. When you take these patients to the operating room, dissect very carefully and be aware of the venous collaterals of the abdominal wall and the retroperitoneum. **Among the many energy device gadgets you are offered in a modern hospital, the bipolar-based LigaSure® is really helpful in this situation**.

During colon surgery in liver patients with ascites, the question of primary intestinal anastomosis versus stoma formation comes up. While I would do an elective colonic anastomosis in the presence of ascites, **an emergency situation (i.e. perforated diverticulitis) calls for diversion or exteriorization — especially if the patient is hypoalbuminemic**. Make sure, however, that the ascites is meticulously controlled with drains when you leave a patient with ascites with a stoma — to allow healing of the stoma and avoid bacterial peritonitis. **Keep the drains *in situ* until the stoma is well healed**.

The protein losses of prolonged drainage in patients with ascites are prohibitive and I would not drain a standard colon anastomosis otherwise, but rather intermittently and regularly tap the ascites (every day or every 2 days) to prevent leakage through the incision and allow early recognition of anastomotic leaks via infected ascites. This holds true for many other operations, including partial hepatectomy, in liver patients with ascites.

At any rate, if your Child C patient survives the first few weeks after surgery, you and the patient have been very lucky. You should present these patients on your weekly M & M as an S & S ('Survival and Success'...).

The liver patient emergency on the ward

Surgeons may be called too, for a very specific emergency — GI bleeding in patients with cirrhosis and an ileostomy or colostomy. Since I have seen a few patients almost die from this, I think it is worth talking about. See the case below.

A patient with chronic liver disease, known portal hypertension, and varices which had never bled, bleeds through his colostomy. At upper endoscopy a source of bleeding was not identified. Next you hear that the patient became unstable with another few liters of blood loss but the source remains mysterious. 'Bleeding scans' are being performed, a trans-stoma colonoscopy scheduled and a capsule endoscopy is planned — which is exactly the time point at which you decide to just go up there and see the patient yourself.

To make the diagnosis, you have to do the unprecedented and really examine the patient and take off the stoma bag — which is a huge effort and you may dirty your hands! You will find a peristomal varicosity that is directly dripping blood into the ostomy bag. Now you ask the nurse for a needle holder and a *Vicryl®* suture and you overrun, with deep locking bites, the bleeding area. Such varicosities may be familiar to the stoma nurses, but they are usually not around when patients bleed. And — as we all know — regular ward nurses do not generally change stoma bags any more. The surgical consult resident long ago lost the habit to thoroughly examine the stoma and the resident who takes over the next shift never actually saw the patient and is only able to tell you that there is a capsule endoscopy scheduled for the next day. **The shift mentality — hallelujah!**

The liver patient emergency in the operating room

We sometimes stumble across patients with portal hypertension in the operating room, either because we were unaware of their liver disease and portal hypertension, because we were led awry by an error in diagnosis or because one of our fellow surgeons calls us unprepared and gives us the honor of consulting the so called 'liver expert'.

You should not miss the fact that a patient has cirrhosis with portal hypertension during the pre-operative work-up. There are too many red lights along the way. If your patient has no stigmata of liver disease like spider nevi, ascites, encephalopathy, edema, cachexia and flapping tremor (when was the last time you have elicited flapping tremor?), he surely must have undergone some routine laboratory test like a platelet count, INR, or bilirubin or creatinine level — which are abnormal. **But remember: when the diagnosis of cirrhosis is missed, laboratory abnormalities are generally not overlooked, but misattributed**. In those cases, the thrombocytopenia is due to immune thrombocytopenic purpura (ITP); the INR is high due to oral anticoagulation for atrial fibrillation (oh, and the patient mentioned that he only had to take 2mg of coumadin once per week); the patient has been told that the hyperbilirubinemia is due to Gilbert syndrome; and there are numerous reasons to have renal insufficiency.

However, the interesting scenario I found myself in several times is when the patient known to you as having cirrhosis but the risk is underestimated (see the case below).

You have a Child A patient who needs a wedge resection of a single hepatocellular carcinoma lesion. According to the Barcelona Clinic Algorithm, you diligently check portal wedge pressures and the gradient with the CVP. At 8mmHg the gradient is absolutely normal in your patients (up to 12mmHg); furthermore, it was done by the new interventional radiology attending who was trained at the big center downtown. Upon entering the abdomen you come across some slightly enlarged veins which are bleeding slightly more than they should. Surprised, you go back to the CT scan on the computer screen and you see that the spleen is around 12cm. Because the venous phase of the CT scan was not well timed, the varices do not seem quite as impressive as they appear in reality.

Comforted by the 'normal' value of the pre-operative portocaval gradient, you decide to continue with the exploration. The omental veins are engorged as well and when you detach the omentum from the gallbladder bed (years ago the patient underwent a cholecystectomy) there is some bleeding. Before you even start your hepatic ultrasound to find the lesion you want to resect, you have lost a liter of blood. Despite these red lights you continue heroically. At the end of the procedure, the patient, who could have had radiofrequency ablation or transarterial chemoembolization, has lost 2L of blood, develops ascites and temporary renal failure, and spends a month in the hospital despite the best peri-operative management. He is lucky to survive!

Remember: single tests may be wrong. And it is not too late to stop a planned operation after the exploratory laparotomy.

Liver trauma (see also ➲ Chapter 30)

Happily enough, the majority of acutely injured livers have a normal parenchyma, unless you work in the old trauma center downtown that receives the homeless alcoholic run over by a car while the posh next door level 1 trauma center receives the photo model who drove over him with her Maserati and has a concussion.

Blunt liver trauma

In blunt liver injury, there are **three different possible mechanisms**:

- Anterior/posterior impact injuries like the typical steering wheel 'bear claw injuries'.
- T-bone impact injuries generally result in lateral serial rib fractures and a transverse rupture of the liver along the division line of the superior and inferior segments, and may result in severe injuries of the right lobe.
- **The most significant injury to the liver results from an extreme deceleration** and vascular avulsion from the vena cava which typically results in massive immediate exsanguination.

Prior to the advent of CT, many patients with blood in their diagnostic peritoneal lavage underwent laparotomy. Frequently, no more was found than a laceration of the liver or the spleen which would have stopped bleeding spontaneously — but they were treated with packing and hemostasis. We know now that the great majority of these laparotomies were non-therapeutic as far as the liver was concerned.

Nowadays, liver lacerations are graded by a CT scan. Grade I or II injuries can be managed conservatively (unless there is an additional injury that is non-liver-related), while injuries above Grade III may require surgical intervention in a little more than half of the patients. **Therefore, you have to know how to distinguish a Grade III or higher injury from a lesser injury.**

What is a Grade III liver injury by CT?

- **Subcapsular hematoma** >50% or expanding.
- **Intraparenchymal hematoma** >10cm.
- **Laceration** >3cm in depth.

If you encounter a ≥Grade III injury, but the patient is well and there is no other reason to take him to the operating room, you may safely observe him. **However, if the patient with a ≥Grade III liver injury 'turns a hair', in terms of hemodynamic stability, it is safer to take him to the operating room. Of course, if the abdomen is distended and there is a lot of blood in the abdomen on CT, you will ignore your laceration grading and explore the patient. The bottom line is that injury grading by CT is a guide only and what matters most is the clinical condition of the patient.**

Now, what are the surgical steps to consider in the injured liver?

- Packing to obtain hemostasis.
- Mobilization of the liver and opening of the lesser sac.
- Surgical control of bleeding:
  - if necessary *resectional debridement*;
  - if necessary control of arterial and portal inflow and selective clamping.
- Re-exploration if the viability of liver tissue is questionable.

As straightforward as this sounds, a recipe like this can result in a disastrous outcome in the hands of surgeons inexperienced with the liver. What has made people underestimate the value of proper training in liver surgery in the management of trauma is **the myth that any liver trauma can be fixed by packing alone** — see the case below.

As a freshly graduated transplant surgeon I worked in Indochina with an American veteran surgeon who had been to many theaters of war and humanitarian disasters, had graduated from several fellowships and might easily have been one of the most experienced surgeons I have ever worked with. I was sure he would never have to summon *me* for help... but one night he called me in: a 16-year-old girl had been involved in a bus injury and was brought in, in an unstable condition, to our little 'trauma center'. On exploration she had a 30cm ruptured subcapsular hematoma from a direct impact injury. My partner had packed the liver well by carefully placing laparotomy pads around the liver; relatives had donated full blood to keep her alive but despite the transfusion of four units she had become unstable in the early morning hours. We re-explored her together; the extensive arterial bleeding from the large capsular defect was obvious to somebody who had just learned how to transplant and resect lots of livers, and a line of running sutures with a large MH needle along the arterial bleeders fixed the ongoing blood loss almost immediately. The girl recovered with one more exploration to remove the packs.

The lesson here is that arterial bleeding from a liver injury cannot easily be fixed by packing alone.

This is why, BTW, many centers routinely perform angiography and embolization — as needed — in all patients undergoing perihepatic packing. However, perihepatic packing usually stops bleeding from low-pressure venous injuries and is the preferred method especially for surgeons not experienced in liver surgery. And the key is to always pack early!

In complex liver injuries, suture ligation of the bleeding source is the key to achieving a good outcome for patients. Similarly, resectional debridement minimizes the amount of necrotic liver tissue that might serve as a source of bile leaks and infections. **Packing liver injuries frequently serves as damage control in patients who are hypothermic and coagulopathic. It is not a mistake to then get the surgeons who have the most experience with liver surgery involved in re-exploration. Or ship out!**

Bleeding that you cannot stop by packing and suture ligation is rare in liver trauma; however, it does occur. There is a common misconception that the hepatic artery may be ligated when bleeding does not stop. Historically, occlusion of the *common* hepatic artery has been described, because collateral flow is maintained through the gastroduodenal artery, thereby bleeding can be slowed or stopped without completely abolishing arterial inflow. This sounds great in theory **but every time I have seen the common hepatic artery injured and not reconstructed, the outcome was dismal**.

Here are some general rules about the vascular supply of the liver in trauma:

- Vascular inflow into the liver should not be occluded once and for all in trauma, neither on the portal venous, nor on the arterial side.
- Complete occlusion of the common hepatic artery may well result in postoperative liver failure, intrahepatic cholangiopathy, cholangitis and abscesses.
- Complete and sudden occlusion of portal venous flow will result in massive liver necrosis with hemodynamic instability and sepsis.

Penetrating liver trauma

Penetrating injuries to the parenchyma are much more problematic when high-velocity missiles are involved due to the large amount of energy deposited and the ensuing cavity with a lot of tissue necrosis.

Usually packing as immediate damage control, hemodynamic resuscitation and, in selected patients, resectional debridement are the way to go. Low-velocity gunshot wounds rarely result in problems, except for hematomas. The associated chest trauma, however, should not be underestimated; while this has already been picked up by the pneumothorax found on the chest X-ray (and treated), remember that gunshot wounds through the liver typically transverse the diaphragm as well.

There are three major scares, that challenge even the experienced trauma surgeon with some liver surgery abilities:

- **Hepatic artery and bile duct injuries** may cause extensive bleeding and make visualization of the not-pre-dissected porta hepatis extremely difficult.
- **Portal vein injuries** may be difficult to visualize and repair, especially if they are behind the pancreatic head. ("I do know that it is harder to control bleeding from the back side of the portal vein than it is to land a 737 with an engine on fire." Richard C. Karl.)
- **Retrohepatic vena cava injuries** may result in massive bleeding if they do not remain contained in the retroperitoneum.

For management of these situations, you may need a temporary vascular occlusion maneuver. You have to have a decent amount of experience with three maneuvers. If you don't — get help early enough. If such help is not available — call the Priest or the Rabbi…or the *Imam*:

- **Pringle maneuver**: rapid placement of an umbilical tape around the porta hepatis to stop vascular inflow and allow the dissection of portal structures. Limit clamping to 15 minutes if you can and isolate injured structures as soon as you can, to avoid global ischemia.
- **Cattell-Braasch maneuver**: to expose injuries to the portal vein and the pancreatic head you have to be able to rapidly perform a complete medial visceral rotation on the right side of the abdomen. The right colon is mobilized and an extended Kocher maneuver performed to mobilize the duodenum. The root of the small bowel mesentery is mobilized up to the superior mesenteric artery and inferior border of the pancreas. Now you may control the portal vein with finger compression and expose the inferior vena cava which is frequently injured as well.
- **Heaney-maneuver**: mobilization of the portal hepatis, the right lobe of the liver, the infrahepatic inferior vena cava and the suprahepatic inferior vena cava to perform **total vascular exclusion** of the liver in extensive vascular injuries of the liver and the vena cava.

Patients with penetrating trauma requiring any of these maneuvers are rare… and so are the survivors!

Emergencies arising from hepatic lesions

A trained surgeon knows how to do it; an educated surgeon knows why you do it.

Rodney Peyton

These are exceedingly rare, but it is good to know them well.

'Ruptured' hepatic cysts

This is one of the most common questions by patients who have been diagnosed with incidental hepatic cysts: will it rupture? Or rather: what happens when it ruptures? The truth is, hepatic cysts almost never rupture.

So you will hear the question from the patient with a large incidentally discovered asymptomatic cyst — whether he/she may continue taking Taekwondo or kick-boxing classes? While some surgeons use scenarios like these to scare people into performing surgery on simple cysts, I have yet to see a hepatic cyst rupture from the practice of martial arts. I would avoid fear-mongering along these lines and tell patients they may continue to do everything they have done in the past even after having been diagnosed with a hepatic cyst.

Despite the above, every 5 years or so, I see a patient with acute abdominal pain who is admitted with a disintegrated hepatic cyst, some free abdominal fluid and a thin membrane hanging from the liver on the CT scan. **My recommendation: check serology for *Echinococcus*, explore the liver laparoscopically, wash out the abdomen, culture the fluid and resect the cyst wall**. Because this is an extremely rare event there are no reliable data on this versus other approaches, but it saves you a lot of headaches. Ruptured echinococcal cysts may present in patients with anaphylactic shock. I saw it once in my life in Switzerland where *Echinococcus multilocularis* is endemic.

Liver abscesses

The diagnosis of hepatic abscess is made by ultrasound or CT in a patient with fevers and abdominal pain. **As usual it is worth looking at the images carefully as your residents may call a hepatic abscess what is actually a 'subphrenic' or 'subhepatic' abscess**. Spilled stones after a previous cholecystectomy, cholecystitis, any source of abdominal infection like appendicitis, deep surgical space infections, perforated diverticulitis and inflammatory bowel disease may cause subphrenic and subhepatic abscesses in the peritoneal spaces above and below the liver that are tightly sealed off by the bulge of liver parenchyma. A thorough work-up of the history of the patient and the laboratory and imaging data should guide you to the diagnosis.

Most true liver abscesses in the western world are pyogenic and amoebic abscesses occur mostly in third-world countries. While amoebic abscesses almost always respond to antibiotic treatment (with metronidazole), pyogenic abscesses are more tricky. While some may simply be aspirated with a needle under US guidance, and resolve with antibiotic therapy, **very large ones and especially loculated ones usually require transcutaneous interventional drainage**.

Surgery is rarely indicated: non-resolving perihepatic abscesses are best addressed through a limited laparotomy (or laparoscopy…) with adequate antibiotic coverage, careful debridement and drain placement. The extraperitoneal approaches (plus/minus rib resection) belong to the skill set of a different generation of general surgeons and are not practiced any more.

When a hepatic abscess is drained surgically, I recommend poking a straight finger into the usually loculated collection to break it up and refrain from tearing apart the inner walls of the loculated collections with a curved finger, since this will invariably destroy the Glissonian structures crossing the abscess and cause bile leaks.

Hemobilia

Hemobilia is most frequently a complication of interventional radiology procedures and is treated by interventional radiologists as well. As a surgeon you simply need to recognize the entity, know how it is diagnosed and pass it on to the specialty who fixes it. **Most frequently, patients present with stigmata of GI bleeding like melena, anemia and sometimes hemodynamic instability and a recent history of instrumentation of the liver — either by transcutaneous biopsy, endoscopic retrograde cholangiography or even a laparoscopic cholecystectomy** — see the case below.

Do you remember the laparoscopic cholecystectomy you did in a diabetic patient a few weeks ago — the one with a baked-in chronically inflamed gallbladder? You got into the wrong plane; there was some bleeding from the gallbladder bed, in the end you asked for the argon beam coagulator. Ultimately it stopped. The patient did fine. He presented with melena, with a negative colonoscopy and upper GI endoscopy. The gastroenterologist did not visualize the papilla, but they might not have seen anything anyways, because hemobilia is frequently intermittent. However, because you are smart, you order a CT arteriogram and there it is: **an intrahepatic aneurysm of the right hepatic artery!**

The pathophysiology is an arteriobiliary shunt causing bleeding into the biliary system and — therefore — GI bleeding. **Embolization of the pseudoaneurysm is the treatment of choice**. Only in scenarios of tumors causing arteriobiliary fistulas and the non-availability of an interventional radiologist, is a surgical resection of one liver lobe or surgical ligation of either hepatic artery required; this is rare.

Hepatic tumors

Liver tumors may present as an emergency because of intra-abdominal bleeding. The "bleeding hepatic tumor" announced by the emergency room crew frequently turns out to be a liver lesion which had been transcutaneously biopsied, although imaging with three-phase contrast CTs or MRIs could have established the diagnosis. **To be fair, there is a risk of spontaneous bleeding in adenomas and hepatocellular carcinomas, but this remains an uncommon presentation**.

Bleeding of hepatic adenomas is more common specifically in pregnant women. **Bleeding hepatic tumors are nowadays managed by transcatheter embolization to stop the bleeding**. Convince your interventional radiologist to embolize the bleeding as selectively as possible and avoid embolizing the entire hemi-liver, because necrosis and intrahepatic cholangiopathy may ensue, which ultimately requires a more extensive resection than initially necessary to remove the tumor. It should be rare that tumor bleeding cannot be controlled by an angiographic intervention.

Only after embolization, **are a thoughtful imaging work-up and staging indicated to establish a surgical treatment plan**. Sometimes an interval of several weeks is required until the hepatic hematoma has resolved to be able to establish a radiologic diagnosis by MRI. **Do not plan elective resectional surgery until the hematoma has completely resolved**. A large central hematoma can compress hepatic veins causing outflow obstruction (Budd-Chiari syndrome!) — operating in such circumstances may prove disastrous!

If no interventional radiologist is available, laparotomy and rapid inflow control of the liver may be necessary. In older, frail patients with comorbidities and limited reserves and a bleeding exophytic hepatocellular carcinoma, I have used a hand-assisted laparoscopic approach and stapler tumorectomy to rapidly remove the bleeding mass.

Should you encounter a bleeding liver tumor causing hemodynamic instability with no local angiographic facilities, no expertise in liver surgery, and no immediate options of rapid transferal — do what you would do with liver trauma: open and pack!

Another emergency scenario is the incidentally discovered liver tumor, either during an emergency exploratory laparotomy or during an elective laparoscopy or laparotomy. You may ask: should I excise the lesion or perform a biopsy? If the lesion is small and peripheral, it is no mistake to excise it, but I wouldn't take any risks, since it is not easy to exclude other lesions in the rest of the liver without cross-sectional imaging by CT or MRI, unless you are a very good ultrasonographer.

I would strongly advise <u>not</u> to perform a direct biopsy into a tumor visible on the liver surface. But if you do, then only do it by driving a core needle through healthy liver tissue and then carefully ablating the needle tract afterwards. You just don't want to spill tumor tissue throughout the abdomen by performing a biopsy with a needle coming through the abdominal cavity. Nowadays MRI diagnosis of liver tumors both in healthy and diseased livers is excellent and tissue diagnosis is not always necessary to decide on further treatment: don't let anybody talk you into a biopsy; the work-up should be performed after the surgery is over.

To sum up

The liver is a quiet organ and doesn't cause many problems unless chronically ill. Patients with chronic liver disease may present with dramatic emergencies and it is important for surgeons to be well prepared for those. Blunt liver trauma can frequently be treated non-operatively; this is also true for hepatic stab wounds and low-velocity gunshot wounds — unless associated with severe bleeding or other injuries. **In emergencies arising with hepatic lesions, it is good to know when not to operate. But isn't this true for anything else?**

> **"Yossarian was in the hospital with a pain in his liver that fell just short of being jaundice. The doctors were puzzled by the fact that it wasn't quite jaundice. If it became jaundice they could treat it. If it didn't become jaundice and went away they could discharge him."**
>
> **Joseph Heller; Catch-22**

Chapter 24

Inflammatory bowel disease and other forms of colitis

Mark Cheetham and Simon Shaw

Save the patient, not the colon.

John C. Goligher

Introduction

There is something innately satisfying about a good dump; the 'right' degree of urgency, the anticipation and then the release of a good stool with a pleasing splash. Pity then the poor person with acute colitis on their 20th trip of the day to the toilet; weak with fatigue and anemia they struggle to reach the toilet in time. Blood and mucus ejaculates from the anus before they struggle back to bed to attempt to rest again.

This accurately reflects the situation of the patient with acute colitis; add in some IV steroids and whatever is the latest flavor of immunosuppression for your gastroenterologists and you have a complication waiting to happen. **Patients with severe colitis are a challenge for the surgeon; they can be extremely ill and yet the usual features of a surgical abdominal emergency are not present**. The unwary or inexperienced surgeon can easily underestimate just how sick these patients are (remember in ➲ Chapter 1 we talked about 'inflamed patients'?). **In this chapter we will discuss how to assess the patient with acute colitis, when to operate and what operation you should do**.

Acute colitis

Many patients with acute severe colitis will be already in hospital under the care of a gastroenterologist by the time you are asked to see them. Some gastroenterologists feel that the need for surgery in colitis represents a personal failure — as depicted in ■ Figure 24.1... We, however, are lucky enough to work with enlightened gastroenterologists who know that surgery is simply another treatment modality necessary in some instances to restore the patient to health.

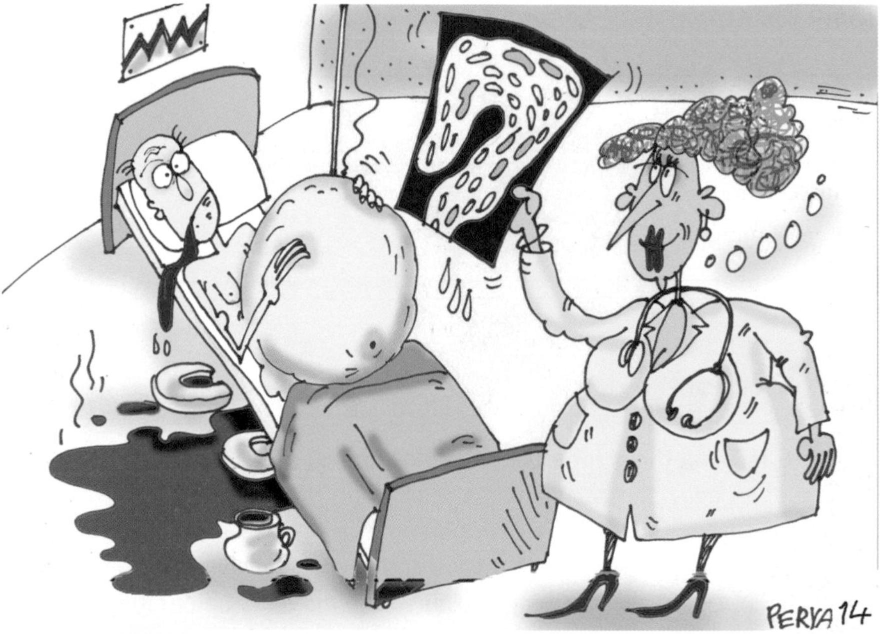

Figure 24.1. "Pancolitis, eh? Shouldn't we increase the steroids and add Imuran®?"

The decision-making around these patients can be complex — this is taken by a joint team of surgeons and gastroenterologists; indeed, we have created a joint medical/surgical GI ward to facilitate this. **We like to meet the patients early in their admission; this facilitates a rounded discussion about surgery and stomas before a crisis arises.**

This chapter deals mostly with acute **severe ulcerative colitis**; we will also discuss the care of patients with other types of colitis, in particular, **Crohn's colitis, *Clostridium difficile* and ischemic colitis**. There is little difference in the decision-making and surgical approach to the management of acute colitis regardless of the underlying cause. However, it is worthwhile discussing some of the differences between ulcerative colitis and Crohn's disease.

When to operate?

Patients with severe colitis may not appear 'ill'; they are often young and fit without the usual comorbidities we are used to seeing in many of our patients. Yet they need to be watched closely; they can deteriorate very quickly. **To identify when and who to operate on with colitis, we need first to provide some definitions**.

Truelove and Witts (*Br Med J* 1955; 2: 1041-8) developed an ulcerative colitis severity index which classifies the acute episode as mild, moderate or severe (see ■ Table 24.1). Although their score is 65 years old it is still valuable. And BTW, some jerks tend to misspell Dr. Truelove's name as "True love"... How witty!

Table 24.1. Truelove and Witts classification of the severity of colitis. *(Adapted from Truelove and Witts. Br Med J 1955; 2: 1041-8.)*

	Mild	Moderate	Severe
Bowel actions per day	4 or fewer	4 to 6	>6
Blood in stool	None or trace	Intermittent	Continuous
Pyrexia >37.8°C	No	No	Yes
Tachycardia >90/m	No	No	Yes
Anemia	No	No	Yes
ESR	<30mm/hr	<30mm/hr	>30mm/hr

But let us ignore mild forms of colitis and focus on the more severe entities:

- **Severe colitis**: >6 bloody bowel movements a day, cramps, fever, heart rate >90, anemia, raised ESR (≥30mm/hour).
- **Fulminant colitis**: >9 bloody bowel movements a day, continuous bleeding, pain, signs of toxic symptoms (anorexia, fever, tachycardia).

- **Toxic megacolon**: a patient with fulminant colitis and radiographic evidence of distension of the colon: transverse colon >6cm in diameter or cecum >9cm in diameter. **Only 1-5% of patients with inflammatory bowel disease ever develop toxic megacolon**. (BTW, *Clostridium difficile* colitis can result in toxic colitis — in up to 3% and the incidence is rising — manifesting with massive colonic edema on CT rather than a megacolon. Other causes of toxic megacolon are CMV colitis, *Salmonella*, *Shigella*, *Campylobacter*, *Entamoeba*, and ischemic colitis. These are all rare.)

So a patient is admitted with severe colitis...

Pre-op diagnostic tests

A limited unprepped flexible sigmoidoscopy should be performed in patients with acute colitis to confirm the diagnosis. We would also advise that a stool sample is sent for testing to exclude *C. diff*, CMV or another infective cause of their symptoms. A patient who has been hospitalized for acute severe colitis should be monitored with serial plain abdominal X-rays to look for signs of toxic megacolon and occult perforation. **Perforation in a patient admitted for the treatment of acute severe colitis should 'never' happen; it implies a failure to monitor properly or operate early enough**.

If toxic megacolon is suspected, an abdominal X-ray or CT scan should be obtained as mentioned above. Particular attention should be paid to the diameter of the transverse colon (not the cecum!). A patient with **colitis, fever, tachycardia and distension of the transverse colon to greater than 6cm is at great risk for perforation and needs to be taken immediately to the operating room. Don't be fooled by a benign abdominal exam; by the time they develop peritoneal signs, it is usually too late and they have already perforated**. The cecum may also dilate, but in acute colitis it is rare; however, a cecum greater than 9cm in diameter is also concerning.

Intravenous steroids are the mainstay of the management. We would expect to see a significant response within 3 days of treatment; if the patient is not getting better then we would consider surgery at this point. Antibiotics are not necessary in all patients — remember that the 'inflammation' alone will cause a fever and a tachycardia. However, in severely ill patients (e.g. fulminant and toxic colitis), we would add intravenous broad-spectrum antibiotics. We would also consider a CT scan here as this may be a sign of subclinical perforation. The waters have been somewhat muddied in the recent past by the use of **infliximab** (Remicade®) for acute severe colitis.

We have noticed that gastroenterologists will often take a stepwise approach and initiate the use of Remicade® after 5 days when it is clear that steroids aren't working (this often seems to be on Friday!). The problem is that it takes about 48 hours to be clear if the Remicade® is working, so as long as you are happy that the patient is safe, take it easy and go fishing for the weekend — you can always do the colectomy on Monday!

With **fulminant colitis** ('severe' on the Truelove scale) we will allow 24 to 48 hours of further medical therapy with close observation, but will recommend surgery after that time or if the patient starts to deteriorate.

Patients with severe colitis not responding to maximal medical treatment require urgent colectomy; this can usually be done the following day. A patient with toxic megacolon needs a colectomy within a few hours!

Surgery for acute colitis

The operation of choice for acute colitis is a COLECTOMY AND END ILEOSTOMY; everything else is not enough (a loop ileostomy) or too much (a panproctocolectomy).

An anastomosis in this situation is plain criminal. We have seen a handful of patients where this rule has not been obeyed and the outcomes were not happy. One young lady had an emergency *panproctocolectomy* for acute ulcerative colitis at the age of 17 because she had told her surgeon that she "only wanted one operation"; years later she is still trawling surgical departments around the country trying to find someone willing to 'reverse' her stoma… Another man had an emergency subtotal colectomy with an ileorectal anastomosis because he didn't want a stoma; the subsequent inevitable leak and its aftermath were devastating for him.

So we will say it again; the operation of choice for acute severe colitis is a COLECTOMY AND END ILEOSTOMY. (In the American literature, surgeons write about a total abdominal colectomy while on this side of the Atlantic we usually refer to a subtotal colectomy. In the rest of the chapter we have decided to refer simply to colectomy and end ileostomy hoping we can satisfy all parties ☺.) In some textbooks you will see reference to dividing the mid rectum — we believe that not only is this more distal resection unnecessary but that it may also make subsequent surgery more hazardous.

The only exception to this is when the indication for surgery is life-threatening rectal bleeding in a patient with colitis; in these circumstances we would consider an emergency panproctocolectomy. Rarely you may have occasion to do an emergency operation for someone with Crohn's colitis — we would still do a colectomy and ileostomy in this situation (this preserves all options including a later ileorectal anastomosis if there is rectal sparing).

Tips for doing a colectomy for colitis

OK look, the key is in the name. **Only remove most of the colon**; leave a long 'rectal' stump! **In fact, the site of distal division should be in the distal colon rather than the true rectum**. But we digress. Here are a few tips:

- First the patient is placed supine on the OR table and a Foley catheter is inserted; an NG (Ryles) tube is not usually needed. Start by making a midline incision deviating to the left of the umbilicus to give more space for the ileostomy. How long to make the incision will depend on the size of your patient and the height of the colonic flexures (tailor the incision to the situation).
- We often use a hand-held Harmonic® or LigaSure™ for this operation as it reduces time and bleeding in these sick patients.
- There is no need to do an oncological resection with high ligation of the named colonic vessels unless the patient is known to have colonic dysplasia or a colorectal cancer.
- We usually take the greater omentum along with the transverse colon (that bloodless plane between colon and omentum is rarely so in our experience; also, sometimes there will be a concealed perforation which is only revealed when dissecting the omentum).
- Divide the distal sigmoid at a convenient point with a linear cutting stapler.

Emergency laparoscopic colectomy for colitis

We know that you are all minimally invasive ninjas and that some of you will want to do this operation laparoscopically. **A few words of advice: there is a vast different between an elective segmental colectomy for cancer and an emergency laparoscopic total colectomy**. The patient with acute severe colitis is unwell, toxic and hypoalbuminemic; he or she needs a swift and safe operation, not several hours of head-down while you show everyone how big your cojones are!

That being said, we do use laparoscopy for total colectomy, but selectively, in patients who are relatively well and where there are no signs of perforation.

Preventing a rectal stump blowout

In days of yore, the dogma was that the rectal stump should be exteriorized as a mucous fistula to prevent the risk of a rectal stump blowout. In modern surgical practice it is usual to close the rectal stump and there is plenty of evidence that it's safe to do so. Nevertheless, the risk of a rectal stump blowout exists. **To reduce the risk of this we oversew the rectal stump staple line with 3/0 PDS® and also leave a 30Fr rectal catheter *in situ* for 48 hours post-op.**

Another way of preventing a rectal stump blowout is to leave the end of the rectal stump subcutaneously in the lower end of the laparotomy wound and tack it onto the fascia; the theory being that if the rectal stump leaks you can simply open the lower part of the wound and have a controlled mucous fistula. We have abandoned this practice — it seems to work although there is a higher rate of wound infection (and of course it's not possible if you did a laparoscopic colectomy).

Rarely you will operate and find that the colon is so friable that it will not safely accept sutures or a stapler; in these patients we would create a mucous fistula by exteriorizing the end of the rectal stump via a small trephine in the left iliac fossa. We use an umbilical cord clamp to hold the end of the rectal stump above the skin level — this then sloughs off in a week or so leaving a sutureless matured mucous fistula.

Postoperative care

The postoperative care of the total colectomy patient is similar to that of any patient after an emergency laparotomy. The return of bowel function is normally fairly swift and we would allow clear fluids as tolerated on the day of surgery, with light diet the following day. **Most of these patients are on steroids and will need i.v. steroid cover until diet is re-established.** At this point we would restart a reducing course of oral steroids at the level of the pre-operative dose and then reducing by 5mg every 7 days until they are off steroids completely. Other drugs including 5-ASA compounds and biologics (the -imabs) can be stopped immediately after the operation without any tapering. We give a 28-day course of subcutaneous low-molecular-weight heparin to these patients (and indeed to all patients having a major resection).

Crohn's disease (CD) emergencies

Depending on where in the world you work, you will see varying numbers of patients with CD presenting as an emergency. As discussed above, the surgical management of Crohn's colitis mirrors that of ulcerative colitis. **In this section, we will consider how to approach surgical problems of small bowel and anorectal CD**.

There are five key scenarios to consider:

- Small bowel obstruction due to CD.
- Perforated small bowel in CD.
- The patient with CD who has acute appendicitis.
- The patient with right iliac fossa pain who is found to have ileocecal CD.
- Anorectal CD.

Obstructed or perforated small bowel CD

Other chapters (see ➲ Chapters 19 and 26) give details of how to manage patients with small bowel obstruction and perforation. **Here are some extra words of advice to help you manage such patients who have CD**.

There is often a tendency to prevaricate in making decisions in this situation, or to defer entirely to the gastroenterologist's opinion. **But remember that a patient with complete small bowel obstruction or perforation due to Crohn's has a 'surgical' disease — you (and your patient) will need the gastroenterologist later on, but for now the decision-making belongs to you!** Increasingly we are recognizing two overlapping phenotypes of Crohn's disease: penetrating Crohn's and stricturing Crohn's. Patients with penetrating disease tend to present with septic complications (intra-abdominal abscesses, internal or enterocutaneous fistulae or free perforation), whereas patients with stricturing Crohn's usually develop obstructive symptoms. Most patients with complete small bowel obstruction due to Crohn's disease have fibrostenotic strictures rather than an area of inflammation — steroids are unlikely to help resolve this; CT scanning or, even better, abdominal MRI in conjunction with the ESR may help you to decide how much of an inflammatory component is present. If the obstruction is incomplete or there is good evidence of an inflammatory component, then we would push for a course of steroids. Although surgeons are rightly keen to conserve small bowel in patients with Crohn's disease, complete small bowel obstruction is one situation when a resection is usually necessary. The worst situation is that the patient is given a few days of IV steroids and then is passed back to you a few days later with unresolved obstruction, malnutrition and all the risks of high-dose steroids.

So if the SBO does not respond to conservative treatment within about 48 hours, or when confronted with perforated CD, have a low threshold to be the one to do the first resection — this establishes the diagnosis and without additional therapy will often induce remission for some years.

Patients with locally perforated Crohn's disease can often be treated with i.v. antibiotics and image-guided drainage of any collections, at least initially. This may be the only 'surgical' treatment needed; at worst you will be able to defer surgery until an elective operation. Obviously, you know that patients with generalized peritonitis will need a laparotomy with resection of the perforated segment.

Operative technique

Small bowel mesentery in CD is thick, stiff and very vascular. When doing a resection in these patients we always suture-ligate the mesenteric pedicles with a 2/0 polyglactin suture — there is a significant risk of bleeding or a mesenteric hematoma if you simply tie these pedicles. We have found that energy devices do not work so well on Crohn's mesentery and we tend not use them here unlike in ulcerative colitis. (Do a conservative resection — this is not a malignancy and your patient may need more surgery in the future.)

Patients with CD may be nutritionally poor and also be on significant doses of steroids and other immunosuppression at the time of emergency laparotomy. This means that you need to have a low threshold for doing a **resection without an anastomosis**, if there are significant risk factors for anastomotic leak (see ■ Table 24.2). In these circumstances, resect the obstructed or perforated bowel and bring the two ends out as a double-barrelled stoma ('an ileocolostomy') (see ➲ Chapter 14).

Table 24.2. Risk factors for anastomotic leak in emergency Crohn's surgery.
Risk factors
■ High dose of steroids (greater than 10mg prednisone per day).
■ Albumin less than 30g/dL.
■ Local abscess cavity.
■ Poor nutritional state.
■ Severe sepsis.

Right iliac fossa pain and Crohn's disease

There are two situations you may come across:

- A patient with known CD and concomitant appendicitis.
- A patient with right iliac fossa pain who turns out to have newly diagnosed ileocecal CD.

The first situation is beloved of examiners — but vanishingly rare in clinical practice. If the base of the appendix appears healthy then simply take the appendix as you normally do. If the base of the cecum is diseased, then consider either treating the appendicitis with antibiotics or doing an ileocecal resection if the appendix is perforated.

The second scenario is something we see every few months. Usually these patients have a more subacute history than 'normal' appendicitis — this should prompt some imaging (i.e. the obligatory abdominal CT scan). **If ileocecal Crohn's disease is diagnosed on CT then what should you do?** This is controversial; we will usually manage these patients together with a gastroenterologist. Conventionally they will be treated medically with an induction course of IV steroids and then some form of immunosuppression. Nowadays we will often offer such patients the choice between this and a primary ileocecal resection. Patients with Crohn's disease who present as an emergency like this have about a 90% chance of having a resection over the next 12 months and operating now will reliably get the patient well without the misery of steroids, etc.

Anorectal disease

We will discuss the emergency management of anorectal CD in ➲ Chapter 28.

Pseudomembranous colitis (*C. diff* colitis)

Pseudomembranous colitis is caused by an overgrowth of the Gram-positive bacterium *Clostridium difficile*. This is almost exclusively due to the indiscriminate use of broad-spectrum antibiotics (even after a single dose!) and is one of the scourges of modern medicine. It can be highly contagious and the rapid isolation of the index patient with careful infection control practices is necessary to prevent an epidemic.

C. diff colitis can be diagnosed by testing the patient's stool for a specific exotoxin expressed by the bacterium. Occasionally it is diagnosed at lower GI endoscopy by the characteristic yellow 'pseudomembranes' which peel off to reveal bleeding mucosa underneath. Histology of a mucosal biopsy is diagnostic.

Most patients with *C. diff* colitis will be treated medically:

- Stop broad-spectrum antibiotics.
- Give oral metronidazole 400mg three times a day.
- Give oral vancomycin 100mg twice a day for severe attacks.
- Consider adding IV metronidazole if there is an ileus.

Other treatments such as IV immunoglobulin and probiotics are used in some institutions but currently lack a strong evidence base. We would advise that you follow the current local policies unless you are performing a research study. **Fecal transplant is gaining popularity for the management of refractory or recurrent *C. diff* colitis**. Drug companies are now jumping on the bandwagon and charge dollars for a gram of s**t. However, there is no role for a fecal transplant in the acute situation — it belongs to the office of the gastroenterologists. (Anyway, we are seeking donors — to apply please email us... [■ Figure 24.2].)

It is fortunately rare to need to operate on a patient with *C. diff* colitis. These patients are often debilitated from a prolonged hospital stay and usually have other comorbidities; the risk of peri-operative morbidity and mortality is consequently extremely high. The conventional surgical approach is to perform a subtotal colectomy as described earlier in this chapter. However, there is emerging evidence that sick patients with *C. diff* colitis can be treated with a loop ileostomy and antibiotic lavage (with vancomycin) via the distal limb of the stoma.

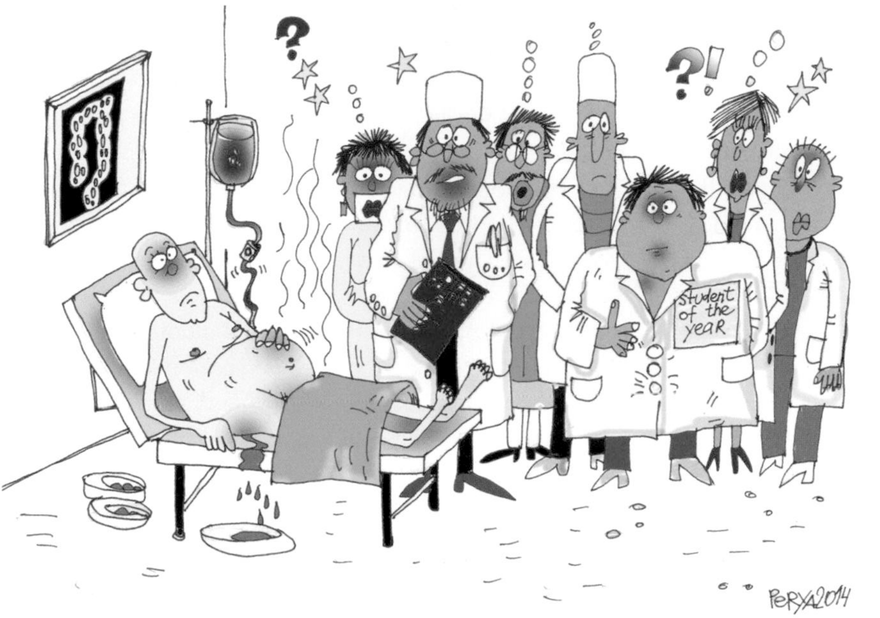

Figure 24.2. Surgeon: "Anyone ready to serve as a st donor for this poor patient." Student of the year: "Sir, what about an autotransplant?"**

Ischemic colitis

Ischemic colitis is a poorly defined entity which encompasses a spectrum of conditions. Paradoxically, occlusion of the named arteries supplying the colon is not associated with ischemic colitis but local vascular changes in the wall of the colon may play a role. **Thus, a patient with sigmoid colon gangrene following repair of an abdominal aortic aneurysm and ligation of the inferior mesenteric artery has colonic ischemia — *not* ischemic colitis.**

Ischemic colitis develops in two different clinical settings:

- **Spontaneous**: in patients with underlying cardiac failure, chronic lung disease, renal failure, diabetes, and collagen disease — probably related to diseased intramural vessels. In fact, we see such cases in otherwise healthy older women with normal mesenteric vasculature on CT-angio and no evidence of atherosclerosis elsewhere.
- **Shock-associated**: in patients who have experienced sustained shock regardless of etiology (e.g. ruptured aortic aneurysms).

Typically, the colonic process involves a varying depth of penetration. **In most cases it represents a transient mucosal involvement which recovers**

spontaneously. In a minority of patients, deeper layers of the colon are involved — and this may progress to full-thickness gangrene. Some patients may develop partial-thickness necrosis which leads to stricture formation. Although most common in the 'watershed' area of the splenic flexure and the left colon, the disease can involve any part of the colon and the rectum and rarely the entire colon; although usually focal it may be patchy or diffuse.

Patients with **spontaneous ischemic colitis** present typically with left abdominal pain and tenderness and hematochezia. Those with **shock-associated ischemic colitis** develop these features on top of their underlying critical disease.

As with mesenteric ischemia (➲ Chapter 22), the clinical picture — as well as laboratory findings — is entirely non-specific as is the commonly associated ileus. Abdominal X-rays may demonstrate an ileus and colonic dilatation proximal to the area of ischemia or a dilated ischemic colon. CT features of a thickened left colon are suggestive; in the rare, advanced transmural cases, pneumatosis coli or free gas may be seen.

Unprepped, fiberoptic flexible sigmoidoscopy is the best diagnostic test, visualizing a spectrum of hemorrhagic and ischemic changes which, although non-specific and may be confused with CD colitis (see above), are highly suggestive in the specific clinical setting.

Treatment

In most cases the process will be self-limiting. Some would treat it with broad-spectrum IV antibiotics and bowel rest. However, we usually prescribe oral metronidazole and a light diet. And expect recovery within a few days. **Rarely, if the patient fails to respond or the ischemia progresses to full-thickness colonic necrosis, you may need to operate**. In these circumstances, perform a Hartmann's procedure, resecting the obviously ischemic colon. A few patients may progress to develop a **colonic stricture** — but this is beyond the scope of our story.

Neutropenic enterocolitis

This is a transmural inflammation of the large bowel in myelosuppressed and immunosuppressed patients — usually suffering from myeloproliferative disorders and receiving chemotherapy. **Profound neutropenia appears to be**

the common denominator. The process involves mucosal damage and alteration in bacterial flora, which then invade the bowel wall. **The cecum is primarily affected but the process may extend to the ascending colon and even the ileum**. The presentation may mimic acute appendicitis; watery or bloody diarrhea is present in only half of the patients. Right lower quadrant tenderness, a palpable cecum, peritoneal signs and features of ileus may be present. Neutropenia is a pathognomonic laboratory finding. Plain abdominal X-rays are usually non-specific, revealing an associated ileus but may show 'thumbprinting' of the right colon and intramural air (pneumatosis) — denoting severe involvement of the cecal wall. **A CT scan of the abdomen is the diagnostic procedure of choice, showing thickening of the cecum and free air if an underlying perforation exists**.

Management should be initially supportive, including broad-spectrum antibiotics effective against colonic Gram-negative bacteria and anaerobes; granulocyte colony-stimulating factor (G-CSF) may be considered. Clinical deterioration, evidence of free perforation and, rarely, severe lower gastrointestinal hemorrhage may necessitate operation. At laparotomy, normal-looking serosal surfaces may hide mucosal breakdown and necrosis. Therefore, the whole involved segment of colon should be resected; anastomosis should be avoided in these debilitated patients. Mortality is obviously high. **The key is to recognize the condition and avoid an operation in the majority of patients**.

Final words

Acute colitis from whatever cause needs careful monitoring and a team approach is necessary. Patients with colitis are usually admitted under the care of the gastroenterologist; make sure that if they are not settling that a surgeon sees the patient early in their hospital stay and keeps a close watch on their progress. The operation of choice for colitis which fails to settle on medical treatment is a colectomy and end ileostomy. Both open and laparoscopic approaches are appropriate, dependent on the severity of the colitis and the overall health of the patient. Don't mess with the rectum. This can be dealt with later at a separate operation.

"We suffer and die through the defects that arise in our sewerage and drainage systems."

William A. Lane

Chapter 25

Colonic obstruction

Adam Farquharson, Simon Shaw and Mark Cheetham

The only time human beings wish they could fart and defecate is when they are not able to do so.

Colonic obstruction is a common presentation for the emergency general surgeon, although in populations where there is screening for bowel cancer it is becoming less common. The striking picture of abdominal distension and absolute constipation is rarely missed.

We will discuss how to diagnose and manage colonic obstruction, of which the commonest cause by far in the Western world is **colorectal cancer** followed by **diverticular disease** — that is only if you include subacute obstruction, since acute obstruction due to diverticular disease is rather rare. Colonic **volvulus** is less frequent and has a different management. Very rarely — but it does happen — the **colon can obstruct-strangulate within a ventral or incisional hernia**. Finally, we will describe the strategy to recognize and manage patients with **acute colonic pseudo-obstruction** — a condition which commonly mimics mechanical obstruction. Table ■ 25.1 lists the entire differential diagnosis of colonic obstruction.

Making the diagnosis

History

Usually, abdominal distension with central or lower abdominal pain and absolute constipation are the dominant complaints. However, when the

Table 25.1. Differential diagnosis for colonic obstruction. This list is a guideline and is by no means exhaustive.

Outside the lumen of the bowel:

- Hernias — internal and external, groin and incisional (rare).
- Adhesions (rare).
- Abscesses — causing external compression or kinking.
- Volvulus.
- Endometriosis (partially in the wall...).

Inside the wall of the bowel:

- Congenital (short segment Hirschsprung's disease).
- Traumatic (hematoma).
- Neoplastic.
- Inflammatory (diverticular stricture; IBD stricture).
- Infectious (tubercular stricture).

Inside the lumen of the bowel:

- Foreign body.
- Fecal impaction.

obstruction is incomplete the patient may pass some flatus and liquid stool. Vomiting occurs late and may be absent; it tends to occur if the ileocecal valve is incompetent and the obstruction is longstanding; in this situation the small bowel fills up and distends — like in small bowel obstruction.

You will also want to ask:

- Has the patient had any preceding bowel symptoms such as rectal bleeding, change in bowel habit or tenesmus?
- **Have they had any prior colonoscopy?** A history of normal colonoscopy within the preceding 5 years (a small polyp or a few make no difference) mostly ('never say never') excludes the possibility of malignant colon obstruction.
- Obviously, you will also want to know about their other medical comorbidities and drug history (best to find out about the apixaban now, eh?).

Examination

Examine the abdomen looking for distension, tenderness and any abdominal masses.

The distended abdomen is tender but **extreme local tenderness and peritoneal signs suggest vascular compromise** of the bowel with impending or actual perforation. A mass in the right iliac fossa may hint at an **obstructing cecal cancer**. Masses elsewhere could signify a malignancy of the colon or ovary, or a diverticular mass.

Remember that the abdominal distension results in increased intra-abdominal pressure, which in turn may lead to incarceration of a pre-excising inguinal or ventral hernia. This situation could confuse the rookie... but luckily, nowadays even the rookie should be able to read the abdominal CT...

Now do a rectal examination. Classically in 'true' large bowel obstruction, the rectum is collapsed around the examining finger — whereas in pseudo-obstruction the rectum is distended and capacious. Extremely rarely the cause of the obstruction is a stenosing rectal cancer — best to feel that before you open the abdomen. A more common scenario is a patient with an obstructing sigmoid cancer and also a synchronous rectal tumor. You operate and resect the sigmoid and a few days later the patient starts bleeding from the rectum. Embarrassing...

Imaging of colonic obstruction

The aim of imaging in suspected colonic obstruction is to establish or refute the diagnosis of obstruction, to exclude pseudo-obstruction and to assess the site of obstruction and the causative pathology.

Plain abdominal X-rays are often done as initial investigations in the ER. Modern CT-addicted docs tend to ignore them but still — they can offer important information especially if your scanner is being repaired or the only scanner in your Banana Republic is 500 miles away:

- **If you see significant colonic distension without any other distension or air fluid levels in the small bowel or stomach**, you can safely assume, given the history and physical exam, that this patient has a colonic obstruction (or pseudo-obstruction). **These observations also imply that the ileocecal valve is competent**

resulting in a 'closed loop' colonic obstruction. This means that you must move fast before the colon dies off and perforates.
- If both the colon and loops of small bowel are dilated you know that the ileocecal valve is incompetent and the obstructed colon is decompressing itself proximally.

In our 'modern' practice (we are not sure what will happen after Brexit ☺), a **CT scan of the abdomen and pelvis with i.v. contrast** would be the next step for most patients. In addition to assessing the level and nature of the obstruction, it also allows an assessment of the degree of spread of any malignancy, if present. We have not found rectal or oral contrast to be necessary in this context; usually the gas in the distended colon acts as a sufficient contrast to visualize the transition point. **However, a CT enema or a Gastrografin® enema (or a flexible sigmoidoscopy) are alternatives which may be needed to supplement the results of the CT scan**. Sometimes it is important to know whether contrast can pass, meaning that we have time to wait, and insertion of a stent is possible. Hip replacements can cause significant artefact which can obscure the details of an obstructing lesion on CT — in these cases rectal contrast is really helpful.

What about adding oral contrast with the CT scan which we recommended above for small bowel obstruction (➲ Chapter 19)? Well, **oral contrast given to these patients can result in a significant increase in fluid and gas buildup within their colon**, with the risk of ischemia and perforation — increasing the urgency for operation.

Decision-making in colonic obstruction

Armed with the results of your clinical assessment, lab tests and imaging, you are now in a position to answer these questions:

- **Is there true obstruction or pseudo-obstruction?** This is crucial. Fortunately, the CT will be the judge. We will dedicate a section to this problematic entity below.
- **Where is the obstruction and what is causing it?** CT will show you the site of the obstruction. But <u>not always</u> will it be able to distinguish between the (more common) obstructing cancer and the (less common) obstructing diverticular mass.
- If it appears to be a malignant obstruction what is the degree of spread?

Next you need to decide, **does the patient need an operation? If so, when do you need to operate — now or in the morning?**

In most patients with large bowel obstruction, surgery can wait, and should wait, a few hours or until tomorrow. **Remember**: those guys have been brewing up their obstruction for many days, during which they were not eating or even drinking much. Some of them will be anemic from chronic blood loss. While waiting for the morning invest efforts in improving their general condition. Now you know how (➲ Chapter 6). And don't forget the NG tube and the Foley before you retire to your call room.

Of course, exceptions to this would be the patient with advanced obstruction and an impending colonic rupture — the one with a very tender abdomen and a cecal diameter of 10cm or greater. A few such patients may even develop an abdominal compartment syndrome (➲ Chapter 31). Here we would operate as soon as the patient is adequately resuscitated.

The next questions to answer — "**Are you going to resect the obstructing lesion and are you going to do an anastomosis?**"— will have to wait until you are inside the abdomen. But before considering these let us bring up our menu of options for the most common scenario you are likely to encounter: **large bowel obstruction due to colorectal cancer**.

Obstructing cancers in the right and transverse colon

Obstructing cecal and right colon cancers would obviously be treated with a **right hemicolectomy** (don't forget that a patient with a cecal cancer may present with small bowel obstruction). **We would do an extended right hemicolectomy for an obstructing lesion proximal to and including the splenic flexure**. Usually you can do a primary ileocolic anastomosis as the obstructed, loaded colon is already in the bucket and joining small bowel to distal, collapsed colon is straightforward. In selected cases, however, you would want to avoid an anastomosis — you know when (➲ Chapter 14.1).

Left colonic obstruction

For this more common scenario, there are three main options:

- **Resect the tumor**:
  - with a Hartmann's procedure;
  - with a primary anastomosis;
  - with a primary anastomosis and a defunctioning stoma.

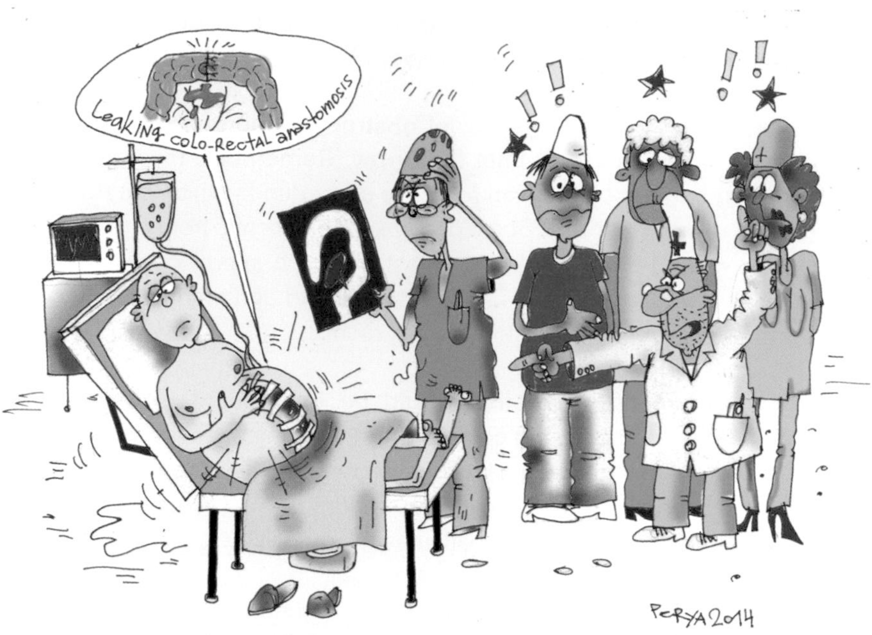

Figure 25.1a. "Idiot! Why did you anastomose?"

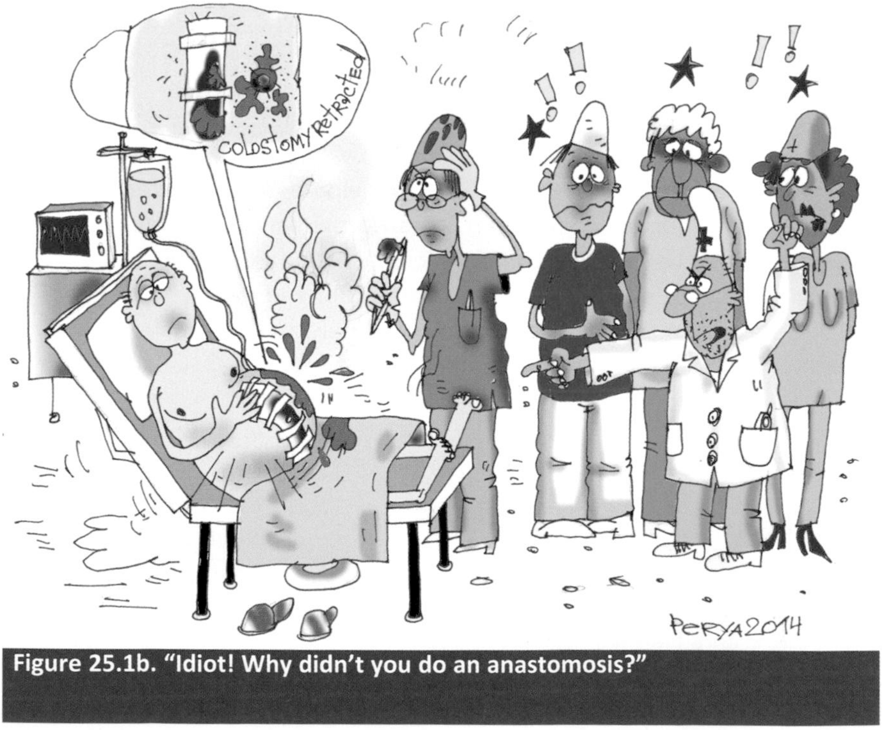

Figure 25.1b. "Idiot! Why didn't you do an anastomosis?"

- **Defunction the tumor with a loop stoma**. We would reserve this for the patient in whom the primary tumor is not resectable, the patient with widespread metastatic disease or the patient with major comorbidities which preclude a resection. It is also relevant in obstructing rectal cancer, as discussed below. About the choice of stoma, whether a transverse colostomy or cecostomy, look up ➲ Chapter 14.2.
- **Insert a colonic stent** (see below).

Resection is the best treatment if possible; it resolves the obstruction and allows a potential cure of a cancer. If the patient is fit, this is what we would aim for in most instances — unless there is widespread metastatic disease. Even if there is a low volume of distant disease, resection of the primary offers the best palliation and together with modern chemotherapy may provide the patient with reasonable survival.

For most patients with a resectable lesion we would at least consider a primary anastomosis unless they had significant comorbidities (wouldn't survive a leak), or they were critically unwell (too high a risk of leak). But you know how things could turn out: if you do an anastomosis and it leaks, they may ask — *why did you do an anastomosis?* (■ Figure 25.1a). If you do a stoma — someone, a smart ass, could ask: *why not an anastomosis?* (■ Figure 25.1b). Life is tough. And indeed, we know that many other surgeons are still hesitant to consider an anastomosis in this situation — some of the co-editors, for example.

The operation for colonic obstruction

We won't insult you by telling you how to do a right or an extended right hemicolectomy — it's going to be a bit more demanding with a loaded, distended colon. But surgery for a left-sided colonic obstruction is even more difficult...

We would avoid a laparoscopic approach where there is complete colonic obstruction; it is extremely difficult to create a useful working space with all the distended colon in the way and additionally the bowel is fragile and vulnerable to trauma from laparoscopic graspers. And anyway, it won't hurt to improve your skills in open abdominal surgery...

Start by making a generous midline incision — you are going to need good access for this. Immediately on opening the abdomen, distended bowel loops will emerge into the incision completely obscuring your view. **The distended loops must be immediately decompressed**; without decompression it is like wrestling an anaconda! To decompress the colon, take a wide-bore (14G) needle and attach it to a 10ml syringe with the plunger removed; the barrel of the syringe is the perfect size to connect the suction tubing. Now insert the needle into the distended colon obliquely through a *taenia coli*. Don't let the tip of the needle block with s#*t, just suck out as much gas as possible. This maneuver would suffice in many cases but not when the obstruction is longstanding with fecal build-up throughout the entire colon producing an associated small bowel obstruction. **In such cases, you will need to insert a large Poole sucker through a colotomy — controlled with a purse-string suture — and suck the crap out**. This may be tedious, as the sucker tends to obstruct. But take your time and try to avoid contamination of the surrounding tissues. The site of the decompressive *colotomy* should preferably be at the site of the planned division of the bowel or a planned colostomy. Obviously, standing at the operating table at 2 a.m. watching suction bottle after suction bottle filling up with thick brown liquid gives us tremendous satisfaction!

Again: avoid spilling any of the fluidly feces — as they say: "An extra hour of shit in the abdomen means an extra day in ICU."

Now withdraw the needle and continue with the operation by **mobilizing the left colon. It may be difficult to know for sure if the obstruction is due to a cancer or a diverticular stricture, but it's wise to assume it's a malignancy and do a 'cancer' operation with a high vascular ligation.**

Assess whether the obstructing mass is resectable or not. Often, in the acute stage such assessment may be difficult. Sometimes your exploring hands are more accurate than the pre-op CT. **A large fixed mass in the pelvis rules out resection; even in doubt do not be an obsessive hero**. In a recent case (that we heard about) an experienced surgeon mobilized the obstructing mass together with the ureter and the iliac artery before deciding that the mass was unresectable. The ureter was repaired and the artery fixed but it later thrombosed resulting in an amputation of the leg 2 days later. Final diagnosis: diverticular disease. **Didn't we tell you already that sometimes a colostomy is your best friend?**

Once the lesion has been mobilized you need to divide the bowel beyond it, either between bowel clamps or using a linear stapler. **Now you need to decide finally if you are going to join the bowel or do a Hartmann's**. Check with the anesthetist about the state of the patient's physiology; if they are hypotensive, acidotic or requiring vasopressors be prepared to abandon dreams of an anastomosis and do a Hartmann's instead. If you are going to do a primary anastomosis, here is where you would do an **on-table colonic lavage** (see below). About how to do a Hartmann's procedure look at ➲ Chapter 26.

On-table lavage

Not everybody believes that on-table colonic lavage is necessary for constructing a safe anastomosis in this situation. Unlike us, some would proceed with an anastomosis when they think that the bowel is relatively empty, and the patient is in reasonable shape.

So, here's how to do on-table lavage:

- First get the surgical team to assemble the kit. You will need:
  - a 16Fr Foley catheter;
  - 2 x 3L bags of warm saline (get the team to steal it from the urology theatre);
  - an i.v. administration set;
  - 2 x nylon tapes;
  - a length of sterilized or disinfected corrugated anesthetic tubing (see ■ Figure 25.2).

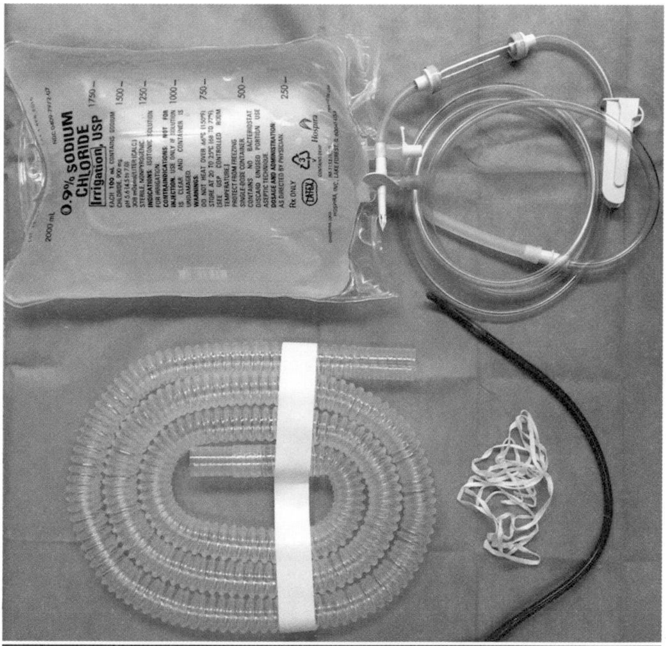

Figure 25.2. Equipment needed for intra-operative colonic lavage: see the text.

- Mobilize the colon so that both the hepatic and the splenic flexures are outside of the wound.
- Now carefully make a colotomy in the colon about 10cm upstream of the obstruction.
- Insert the anesthetic tubing into the colotomy and tie it in place with the two nylon tapes, drop the other end of the tubing into a bucket between the patient's legs. (It is useful to tape large polythene bags to the end of the tubing inside the bucket to create a 'closed' system…).
- Next divide the mesoappendix and cut off the tip of the appendix.
- Pass the Foley through the appendix.
- Blow up the balloon and tie the Foley into the appendix with two heavy silk ties.
- Now connect the administration set to the Foley and run 4-6L of warm saline through the colon until it comes out clear into the bucket (■ Figure 25.3).

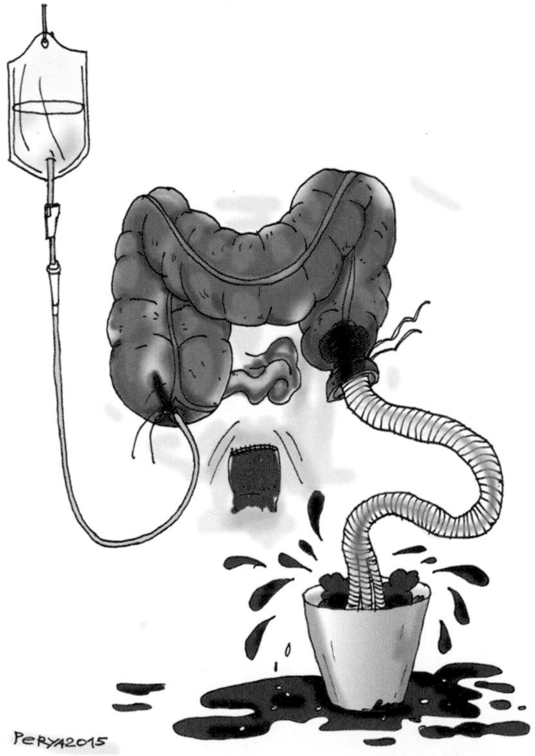

Figure 25.3. Intra-operative colonic lavage.

- Now remove the Foley and complete the appendectomy.
- We have trained our best junior resident to perform the lavage. It may take some time which allows us a good cup of Shrewsbury tea.
- Now we return fortified to complete the sigmoid resection and the anastomosis of our choice.

(BTW, in practice we often use a proprietary system called Retrowash™; this contains all the kit you need in a sterile package together with a set of cable ties to secure the tubing. This kit is more secure, the washout is contained in a sealed system and it does not require an appendectomy.)

Now, after the anastomosis is completed **should you add a proximal stoma to divert your 'high-risk' anastomosis?** The answer is the same as in ➲ Chapter 26.

The role of stenting

Whether you will be able to stent a patient with large bowel obstruction depends on the level of obstruction and also your local facilities. If you work in an ivory tower with ready access to a 'stentologist' then great; but in many hospitals this skill set is not readily available (maybe you should transfer your patient to someone somewhere who has the skills?).

There are two situations when stenting may have a role to play:

- As definitive treatment for obstruction in a patient with widespread metastases or who is too frail for a resection.
- As a 'bridge to surgery' — resolving the acute obstruction and then allowing a planned resection later.

Stenting can be carried out in the endoscopy suite or in the OR and is usually done under i.v. sedation. **Here are some tips**:

- Obtain a water-soluble contrast enema beforehand to delineate the site and length of the stricture. Some endoscopists will do this at the time of stenting. **If contrast won't pass through the stricture then it's not possible to pass a guidewire to stent the obstruction**.
- Stenting is most successful for obstruction caused by a primary bowel cancer. It is less successful if the obstruction is due to diverticular disease or infiltration from another cancer.
- Stenting is usually most feasible for obstruction in the left colon located between the splenic flexure and the rectosigmoid junction.

- Stenting a tumor proximal to the splenic flexure may be possible depending on the skills and experience of the team. **Placing a stent distal to the rectosigmoid junction will often cause unbearable symptoms of tenesmus and carries a high risk of stent migration.**

The obvious advantages to stenting include avoiding the risk of anesthesia and a major operation in an acutely ill patient. On the other hand, there is a risk of the stent causing a perforation which may render the tumor incurable. **The greatest advantage will be achieved in properly selected patients, operated upon within 5-10 days after stenting.**

Obstructing rectal cancer

Rectal cancers rarely cause obstruction; the wider diameter of the rectum and the more obvious symptoms mean that a cancer in the rectum is usually diagnosed before it causes large bowel obstruction.

However, occasionally you will come across an obstructing rectal cancer and we believe that this should be managed differently. Modern management of rectal cancer relies heavily on MRI imaging of the primary to select a suitable multimodal neoadjuvant treatment plan. Rectal cancers which obstruct are typically advanced and are likely to need chemoradiotherapy before a resection.

For this reason, we would initially treat an obstructing rectal cancer with a defunctioning loop stoma (usually a transverse loop colostomy) — remember to biopsy the rectal tumor during the operation. Once the obstruction has resolved we would arrange a pelvic MRI scan to stage the cancer and then administer suitable neoadjuvant treatment before any planned resection.

Volvulus of the colon

Sometimes a bowel-coil gets out of place
By twisting round a narrow base
With gradual strangulating of the blood supply
And danger that th' affected coil will die
This is VOLVULUS which you should learn
Is from the Latin — volvere — to turn.

Zachary Cope, The Acute Abdomen in Rhyme

The sigmoid colon is the most common site for a colonic volvulus to occur (see below); volvulus of the caecum and at other sites in the colon is much less common.

Sigmoid volvulus

This condition most frequently afflicts the infirm and elderly, often in institutionalized care; many have dementia or learning difficulties and they are often frail. It is associated with chronic constipation and a redundant sigmoid loop.

The classic presentation is of massive abdominal distension with absolute constipation. There is often a past history of previous episodes of volvulus as many of this group are 'frequent flyers'.

On examination, the abdomen is usually tensely distended. A finding of tenderness or guarding in the left iliac fossa may signify gangrenous volvulus. **A plain abdominal X-ray is usually diagnostic: the sigmoid volvulus is visible as a large 'coffee bean'-shaped gas-filled loop of bowel occupying the whole abdomen**. Classically the concavity of the bean points towards the base of the sigmoid mesentery. In most instances, no further imaging is needed; if there is doubt about the diagnosis then we would arrange for a CT (showing a huge loop of sigmoid and the 'whirl' sign, typical of intestinal volvulus developing at the twist point of the mesentery). An alternative would be a Gastrografin® enema, showing obstruction at the rectosigmoid junction — where the contrast ends with the characteristic *bird's beak sign*.

Treatment

In most cases, a sigmoid volvulus is treated with endoscopic deflation. Emergency surgery is reserved for patients with an irreducible or gangrenous volvulus. Planned surgery may be arranged for some fit patients after their first attack of volvulus.

Endoscopic decompression of a sigmoid volvulus

Classically, deflation of the volvulus is achieved with a flatus tube inserted through a rigid sigmoidoscope on the ward.

To do this you need a light source, a sigmoidoscope and a flatus tube (Americans would call it a rectal tube). Wear an apron! With the patient in the left lateral position, advance the lubricated sigmoidoscope to the top of the rectum. The twist in the bowel should be visible — now pass the flatus tube through the twist. **Try to delegate the procedure to someone more junior**

than you (but stay at his side), as success is indicated by a tsunami of liquid stool and flatus! If the tube cannot be easily passed then stop — an inability to reduce the volvulus may indicate gangrene. If deflation with a rigid sigmoidoscope is not successful then try a **flexible endoscopy** — the view is better and the ability to use suction means that this is more successful. And anyway, the good old rigid sigmoidoscope has been gradually disappearing from sight — replaced by useless disposable plastic tubes. And when was the last time that you found a good-sized rectal tube in your hospital?

Don't delay in arranging for endoscopic decompression; we have seen deaths due to gangrene and perforation of the volvulus when this has not been done promptly.

Surgery for sigmoid volvulus

It is rare to need to operate as an emergency for sigmoid volvulus because endoscopic decompression is commonly successful. **However, you will need to operate if the volvulus is irreducible, gangrenous or perforated. We would approach these patients via a midline incision and would resect the sigmoid colon and either do a Hartmann's or a double-barrelled colostomy**. In selected cases, however, primary anastomosis would be acceptable — use your judgment.

More commonly we operate on a planned basis to prevent further episodes of volvulus. Be careful, as this is a group of patients with a very high rate of comorbidities and many are not fit for major surgery. Laparoscopy in the situation is pointless — *surgical masturbation*. Our preference is for a small muscle-splitting left iliac fossa incision, although some prefer a lower midline incision (we think that is unnecessary in this situation). No mobilization of the sigmoid is needed — it is 'pre-mobilized'. Given the benign nature of the condition, vascular ligation does not have to be 'high', and the anastomosis can be safely undertaken at the top of the rectum. There is often a degree of size discrepancy here and we often use a side-to-end anastomosis.

While the concept of **'pexy'-fixation instead of resection** has gained a bad reputation, recently there has been a revival of this approach, with 'retroperitonealization' of the mobile colon — even by laparoscopy. Early results are promising, but solid data are still lacking and sigmoidectomy remains the gold standard.

Cecal volvulus

Cecal volvulus is rare and you will only see a handful of such cases in your whole career. The underlying cause is a redundant mesentery and lack of fixation of the cecum: it flips and twists (usually) clockwise, which results in obstruction and compromise of the blood supply. A rare variant of cecal volvulus is **cecal bascule** — involving upwards and anterior folding of the right colon. **These patients have clinical and radiographic signs of small bowel obstruction. In addition, typically, the cecal 'shadow' is absent from the right lower quadrant. Instead, the poorly attached and redundant cecum has flipped to the left and upwards to the left upper quadrant**. It is visualized on abdominal radiographs as a coffee-bean sign in the epigastrium or the left hypochondrium, with its concavity pointing to the right lower quadrant. It contains a single fluid level representing the dislocated cecum which is often confused with the gastric shadow. If in doubt (there is always some 'doubt') and in the absence of peritoneal signs, you may order a Gastrografin® enema, which will demonstrate the characteristic 'beak' in the right colon. **But today a CT is the easiest and most accurate route to a diagnosis**.

In our hands the treatment of choice is a right hemicolectomy; we would do this urgently as there is a high risk of cecal necrosis. If the volvulus is gangrenous and the patient is in poor condition, we would do a double-barrelled stoma rather than an anastomosis. Yes, previous editions of this book mentioned the options of *cecopexy* and even (God forbid) *tube cecostomy* — options that have become less popular. However, laparoscopic retroperitoneal fixation has been presented as a successful alternative but is still controversial.

Acute colonic pseudo-obstruction

This is also known as **Ogilvie's syndrome**.

William Heneage Ogilvie (1887-1971) was not only a great British surgeon but also a keen surgical aphorist. For example: "Personal statistics are at the bottom of all unsound teaching; they are either too good to be true or too true to be good."

Quite frankly, this is a disheartening situation to manage. The patient is usually referred for a surgical consult to 'exclude a bowel obstruction' from other subspecialties in medicine or orthopedics and will usually be frail with significant comorbidities. At the bedside, you will see a debilitated patient with a grossly distended abdomen. The arrival of the surgical team prompts concerns from the patient and their family that there will be the need for (another) major operation. Fortunately, this is unlikely to be necessary.

Nobody really knows the exact etiology of this syndrome (we suspect that in the background there is sympathetic overactivity which paralyses the colon), but here's how we would approach such patients:

- Take a history and examine the patient (yes, old fashioned we know).
- Do a rectal examination yourself (in 'true' obstruction the rectum is collapsed whereas in pseudo-obstruction the rectum is capacious and you cannot 'touch the sides').
- Look at the patient's recent lab results and fluid balance charts (dehydration and electrolyte disturbances are common in this group of patients — both cause and effect…).
- Do some imaging to exclude a mechanical obstruction. This will usually be the ubiquitous CT scan, but a water-soluble contrast enema is a good alternative if you don't have access to CT scanning.
- Make sure that they do not have *C. diff.* colitis (which may rarely cause abdominal distension without diarrhea).
- Look for factors which could cause or perpetuate acute colonic pseudo-obstruction (■ Table 25.2).

Table 25.2. Causative factors in acute colonic pseudo-obstruction.
■ Dehydration.
■ Acute kidney injury (AKI).
■ Hypokalemia.
■ Hypomagnesemia.
■ Infection (commonly chest or urinary tract).
■ Recent hip or spinal surgery.
■ Malignant infiltration of the retroperitoneum.
■ Drugs.

So, you will find the patient on the far distant non-gastrointestinal surgical ward where they will have been an inpatient for a period of time. **Frequently they will have another predominant problem such as a pneumonia, urinary tract infection, major joint reconstruction or spinal surgery**. There may be an associated low-grade sepsis, electrolyte imbalance and suboptimal fluid management, potentially with an acute kidney injury. There will be a history of the bowels not being open for a variable period but vomiting may not be a predominant feature.

Clinical examination demonstrates a generally distended but soft and non-tender abdomen without tension. Digital rectal examination identifies a dilated rectum, often with an amount of stool but no palpable rectal cancer. The clinical diagnosis can be clarified with a CT scan of the abdomen and pelvis with intravenous contrast. The only concern about achieving this is the status of renal function to allow administration of intravenous contrast. **The scan will usually identify a globally distended colon down to the rectum with or without an amount of feces**. If there is any doubt regarding a true obstruction, then supplementary tests such as a Gastrografin® enema or a flexible sigmoidoscopy may be needed. Some people claim that the Gastrografin® enema is also therapeutic. We suspect they are right...

Management

After excluding mechanical obstruction... do the following:

- Correct any electrolyte disturbances by infusing i.v. Hartmann's solution or normal saline with potassium/magnesium as necessary.
- Stop any drugs which may be affecting bowel motility or are nephrotoxic.
- Identify and treat any focus of infection.
- Deflate the colon. Like the heart, **once the colon is stretched beyond a certain point it ceases to function adequately** (Cheetham's Law of the Colon) leading to fluid and gas building up. **A flatus tube may help initially but endoscopic deflation with a colonoscope is more effective (you may need to repeat this)**.
- Stimulate the rectum to empty. Try stimulant suppositories such as bisacodyl or a phosphate enema.

In most case the measures described above will allow the pseudo-obstruction to resolve over a few days. In refractory cases there are two other options to consider:

- i.v. neostigmine.
- Blowhole cecostomy.

i.v. neostigmine

Randomized trials have demonstrated good rates of resolution of colonic pseudo-obstruction following i.v. neostigmine. We have not had quite such successful results, although when it does work it's spectacular. We have found that many patients with pseudo-obstruction have contraindications to neostigmine (which has a lot of side effects). **If you are going to give i.v.**

neostigmine we would recommend that the patient is on a continuous EKG monitor as this often results in profound bradycardia. Give 2mg of neostigmine as a slow i.v. bolus. The patient will usually feel awful, drool saliva and the EKG trace goes flat for frightening amounts of time. Then, if you are lucky, there is an enormous explosive fart and the patient is better. If you have missed a mechanical obstruction, the patient will explode...

Blowhole cecostomy

Rarely all the methods above fail (including repeated endoscopic decompression) and you are stuck with a patient with refractory pseudo-obstruction. Without resolution the patient is condemned to deteriorate through poor nutrition or respiratory embarrassment. **In this situation you should consider surgery.**

The least invasive approach is to create a **blowhole cecostomy** in the right iliac fossa via a small muscle-splitting incision; you can do this under local anesthetic (➲ Chapter 14.2). The distended cecum will pout into the wound where you can create an opening and suture the cecal wall to the skin (see ■ Figure 14.5). You don't need to mobilize the bowel or create a formal colostomy — remember all you are creating is an opening in the colon to allow flatus out. Tube cecostomies frequently block and are not as effective.

To recap...

Large bowel obstruction usually causes florid symptoms of abdominal distension and complete constipation. The majority of patients will have an obstruction due to a colorectal cancer. **You must ensure that the patient doesn't have a rectal cancer or a pseudo-obstruction before you operate.** Usually surgery can be delayed until the following day, but beware the patients with a closed loop obstruction (remember who will have closed loop obstruction and why? [1]) who need surgery within a few hours to avoid the risk of cecal necrosis and perforation.

> **"If you don't eat, you don't shit**
> **If you don't shit — you die!"**
>
> **Barry (Baz) Alexander**

1 Answer: those with a competent ileocecal valve...

Chapter 26

Acute diverticulitis

Simon Shaw and Mark Cheetham

The British have such trouble with their diverticula because no one is allowed to fart!

Harold Ellis

Diverticulosis (like hypertension and obesity) is endemic in Western countries where the diet of some people seems to consist entirely of burgers and fries washed down with high-sugar drinks. Diverticular disease, along with gallstones and hernias, is bread and butter to the general surgeon; it puts food on the table and fills the Merc's gas tank. **In this chapter we will discuss the common emergency presentations of diverticular disease and give you some tips to manage each situation**.

The word diverticulum comes from a Greek word meaning "a wayside house of ill repute" (you know the kind of place where some of the readers of this book might hang out...). Colonic diverticula are protrusions of the colonic mucosa through the muscularis layer of the colon where the vasa recta enter the bowel wall. **They can occur anywhere along the colon but are most common in the sigmoid colon and never occur in the rectum**.

Diverticular disease is very common in patients older than late middle age. Well, it would be hard to find a 'healthy' elderly Brit or American who does not have any diverticula in his colon (■ Figure 26.1). And with the epidemic of junk food we see an increasing number of patients in their 30s with complicated diverticular disease. They are even more common in certain patient groups,

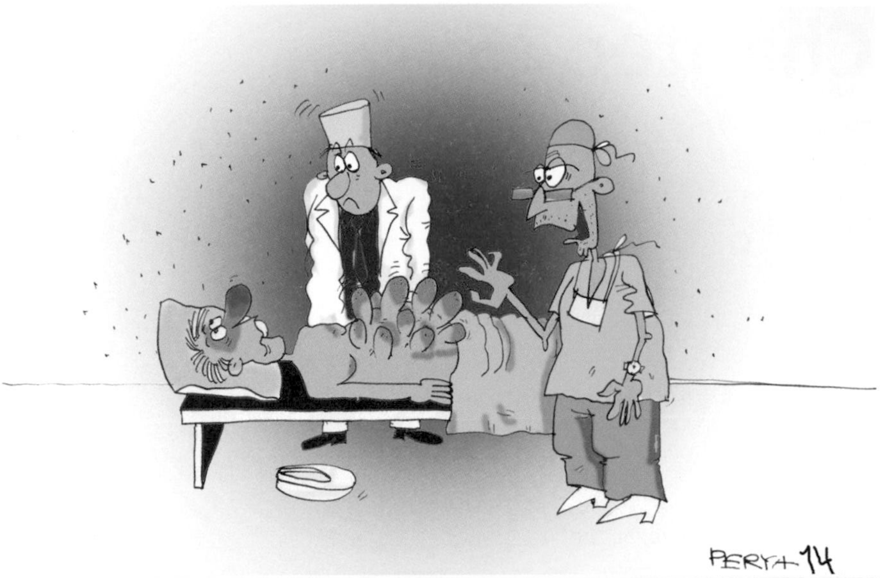

Figure 26.1. "Which of these do we have to remove?"

such as the obese, inactive, elderly and seemingly anyone on our colonoscopy lists!

The vast majority of diverticula cause no symptoms; of those that do cause symptoms, there are three common emergency presentations:

- Acute diverticulitis or perforation.
- Bleeding (see ➲ Chapter 27).
- Obstruction (see ➲ Chapter 25).

Acute diverticulitis

Like acute appendicitis, we divide the clinical scenarios of acute diverticulitis in order of increasing severity:

- **'Simple' (uncomplicated) acute diverticulitis.**
- **'Complicated' acute diverticulitis:**
  - **local perforation with pericolic or pelvic abscess;**
  - **'free perforation'.**

Simple acute diverticulitis

Acute diverticulitis is such a common presentation in the West that **we do not believe there are any surgeons who will not immediately recognize a combination of left iliac fossa pain, tenderness and guarding, loss of appetite, low-grade pyrexia and a degree of relative constipation**. Add to this blood tests revealing elevated inflammatory markers and you have an unmistakable clinical picture.

To image or not to image?

We believe that in a typical patient who is not unwell, imaging is unnecessary. **And, of course, there is no reason to rescan patients who return with yet another mild attack of recurrent diverticulitis**. Our American friends tell us however that all their patients get a CT — to document and stage the process and to exclude other diagnoses — and anyway in the USA such patients cannot be transferred from the ER to the wards without passing through the scanner. They call it 'defensive medicine'. Well we think, let them make America great again…

Let us not forget however, that on occasion, **a loop of sigmoid colon can flip over to the right and present with a right iliac fossa pain and tenderness, mimicking acute appendicitis** — you don't want to operate on these patients, do you? A similar presentation, with bloody diarrhea, may herald an attack of ischemic colitis. And of course, there are other causes of left iliac fossa pain (some of which will need emergency intervention; see ■ Table 26.1).

Table 26.1. Some mimics of acute diverticulitis.

- Ischemic colitis.
- Inflammatory bowel disease.
- Perforated colorectal cancer.
- Leaking abdominal aortic aneurysm.
- Renal colic.
- Aortic dissection.

So, whenever the clinical picture is not 'classical' of acute diverticulitis and we have some doubts, we may become a little American-like and admit that:

CT scanning can be useful in this setting, to get things right.

How do we manage simple acute diverticulitis?

Many of these patients can be treated on an ambulatory basis with oral antibiotics. However, patients who are sicker or who do not tolerate oral intake are best admitted and placed on i.v. antibiotics (no need to tell you which antibiotics to use, eh?). We do not restrict diet in these patients but many will feel off-color and will not want to eat much anyway. Often, we find that someone else has told the patient that they need to eat a high-fiber diet and avoid seeds. Whilst there is good evidence to support a high-fiber diet preventing the development of diverticulosis, we do not believe that adding fiber after an acute attack reduces the risk of another attack. And seeds? Well, we have yet to come across any seed clever enough to seek out and lodge in a diverticulum...

With conservative management, uncomplicated diverticulitis will usually settle. **It is our practice to undertake colonoscopy some 6-8 weeks following resolution** as the frequency of a cancer, although small (approximately 2%), is not insignificant (we are sure that if you work in a fee-for-service system that your patient will undoubtedly have a colonoscopy...).

Does simple diverticulitis need to be treated with antibiotics?

Antibiotics have been an established part of the management of diverticulitis for so long, that it seems difficult to imagine they would not have a role to play. Yet this is what an increasing body of evidence suggests. So, what are the implications for practice? We suggest that well, immunocompetent patients with a clinical diagnosis of simple diverticulitis can be treated safely without antibiotics, providing they have good access to medical care; for the rest (sick patients, diabetics or those who are immunosuppressed), we would continue to treat them with antibiotics. Bear in mind however that this topic is also subject to a 'transatlantic divide', based on fear of litigation and 'failure' to follow the so called 'standard of care' on one of the side of the Atlantic — you know which side it is...

What about elective, interval sigmoid resection to prevent recurrent attacks? Be patient. This will be discussed below.

Complicated acute diverticulitis

OK, now we are getting to the crux of the matter, what you have been waiting for; those **situations which may need emergency surgical intervention**.

Perforated diverticulitis

If your patient is sicker than described above, or there is more than 'just local tenderness', then you will want to perform the 'obligatory' CT to confirm the diagnosis and stage the disease.

We believe that, as with appendicitis, perforated diverticulitis is a distinct entity when compared to simple diverticulitis. Having said that there is a wide spectrum of disease seen in acute diverticulitis and this is also reflected in the diversity of opinions as to how to treat different clinical situations. The **Ambrosetti classification** (■ Table 26.2) is based on the CT findings and is a useful guide as to how the patients can be treated. It is in some way analogous to the older **Hinchey classification** (■ Table 26.3) which is based on the operative findings and is focused on the 'complicated' cases.

Table 26.2. The Ambrosetti CT classification of diverticulitis. *(Ambrosetti P, Becker C, Terrier F. Colonic diverticulitis: impact of imaging on surgical management — a prospective study of 542 patients. Eur Radiol 2002; 12: 1145-9.)*

Moderate diverticulitis	Localised sigmoid wall thickening Pericolic fat stranding
Severe diverticulitis	Abscess Extraluminal air Extraluminal contrast

The combination of clinical and CT findings will allow you to allocate your patient to one of the following groups:

- **Simple — 'smoldering' diverticulitis.**
- **Pericolic or pelvic abscess.**
- **Generalized peritonitis.**

Table 26.3. The Hinchey classification of acute diverticulitis. *(Hinchey EJ, Schaal PG, Richards GK. Treatment of perforated diverticular disease of the colon. Adv Surg 1978; 12: 85-109.)*

Classification	Description
Hinchey 1	Pericolic abscess or phlegmon
Hinchey 2	Pelvic, intra-abdominal or retroperitoneal abscess
Hinchey 3	Generalized purulent peritonitis
Hinchey 4	Generalized feculent peritonitis

Simple — 'smoldering' diverticulitis

This means that a patient diagnosed with simple acute diverticulitis is not improving after 3-5 days of conservative management.

Consider repeated imaging to see if there has been progression to complicated disease, in which case 'salvage' can often be achieved via radiological drainage (if there is a localized collection, for example). **In the absence of radiological progression, be patient and try to continue antibiotics for a few days.** If the patient was on oral antibiotics until now then surely he has to receive them intravenously. (Although some of us doubt that, in a patient with a normally absorbing gut, intravenous antibiotics represents 'stronger' medicine…). In addition, perhaps consider switching antibiotics in response to any available blood cultures or advice from your local microbiology service. **At the same time, warn the patient that if he won't improve within 48-72 hours then resection will have to be considered.** In this situation we would consider a planned sigmoid resection within a few days to obtain source control; whether or not the resection should include a primary anastomosis we will discuss below.

There is also a group of patients who seem to recover after a course of antibiotics, only to flare up again when the antibiotics are stopped. **We consider this to be *smoldering* diverticulitis and the correct course of action is to proceed with resection.**

Pericolic/pelvic abscess

When acute diverticulitis presents with a localized, contained perforation, the clinical presentation tends to be indistinguishable from a non-perforated diverticulitis. We remember that in the good old pre-CT days many such patients were successfully treated with antibiotics alone. What about these days?

- When the CT shows a small pericolic abscess, you should not jump off your couch. **Abscesses of less than 4-5cm in diameter should resolve with antibiotics alone; but a prolonged course of up to 2 weeks may be needed**.
- **Larger abscesses will need to be drained**. This should be done, if possible, percutaneously by the radiologist.

Generalized peritonitis

If there are clinical and/or radiological features of diffuse peritonitis suggesting disseminated contamination of the abdomen, surgery should be considered.

Even in this situation, there is a spectrum of disease from the 'quiet' patient to the critical ill patient with fecal peritonitis.

Remember: the mere presence of free air on CT is not an absolute indication for an operation. In the 'well patient', with a few bubbles of air surrounding the sigmoid, or even a sliver of free air under the diaphragm, you can try conservative treatment — as long as they are not overtly 'septic' and their abdominal signs are localized. **We have frequently treated this group of patients with antibiotics and MICLO (masterly inactivity and cat-like observation)**.

The emergency operation for acute diverticulitis

> *The operative approach should be individualized and depends on the stage of the disease present, the general condition of the patient, the experience of the surgeon in colon surgery and the availability of facilities and personnel to provide intensive care.*
>
> **E. John Hinchey**

Let us recap the indications for surgery in acute diverticulitis:

- Refractory 'simple' diverticulitis ('smoldering').
- Localized perforation with pericolic or pelvic collection (not treatable percutaneously).
- Purulent diffuse peritonitis.
- Fecal diffuse peritonitis.

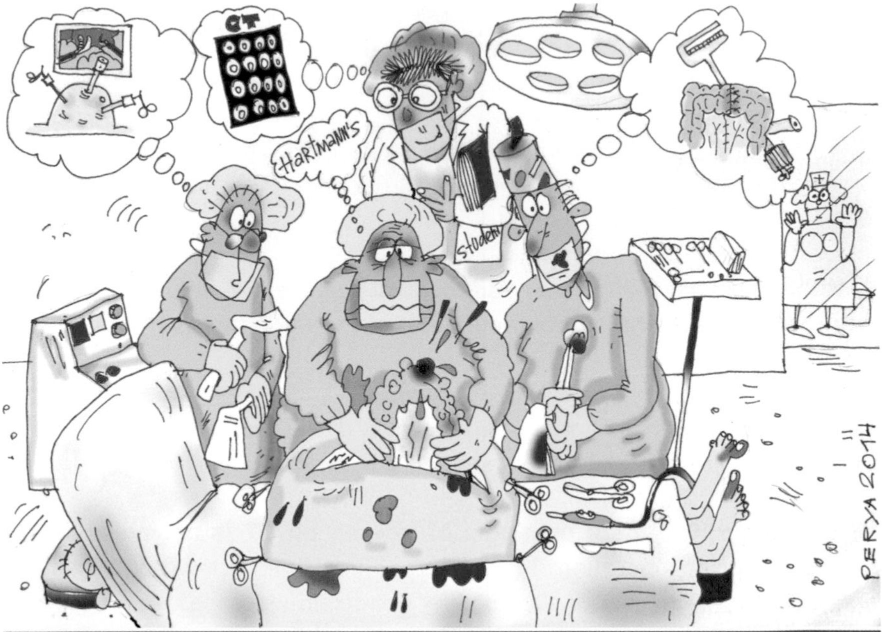

Figure 26.2. Chief surgeon thinks: "Hartmann's..." First assistant thinks: "Resection and anastomosis..." Second assistant thinks: "They should have done laparoscopic peritoneal lavage..." Medical student (the one with big glasses): "Why didn't you get a CT? This would have responded to antibiotics..."

So, you decided to proceed with an emergency operation for acute diverticulitis. What are your options? (■ Figure 26.2).

We have summarized the surgical options for various situations and grades of acute diverticulitis in ■ Table 26.4. You can see that there is a wide spectrum of conditions, ranging from a simple phlegmon to fecal peritonitis, and there is an equally wide spectrum of opinions as to how to approach each situation.

Herein we will bring our opinion on how to tailor the 'optimal' procedure to your patient, under three main headings:

- Sigmoid resection without an anastomosis.
- Sigmoid resection with an anastomosis +/- a diverting stoma.
- Laparoscopic lavage (no resection...).

Table 26.4. A suggested scheme for the emergency surgical treatment of acute diverticulitis.

Clinical situation	Hinchey grade	Ambrosetti grade	Surgical options
'Smoldering' diverticulitis	1	Moderate	• None • Scheduled diverticular resection with primary anastomosis
Locally perforated diverticulitis with pericolic, pelvic or retroperitoneal collection	2	Severe	• Radiological drainage • Laparoscopic drainage • Resection with anastomosis (+/- defunctioning stoma) • Hartmann's procedure
Purulent peritonitis	3	Severe	• Laparoscopic washout • Sigmoid resection with primary anastomosis (+/- defunctioning stoma) • Hartmann's procedure
Fecal peritonitis	4	Severe	• Hartmann's procedure

Sigmoid resection without an anastomosis (Hartmann's procedure)

This procedure has the advantage of avoiding the risks of anastomotic leakage.

The classic indication for Hartmann's procedure is a patient who is acutely ill with a free perforation leading to fecal peritonitis.

Hartmann's procedure is considered by some an 'easy operation' and thus may be delegated to an inexperienced surgeon. This can result in the **Hartmann's triad of doom: a blown rectal stump, a deep-space infection and a retracted colostomy.** Avoid this by ensuring that there is adequate surgical experience in the room. We wish we could offer tips and tricks into how to make this an easy resection, deftly mobilizing the sigmoid colon with one hand, whilst flashing a winning smile and chatting to the anesthetist/scrub staff at the same time. In reality, these are difficult, sweaty and often 'sweary' operations with an acutely inflamed, adherent colon seemingly stuck to everything and a thickened, foreshortened mesocolon. And with obesity being a known risk factor for acute diverticulitis things are not getting easier...

Some tips for performing a Hartmann's procedure:

- **Make a long midline incision** — you will need good exposure and you may (although not very often) need to take down the splenic flexure.
- Start mobilizing the descending colon first.
- Continue the mobilization of the sigmoid to the upper rectum, and (you hope!) healthy-looking tissues.
- Use a combination of blunt dissection ('finger fracture') and sharp dissection to complete this mobilization.
- You don't need to radically remove every single diverticulum — resect the perforated segment and any 'hard' bowel and make sure that you have supple bowel at either end of your resection.
- Oversew the cross-stapled rectal stump to reduce the risk of a stump blowout. (BTW, if you wish — you can suture-close the rectal stump.)
- Rarely, if the rectal stump is very friable use a purse-string suture to tie a 30Fr Foley catheter into the end of the rectal stump; bring the catheter out through the lower abdominal wall. We would also place a wide-bore tube drain in the pelvis. (Yes, we know that some of the Editors would think that this is unnecessary...).
- By the way, Henri Albert Hartmann was a French Surgeon of Paris (1860-1952).

When we discuss the planned Hartmann's procedure with patients and their families we usually declare that this will be a 'temporary colostomy'. **But in real life fewer than half of these patients are assessed as fit enough to undergo restoration of bowel continuity**; the latter being a major procedure associated with significant morbidity. **Remember: the Hartmann's procedure can save life. But it condemns the patients to living with a colostomy or to yet another major operation with all its potential morbidity. Do not undertake it lightly**.

Sigmoid resection with an anastomosis with or without a diverting stoma

This procedure has the advantages of avoiding the morbidity of a stoma and the difficult subsequent operation to reverse the Hartmann's procedure.

We would consider doing a primary anastomosis under the following circumstances:

- The patient is in a relatively good general condition (he is likely to survive an — God forbidden — anastomotic leak…).
- Local conditions are favorable: Hinchey 1 or 2 and selectively in some patients with Hinchey 3 peritonitis. **Never in fecal peritonitis.**
- Systemic factors are favorable (e.g. the patient is hemodynamically intact and not malnourished).

One should not be surprised that as most of our patients in need of an emergency operation suffer from diffuse peritonitis we rarely have the opportunity to do a primary anastomosis. **Those who do many such cases must surely be operating on patients who should have been treated conservatively…**

Obviously, you will know all the technical rules about doing a good colorectal anastomosis (no tension, well-perfused bowel and good anastomotic technique — see ➲ Chapter 14).

Should you add a proximal stoma to divert your 'high-risk' anastomosis? We would be selective about this as well. If the 'resection cum anastomosis' has gone well and you are not too worried, then we wouldn't be adding a stoma.

Remember that this is a very different situation to an elective anterior resection when the patient has had oral bowel prep; here, instead, the colon is going to be full and your diversion will be less effective. So, if you are going to do a stoma it is probably worth considering doing an on-table colonic lavage too (we have covered this in more detail in the preceding chapter on large bowel obstruction — ➲ Chapter 25).

Laparoscopic lavage (no resection)

Laparoscopic lavage for acute diverticulitis was first reported a decade ago and initially it showed great promise. It offers the obvious advantages of avoiding both a stoma and the risks of an anastomotic leak. The downside is that the source of sepsis is not completely removed, and some patients will need a later resection. Maybe that's a good thing if at worst the patient's resection is deferred to a later, planned operation!

We would consider doing a laparoscopic lavage in patients with Hinchey 2 or 3 acute diverticulitis. **We think it to be pointless in patients with Hinchey 1 disease and futile in patients with fecal peritonitis (the latter group need a Hartmann's)**.

At laparoscopy you initially examine the inflamed colon. Usually you see a perforated abscess cavity and no opening to the colon. Sometimes you see no cavity and just the inflamed bowel. **If you don't see an obvious hole in the colon, for God's sake do not go poking around for it! In other words, don't mobilize the colon unless you plan on resecting it**. Most of the time you just see the inflamed colon with a part of the abscess cavity; in these cases you irrigate the abdomen — all four quadrants and the pelvis until clean and then leave a round 19Fr Jackson-Pratt drain in the abscess cavity or near the colon, bringing it out through the suprapubic trocar site. The purpose of this drain is not to drain the general peritoneal cavity, which is a 'mission impossible', but to drain any colonic hole which you may have missed. **The truth however is that we almost never see any feces from such drains after lap lavage for purulent peritonitis — the reason being that the perforations in such cases are minute and self-sealing rapidly; this explains why lap lavage is successful... In the rare case when you see a colonic perforation consider proceeding with resection**.

Please watch these patients carefully after the lap lavage. They should improve within 24-48 hours. Do not procrastinate with those who continue to be 'septic' — **they must go back to the OR for resection**.

By now, you may have realized that we, as many others, are still not entirely sure about the role of peritoneal lavage in perforated diverticulitis. It seems that the main role is in patients with diffuse peritonitis who turn out to have widespread pus due to intra-abdominal abscess rupture; they need surgery but many can avoid a stoma. On the other hand it appears to us that non-selective use of lavage is mainly successful in patients who could have been treated conservatively. However, it surely gives you something to do, to be active, when the patient is not improving fast enough on conservative treatment — perhaps even accelerating recovery. At the same time, it avoids a few colostomies, which may however still be needed if the 'lavage' fails. **Sorry, not much science here... you can consider this option based on your local circumstances**.

What about laparoscopic colectomy?

Laparoscopic colectomy for acute diverticulitis is controversial. Even elective diverticular resections can be really challenging due to adhesions and loss of tissue planes. If you are a technical whizz-kid with your own YouTube channel, we are sure that an emergency laparoscopic sigmoid colectomy is feasible for you. **Whether it is desirable to put your sick, septic patient with complicated diverticulitis in a steep head-down position for hours is another matter. For these patients it is the degree of 'sepsis' which determines outcome, rather than the trauma of surgical access**. However, when successful, feel proud you have significantly reduced the common risks of SSI and incisional hernias.

Even to us mortals, who do perform a significant volume of elective laparoscopic colorectal surgery, the open surgical approach appears to be the safest in this context.

A few words about diverticular fistulas...

The most common fistulas are either to the urinary bladder (colovesical) or the vagina (colovaginal). In some cases, the colon may fistulate to the skin, the uterus, Fallopian tubes, small intestine or even another segment of the colon. Such fistulas are usually evaluated and treated electively — with resection of the origin in the sigmoid colon.

Occasionally, however, you may have to operate on patients with either colovaginal or colovesical fistulas urgently. If a **colovaginal** fistula forms *immediately* after an acute perforation, the patient will experience a sudden release of pus, blood, and stool from the vagina that, in most instances, stops quickly. However, if the fistula is large and persistent, stool continues draining from the vagina. If this happens we perform a (laparoscopic) loop ileostomy to divert the fecal flow. **Let the acute disease settle down and remove the offending colonic segment a few months later**.

Colovesical fistulas very rarely need an emergency procedure except perhaps if developing in transplant patients (particularly kidney transplants) who develop persistent urosepsis. Early diversion or resection may be indicated to stop the flow of s**t into the bladder. In patients who respond initially to antibiotics we would keep them on maintenance antibiotics for 6 to 8 weeks until the 'elective' operation.

After the resolved attack: elective interval resection

Most patients with acute diverticulitis respond to conservative therapy. It is estimated that around one-fourth of them will experience a

recurrence. This is interpreted by knife-happy surgeons as confirming the need for elective surgery, **while for the more conservative surgeons it indicates that most patients do not require an operation**. To which of the two groups do you belong?

According to tradition, the second (or third) attack has been considered an indication for an elective sigmoidectomy, this being particularly preached for the younger patient. However, this approach too has been questioned by not a few studies showing that **patients undergoing such elective interval sigmoid resections do not fare symptomatically better compared to patients who have no surgery**.

In general, it is the initial attack which tends to complicate — with free perforation, abscess formation or a fistula. Recurrent attacks tend to be relatively benign and to respond to medical treatment.

The reasonable approach is to individualize the management and offer elective resection under the following 'talking points':

- Multiple recurrent and frequent attacks greatly interfering with quality of life.
- Prolonged, 'smoldering' attacks with the patient never really having completely recovered.
- Following attacks of complicated diverticulitis; e.g. pericolic abscess managed percutaneously.
- Immunocompromised patients (e.g. post-liver transplant) who are highly susceptible to develop a free perforation.
- In patients developing fibrotic stenosis of the colon with symptoms/evidence of colonic obstruction.
- Patients who developed fistulas.

By 'individual approach', we mean that you should not be dogmatic. So, while a 30-year-old guy who had suffered five attacks over the last year deserves an operation, an 80-year-old lady who had a few mild attacks does not. And a 90-year-old gentleman who has percutaneous drainage of a diverticular abscess can live on without having his sigmoid removed.

Of course, there are those whose opinion may drastically differ from ours. In their 'modern' view, the mere fact that they can do laparoscopic, nay, robotic, sigmoidectomy, proves that sigmoid resection is a 'walk in the park' and indications should be relaxed. The choice of which camp to belong to... depends on your own *weltanschauung*.

When the chips are down, Hartmann's is your friend!

Other forms of acute diverticulitis

Although sigmoid diverticulitis is common in our daily practice, other forms of diverticulitis should be kept in mind:

- With the horrendous amount of junk food consumed by 'western societies' we see a growing number of younger patients with colonic **pandiverticulosis** extending from the rectosigmoid junction to the ileocecal valve. Some of these present with **acute diverticulitis in the right or transverse colon**, which may mimic acute cholecystitis or acute appendicitis. The key to diagnosis here is an abdominal CT scan finding of a localized colonic phlegmon. This avoids an unnecessary operation and the temptation to proceed with colonic resection when they almost all would respond to conservative treatment with antibiotics.
- **'Solitary' cecal diverticulitis.** This is a different entity: young, mostly male, patients with one or two diverticula in the cecum — in the absence of diverticula distally. Once or twice a year you will see a patient presenting with what you think to be 'classic' acute appendicitis but at operation you'll find a cecal inflammatory mass or phlegmon of variable size. Free perforation and generalized peritonitis are uncommon. **This misadventure will happen to you only if you skip the CT, on which a good radiologist should be able to distinguish cecal diverticulitis from acute appendicitis.** If this is the case, you can treat conservatively as these patients would respond to antibiotics exactly like those with sigmoid diverticulitis. And, of course, recurrent cecal diverticulitis has been reported in conservatively treated patients. Many patients, however, come to operation, either because CT is not done, or its findings are mistaken for acute appendicitis. **What to do at operation depends on the magnitude of the process (i.e. how bad it looks)**, ranging from diverticulectomy (place a linear stapler across the base of the diverticulum — including healthy cecal wall — and fire) to partial cecectomy (again, fire a stapler across and be careful not to narrow the ileocecal junction). Occasionally, when the diverticulum is situated just off the ileocecal valve it is safer to excise and close the cecal hole by hand. Surgeons who are not aware of this condition, or cannot recognize it, are often carried away and perform right hemicolectomy.

For the sake of completeness let us mention here that acute diverticulitis *very rarely* affects patients with **jejunal diverticulosis**. These patients present with systemic signs of inflammation as well as with local peritoneal signs in the center of the abdomen. **The key to diagnosis and subsequent non-operative management and treatment with antibiotics (usually successful) is a CT scan — showing an inflammatory mass affecting a segment of the jejunum and its mesentery**. If forced to operate, all you need do is a segmental small bowel resection and anastomosis.

Final thoughts

Looking at the 'whole picture' it appears that we operate too early in acute diverticulitis, perform too many CTs, carry out too many PC drainage procedures, remove too many colons, raise too many colostomies, reoperate electively on too many patients, treat too many with antibiotics, and perform too few randomized controlled trials in order to know what is right and what is wrong.

"In the heart of Africa you will rarely see a case of acute diverticulitis: people there do not yet eat the junk that we do."

Chapter 27

Massive lower GI bleeding

Ghaleb Goussous and Mark Cheetham

Bleeding in the belly is like fire on a ship — you run towards it.
Jeffery Young

All bleeding stops — eventually.
Anon

In this chapter, we are not talking about people who have a little bit of rectal bleeding. We know that you can handle these patients (see ➲ Chapter 28 about anorectal disorders). No, here we are talking about that rare patient who is trying to exsanguinate via the anus.

We all know the heart-sink moment answering a phone call from the Emergency Department asking us to attend to a patient with a '**massive rectal bleed**'. Luckily, in almost all such cases it isn't that massive! Those of us who shave know that a drop of blood can stain a whole sink red and the same applies to blood dripping in the toilet: it can look catastrophic indeed.

Presentation and definitions

Lower GI bleeds (LGIB) present with passage of either fresh or maroon-colored blood per rectum (aka hematochezia). Anatomically, it is a bleed originating from beyond the ligament of Treitz. *Politically*, it is a bleed that the gastroenterologist won't take until seen by a surgeon — which, as we know, is not such a bad idea... (unless this happens after midnight ☹).

There is, however, no universally agreed definition for a *massive* lower GI bleed. Some say it is a bleed requiring more than 4 units of RBCs or a hemoglobin concentration (Hb) of 6g/dL or less.

We feel this is not very useful as Hb concentration will take time to dilute and most of the time we don't know the starting concentration. We know that it is rather difficult to 'guestimate' how much blood a person will need from the outset and transfusion requirements are subject to the patient's response; a younger patient may need less blood than an older patient on antihypertensives to remedy the same blood loss. **Put simply, if the bleeding is associated with a degree of hemodynamic instability then it is most likely massive enough and will need your undivided attention**.

Now, going more into detail we should mention that the individual patient matters as well (surprise!). So, you should take the bleeding seriously also in the following particular situations:

- Older patients (>60 years) with comorbidities.
- Gross ongoing bleeding.
- Patients on 'blood thinners'.

Such patients should be admitted, monitored and investigated as discussed below.

Causes

Diverticulosis and arteriovenous malformations (AVMs) are the two most common causes of LGIB and vie for the number one spot. As you probably remember from your medical school, diverticular bleeds tend to be more commonly seen than AVMs. **Diverticular bleeds are more common on the left, while AVMs are more common on the right**. AVMs are thought to be associated with cardiac valvular disease so be vigilant and check those patients are not on antiplatelet medications or anticoagulation.

We won't bore you by going through all the causes of hematochezia (see ■ Table 27.1). Instead, we will focus on discussing how to deal with the common causes of massive LGIB.

Table 27.1. Causes of LGIB.

Causes of massive LGIB

- Diverticulosis.
- Arteriovenous malformations.

Other causes of LGIB

- Inflammatory:
  - IBD (ulcerative colitis and Crohn's disease);
  - infectious;
  - ischemia;
  - radiation (proctitis).
- Anorectal:
  - hemorrhoids;
  - fissure-in-ano;
  - fistula-in-ano.
- Neoplastic:
  - cancer of the colon or rectum;
  - polyps.
- Iatrogenic:
  - foreign bodies;
  - post-polypectomy (especially after clever procedures such as endoscopic mucosal resection [EMR] or endoscopic submucosal dissection [ESD]);
  - anastomotic bleeds.
- Small bowel causes:
  - Meckel's diverticulum;
  - small bowel tumors.

Management: resuscitate — localize — control

Initial assessment and early management

When you come to see the patient make sure that adequate resuscitative measures have taken place. You don't want us to nag you again with the ABC of resuscitation. Only that... **as a rule of thumb replace blood with blood and avoid over-resuscitation with salty water**. We usually give a dose of i.v. tranexamic acid to patients with a significant GI bleed. Remember to ensure that clotting factors are replaced along with red cells.

At an early stage it is paramount to establish whether the patient is anticoagulated. If they are, then normalize their clotting as a matter of priority. Patients on novel oral anticoagulants (NOACs) are very tricky to deal with when compared to patients on the good old warfarin. Most of those new agents do not currently have an antidote (apart from dabigatran) and are challenging to reverse. It is wise to involve your friendly hematologist in the management of any patient who is anticoagulated and particularly if on a NOAC.

After you have dealt with the immediate ABC, take a focused history and examine the patient thoroughly and perform a digital rectal examination and proctoscopy to rule out anorectal causes (■ Figure 27.1 and ■ Table 27.1). (Don't smile; we have seen colectomy performed for bleeding piles...).

If the examination is negative or inconclusive, **it is vital at this stage to determine whether the bleeding is genuinely a LGIB or a massive upper GI hemorrhage presenting per rectum** (see ➲ Chapter 16.2). **Insertion of a nasogastric tube should be mandatory for all large GI bleeds as a**

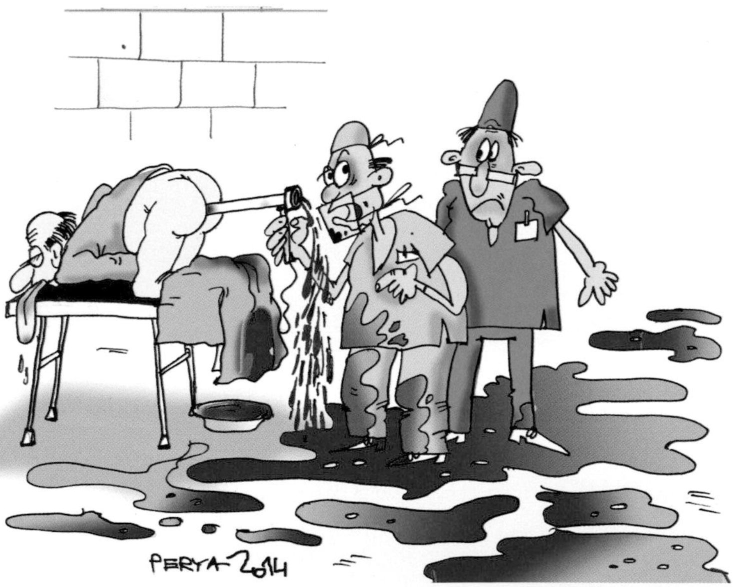

Figure 27.1. "Hey, are you sure that all of this is coming from the rectum?"

diagnostic tool. No one will accuse you of being over cautious, but you will have a lot to answer for if you chop out a patient's colon and they continue to hose blood from their end ileostomy. So insert a NG tube and irrigate the stomach; if no fresh or old blood appears in what you suck back then it is extremely unlikely the source of the massive GI bleed is in the foregut. If, however, an upper GI bleed cannot reliably be ruled out then an upper GI endoscopy is mandatory.

After the initial period of resuscitation, you should be able to tell if the patient is responding or not — most will do so. If, however, the patient is crashing, then they need to be transferred either to the operating theater or (preferably) to the angiography suite, where adequate anesthetic support must be available.

Localize...

A bit like buying real estate, in this situation there are three priorities: location, location, location.

Localizing the source of the bleeding is crucial in providing the optimal treatment — you don't want to chop out the whole colon if you can avoid it, right?

How you find the location of the bleeding will depend on the clinical setting (has the patient had a recent procedure or is this a *de novo* bleed?) and the capabilities of your hospital (principally the availability of skilled endoscopists and interventional radiologists). What works and is available around the clock in an ivory tower may not be applicable to other settings with fewer resources. Below we have described the pros and cons of the available diagnostic modalities. However, the practicing surgeon needs a simple scheme to manage these patients which we describe in ■ Figure 27.2.

Briefly:

- If the patient presents with rectal bleeding without any preceding intervention, we would start off with a CT angiogram.
- Patients presenting with massive rectal bleeding after a colonoscopic intervention or a colorectal resection should go straight to colonoscopy.

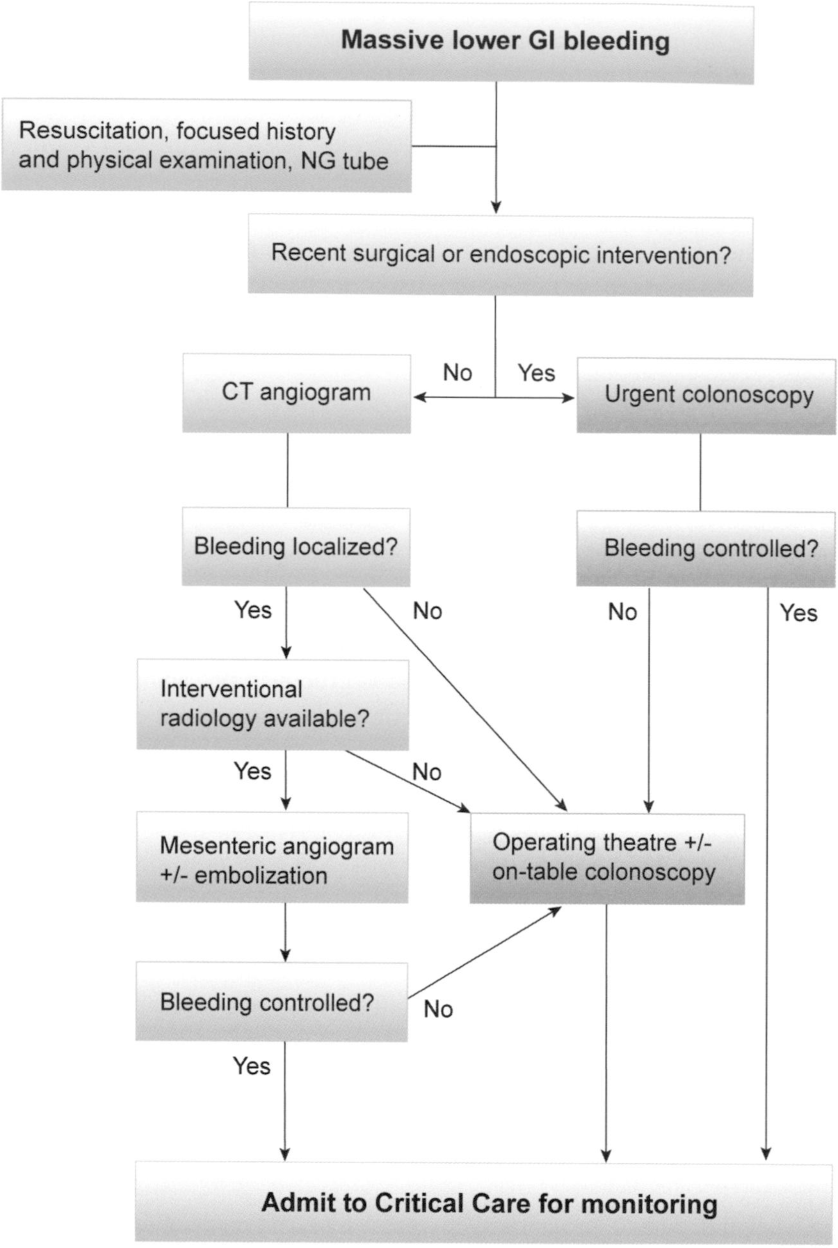

Figure 27.2. The management of massive lower GI bleeding.

CT angiogram (CTA)

If the patient is reasonably stable — even on the hypotensive side — we would get a CTA. (If you have time to scan a ruptured AAA there is no reason you cannot scan a GI bleeder.) It is quick and very accurate. **If the bleeding is brisk enough the scan is likely to localize the culprit (contrast blush, bowel wall hyper-enhancement or thickening) and guide further treatment be it surgical, endoscopic or radiological**. Even if the scan does not localize the bleeding, the images could provide important information on the possible pathology and its extent. We are sure you'd agree that if the CT scan shows extensive portal varices or disseminated malignancy you would want to know.

Radionuclide scan

Radionuclide scans with tagged RBCs in the context of massive bleeds are of very little benefit as they are both time-consuming and poor at localizing a bleeding vessel; for this reason we tend to avoid resorting to this modality in the emergency setting. The logistics of arranging the relevant staff and the radionuclide in an emergency are beyond most hospitals. **These scans however are useful in slower bleeds in stable patients as they can show bleeds at much lower rates of bleeding** (as low as 0.1ml/min) as opposed to a CTA that requires a brisker bleeder (around 2ml/min). Of course, you will know that a Meckel's scan is a useful test to identify ectopic gastric mucosa in the more stable patients with classic brick-red rectal bleeding.

Urgent colonoscopy

Urgent colonoscopy is a great adjunct to diagnose and treat bleeding patients. We would recommend attempting a colonoscopy on any patient with a LGIB. A colonoscopy is particularly useful and, in our opinion, should be the first line of managing a bleeding patient who has recently undergone a colonoscopic or surgical intervention.

Tips for colonoscopy for massive LGIB:

- We strongly recommend enlisting the services of the most experienced colonoscopist available in the hospital at the time.
- If the patient is stable enough, perform the procedure in a dedicated endoscopy suite where access to all the gadgets (e.g. clips, adrenaline, APC [argon plasma coagulation] etc.) is within reach. If the patient is unstable or transiently unstable, we would perform the

colonoscopy either in the operating room or in the angiography suite, wherever anesthetic support is available.

- We advocate using an irrigation pump (a mechanical water-jet device) to wash out clots and aid identification of bleeding points (squirting syringefuls of water through the scope's irrigation channel is hardly efficient).
- Using a magnetic endoscope imaging system (e.g. ScopeGuide, Olympus) when available is great to aid understanding of the scope position in the colon as we all know that luminal guesswork is seldom accurate especially when views are poor.
- **Bowel prep is obviously not possible in acutely bleeding patients**. We are happy to proceed with colonoscopy in an unprepared bowel. Blood is an excellent cathartic and the colon is usually free of solid matter by the time colonoscopy is attempted.
- If time allows, however, and the patient is stable (indicating a slow bleed), rapidly prepping the colon with a volume cathartic such as polyethylene glycol given via an NG tube might improve the view. Be cautious about potential fluid shifts and the potential for causing hypotension. There is no evidence that bowel prep is associated with more adverse events in bleeding patients than with non-bleeding patients.

Tips for <u>therapeutic</u> colonoscopy for massive LGIB:

- If the patient is bleeding after a previous colonoscopic procedure, the endoscopist who performed it should be present.
- Bleeding from a previous polypectomy site can usually be controlled with either clips (if a sessile polyp has been removed) or endoloops applied around the residual stalk of a pedunculated lesion.
- Bleeding from a new colonic anastomosis is best controlled with endoscopic clips or injection of adrenaline. Be careful — this is a fresh anastomosis!
- Use diathermy sparingly to gain temporary control (be cautious on an anastomosis) before deploying a mechanical device (loop or clip).
- **If the bleeding is arising from a diverticulum (the most likely cause)**, then we would attempt to clip the base of the bleeding vessel or if the vessel is not visible, we would inject adrenaline solution.
- **Bleeding from angiodysplasia is trickier to control** and our method of choice would be APC. If APC is not available, injecting the bleeding point with adrenaline can be efficacious in halting the bleeding.
- If a bleeding point is identified and dealt with (or not) **it is wise to tattoo the bowel with India ink distal to the bleeding point so that if surgery is needed the relevant segment of colon can be**

identified (this needs to be clearly documented on the report especially if the surgeon is not the one performing the colonoscopy). We also place a metal clip in case further intervention (endoscopic or angiographic) is required or if the patient ends up needing surgery.

Interventional radiology (IR)

Modern day interventional radiology suites are like operating rooms; this is where we would like our patient to be if they are having a significant bleed. Treat these patients as if they are having an operation; that means an anesthesiologist and surgeon in the room during the procedure. The interventional radiologist will be focused on the technical aspects of the procedure (identification and embolization of the bleeding point) while the anesthesiologist ensures that the patient is adequately resuscitated. You (the surgeon) are there to coordinate care and make strategic decisions about management. **The best chance of identifying and stopping the bleeding is when the patient is *actively* bleeding** — so get the patient and radiologist to the IR suite when the bleeding is occurring (i.e. tonight not tomorrow morning).

Once the patient is in the IR suite and the site of bleeding has been identified, then an attempt to embolize the feeding vessel should be made. The most commonly used products are metallic coils, micro coils, polyvinyl alcohol and gel foams. Micro catheters allow for accurate highly selective embolization of the vessels responsible for the bleed. This is successful in diverticular bleeds about 85% of the time with a low rate of rebleeding. The success rate of embolization for AVMs is lower — at about 50% with a higher risk of rebleeding.

If angiography has localized the bleeding point but embolization has not been successful, then take the patient to the operating room and do the appropriate segmental colectomy with an anastomosis or stoma depending on the patient's physiological state and comorbidities.

If the embolization has been successful, consider leaving the catheter in place for 24 to 48 hours to allow easier access to the site if reintervention is needed. Vasopressin infusion or embolization can be used through the catheter in the event of a rebleed.

The main complications related to embolization are: injury to the femoral artery where the access sheath was inserted for the angiogram (most commonly a pseudoaneurysm); acute kidney injury from the contrast agent used (10% or less); or ischemia of the embolized colon. Ischemia is rare with highly selected angiography and can be treated with i.v. antibiotics and observation. Intervene if the patient deteriorates or has persistent symptoms of ischemia. **We observe the patient for 3 days after embolization to ensure that they do not have signs or symptoms of ischemia**. Perforation is rare and should not happen.

Surgery

When the patient is on his fifth or sixth unit of blood and blood is still dripping from his rectum — after all your radiological or endoscopic hemostatic efforts — it is time to take him to the operating room.

Fortunately, the need for surgery in massive LGIBs is becoming rare but if all else fails and the patient's instability persists, be prepared for an expeditious laparotomy. Don't forget that at this stage you are probably dealing with a sick patient who already has been massively transfused, prodded and pushed in every orifice and filled to the eyeballs with vasopressors. What this patient needs now is a quick single life-saving operation.

The best operation a bleeding patient can have is a segmental resection following accurate endoscopic or angiographic localization. If localization failed (for f##k's sake, I'm not sure where the bleeding is coming from...) then a total colectomy with an end ileostomy is the operation of choice.

If you are not certain of the location of the bleed in the colon, and we mean 100% sure, then do not take any chances with blind segmental colectomies. Any 'blind' segmental resection of the colon without definitive localization of the bleeding is gambling with the patient's life and wellbeing.

Position the patient in the lithotomy position and **perform rigid or flexible anoscopy, proctoscopy and sigmoidoscopy**. It takes a few minutes to look in the rectum and the anus and will avoid you making a terrible mistake (as alluded to above). **Remember that bleeding from the upper anal canal and lower rectum will reflux at least to the rectosigmoid junction, so do not be fooled by finding fresh blood at that level.**

If still none the wiser about where the bleeding is coming from, you have no choice but to perform a midline laparotomy (sorry, no role for laparoscopy…). Inspect the peritoneal cavity systematically and walk the small and large bowel for clues. Blood seen in the small bowel suggests that it's not coming from the colon. **Look specifically for obvious culprits such as a Meckel's diverticulum or a tumor.**

If you suspect that bleeding is from the small bowel (i.e. altered blood PR or the small bowel is blood-filled at laparotomy) and you cannot see or feel a source, then consider doing an **on-table enteroscopy** at this point. To do this, get an upper GI scope in theatre and place the scope in a laparoscopic camera sleeve (you need at least two people — a scrubbed operating surgeon to control the distal end and an unscrubbed one to handle the scope controls). If you find a source endoscopically, then resect this segment of small bowel.

If you believe that the colon is the culprit (it usually is) you can start mobilizing it. Don't be tempted to do sequential bowel clamping to find the bleeding segment; it is time-consuming and not accurate. Proceed to controlling and dividing all the named vascular pedicles which allows you to complete a total colectomy. **Don't be tempted to add an ileorectal anastomosis in any patient who needed more than a few units of blood, for it will leak!**

Now a few words about segmental colectomies — how much to resect if you are sure where the source is:

- **If on the left side**, and the bleeding is from diverticulosis, we would perform a resection as for a patient with diverticulitis. Resect the bleeding site and anything distal to that point down to the upper rectum. Whether to anastomose or perform a Hartmann's procedure — use your judgment…
- **Right hemicolectomies** are adequate for bleeding from a site in the cecum or ascending colon. We would do an extended right colectomy for those patients with bleeding from anywhere in the transverse colon. Ileocolic anastomosis vs. ileostomy? Again, by now you know how to decide…

Some other specific etiologies of LGIB

Malignancies

Colon or rectal cancers are common bleeding entities, but rarely cause massive bleeding. Rectal cancer may be associated with other symptoms and will be seen at proctoscopy. The obvious management for a colon cancer presenting with massive rectal bleeding is resection.

The situation with rectal cancer is different; an emergency rectal resection is a big undertaking and besides in modern rectal cancer surgery we want to stage the tumor to tailor neoadjuvant treatment. For these reasons, we would make strenuous attempts to stop the bleeding from a rectal cancer before resorting to resectional surgery.

Bleeding from a rectal cancer that cannot be controlled endoscopically with fulgarization often must be managed in the operating room. If a distal tumor is present then a transanal approach to cauterize-fulgarize, or suture the bleeding point should be used. **If the bleeding cannot be stopped in this manner, then packing the rectum with epinephrine-saturated gauze will almost always control the bleeding**. We use vaginal packing for this, and have found that this will often stop the bleeding to allow an elective resection. Ultimately, the best therapy for a bleeding rectal tumor is to remove the tumor, and if bleeding cannot be stopped by the above methods, then an emergency resection is required. **If the acute bleed can be stopped or slowed, then treating with neoadjuvant radiation therapy will stop any chronic bleeding, prevent a massive rebleed, and allow for a less urgent resection**.

Inflammatory bowel disease

It is very rare for bleeding to be the initial presentation of either Crohn's or ulcerative colitis and equally rare for these afflictions to be the cause of significant LGIB. Most patients will present with a history of IBD and if they do sustain massive bleeding from colitis the treatment of choice is total colectomy with ileostomy (➲ Chapter 24). **A massive bleed in the face of colitis signifies a failure of medical management and the colon belongs with the pathologist**. Ensure the patient does not have an infectious condition causing the bleeding, especially if it is intermittent.

Ischemic colitis

Ischemic colitis (➲ Chapter 24) may present with a massive bleed, although it usually occurs at a slower and steadier pace. Diagnostic steps are as mentioned above but this group of patients, if stable, benefits from a pre-operative CT angiogram. Colonic ischemia may be related to other mesenteric vascular insufficiencies and the angiogram may help identify this. At operation just resect the ischemic segment of colon. Of course — a stoma!

Anorectal conditions (see also ➲ Chapter 28)

All these conditions can bleed profusely and may be difficult to deal with. **If your patient is hypotensive from a distal rectal or anal site of bleeding and you need to obtain temporary control, place a 30cc balloon Foley catheter in the rectum, blow up the balloon and pull tight against the anus**. This should tamponade the bleeding until the patient can reach the operating room. Have a medical student or resident hold the pressure while you get the patient to the OR. **We would approach all of these patients in the prone jackknife position**. It gives you a better ability to suction away the blood, thereby giving you better visibility, and a better ability to ligate the bleeding source.

Radiation proctitis

The history of radiation therapy to the prostate or cervix should lead you to identify these patients. Bleeding can be brisk at times and may require intervention with either cauterization or suture. Simple pressure can often stop the bleeding although for massive bleeding a stitch is usually required. If the bleeding is coming from a source high in the rectum, an endoscopic approach may be required. **Topical formalin** therapy for less severe bleeding from radiation proctitis works well, but it will not work for a massive bleed. For lesser bleeds treated with formalin, several applications may be required, and we perform this in the office using an anoscope and a large Q-tip applicator and 4% formalin. Coagulation may also be used for bleeding from radiation proctitis. **Argon plasma coagulation (APC)** applied at colonoscopy has been used by some effectively.

Last words...

- Most lower GI bleeding stops spontaneously.
- Massive lower GI bleeding is defined as bleeding distal to the ligament of Treitz which requires more than 4 units of blood (oh well, there are other 'definitions'...).
- CT angiography is quick and easy and can accurately localize heavy bleeding.
- Don't operate without having done an upper GI endoscopy and a rigid sigmoidoscopy as a minimum.
- If you can localize the bleeding, do a segmental colonic resection (think very carefully before doing an anastomosis in this context).
- If you cannot localize the bleeding do a total colectomy and end ileostomy.

Beware: in lower gastrointestinal bleeding, removing the wrong side of the colon is embarrassing. Removing any segment of the colon while the bleeding source is in the anorectum — or the small bowel — is shameful.

"The only weapon with which the unconscious patient can immediately retaliate on the incompetent surgeon is hemorrhage."

William Stewart Halsted

Chapter 28

Anorectal emergencies

Mark Cheetham and Simon Shaw

> *We suffer and die through the defects that arise in our sewerage and drainage system.*
>
> **William A. Lane**

OK you guys, we know that the anus is not strictly part of the abdomen... However, people with ass pain are commonly seen by the team dealing with abdominal emergencies, so on the grounds of common sense we have included a chapter on anorectal emergencies here.

Most people do not spend a lot of time thinking about their anus, but when it goes wrong the anus can cause a disproportionate degree of pain and distress. To many patients and not a few doctors, any anal symptoms are attributed to hemorrhoids. **It seems that the only doctors with a reasonable understanding of the anus and its environment are general surgeons. In this chapter we will help you to become an astute *assologist*.**

Assessing the patient

You will save yourself a lot of time by listening to your patient. There are only a few symptoms of anal disease and they form classic combinations, which means that usually you can guess the diagnosis from the history alone — before even examining the sufferer. Most patients will present with a

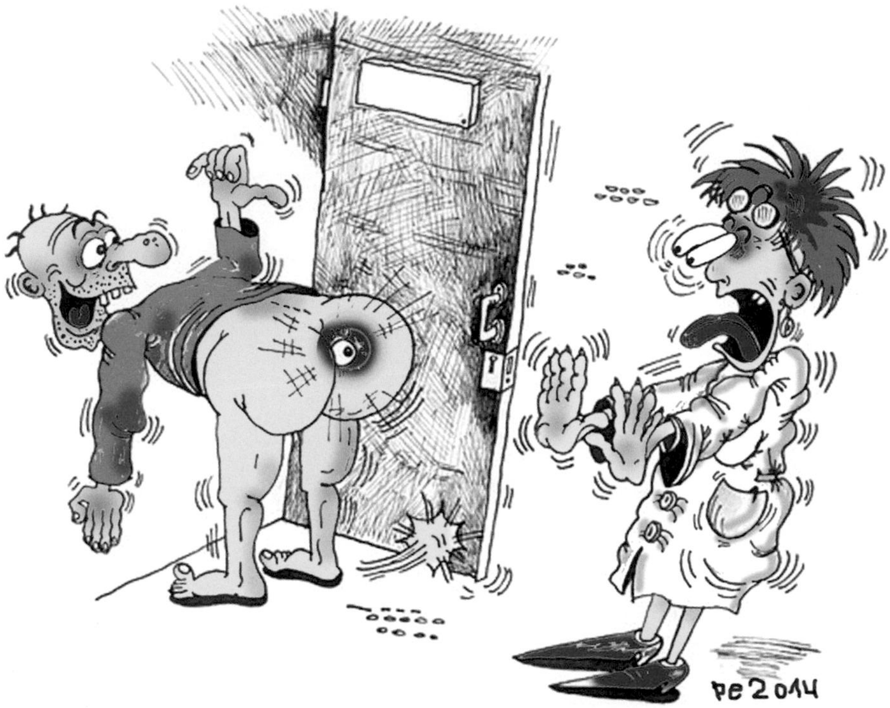

Figure 28.1. "I know I'm a pain in the ass, but please help me!"

combination of anal pain (■ Figure 28.1), rectal bleeding, a swelling or discharge. The character and periodicity of the pain are important clues to differentiate between the various causes of anal pain, as depicted in ■ Figure 28.2:

- Throbbing pain, increasing over a few days, and associated with a lump is likely to be a **perianal abscess**.
- Sharp pain during defecation, often associated with bleeding, is classical of an **anal fissure**.
- Pain which improves over a few days, associated with an anal lump suggests a **perianal hematoma** ('thrombosed external pile' — as it is termed across the ocean from us).
- A very painful anal lump which is not improving over a few days suggests **strangulated *internal* hemorrhoids**.

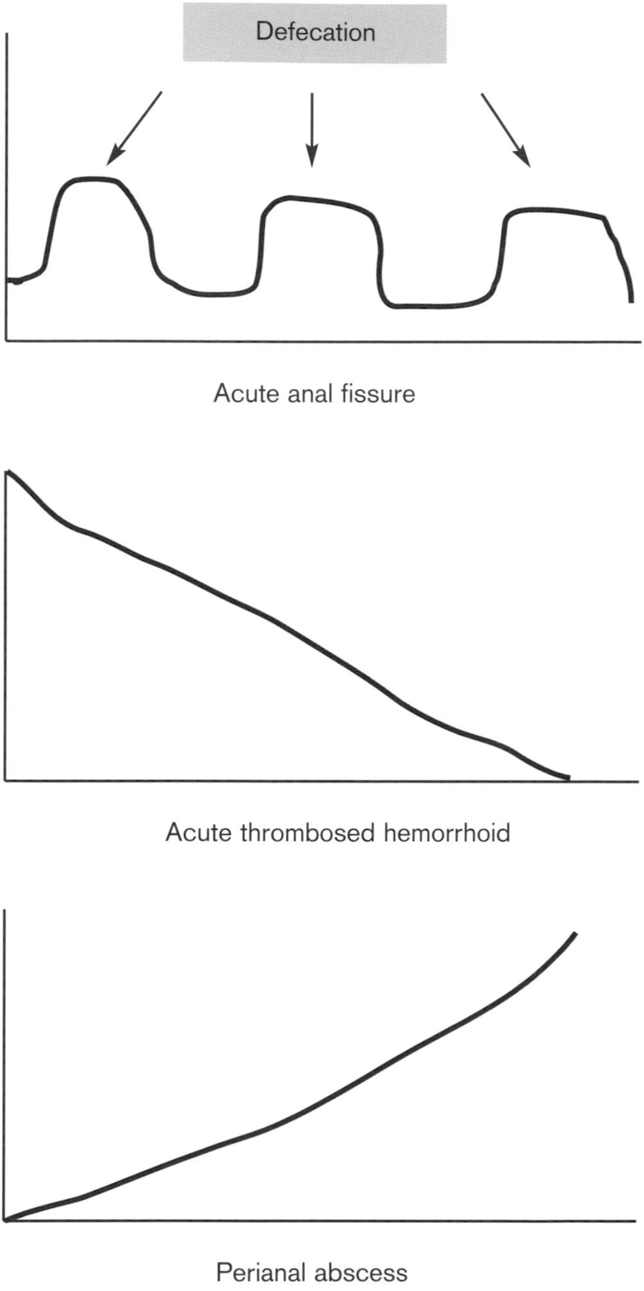

Figure 28.2. Pattern of acute anal pain.

Examination

Examination of the patient in the left lateral position will often give the diagnosis. **Don't shove in your gloved index finger straight away unless you want the patient to kick you in the head!** First retract the buttock cheeks and inspect the anal margin; then using both hands gently part the anus to look for signs of an anal fissure. In the setting of severe anal pain, it is usually impossible to evaluate the anorectum with digital examination and anoscopy. The liberal application of lidocaine gel and a few minutes wait may be helpful, although we have a low threshold for examining the patient in the operating room under (general or spinal) anesthesia if necessary.

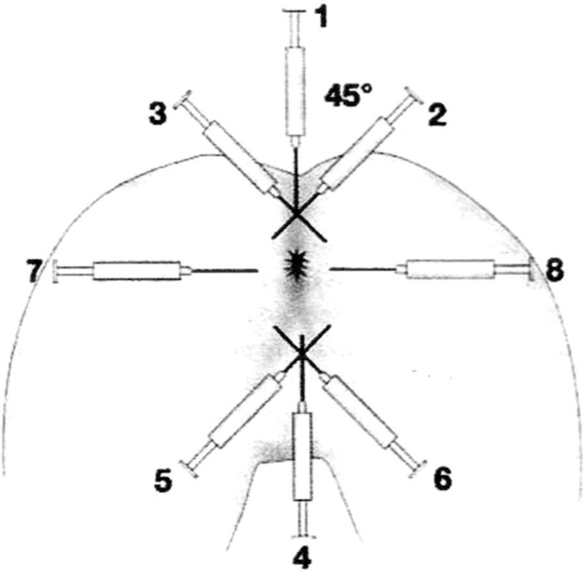

Figure 28.3. Perianal local anesthesia. With the patient in a position of your choice, using a local anesthetic mix of your choice (we like to mix short- and long-acting agents), inject 5cc of the mixture deeply behind the anus, peripheral to the external sphincter. Then without totally removing the needle, repeat the injection on both sides, with a 45° inclination (steps 1, 2, 3). A second injection is done anteriorly (steps 4, 5, 6), with the same fanning. And finally, two more injections following a similar pattern at 3 and 9 o'clock (steps 7, 8). ***Courtesy of Professor Luis A. Carriquiry.***

An alternative in some circumstances is to use local anesthesia. A few milliliters of lidocaine injected under an acute anal fissure abolishes the pain completely. For how to achieve complete anal local anesthesia look at ■ Figure 28.3. A pudendal nerve block may allow you to disimpact a painful rectum after hemorrhoidectomy.

Anal fissure

The most common cause of anal pain is an anal fissure. Fissures hurt and most patients describe it as the worst pain they have experienced. The pain is exacerbated by defecation and continues sometimes for hours afterwards. The pain is not limited to bowel movements but also occurs with sitting or walking. Always suspect a fissure when a patient's main complaint is pain. **However, associated bright rectal bleeding is not uncommon. There is usually a characteristic ('diagnostic!') story of excruciating defecatory anal pain ("like passing broken glass, doc") associated with small amounts of fresh anal bleeding**.

Don't be in a hurry to do a digital exam if you suspect a fissure; look first. Inspection of the anus with the patient in the prone jack-knife position (or the lateral decubitus one), while spreading the buttock cheeks will, most of the time, allow you to see the fissure. The common ('primary') fissures are usually (90% of the time) posterior, situated at anal six o'clock, but they may be anterior as well (9% of the time); this is more common in females and may be associated with childbirth. **If the patient has a painless anal ulcer, a lateral fissure or multiple fissures, be suspicious — this is probably not an idiopathic anal fissure (think of a sexually transmitted infection or Crohn's disease or a skin disorder). If you see a lateral fissure, beware! These are mostly from a more sinister pathology than the usual tight ass**. (See ■ Table 28.1 for etiologies of lateral, 'secondary' fissures.)

Table 28.1. Alternative causes of fissures.
■ Inflammatory bowel disease.
■ Infections.
■ HIV.
■ Cancer.
■ Trauma.

We divide anal fissures into acute and chronic fissures. These differ in the duration of symptoms and the clinical appearances:

- Patients with **acute anal fissures** give a short history (a few days or so) of severe pain. There is often intense anal tenderness and it can be impossible to examine the anus properly. On anal inspection — if the patient will let you — you will see a linear superficial tear extending from the anoderm to the dentate line without a sentinel tag or visible internal anal sphincter muscle fibers.
- **Chronic anal fissures** present with a longer history (at least 6 weeks) of pain and fresh anal bleeding. The pain and tenderness is not as severe making examination easier, that is if you are careful and gentle as described above. Typically, chronic fissures are often associated with a sentinel tag or 'pile' (below the fissure) and a hypertrophic anal papilla seen above. Chronic fissures are deeper and there may be visible fibers of internal anal sphincter in the base.

After diagnosing a 'benign' fissure don't bother performing a digital exam, unless you wish to torture the patient. However, if you are unsure — sometimes the anal spasm and pain elicited by the simple separation of the buttocks make visual confirmation difficult, especially in obese patients — or feel the need to perform a digital exam or anoscopy, then apply some lidocaine jelly 2% at the site of the anal verge tenderness, leaving it for several minutes. This usually provides enough anesthesia for a humane exam or anoscopy.

Treatment of anal fissures

Primary anal fissures are caused by hypertonicity of the internal anal sphincter — 'a tight ass'. Thus, all therapies are geared towards decreasing the anal tone and breaking the cycle of anal spasm and pain.

Acute fissures

Most of the fissures we see as emergency presentations are acute anal fissures and although these are very painful the vast majority of them will heal spontaneously within a few days.

Our initial treatment is to keep the stool soft with a fiber supplement and stool softeners, warm sitz baths, and a topical cream to decrease internal anal sphincter tone — such as 2% diltiazem or 0.2% nifedipine cream. Glyceryl trinitrate (GTN) ointment is also effective in healing anal fissures but its use is limited by a high incidence of headaches.

Occasionally, you will encounter a patient who screams because of the anal pain. Your task is to interrupt the pain-spasm cycle; the pain caused by the fissure — resulting in spasm of the internal sphincter — which in turn increases the pain. I would inject, using a fine needle, a few milliters of local anesthetic solution (e.g. Marcaine®/bupivacaine) just under the fissure. The pain will disappear instantly and with it the anal spasm. Now the patient will allow you to gently insert a gloved finger into the anus. Use a generous dose of local anesthetic gel as a lubricant and gently dilate the anal canal. Do not try to make a further dilatation. Continue as above... **Moshe**

Chronic anal fissures

About half of chronic anal fissures will heal with medical management as described above. The management of chronic fissures which have persisted despite conservative treatment depends on the patients and their anal sphincters.

Botox® injections

In some situations, we are concerned about the risk of permanent fecal incontinence, typically in women (who have a shorter anal sphincter) and in people who have had previous anal surgery. Here we would consider using Botox® injections temporarily to reduce the anal sphincter tone

The Botox® is injected into the internal anal sphincter at 3 and 9 o'clock. The dose used varies in the literature. We use 50 units of botulinum toxin, mixed in 2ml of normal saline. Botox® can be given in clinic using a 25-gauge needle and no local anesthesia. In the UK we often inject Botox® under anesthetic and will combine this with excision of any sentinel tag or hypertrophic papilla and curettage of the fissure base. A small percentage of these patients may develop post-injection fecal incontinence; however, this will resolve in approximately 6-8 weeks when the Botox® wears off. This approach heals about three-quarters of fissures but around a quarter of patients may develop a recurrence when the sphincter tone returns to baseline.

Lateral anal sphincterotomy

A lateral anal sphincterotomy will heal about 90% of anal fissures and relieve the pain almost immediately. The risk of incontinence to stool in patients with hypertonicity is small; however, up to 20% of patients may have trouble controlling flatus (this will not be noticed by some patients!). **The incision is made at 3 or 9 o'clock and can be done through either an open or closed technique. It is important to tailor the length of the sphincterotomy to the length of the fissure; don't divide the internal sphincter all the way up to the dentate line as this significantly increases**

the risk of fecal incontinence. As hinted above, we are hesitant to do a lateral anal sphincterotomy in a woman and will have a really good go at other treatments before resorting to this.

A catch to be aware of is a **chronic intersphincteric abscess**. This presents with symptoms very similar to a chronic anal fissure, although there is sometimes some purulent discharge. The key is that at rectal examination there is a small pea-sized lump posteriorly in the anal canal where you would expect an anal fissure to be. These need to be laid open — lotions and potions will not help here!

Hemorrhoidal emergencies

Perianal hematoma

This very common condition is often called by our dear American buddies a "thrombosed external hemorrhoid". There is a characteristic firm, bluish, round tender swelling next to the anal margin. If you see this soon after the onset of symptoms (say up to 3 days) it's a pretty simple matter to inject a small amount of lidocaine and then incise the swelling; the hematoma (actually little dark clots) should shell out easily. In patients presenting after a few days the clots may become adherent and not shell out as easily; here we would advise conservative treatment. The process should resolve within a few days with or without drainage.

Acute strangulated internal hemorrhoids

Despite the commonly held opinion of family doctors, internal hemorrhoids do not cause acute anal pain. In most cases when a patient tells you that he has painful hemorrhoids you know he has an acute fissure. But there is an exception to this rule: **acute strangulated internal hemorrhoids**.

This occurs in patients with grade III or IV hemorrhoids. The prolapsed hemorrhoids become irreducible because of swelling and thrombosis. The patient experiences intense pain and has serious difficulties sitting and walking. On examination you see the prolapsed piles (this is what we Brits call hemorrhoids) — blue with areas of mucosal necrosis. Like rotten grapes.

Most surgeons, including us, would treat this situation conservatively as they are aware of the danger of removing too much tissues — ending

up with anal stenosis. If you do operate, the patient will have pain and need time to recover; if you don't operate the patient will have pain and need time to recover — **either way they have pain so why operate?**

Conservative management allows the process to resolve within a week or so — permitting the swelling to decrease and then we can consider an elective procedure if needed. Conservative management would include: bed rest (with the buttocks elevated), potent analgesia, laxatives, local application of diltiazem cream to reduce anal spasm and warm sitz baths. **Application of plain white sugar to coat the prolapsed tissue is effective in the early stages**. The hygroscopic sugar rapidly reduces the tissue edema — shrinking the prolapsed tissues and allowing manual reduction. Simply place the patient prone and pour a generous quantity of sugar on the strangulated parts until the tortured anus looks like a cake covered with icing. Repeat as necessary following any sitz bath — you won't believe how fast the swelling subsides.

Now if you are a cowboy, you may want to take those patients directly to the OR. But you may fall off the horse....

Bleeding after hemorrhoidectomy (and other anal surgery)

We have covered this in the chapter on lower GI bleeding (➲ Chapter 27). Suffice it to say here that pooling of blood in the rectum can cause the treating surgeon to significantly underestimate the degree of bleeding!

Perianal abscess (and the associated fistula-in-ano)

> *"An untrained surgeon with a fistula probe is more dangerous than a gorilla with a machine gun."*
>
> **Robin Phillips**

Patients with acute anorectal sepsis complain of a characteristic, progressive throbbing anal pain; they may have noticed a swelling at the anal margin and, if the abscess has burst, there will also be purulent or blood-stained discharge. **It is important to note if the patient has had previous anorectal surgery or if they have Crohn's disease which may modify your approach**. Beware the patient with pain and signs of sepsis but no visible or palpable abscess — **these patients may have an intersphincteric, postanal or supralevator collection which is hard to demonstrate without imaging or surgery**. In such patients, with clinical features of perianal abscess but nothing to see or feel, we advocate imaging pre-operatively as discussed below.

To treat perianal abscesses successfully, you must understand the etiology, pathology and anatomy. **Most of the patients suffer from 'idiopathic' perianal abscesses, which arise within one of the 12 to 20 anal glands**, which lie in the intersphincteric plane at the level of the dentate line. A blocked duct allows the build-up of pus in the intersphincteric plane. If this doesn't resolve, the collection may spread, initially within the intersphincteric plane. Spread caudally may result in a visible ('superficial') abscess at the anal verge, while spread cranially will result in a collection above the pelvic floor (a supralevator collection). If the initial intersphincteric collection penetrates the external anal sphincter, it will result in an **ischiorectal fossa abscess**. The other pattern of spread of infection to be aware of is 'horseshoeing'. This is the circumferential spread of pus within the ischiorectal fossa, the **intersphincteric plane** or the **supralevator space**.

Examine the patient lying on their left side and first look for any swellings, discharging sinuses or scars from previous surgery. An ischiorectal abscess is usually visible as a brawny swelling of one side of the buttock. Next gently feel the anal margin with a gloved and lubricated index finger, but cautiously — a perianal abscess will be characteristically tender and fluctuant. Finally, do a rectal examination. **But in all honesty in this situation a rectal examination may not give you much more information**. If you have already decided to operate then you may skip this and do it under anesthetic. Some patients with an intersphincteric collection for instance will not let you do a rectal examination because of intense pain and sphincter spasm.

In most instances, you will not need any imaging tests; the combination of physical examination with operative finding is enough to define the anatomy and allow you to plan the operative approach. **If you cannot see, feel, understand or localize the abscess then cross-sectional imaging is needed**. The best test is an MRI, although this may not be easy to arrange in an emergency in most hospitals. CT is less accurate but in an emergency it will help you to locate where the problem lies.

Treatment

We think it is best to drain anorectal abscesses under general or regional anesthetic — this allows a better examination and is more comfortable for the patients. Sure, it is possible to drain a small perianal abscess under local anesthetic, in the office or in the emergency room, but it is very painful! As always, the patients should be offered the various options. Sometimes individual or institutional constraints prevail.

How to position the patient seems to be a matter of geography — in the UK most anal surgery is performed in the lithotomy position which gives good access and allows the surgeon to sit; in the USA the prone jack-knife position is often used — this gives especially good exposure to the anterior anorectum but can cause some moaning from the head end of the operating table if the patient is under general anesthetic! (Brits like to sit between the legs; Americans prefer to stand over the ass.)

Initially, before you cut anything, assess the situation:

- Where is the abscess in relation to the sphincters?
- Is there an obvious anal fistula?
- Is there evidence of a horseshoe collection? (A supralevator collection will feel hard on digital rectal examination — like too much bone — whereas a horseshoe collection within the ischiorectal fossa is usually visible.)
- Are there any scars from previous anorectal surgery?
- Is there any evidence for Crohn's disease?

Only now proceed with drainage:

- **Make an incision** at the point of maximal fluctuance and evacuate any pus. Generally, we use a curved incision outside the external sphincters if possible (although a radial incision towards the anal canal will be needed to treat an intersphincteric abscess). Make sure that the skin incision is big enough (as long or as wide as the abscess cavity) to drain the collection adequately and break down any loculi within the cavity. We don't believe that it is necessary to make a cruciate incision or to excise any skin — unless it is necrotic and in need of debridement.
- **Horseshoe collections** need particular attention to ensure adequate drainage ("like a small shark has bitten the ass"). These originate from a postanal space infection which has spread laterally to one or both ischiorectal fossae. **There is always a posterior anal fistula**. Treatment involves widely laying open the involved ischiorectal fossa and the postanal space via a long curved incision immediately posterior to the anal canal. The primary anal fistula will need to be addressed on a planned basis later.
- **To drain an intersphincteric collection** adequately you will need to divide the internal anal sphincter (i.e. do an internal sphincterotomy as you would do for an anal fissure but placed over the collection).
- **Supralevator collections** should be laid open into the rectum via a transanal approach. In general terms, **don't divide any skeletal**

muscle (the external sphincter or the levator ani), but if you need to, divide smooth muscle (the internal anal sphincter or the rectal muscle). Now stop the bleeding and get out.

- **We infiltrate the wound with bupivacaine** at the end of the procedure. We usually don't pack these wounds unless this is needed for hemostasis. And if your skin incision is adequate there is no need for drains.

After the operation

Postoperatively, most patients can go home the same day or the day after. There is a ritual of regularly packing perianal abscess wounds which is not necessary — and it delays healing. An alternative is to teach the patient to digitate the wound with a soapy finger in the shower or bath. **Up to half of patients with a perianal abscess will develop an anal fistula later**; **either follow up these patients or ensure that they can easily get to see you if a fistula develops**.

What to do if you find an anal fistula? In the acute setting we would not search too hard for an anal fistula — the anatomy is distorted, and the tissues are friable making this a high-risk situation even for an experienced fistula surgeon. However, if there is an obvious trans-sphincteric fistula, insert a loose, draining seton if you have the skills to do so rather than laying the fistula open at this point.

Abscesses you cannot see or feel

These patients present with progressive, dull anorectal pain. On inspection of the anus you will see nothing; on rectal exam there will be tenderness but no discrete 'mass-to-be-drained' can be localized. Two entities are responsible for such a scenario:

- **Post-anal space abscess**. These are difficult to diagnose and identify but when suspected, an examination under anesthesia in the operating room to define and drain these abscesses is needed. **A pre-operative CT scan (or even better an MRI scan) is helpful in providing the diagnosis and a roadmap for drainage**. At operation place the patient in the lithotomy position, perform an anoscopy and then pass a wide-bore needle into the post-anal space at the level of the dentate line. Once you aspirate some pus, enter the space by incising the internal sphincter followed by poking your finger into the cavity. **For an**

isolated post-anal space abscess DO NOT make a counter incision on the skin between the anus and the tip of the coccyx. This is because transrectal drainage avoids the creation of a 'high' posterior fistula-in-ano, which always develops after transcutaneous drainage of such an abscess.

- **Extrasphincteric fistula.** These generally are not caused by cryptoglandular infections. Instead, they usually develop secondary to an intra-abdominal pathology that has formed an abscess deep in the pelvis at the level of the anorectal ring (e.g. from appendicitis or diverticulitis). **CT is required for diagnosis; and drainage, if not amenable to the CT-guided route, can be performed transrectally.** You may also need to remove the abdominal source of such collections by doing a laparotomy.

The Crohn's anus

Septic complications of anal Crohn's disease can present with a wide spectrum of disease: from an isolated perianal abscess to a destroyed anus with multiple collections and fistulae. **Your role in the emergency setting is only to drain the pus.** Perform an examination under anesthetic and drain any collections widely. If an anal fistula is identified at the time of surgery, insert a loose draining seton into the primary track. These patients need close liaison with a gastroenterologist, and many will need to start Remicade® (infliximab) early in order to preserve the anus.

Necrotizing perineal infections (*Fournier's gangrene*)

Necrotizing perineal infections may be the consequence of neglected anorectal infections but they also arise from trauma, skin infections and urethral instrumentation. A urethral source implies *Fournier's gangrene* — an eponym that has been incorrectly extended to the whole spectrum of this entity. **But more important than etiology is prompt diagnosis and treatment.**

These patients are commonly diabetic, very obese or immunosuppressed. The synergistic action of Gram-negative bacteria, anaerobes and *Streptococcus* causes rapid dissemination of the infection along superficial fascial and subcutaneous planes, with secondary ischemic involvement of the skin. Pain may be the first symptom, but it may be vague. **Swelling of the perineum, crepitus, local tenderness and erythema of the skin — followed by its necrosis — are the typical elements found on examination.**

There is no need for X-rays or CTs, unless one suspects extension to fascial abdominal or retroperitoneal tissues. **Only prompt treatment can prevent a fatal evolution; it should include supportive care, high-dose i.v. antibiotics to cover aerobic and anaerobic bacteria and prompt surgical debridement — which is the mainstay of treatment**.

Necrotic skin must be resected, but as fascial and fat necrosis extend much further, extensive skin incisions are usually necessary to allow radical excision of superficial fascia and fatty tissue until well-perfused and viable fat is found. If the infection extends to the perineal muscles, they must be sacrificed following the same criteria. **Debride as much as necessary at your first operation but plan on taking the patient back to the operating room the next day(s) until you are satisfied that the infection is under control**. Concerns about future reconstruction should be left to the plastic surgeon, but if it is necessary to excise scrotal skin, it is convenient to wrap the testicles, which are rarely compromised, in healthy tissues in the abdominal wall or the thigh.

So chop out everything that stinks, is dark, gray or dead — irrespective of how large and horrendous the wound you create. And do it again and again — as many times as necessary. Eventually it will all pink-up, granulate, contract and heal.

Two controversial issues remain: the necessity of a colostomy and the use of hyperbaric oxygen. Most authors think a diverting stoma is generally not necessary even in the case of a free-floating anus. Nevertheless, when ongoing fecal contamination is not easily manageable (e.g. incontinent patient, poor nursing facilities), consider proximal fecal diversion. The use of hyperbaric oxygen has been strongly recommended based on the action of oxygen free radicals against anaerobic bacteria, but it remains controversial, cumbersome and expensive and so cannot be considered a necessary component of the 'standard'. **At the end of the day your knife should be the instrument to provide oxygen to the wound**.

Full-thickness rectal prolapse

We see two principal emergency presentations of full-thickness rectal prolapse:

- **The more common variant is an elderly patient (often from a nursing home) with a prolapse which has been out for a short**

period — a day or so. In this situation it is best to reduce the prolapse with osmotic assistance using sugar therapy: tip a pound of sugar on the prolapse and have the patient sit in it until you finish your rounds. When you come back the sugar will have sucked all the edema out of the prolapse and you should be able to easily reduce it. (A word of warning, you do need to be specific about the dose of sugar needed; last time we tried this we asked a nurse to fetch a bag of sugar, she came back with a small sachet of 5 grams of sugar!) Once the prolapse has been reduced, plan for elective definitive prolapse surgery — whatever is your operation du jour. We usually operate on the next available elective list.

- The second situation is fortunately rare, and this is when the **prolapse is gangrenous or irreducible by any means**. In these circumstances one must proceed directly to an emergency resection of the prolapsed rectum. In our hands, this means doing an Altemeier's perineal rectosigmoidectomy. It requires a degree of experience in elective colorectal surgery — if you don't have such experience, we would recommend that you either get help or ship the patient out to another hospital.

Anorectal trauma

In civilian practice, anorectal trauma is most likely to occur following an assault (stabbing or shooting), impalement injury or a fall astride a bicycle bar.

Obviously in a major trauma situation do not initially focus on the anorectal injury (as you probably know, the A of 'trauma ABC' does not stand for ass!).

For many years the dogma for managing injuries to the rectum included a triad of a diverting colostomy, rectal washout and insertion of presacral drains. However, nowadays we are more flexible. How you will manage these injuries depends on the site and type of injury and the general status of the patient:

- **Injuries to the rectum above the peritoneal reflection** are accessed at laparotomy where the defect is debrided and closed primarily — just as you would do for 'early' — non-destructive — colonic injury. If the defect is large you may need to consider performing a rectal resection — then you need to consider carefully whether to do an anastomosis or more likely a Hartmann's procedure.
- **Injuries to the lower rectum/anal canal** may be approached transanally where they can often be suture repaired. If you cannot adequately close the hole in the lower rectum, then leave it alone but add a colostomy.

- Low rectal **injuries to the anal sphincter** should be debrided and repaired with fine PDS® sutures. In severe destructive anal injury, just clean, drain and divert — leave late attempts at sphincter reconstruction to the experts. Leave the skin open.
- **A loop colostomy is not mandatory** — but should be considered for patients with severely destructive injuries, delayed presentation or when you cannot fix the rectal hole.

Anorectal foreign bodies

All general surgeons (should) have a ready repertoire of stories about objects they have fished out from the rectum. For the record here are a few of our favorites:

- A double-ended dildo (very hard to grasp).
- Vibrators (including one which was still running; we asked the cardiology resident to see this patient with a new machinery murmur...).
- Water-pipe foam insulation.
- A broken glass (ouch).
- A bath plug.
- Sundry fruit and veg from a frequent flier we named "ratatouille man".
- A cellphone.

Although these episodes are a ready source of humor for us, there is a serious aspect to rectal foreign bodies which can cause rectal bleeding, perforation or obstruction if left too long. **Here are some tips for a successful removal**:

- Use a combination of clinical examination and plain X-ray to locate and characterize the foreign body before removal.
- Be cautious when performing a digital rectal examination in this context (you don't want to do a rectal examination for the guy with a broken glass in his ass).
- Have a go at removing the object in the emergency department if feasible; this may remove all the hassle of an anesthetic and an admission.
- **If you cannot feel it *per rectum*, you are unlikely to be able to remove it without a colonoscopy or a laparotomy.**

- Consider an unprepped colonoscopy to remove the foreign body (if you don't do colonoscopy you may need to persuade your local GI guy to do this). Have a selection of rat tooth forceps and various snares available to grab the object.
- Vibrators usually have an on/off lever switch on their base; this can be a useful grip point for a clip or an endoscopic snare.

Summary

Anal emergencies do not kill (except necrotizing fasciitis and severe trauma) but they are a real pain in the ass to the patient. Know how to solve the problem promptly and simply... and you will be a greater hero to the patient than a surgeon performing a robotic Whipple operation for pancreatic cancer.

You have to realize that most of what you have read above is as old as medical history. What for you may appear novel has been recycled for thousands of years. For example:

"An abscess near the anus should not be left to burst by itself, but... be boldly opened with a very sharp lancette, so that pus and the corrupt blood may go out. Or else... the gut which is called rectum... will burst... for then may it... be called fistula. And I have seen some who have seven or nine holes on one side of the buttocks... none of which except one pierce the rectum."

John of Arderne, 1306-1390

Treatment of hemorrhoids: "Force out the anus as much as possible with the fingers and make the irons red hot, burn the pile until it be dried up and so that no part may be left behind."

Hippocrates, 460?-377? BC

Chapter 29

Surgical complications of endoscopy

Ahmad Assalia and Anat Ilivitzki

If you are too fond of new remedies, first you will not cure your patients; secondly, you will have no patients to cure.

Astley Paston Cooper

Complications of endoscopy may be defined as *immediate*, occurring during the procedure or before the patient leaves the endoscopic suite, or *delayed*, occurring up to 30 days after the procedure. In recent years, gastroenterologists have become more daring, especially with the advent of endoscopic techniques for resecting lesions along the GI tract (e.g. endoscopic mucosal resection [EMR] and endoscopic submucosal dissection [ESD]) and other endoscopic interventions including new generations of stents, endoscopic ultrasound interventions and more. Therefore, we should expect to see more and more complications following visits at the GI suite.

Some basic points

- In the real world, complications are much more frequent than is suggested by the 'beautiful' figures quoted in the books!
- Complication rates vary with expertise and case volume; expect more with less experienced endoscopists — those still climbing the learning curve, or those who continue climbing forever.
- The risks associated with endoscopy are higher when the pathology is more complex and in *therapeutic* as opposed to *diagnostic* procedures.

- With complications of endoscopy **it's particularly important to know when not to operate rather than when to operate**; many episodes of post-endoscopy bleeding and perforation are best treated conservatively. It is unhelpful to carry out a laparotomy for post-endoscopy complications and then be unable to identify the perforation or bleeding source.

When called to see a 'sick' patient after an endoscopic procedure:

- **Suspect catastrophe!** And until proven otherwise, assume the patient has the most dreadful surgical complications.
- **What's common is common!** Adverse events following immediately after endoscopy are likely to be due to the procedure itself.
- **Always transfer these 'sick' patients to the surgical service** regardless of the immediate need for surgical intervention. In the interests of everyone, *especially the patient*, the best environment is the surgical floor where patients can be monitored and treated appropriately.
- **Recognition and early management of complications is the key for a successful outcome**. So... if you don't think about it, you won't diagnose it.
- **Regardless of the etiology, always treat shock immediately and prepare the patient with obvious peritonitis for urgent laparotomy or laparoscopy**.
- Always **READ** carefully any admission and progress notes and the endoscopic report; **TALK** to the patient, his doctor and **directly contact the GI specialist who performed the 'uneventful' procedure** (many clues for the nature of the complication are there) and **VIEW**, personally, all images taken at the endoscopy and thereafter.

Complications of upper gastrointestinal endoscopy

Flexible esophagogastroduodenoscopy (EGD) is a relatively safe procedure with few complications. Almost half of the serious complications that occur are cardiopulmonary, related to aspiration, hypoxemia, vasovagal reflexes, and endocarditis. The surgical complications are outlined below.

Esophageal perforation

The cervical esophagus is the area most at risk. Risk factors include anterior cervical osteophytes, Zenker's diverticulum, esophageal stricture or web and a cervical rib. **Most cervical esophageal perforations occur during rigid endoscopy or with blind passage of a flexible endoscope**. Retching with an over-inflated stomach, and the endoscope occluding the gastroesophageal junction, can result in Mallory-Weiss tears or transmural perforation.

Cervical pain, crepitus and cellulitis are all signs of high esophageal perforation. *Halitosis* develops rapidly due to overgrowth of anaerobic bacteria. Distal perforations cause chest pain. A cervical soft tissue X-ray and chest radiograph may be helpful in the initial stages for the detection of cervical air, pneumomediastinum and pneumothorax or pleural effusion.

The diagnosis is confirmed with water-soluble esophagography or a CT scan. Don't waste time — get an urgent CT scan with an oral, water-soluble contrast medium — it will detect minimal perforations and provide additional valuable information as to the location and extent of the inflammatory process. Esophagoscopy is accurate in visualizing clinically significant perforations. However, it may miss tiny tears hidden under a mucosal fold and could convert a mini-perforation into a larger one. Thus, endoscopy is not considered a primary diagnostic tool but may be useful in management.

The management of esophageal perforation is beyond the scope of this brief chapter. If you can, try reading the excellent Chapter 15 on "Esophageal emergencies" in the previous 4th edition of this book (or e-mail Moshe at mosheschein@gmail and he will send you a copy of that chapter).

Post-EGD upper gastrointestinal bleeding

This is approached and treated according to the principles presented in ➲ Chapter 16.2).

Other complications

Following **sclerotherapy**, and less frequently after *band ligation* for esophageal varices, up to half of patients will experience one or more of the following: chest pain, pleural effusion, pulmonary infiltrates and bacteremia (without perforation).

Esophageal placement of stents for malignant strictures may cause erosions, bleeding, migration, tumor ingrowth with recurrent obstruction, food impaction or (if they are inserted across the gastroesophageal junction) reflux with aspiration. Bacteremia is especially common after esophageal dilatation, so antibiotic prophylaxis should be considered to reduce the risk of bacterial endocarditis in susceptible individuals.

Remember: most patients treated with esophageal stents have a short life expectancy; do no more than the minimum required for palliation. This may include repeated endoscopies for ablation of the tumor ingrowth or placement of a second stent.

Complications of percutaneous endoscopic gastrostomy (PEG)

PEG tubes are commonly used as a feeding route in elderly and debilitated patients. In some cultures and places it seems that patients are not allowed to die without having a PEG tube inserted! (Hurrah! No need to spoon feed the poor old chap — more time for the modern nurse to stare at the computer screen.) **This is an invasive procedure and complications after PEG insertion are not uncommon**.

Leakage

This is by far the most important complication. It tends to present in the first few days following the procedure. The clinical scenario ranges from asymptomatic leakage *around* the gastrostomy tube to overwhelming peritonitis and sepsis. **The reason is inadequate fixation of the stomach against the inner abdominal wall or separation of the two** due to various factors, especially ischemia and necrosis of the gastric wall due to excessive tightness of the fixing device — whatever method is used.

Clinical features

These depend on whether the leaking gastric juice or feeding solution leaks only to the outside around the tube, or whether the leak is into the peritoneal cavity. In the latter case the clinical picture may range from mild pain and abdominal distension due to ileus to full-blown peritonitis and 'sepsis'.

Diagnosis

The finding of free intraperitoneal air is not diagnostic because pneumoperitoneum may be present for 1-2 weeks after uncomplicated PEG insertion. However, large amounts of free air are extremely unusual and should hint that there is a problem. Intraperitoneal leak should be excluded by a contrast study (preferably under CT) — with contrast instilled through the PEG tube. It will delineate the extent of the leak, as well as the amount of intraperitoneal fluid, peritonitis, ileus, etc.

Management

If a contrast study *excludes intraperitoneal leakage*, then the PEG tube has to be 'rested' — allowing the tissue around it to seal. Attach the PEG tube to gravity drainage, administer i.v. fluids and antibiotics, and follow the patient closely. Wait a week and then repeat the contrast study before attempting PEG feeding. **This, with the addition of a nasogastric tube, should also be the approach when the PEG tube is pulled out inadvertently less than 2 weeks after insertion, and there are no signs of peritonitis or sepsis and no evidence of intraperitoneal leak on contrast study**. In cases with *obvious leakage into the peritoneal cavity*, your management should be guided by the clinical scenario. **While minor and asymptomatic leaks can be treated conservatively, operative treatment is mandatory with free intraperitoneal leaks and signs of infection**.

Operation

Early on, in the absence of significant tissue edema, place a purse-string suture around the PEG tube and (carefully and all around) refix the stomach to the abdominal wall. But if the surrounding tissues and the hole in the stomach look 'bad', then take out the tube and carefully suture or staple off the hole. Based on the condition of the patient and the degree of peritonitis consider whether you wish to insert a gastrostomy (or jejunostomy) tube in another, healthier location. Needless to say, thorough 'peritoneal toilet' is mandatory (➲ Chapter 13). This procedure can be accomplished laparoscopically if you have enough skills or by a limited upper abdominal midline laparotomy.

Late leaks

Less frequently, leaks may occur long after PEG insertion, particularly in patients with poor healing capabilities and occasionally also after inadvertent or planned removal of the tube. Most often such late leaks behave like a *controlled gastric fistula* and will eventually seal spontaneously with conservative measures. However, an uncontrolled leak into the peritoneal cavity may occur and should be managed according to the above principles.

Perforation of a viscus

Rarely, the colon or even small bowel can be 'impaled' by the PEG tube during its placement. This could present early on with a free leak and peritonitis or later with an abscess or colonic fistula (external and/or communicating with the stomach). The management (conservative vs. operative) depends on the acuteness of presentation, the anatomy of the complication and the patient's general condition. Free leaks must be controlled and abscesses drained, while controlled fistulas are managed conservatively. **PEG-associated gastrocolic fistulas may subside when the tube is pulled out — but not necessarily so.**

Complications of endoscopic retrograde cholangio-pancreatography (ERCP)

ERCP carries a relatively high incidence of complications. Were we not constrained by the Editors, who forbade mention of percentages in this book, we would have told you that in decreasing order of frequency, the complications include: pancreatitis (2%-5%), bleeding (2%), cholangitis (1%-2%) and perforation (0.5%-1.2%). **The mortality rate of the last-mentioned complication may be as high as 15%. Therefore, ERCP — especially therapeutic ERCP — should be viewed as a potentially risky endoscopic procedure that shouldn't be embarked upon lightly**. We have seen disasters developing after unnecessary ERCP, ordered, for example, because of transient elevation of liver function tests after laparoscopic cholecystectomy. Remember that advanced imaging (MRCP, high-quality CT scans) and, particularly, endoscopic US (EUS), has removed the need for most diagnostic ERCP! **Therefore, keep ERCP just for the therapeutic option, namely extraction of CBD stones and drainage of the biliary tree**.

Pancreatitis

While hyperamylasemia may be seen in up to two-thirds of patients, clinical pancreatitis occurs rarely. It may occur both during diagnostic and therapeutic procedures, albeit with a higher incidence in those with any kind of intervention. The severity in most cases is usually mild to moderate and self-limiting. **Unfortunately, however, severe post-ERCP pancreatitis, and even fatalities, can occur**. Interestingly, pancreatitis is more common in younger patients and has its highest incidence in patients having ERCP for suspected 'sphincter of Oddi dysfunction' (one of those mystifying diagnoses seen only by those who write the articles).

Diagnosis

Any significant upper abdominal pain coupled with hyperamylasemia after ERCP should raise the suspicion of pancreatitis. Sometimes the diagnosis is difficult to make, since **perforation** (see below) may give a similar clinical presentation. If cannulation of the duct was easy and no 'precut' or therapeutic interventions were attempted, the likelihood of duodenal perforation is low. **Even so, whenever you suspect a perforation, order a Gastrografin® UGI study, or preferably and much better, a CT scan with *oral* and i.v. contrast, to exclude the perforation and to confirm the pancreatitis**.

Management

Intravenous fluids and NPO until the symptoms abate are usually all that is required. In a minority of patients, a more severe and protracted course may follow. The management strategy in such cases is discussed in ➲ Chapter 17. Obviously, impacted common bile duct stones may precipitate pancreatitis and prolong its course; if so — repeated ERCP or operative common bile duct exploration may be indicated. BTW, do not rush in with a laparoscopic cholecystectomy following the ERCP before making sure that the pancreatitis has totally resolved. Do we need to explain why?

Hemorrhage

Clinically significant hemorrhage may occur after endoscopic sphincterotomy (ES).

Diagnosis

Bleeding may present as upper GI bleeding or mimic lower GI bleeding; the patient may develop hemodynamic compromise before hematemesis or melena appears. Admit the patient to the ICU or the surgical floor for close monitoring and apply all the principles of management of UGI bleeding (➲ Chapter 16.2).

Management

Repeat endoscopy is indicated for accurate diagnosis and to confirm if the bleeding is in the form of oozing or brisk arterial 'pumping', and also to achieve hemostasis.

If endoscopic hemostasis fails and the patient's condition is still stable, and an experienced interventional radiologist is available, then *celiac angiography* with **selective embolization** may prevent operative intervention. However, if this in turn fails or is unavailable, and the bleeding continues or the patient is unstable, then **operative intervention must be undertaken**. After full mobilization (*Kocherization*) of the duodenum, a longitudinal duodenotomy (some would prefer an oblique one to prevent narrowing) in the second part will allow access to the papilla of Vater. The bleeding is controlled by suture ligature, being careful not to stenose the opening of the papilla or the *sphincterotomy* site (it may be safer to cannulate the papilla before suturing!).

In a 'stable' patient in whom ERCP and ES has failed, one can proceed with a definitive surgical correction of the problem for which the ES had been attempted — e.g. common duct exploration for impacted stones. **Otherwise, the minimum should be done that allows drainage of the obstructed biliary system** (e.g. cholecystostomy or a T-tube). **Care must be taken not to stenose the duodenum with closure of the duodenotomy site**.

Perforation

This is by far the most serious complication of ERCP with up to one-fifth of patients dying. **Most perforations are into the retroperitoneum in the peri-ampullary area**. They are caused by the 'precut' or ES. Less frequently, guidewire perforations of the common bile duct and the pancreatic duct may occur. **Only a tenth of perforations are intraperitoneal and are caused by the endoscope itself — usually in the anterior wall of the second part of the duodenum**. Risk factors for this include limited experience of the endoscopist, too generous precut or ES, therapeutic procedure, intramural injection of contrast material, repeated ERCP, and patients with a Billroth II gastrectomy (in whom the access to the papilla is in 'reverse' through the afferent loop).

Diagnosis

This is often apparent during the procedure or at the conclusion of it when the endoscopist suspects that something went awry. Abdominal and back pain during or immediately after ERCP, together with the presence of **retroperitoneal air on plain X-ray**, will confirm the diagnosis. If suspected already during the procedure, then injection of contrast medium by the endoscopist can demonstrate the leak. **The preferred single modality for the diagnosis is an abdominal CT scan (don't forget oral contrast!) detecting retroperitoneal or intraperitoneal air and contrast leakage**. This prevents a mistaken diagnosis of pancreatitis, which could delay the appropriate management. **Even more importantly, what you see on the CT helps you to decide how to manage the patient!**

Management

Patients with evidence of a free leak into the peritoneal cavity should undergo an emergency laparotomy (yes, of course after adequate resuscitation and administration of antibiotics). Only those who are blessed with highly motivational and skilful endoscopists, who will close the perforation using 'ovesco' (over-the-scope) clips or sutures, are exempted from surgery. Free leak is usually a result of 'rough' endoscopy with the endoscope gashing the duodenum. Clinically it manifests with peritonitis and a spectrum of systemic sepsis. When abdominal X-rays show a significant pneumoperitoneum, you can take the patient to the OR without a CT. **But if the diagnosis is not clear, CT would show intraperitoneal air and leaking contrast.**

At operation — 'Kocherize' and simply repair the duodenal rent. You can do it in one or two layers but try not to narrow its lumen. Most of these cases are operated upon within 24 hours (those who are neglected longer tend not to survive), thus there is absolutely no need to add any maneuvers (such as a 'duodenal exclusion' or feeding jejunostomy) to the repair. **This is, however, one of the rare indications for leaving a drain behind.**

Most patients, however, experience mini-perforations into the retroperitoneum at the site of the 'precut' or sphincterotomy. Sepsis may be mild or moderate and abdominal tenderness confined to the upper abdomen. X-rays and CT will show air only in the retroperitoneum and contrast won't be seen leaking into the peritoneal cavity (a few bubbles of air leaking into the peritoneal cavity should not make you rush to the OR...).

There is ample evidence that most of these patients can be successfully treated non-operatively if the following conditions are met:

- **Absence of clinical peritonitis and/or systemic inflammation** (hemodynamic compromise, high fever and leukocytosis).
- **Absence of large pneumoperitoneum.**
- **Absence of free leakage of contrast.**

If such conditions are met, a nasogastric tube is inserted and broad-spectrum antibiotics with adequate Gram-negative coverage are administered. Patients should be followed closely (by one observer — YOU!) and improvement should be expected within 12-24 hours. Normally, these patients recover within 7-10 days; any repeated procedures, if still indicated, should be postponed until well after that time.

The lack of significant clinical improvement, with the appearance or worsening of peritoneal irritation or signs of ongoing sepsis mandate an operation. After fully 'Kocherizing' the duodenum, the site of perforation is usually revealed at its posterior aspect. Depending on the degree of induration and inflammation of the tissues, either primary closure or an omental patch repair is performed and a drain left *in situ*.

The next step depends on the patient's condition, underlying pathology, failure or success of the 'index' ERCP and the adequacy of the duodenal closure.

The principles are: if the patient's condition is stable and the repair looks adequate (this occurs with early diagnosis), there is no need for a pyloric exclusion procedure. An obstructed biliary system should be decompressed preferably by a T-tube (after cholecystectomy and common bile duct exploration and clearance). **If you are already there, please do not leave the patient at the mercy of the endoscopist again!**

If you are worried about the quality of duodenal repair, or its lumen, you may want to add a *pyloric exclusion* procedure. This is accomplished either by simply and safely stapling of the antrum-pyloric junction or by making a gastrotomy just proximal to the pylorus and suturing the pylorus from the inside (PDS® would be fine) — then forming a gastrojejunostomy. Finally, you may want to feed a narrow-bore nasogastric tube deep into the efferent loop of the gastrojejunostomy to feed your patient distal to the anastomosis and the duodenal repair. **And leave a periduodenal drain!**

In highly specialized centers, a repeat ERCP with insertion of a stent, to 'seal' the perforation, may be attempted, but most endoscopists are understandably reluctant to have another go at these patients after endoscopy has caused the problem in the first place.

Yes, severe complications and deaths after ERCP are heartbreaking. But what is tragic is that in many such cases it is clear in retrospect that the original procedure was not really indicated (for example, EUS or MRCP could have excluded the suspected choledocholithiasis). Make sure <u>your</u> requests for ERCP are solidly indicated.

Complications of colonoscopy

Colonoscopy is relatively a safe procedure, with the main complications again being perforation and hemorrhage. The complication rate is very low for diagnostic procedures but rises when the procedure is therapeutic — especially after polypectomy. With the rising boldness of the gastroenterologists and the use of endoscopic submucosal dissection (ESD) and endoscopic mucosal resection (EMR) in recent years, be prepared to see more 'troubles' after colonoscopy!

Bleeding (see also ➲ Chapter 27)

Bleeding might occur immediately after the procedure or may be *secondary* or *delayed*, from an ulcer developing at the site of the polypectomy or biopsy. The risk is higher with resection of polyps larger than 15mm, recurrent or difficult procedures, or a bleeding tendency. Rarely, bleeding may occur due to mucosal injury caused by traumatic insertion and manipulation of the scope. Very rarely, vigorous manipulations in the region of the splenic flexure of the colon result in a *splenic injury* and intra-abdominal hemorrhage.

Management

This includes resuscitation and correction of any coagulopathy followed by an **endoscopic attempt to treat the bleeding**. When considering repeated colonoscopy for hemostasis, insist on tattooing the bleeding site for possible subsequent surgical intervention in case of endoscopic failure. If, after replacing fluids and correcting coagulation deficits, the patient has clearly stopped bleeding, one may elect not to repeat the colonoscopy to minimize the risk of a perforation at the biopsy site. In selected stable patients who continue to bleed following failed endoscopic hemostasis and whose pathology (diagnosed during the colonoscopy) doesn't require resection, an **angiographic selective distal embolization** may be attempted provided a highly skilled interventional radiologist is available. Just remember the (rare) possibility of bowel ischemia following such an intervention!

The persistence of bleeding after unsuccessful colonoscopic or radiological management mandates an immediate abdominal exploration. **Always have the endoscopist ready in the operating room to perform an intra-operative colonoscopy** (or even better — master the technique yourself). **Remember — finding the bleeding spot could be a difficult task: an intra-operative colonoscopy will minimize blood loss and prevent unnecessary bowel resections**. In most instances, after localizing the bleeding source, all you have to do is to place a colotomy and achieve hemostasis by oversewing the site of bleeding; then close the colotomy. **Of course, if bleeding originates from a source that requires resection (e.g. a large polyp or carcinoma) then an appropriate colectomy should be performed**.

Perforation

The mechanism of perforation determines the size of the hole, which, occasionally, can then be managed selectively by the smart surgeon — not the gastroenterologist.

Difficult, traumatic, and therapeutic colonoscopies are associated with an increased risk of perforation of the colon. Barotrauma from excessive insufflation of air, 'looping' the scope, excessive use of cautery, or overzealous dilatation of strictures are common causative factors. In addition, prior surgery, diverticulitis, or pre-existing intra-abdominal adhesions, large abdominal wall hernias and a poorly prepared bowel may increase the difficulty of the procedure and the risk of perforation.

When a colonic perforation occurs, the spectrum of consequences is wide and unpredictable.

The *mechanism* of perforation matters:

- **Perforations following diagnostic colonoscopy** often result in sizeable rents in the colonic wall and thus require prompt surgical treatment (luckily these are really rare, so the overall risk is small).
- **Perforations that follow therapeutic colonoscopy** (at a biopsy or polypectomy site) are usually small and more amenable to non-operative treatment.

Diagnosis

The key to diagnosis is to suspect it. Think about the possibility of perforation in any patient who develops abdominal discomfort or unusual pain at any time after colonoscopy. We have seen patients dying from neglected intra-abdominal infection — having their 'non-specific' complaints attributed to 'gas pain' by their super-busy and ultra-confident gastroenterologists.

Presentation is wide-ranging: abdominal complaints and signs may develop immediately after the colonoscopy when there is a large colonic tear. On the other hand, patients may present a few days later with gradually increasing local and systemic manifestations of infection. Such delayed presentation is typical of perforations that are initially contained within the retroperitoneum or the mesenteric leaves, and gradually leak or rupture into the free peritoneal cavity. Polypectomy with cautery necrosis of the bowel wall may also result in delayed perforation.

The abdominal-peritoneal signs and systemic repercussions of colonic perforation are well known to you. But remember that loops of bowel — pumped up with air during colonoscopy — may still be tender many hours after the procedure.

Start with a plain upright chest X-ray or left lateral decubitus films of the abdomen and look for free air. The findings of free intra-abdominal air together with a clinical picture of local or generalized peritonitis are diagnostic of perforation. **However, remember that small amounts of pneumoperitoneum may be seen after colonoscopy with minimal or no clinical evidence suggesting perforation ('benign' post-colonoscopic pneumoperitoneum)**. Conversely, free air may be missing when the perforation is initially contained or retroperitoneal. **Basing decision-making on the absence or presence of free air reflects naivety common to non-surgeons (e.g. gastroenterologists) attempting to treat abdominal surgical emergencies**.

Obviously, clinical signs of perforation and free air on abdominal X-ray are diagnostic of perforation. **In the absence of free air insist on obtaining a CT scan (or a Gastrografin® enema if CT is not available)**. Not only is CT able to show free air not visualized by plain X-rays but it may also show other details suggestive of injury such as intra-abdominal fluid, colonic wall hematoma or air

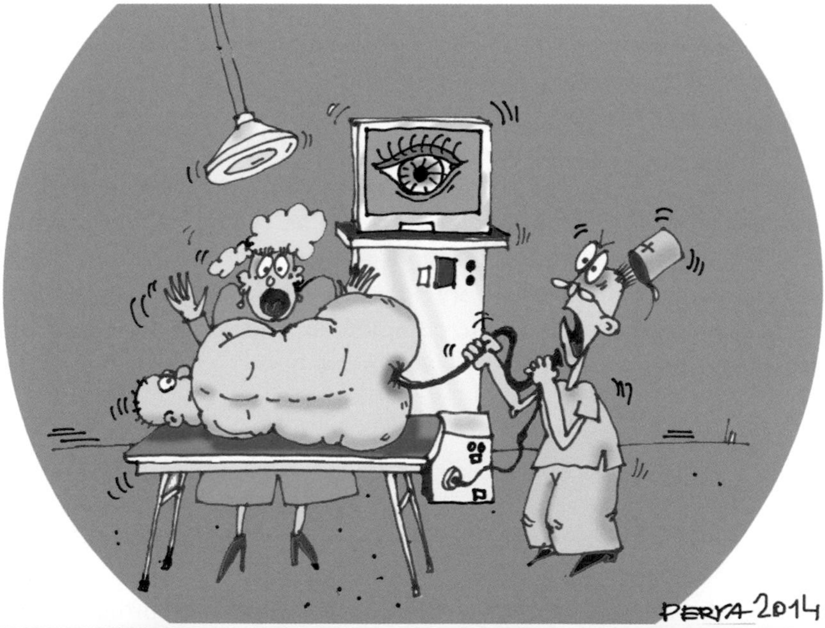

Figure 29.1. "Nurse, is that the omentum?"

in the colonic wall, the mesentery or the retroperitoneum. When combined with rectal contrast, CT usually demonstrates the site and size of the leak and whether it is *contained* or not. **Free fluid may reflect spillage of bowel contents or developing peritonitis.**

The chief cause of death following colonoscopic perforation is a delay in diagnosis and a consequent delay in treatment. This hold-up usually results from the failure of the responsible clinician (it is usually the colonoscopist himself to whom the patient presents with the complication) to consider such a diagnosis. Remember the 'surgical ostrich' who can't diagnose his own complications? Well, some endoscopists are no different (■ Figure 29.1). We have to help them pull their head out of the sand.

Non-operative management

Not all patients with colonoscopic bowel injury need an operation. Patients who are minimally symptomatic, without fever or tachycardia, and in whom the abdominal exam is benign (i.e. no features of peritonitis), can be managed non-operatively with nil per mouth and broad-spectrum antibiotics (as you would manage acute diverticulitis — ➲ Chapter 26). Patients who respond to conservative treatment typically have no, or minimal pneumoperitoneum and no, or minimal leak of contrast on CT.

As stated above, perforation at the site of a polypectomy is more amenable to a trial of non-operative management. Such an approach is often successful because these patients have had bowel preparation prior to colonoscopy and therefore the potential for abdominal contamination is reduced. All such patients should be closely monitored for local and systemic progression of the process or failure to improve. Deterioration should prompt an urgent surgical intervention. **If the perforation is at the site of pathology for which a colectomy will be recommended anyway, what's the point of sweating through conservative management? Go ahead and do the definitive surgery right away. However, this is true only if the local conditions allow you to complete an oncologic dissection and a safe anastomosis. Otherwise — what's the hurry?**

Operative management

Patients who look sick, complain of localized or spreading pain, with systemic sepsis and localized or generalized peritonitis — associated with the aforementioned radiological features — should receive antibiotics and undergo an emergency laparotomy. In most patients undergoing early exploration the findings are those of peritoneal *contamination* rather than established *infection*; all that is required is 'peritoneal toilet' (➲ Chapter 13) and **primary suture of the perforation** as you would do with any traumatic colonic injury, unless you have to resect the associated polyp or cancer. The absence of feces in the colon helps to minimize the severity of contamination/infection. A diverting or exteriorizing colostomy may be indicated in selected patients, e.g. with neglected established peritonitis or severe debilitating comorbidities such as malnutrition or steroid dependence.

Endoscopic or laparoscopic management

With modern endoscopic equipment, and advanced laparoscopic capabilities, less traumatic options exist for some colonoscopic perforations. **When a perforation is diagnosed at the time of the procedure, the endoscopist may try to approximate the edges of the tear using endoscopic clips**. The (now dwindling) interest in 'natural orifice transluminal surgery' (NOTES) had led to the development of even more advanced solutions for endoscopic suturing and other forms of tissue approximation but the availability of these investigational devices is still limited.

When an operation is mandatory, most injuries can be approached laparoscopically provided an experienced surgeon and appropriate instruments are available. Colonic perforations can be sutured or stapled, if local conditions allow for a primary repair. Alternatively, laparoscopic exteriorization and stoma construction for late, neglected cases, is a valid option.

Complications of endoscopic ultrasound (EUS)

In recent years we are witnessing an increased use of EUS for diagnosis as well as for various kinds of therapeutic intervention. EUS-guided interventions have replaced many ERCP, percutaneous and surgical procedures. Therefore, we should be familiar with this procedure and its associated complications. Depending on the nature of the procedure and the site of intervention, the complications include bacteremia, bleeding (intraluminal, extraluminal and inside pancreatic cystic lesions), perforations of hollow viscera, bile and pancreatic leaks, and pancreatitis. In most cases, non-operative measures will suffice, but in cases with uncontrolled hemorrhage or peritonitis, surgical intervention is inevitable. The same principles that we have discussed earlier should guide us in managing these complications.

To re-cap

The management of endoscopic injury to any hollow gastrointestinal viscus, from the esophagus down to the rectum, can be summed up as follows:

- Always suspect disaster.
- Image for diagnosis.
- Those who are missed and neglected tend to die.
- Some can be managed conservatively.
- Some can be managed endoscopically.
- Some need an immediate operation.
- Some who are managed conservatively may eventually need an operation.
- **To achieve optimal results — be selective, alert and always ready to change your mind. You are not a politician — you can be proud to be a flipflopper!**

"A fool with a tool is still a fool."

Chapter 30

Abdominal trauma

Roger Saadia

This chapter has been subdivided into the following three sections:

1. Penetrating abdominal trauma.
2. Blunt abdominal trauma.
3. Operative management of individual organ injuries.

For a more detailed discussion of the general management of trauma and its complications we recommend that you look at Chapter 24 by Ari Leppäniemi in our other book [1].

1 Penetrating abdominal trauma

It is absolutely necessary for a surgeon to search the wounds himself, which are not drest by him at first, in order to discover their nature and know their extent.

A. Belloste

[1] *Schein's Common Sense Prevention and Management of Surgical Complications.* Shrewsbury, UK: tfm publishing, 2013: Chapter 24.

General principles

The crucial decision faced by the surgeon managing penetrating abdominal trauma is whether an exploratory laparotomy is indicated. The decision to operate rests solely on the high likelihood that a significant injury is present; it does not require a precise inventory of all the possible intra-abdominal visceral injuries. **In penetrating trauma, the role of clinical evaluation is primordial.** Depending on the circumstances, it needs to be complemented sometimes by adjunctive diagnostic measures.

> **The surgeon's initial objective is to identify the patient requiring surgery while avoiding unnecessary laparotomies.** These are termed 'negative' when no injuries are present and 'non-therapeutic' when the identified injuries would have healed spontaneously if left alone (for example, a minor hepatic laceration associated with a small hemoperitoneum but no active bleeding).

In order to fulfil this ideal requirement of timely necessary surgery with a zero rate of unnecessary laparotomies, numerous algorithms, some very complicated, have been devised incorporating various diagnostic tests. **Not a single one is fool-proof or has gained universal acceptance. In fact, even the most experienced trauma surgeon, from time to time, does perform an unnecessary laparotomy. While such surgery is attended by some morbidity, this is a fair price to pay for not missing a significant intra-abdominal injury, provided that the frequency of such laparotomies is not unreasonably high.**

In **civilian practice**, there are two main mechanisms of penetrating abdominal trauma: **stab wounds** and **gunshot injuries**. Owing to surgical tradition, these two categories have been treated differently, with mandatory surgery being advocated for gunshot wounds. More recently, there has been a tendency to apply the same management principles irrespective of the injury mechanism.

After penetrating abdominal trauma, two possible clinical pictures can be found, in isolation or in combination: hypovolemic shock and peritonitis. The former is the result of bleeding from an injured solid organ (e.g. spleen, liver) or a sizable vessel. The latter is the consequence of soiling of the peritoneal cavity caused usually by an injured hollow viscus (gut, biliary system, urinary bladder).

Abdominal stab wounds

Though shock may be temporarily alleviated by transfusion, it cannot be arrested or overcome; resuscitation divorced from surgery is folly.

William Heneage Ogilvie

The diagnosis of a stabbed abdomen is straightforward in most cases: there is a visible wound on the abdominal wall and the patient or witnesses usually confirm the circumstances of the assault. **Don't be taken in by fishermen's tales about how long the steak knife was but remember instead the adage**: "**Treat the patient not the weapon**."

It bears repeating that clinical evaluation of the patient (supplemented by an upright chest X-ray) is the most important step in the diagnostic work-up. There are scenarios mandating an exploratory laparotomy without the need for additional confirmatory diagnostic procedures. The only required tests are those in preparation for a laparotomy (basic blood work, blood group and match, and when necessary EKG, βHCG...).

The following are indications for immediate surgery:

- **Hemodynamic instability** in the absence of an associated extra-abdominal injury that could, by itself, account for shock. Fluid resuscitation must be started immediately. **However, remember that the patient is not bleeding Ringer's lactate!** Blood and its components should be started as soon as available to reduce crystalloid loading or 'salt-water drowning'. **'Permissive hypotension'** should be maintained until surgical hemostasis has been achieved. (Patients in extremis should be transferred expeditiously to the operating room since emergency room thoracotomy is not a useful maneuver in this context; as for emergency room laparotomy, it is extremely efficient in transferring the patient's total blood volume from the abdomen to the floor...).
- **Peritonitis** is frequent and there is little diagnostic value in eliciting tenderness and even guarding on abdominal palpation in the immediate vicinity of the laceration. **Signs of peritonitis need to be found at a distance from the wound in order to confidently establish the diagnosis**. Always ensure that the bladder is empty before you prod for abdominal tenderness (these patients often arrive to the emergency room with a bladder ready to burst, courtesy of over-enthusiastic paramedics).

- The demonstration of **free intraperitoneal air** on the upright chest X-ray. Abdominal X-rays are unnecessary in stabbed abdomens except for the lateral decubitus film in a patient that cannot sit up for a chest X-ray.
- **Omental or intestinal evisceration**. A laparotomy is advisable because of the high likelihood of visceral injury. Even if the laparotomy turns out to be negative, it would have served the double purpose of safely reducing the herniated viscera and allowing for a meticulous closure of the lacerated abdominal wall, preventing hernia formation.
- **A retained stabbing instrument**. This could be tamponading a sizable blood vessel and therefore should be removed in the operating room.

Abdominal stab wounds: when to observe? How to investigate?

Reading the standard textbooks, one gets a little confused about how to manage the asymptomatic patient with, typically, an anterior abdominal wall laceration. In about one-third of these, the wound does not extend into the peritoneal cavity and in another third it does — but there are no significant visceral injuries. Exploring all these patients would not be a good idea.

Diagnostic procedures are sometimes advocated. Diagnostic peritoneal lavage is cumbersome and lacks accuracy; it is attended by a high rate of non-therapeutic laparotomies. **Exploration of the wound** under local anesthesia aims at identifying a breach of the parietal peritoneum. It is often difficult though to determine with certainty the extension of the track — try it in an obese or combative patient in the rough-and-tumble atmosphere of a busy emergency department! **Laparoscopy** is a logistically demanding test since it requires general anesthesia. Here, its main value is to ascertain intraperitoneal penetration. **Don't be fooled by overconfident minimally invasive surgeons**; a negative laparoscopic assessment of the peritoneal cavity cannot exclude a small intestinal laceration with minimal spillage, nor can it assess the retroperitoneum. **In addition, post-procedure clinical or radiological abdominal assessments are made unreliable**. About the selective role of laparoscopy for a suspected diaphragmatic injury see below.

There remain two (we believe, complementary) approaches to the asymptomatic patient with an anterior abdominal stab wound: clinical reassessment and helical computed tomography (CT) scanning.

Serial clinical reassessment of the patient

This policy has been dubbed 'selective conservatism', and has proved its worth in many centers. The patient is admitted, kept nil per os and given an i.v. infusion. The vital signs and urine output are closely monitored. **The abdomen is re-examined at frequent intervals checking for the development of peritonitis; the initial area of tenderness around the wound can be circumscribed with a marker and spreading tenderness is watched for over the observation period**. Analgesia, antibiotics or nasogastric decompression are not required.

If, after an observation period of 18-24 hours, no signs of hypovolemia or peritonitis are elicited, it is highly unlikely that a significant intra-abdominal injury is present. **A very good indicator of this is a patient angrily demanding a meal tray**. In applying this policy, always keep an open mind and do not persevere stubbornly with non-operative management in the face of even subtle deterioration. **Having to operate in a delayed fashion in a well-monitored patient is not a sign of personal failure but a tribute to your clinical acumen**. An occasional unnecessary laparotomy will be performed: this is nothing to be ashamed of and when in doubt it is safer to err on the side of surgical exploration.

Abdominal CT scan

In recent years, both the access to CT scanning and the quality of the images have improved dramatically. **In many centers, the asymptomatic stabbed patient is often sent to the scanner by the emergency physician before the surgeon is even consulted**. Whatever seasoned trauma surgeons may think of this practice, the train has long since left the station...

Undoubtedly, this investigation is often valuable, even though its shortcomings in early intestinal perforation are well known. Some patients are shown to have only a superficial wound with greater ease and accuracy than by local tract exploration. They can be safely discharged from the emergency department. A small minority of asymptomatic patients are diagnosed with a significant visceral injury (that would have eventually declared itself under observation). Their trip to the operating room is thereby expedited. The remaining majority of the patients with a negative or equivocal CT scan need to be admitted and observed as described above.

The primacy of clinical evaluation is unquestioned. However, as in the management of acute appendicitis, its interplay with the judicious use of the CT scanner can refine one's decision-making a little further.

Abdominal gunshot wounds — dogma versus modern imaging

It is highly desirable that anyone engaged in war surgery should keep his idea fluid and so be ready to abandon methods which prove unsatisfactory in favour of others which, at first, may appear revolutionary and even not free from inherent danger.

H. H. Sampson

Traditional wisdom inherited from war experience has held that an exploratory laparotomy is always indicated in these patients irrespective of their clinical condition. This policy has been predicated on the higher likelihood of significant intra-abdominal injuries in gunshot than in stab wounds. This premise, if true, implies merely that shock and peritonitis are more frequently associated with the former than with the latter. Decision-making is then easy. **But what about the benign-looking abdomen with a gunshot wound that is encountered nowadays not that infrequently in many large urban trauma centers?**

There is accumulating evidence to suggest that initially asymptomatic gunshot victims can be managed safely along the same broad lines as stabbed patients. While the role of initial and serial clinical reassessments is here again very important, **we contend that an early CT scan of both the abdomen and chest is mandatory, not only in asymptomatic patients but in all gunshot victims who are stable enough to go to the scanner**.

Bullets tend to travel longer distances than the length of a knife blade. Imaging of the whole torso is essential to document the trajectory of the bullet(s), which could extend beyond the confines of the abdominal cavity. A missing bullet should prompt the search for an extra-abdominal location or a hidden exit wound. Furthermore, a bullet entering the abdomen can significantly damage bony structures (thoracolumbar spine, pelvis, hip, etc.). The information gleaned from these images is often invaluable despite the occasional 'scatter' caused by a retained metal fragment. **Sometimes, it will be seen that the missile's trajectory is tangential, missing the peritoneal cavity: a laparotomy can be avoided** but semi-elective debridement of the abdominal wall may prove necessary in some of these cases.

So, if you have immediate access to the scanner and the patient is not exsanguinating, then use it! The findings can modify your operative approach and even help you to avoid an operation altogether.

Difficult scenarios: the CT scan reigns supreme

Stab wounds to the lower chest, the flank or the perineum pose the problem of possible but clinically occult injury to intra-abdominal viscera:

- **The diaphragm**. An isolated diaphragmatic laceration is often at first clinically silent but is sometimes complicated by a secondary diaphragmatic hernia. This complication is more likely to occur on the left than on the right side which is relatively shielded by the bulk of the liver. Little is known about the natural history of diaphragmatic wounds but very small ones are probably often missed with impunity. **It is, however, the standard of care to look for them whenever a stab wound is located in the lower chest or upper abdomen (especially on the left side). In this scenario, if there are no other clinical reasons to operate, then a thoracoscopy or a laparoscopy should be performed during the patient's hospital stay to check the integrity of the diaphragm**; if a laceration is identified, it should be repaired at laparotomy (or laparoscopically if you are able to do it). Reconstructed coronal CT scan views of the diaphragmatic domes can also be very helpful and, if available, are already supplanting laparoscopy.
- **The flank**. A stab wound to the flank can involve the retroperitoneal portion of the duodenum or colon and the kidney. Peritoneal signs are present only at a late stage (sometimes too late, associated with advanced retroperitoneal infection). Therefore, a CT scan must always be obtained early (there is no longer any need for a combined contrast enema). An injury to the kidney is often benign and is usually associated with frank hematuria. The possibility of a ureteric injury is more serious and must be entertained in the presence of microscopic hematuria. Nowadays, the CT (with i.v. contrast of course) scan has supplanted the intravenous pyelogram (IVP) as the screening investigation of choice in suspected injuries to the urinary tract.
- **The perineum**. Abdominal penetration must always be suspected. **A digital rectal exam looking for rectal bleeding is a mandatory component of the clinical examination**. A CT scan is helpful and may need to be supplemented by rectosigmoidoscopy.
- **Patients with multiple stab or gunshot wounds to both the chest and abdomen** may constitute a dilemma in the choice or sequencing of the operations if both the chest and abdomen are possible candidates for the source of severe hemorrhage; this is particularly the case if they are unstable and unfit for transfer to the CT scanner. Alternatively, one can come across a patient with a high epigastric stab wound and hypotension in whom the possibility of a cardiac tamponade should be entertained. **In these cases, an ultrasound scan in the emergency room (focused assessment with**

sonography for trauma [FAST]) may help to formulate a logical management plan. FAST is used more frequently in blunt trauma and will be discussed in the next section.

What to do when CT scanning is not available?

Some of you readers from developing countries may not have unrestricted access to emergency CT scans. **The great majority of penetrating trauma victims can be managed by the combination of three diagnostic modalities: clinical examination, an upright chest X-ray and, yes, exploratory laparotomy**, the latter being resorted to more liberally whenever in doubt. Keep the threshold for intervention low. The acceptable price to pay, in this context, is a higher rate of unnecessary laparotomies rather than missed injuries. In patients with a flank injury or hematuria, a one-shot IVP in the emergency room is easy to perform and very useful (especially in confirming the presence of a functioning kidney on the *uninjured* side).

To recap...

Clinical evaluation (including vital signs assessment and abdominal examination) retains to this day its primacy in the management of penetrating

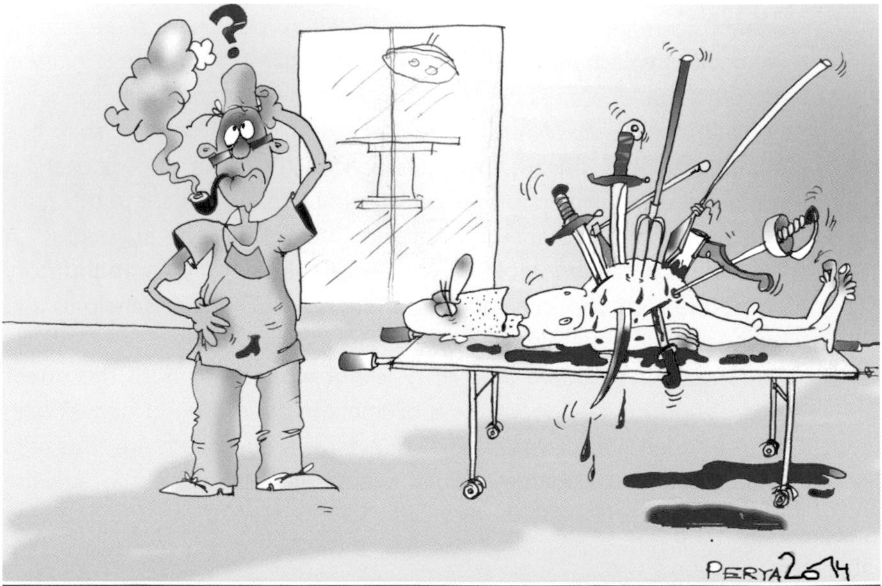

Figure 30.1. "Let's be conservative!"

abdominal trauma. There are clear-cut clinical scenarios requiring immediate laparotomy. In other situations, clinical observation remains extremely valuable. In recent years, abdominal CT scanning has established itself as the best diagnostic adjunct. **Know when to operate and when not to** (■ Figure 30.1)!

> *Failure to promptly recognize and treat simple life-threatening injuries is the tragedy of trauma, not the inability to handle the catastrophic or complicated injury.*
>
> **F. William Blaisdell**

Special forms of penetrating trauma [2]

I would like to mention here three 'special forms' of penetrating trauma which may need a different approach:

- **Impalement injuries.**
- **Shotgun injuries.**
- **Pellet gun injuries.**

Impalement injuries

Impalement injuries are caused by penetration of the body by an object that usually is retained *in situ*. It can be a steel rod (■ Figure 30.2), piece of wood, or even an AK-47 (■ Figure 30.3). The most common causes are accidental falls or collisions, violence or sexually perverted acts. Typically, they cause complex and multiple organ injuries, and require some special attention during transport and at treatment in the hospital.

The basic rule is that the impaled object should not be manipulated or removed during transport or at the ER, but it is important that it is stabilized securely. If possible and needed, it can be shortened. Because they are always contaminated, antibiotic and tetanus prophylaxis should be administered.

Virtually all patients require surgery; those in shock need to go to the OR immediately. The positioning of the patient may require special supports and modifications of the standard techniques. **The object must remain secured and in place until everything is ready; premature removal of the object may cause the release of a tamponade from a major vascular**

2 Ari Leppäniemi, MD, contributed this section.

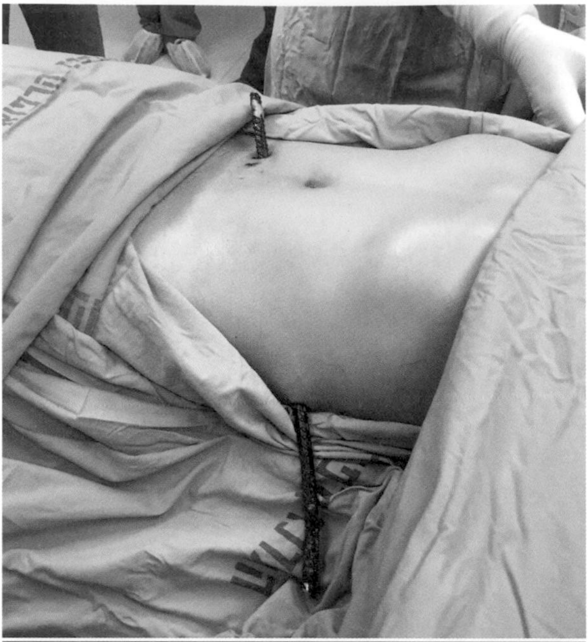

Figure 30.2. Impalement injury: steel rod.

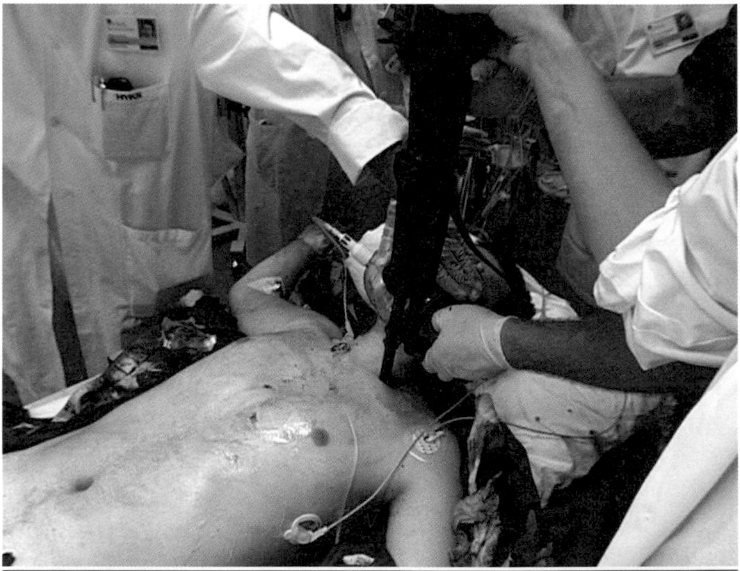

Figure 30.3. Impalement injury: AK-47.

structure! Use unconventional incisions if needed. Once the object has been removed, the standard routine for exploration and repair of all injuries is performed like for any other trauma.

Shotgun injuries

Shotgun injuries form a special type of penetrating injury because of the unique ballistic properties resulting in a wide range of injuries from trivial to the most severe ones. **Although there are many things that affect the severity, the range is the most important**. The point-blank or close-range shotgun injuries (less than 3 yards... a yard being almost a meter) cause massive tissue destruction in a fairly tight pattern and are often fatal, if hitting vital structures. **Surgery, even only for debridement, is mandatory**. Often it also involves removal of the embedded foreign material such as the victim's clothing.

Injuries from close to middle range (3 to 7 yards) will usually penetrate the abdominal wall and cause injuries to the internal organs. Laparotomy is nearly always the safest option.

Shotgun injuries from 7 to 20 yards usually produce a scattered wound and can penetrate the skin and fascia. These patients need close observation, whereas asymptomatic patients with long-range shotgun injuries (more than 20 yards) seldom need treatment other than managing the superficial wounds.

In patients needing urgent surgery (close-range injuries, usually lateral in those surviving to the hospital) and where evisceration is often present, a transverse incision is preferred to facilitate later abdominal closure, because of the extensive debridement required. In middle-range injuries a formal midline laparotomy can be performed, the abdomen explored, and injuries repaired like in other penetrating gunshot wounds. **Special care must be taken to run the whole small bowel completely and repair all perforations, because small pellets can travel between the leaves of the mesentery and cause small perforations that are difficult to see**.

Air gun pellet injuries

Air and paintball gun activities have become very popular among the Rambo-generation adolescents and like-minded grown-ups. More than 30,000 air gun injuries occur annually in the United States — where in some states killing innocent squirrels seems a national hobby. These non-powder guns employ the power of compressed air to launch a projectile, mostly of a low-velocity nature. **Although deemed harmless, there are many reports of serious morbidity or even deaths after air weapon injuries**.

While the injuries were seldom dangerous in the past unless hitting the eye or other poorly protected areas in the head, **modern air guns have the capability of causing penetrating abdominal injuries with hollow organ perforations**.

The management of patients with one or multiple pellet injury signs over the abdomen must undergo a thorough clinical examination. It is useful to know the type of gun used as well as the distance from which the shots came. The longer the distance, the less likely there will be a penetrating injury because pellets, due to their ballistic properties, rapidly lose velocity. Any signs of severe (intra-abdominal) bleeding or generalized tenderness should alert to the possibility of a penetrating vascular or hollow organ injury best treated with early laparotomy. Other (stable) patients should undergo radiological imaging like regular penetrating trauma patients.

Obvious subcutaneous pellets can be removed. Patients with suspected or verified intra-abdominal pellets should be admitted for observation unless urgent surgery is indicated for shock or peritonitis. Although there are reports of successful 'expectant observation' of asymptomatic patients with pellets penetrating the colon and passing per rectum 12 hours later, the post-traumatic phase after pellet injuries can be subtle with signs of infection appearing later than with more powerful gunshot wounds of the abdomen. **Most surgeons do not want to wait and take the risk but prefer early laparotomy to explore and repair the injuries**.

2 Blunt abdominal trauma

Definition of a heavy trauma: somebody who arrives at the hospital in more than one ambulance.

John Edwards

He should have a special love for the wounded persons as for his own body.

Hans von Gersdorff

Differences between blunt and penetrating trauma

There are several differences between these two types of injury:

- **Penetrating abdominal trauma is made obvious by the presence of a wound**. Blunt abdominal trauma is sometimes unequivocally identifiable by the presence of a visible contusion of the abdominal wall (e.g. seat belt sign) but, more frequently, it is only suspected from the mechanism of injury.

- **Penetrating abdominal trauma is usually confined to the abdomen**. Common mechanisms of blunt trauma (vehicle accidents, falls, beatings…) often result in polytrauma, the abdominal component being associated with other cavity or system injuries (head, chest, pelvis, vertebral column, long bones).
- **The patterns of intra-abdominal visceral injuries are different**. Hollow visceral injuries are common in penetrating trauma. They are very rare in blunt trauma where solid organ injuries (to liver, spleen, and pancreas) predominate.
- **Clinical evaluation is unreliable** in blunt trauma. This is due to several factors:
  - the frequent presence of a **head injury** with decreased level of consciousness;
  - the nature of **multi-system trauma** results in 'distracting' injuries whereby the pain experienced at other sites (chest, long bones, pelvic fracture…) masks or distorts the patient's perception of abdominal pain and tenderness;
  - while **hypotension** is frequently caused by an injured intra-abdominal solid organ, it is as frequently due to an associated long bone or pelvic fracture or a hemothorax. It may not even be the result of hypovolemic shock but represent a sign of cardiogenic (due to cardiac contusion, pericardial tamponade, tension pneumothorax) or spinal shock;
  - tenderness on palpation may be the result of bruising of the abdominal wall rather than reflect a more severe intra-abdominal injury.

In blunt abdominal trauma, unlike in penetrating injuries, the reliance on a clinical picture of shock or peritonitis cannot constitute the sole justification for a laparotomy. The abdomen in blunt trauma has come to be seen as a 'black box' (■ Figure 30.4), in other words, an uncertain source for the patient's current instability or subsequent deterioration. It is, therefore, imperative to resort to additional diagnostic tests. **The aims of these investigations are not only to confirm the presence of abdominal trauma, but also, whenever possible, to document as precisely as possible the nature of the visceral injuries since their treatment is not invariably surgical**.

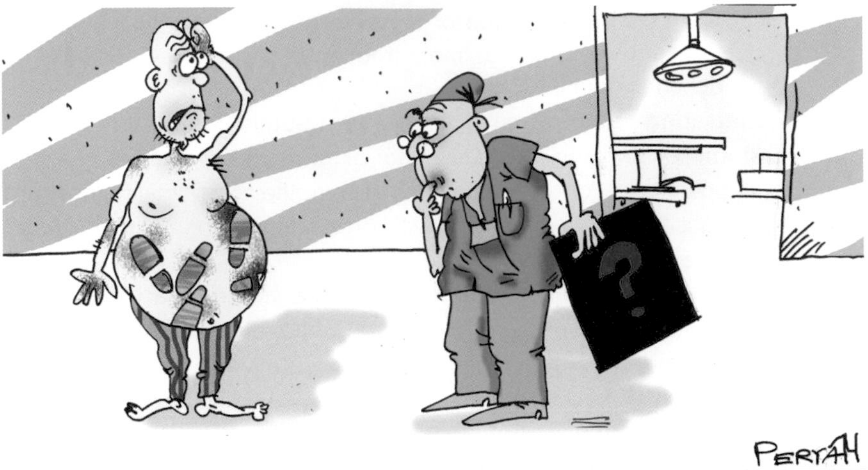

Figure 30.4. "So what's wrong inside your black box?"

Adjunctive diagnostic tests

There are three main diagnostic tests used in blunt trauma: helical computed tomography (CT) scan, ultrasound scan (referred to as FAST — focused assessment with sonography for trauma) and diagnostic peritoneal lavage (DPL).

In modern, well-equipped centers, an abdominal CT scan is the investigation of choice in the stable patient, while FAST or DPL (if FAST is not available) are more frequently employed when the patient is hemodynamically unstable. The latter two tests could also be used more liberally in facilities that cannot offer unrestricted access to CT scanning.

Diagnostic peritoneal lavage

Both a nasogastric tube and a Foley catheter are first inserted in preparation for the DPL (it would be a pity to puncture the stomach or the bladder!). The technique entails the placement, under local anesthesia, of a catheter into the peritoneal cavity. One liter of warmed saline is thereby infused, given a moment to mix with the intraperitoneal contents and recovered by laying the bag on the floor.

The DPL is deemed positive in cases of:

- Aspiration of blood from the catheter on insertion (grossly positive DPL).

- Presence of more than 100,000 red blood cells per mm^3 in the effluent (microscopically positive DPL).
- Presence of bile, intestinal contents or urine in the effluent.
- Presence of more than 500 white blood cells per mm^3 in the effluent (this is controversial).
- Flow of the DPL fluid through the urinary catheter or the chest tube, indicating a bladder or diaphragmatic injury, respectively (these scenarios are rare).

Historically, DPL was the diagnostic gold standard for blunt abdominal trauma but, in recent times, it has lost its shine for the following reasons:

- It is cumbersome and difficult to perform in a combative or obese patient.
- It has absolute or relative contraindications: previous surgery, pregnancy.
- It is invasive and attended by a small complication rate (e.g. bowel perforation).
- **Most importantly, if laparotomies were to be performed for all instances of microscopically or even grossly positive DPL, the rate of non-therapeutic laparotomies would be unacceptably high because, in most cases, the source of bleeding could have been treated non-operatively. Of course, an unnecessary laparotomy carries a significant morbidity in the context of multi-system trauma.**

In modern centers, DPL is used only in the very unstable patient to confirm, pre-operatively, the presence of a large hemoperitoneum. But if your hospital lacks access to the more sophisticated investigations, do remember that a negative DPL is a crucial piece of information in ruling out the abdominal 'black box' as a source for concern in a severe, multi-system trauma patient.

Focused assessment with sonography for trauma

The aim of FAST is to detect the presence of free fluid in the following areas:

- The pericardial sac.
- Morrison's (hepatorenal) pouch in the right upper abdominal quadrant.

- The splenorenal recess in the left upper abdominal quadrant.
- The pelvis.

FAST can assist in the diagnosis of pericardial tamponade (a rather rare finding in blunt trauma). In the evaluation of the abdomen, it duplicates somewhat the role of DPL with the advantages of being relatively cheap, totally non-invasive and applicable at the patient's bedside. FAST is reliable only in the hands of personnel specially trained in the technique (surgeons, emergency room physicians, radiologists) and in centers with a high case volume. **In modern centers, FAST plays an important role in the assessment of the unstable trauma patient — a laparotomy is usually indicated in a hypotensive patient found to have a large amount of free intraperitoneal fluid**. It is also commonly used in stable patients, but more as a practice exercise rather than a test allowing for definitive decision-making. The use of FAST as a screening tool for abdominal CT scanning is more controversial.

Computed tomography

CT scanning has become an essential part of modern management of the stable, blunt, multi-trauma patient. It is very common nowadays to dispense with cervical and thoracolumbar spine X-rays, the pelvic X-ray and even sometimes the chest X-ray: the patient is taken instead to a radiology suite adjacent to the resuscitation room and a quadruple scan of the head, neck, chest and abdomen (including the vertebral column and the pelvis) is obtained in a few minutes.

The abdominal component of this diagnostic work-up is extremely valuable because:

- Both the peritoneal cavity and the retroperitoneum can be assessed.
- The integrity of bony structures (lumbar spine, pelvis) can be ascertained.
- A precise inventory of injuries to solid intraperitoneal (liver, spleen) and retroperitoneal (pancreas, kidneys) organs can be made; these injuries can be accurately graded.
- The new generation scanners can also detect intestinal injuries (suggested by mesenteric stranding, bowel thickening or extraluminal air).
- Free fluid (with radiological blood density) in the absence of solid organ injury can be detected, suggesting the presence of a significant mesenteric injury.

In equivocal CT scan findings, clinical judgment is essential; a repeat CT scan 24 hours later, clinical observation or immediate laparotomy are the main options to be weighed.

The recourse to 'total body scanning' has become so unregulated in some 'high-tech' centers that a note of caution needs to be sounded:

- Cost aside, liberal trauma 'scannograms' deliver a very high dose of radiation; this, combined with the recurrent need for CT scanning through an entire life-time carries a significant long-term cancer risk. Always ask yourself when sending a trauma patient to the scanner whether a quadruple test is essential in this particular patient. Could not, for example, the chest CT be replaced by a simple chest X-ray? **An easy way to keep in mind this danger is to remember the acronym, VOMIT (Victims of Modern Imaging Technology), coined by R. Hayward (*BMJ*, 2003).**

Only stable or well-resuscitated patients can be put through the scanner. Borderline patients can decompensate catastrophically in the radiology suite — especially in slow machines placed remotely from the trauma room.

- CT images are as good as their interpreter. In the middle of the night, expert radiologists are sometimes not available. Always keep your clinical judgment on high alert, especially when there is discordance between the clinical picture and CT images. **Remember BARF (Brainless Application of Radiological Findings) and reach for an anti-emetic.**

Non-operative management of solid organ injuries in blunt trauma

Most patients with blunt splenic or hepatic injury (and almost all patients with an isolated blunt renal injury) can be treated conservatively. Once such an injury has been identified on CT scan, and provided there is no clinical or radiological evidence of an associated hollow viscus injury, non-operative management can be attempted.

The hemodynamic status rather than the radiological grade of the injury constitutes the basis for therapeutic decision-making — treat the patient and not the images — the grade of injury has merely predictive value in the success of conservative management. The patient is admitted for the first 24 hours to a high care unit for close observation. Continuous vital signs and urine output monitoring, serial abdominal examination and repeated hemoglobin evaluation are conducted. Then, with every passing day on the ward with no sign of ongoing bleeding, the success of the conservative approach becomes more likely.

Repeat CT scans are not required routinely on this admission but only if complications occur. On discharge, the patient is cautioned to avoid putting the injured organ at risk of a secondary rupture (e.g. contact sports, bar-room brawls) until a CT scan 8-12 weeks later documents complete healing.

More subtle differences between splenic and hepatic injuries should now be pointed out.

Spleen

Non-operative management of a splenic injury should not be stubbornly continued in the face of an increased requirement for blood transfusion. When there are episodes of hypotension (unexplained by extra-abdominal injuries) or a sustained drop in hemoglobin (not accounted for by hemodilution), there should be a low threshold for splenectomy especially in an adult. It is a real tragedy to lose a patient from splenic hemorrhage when definitive control of the bleeding can be achieved by a simple surgical procedure, namely a splenectomy (**acrobatic splenic salvage procedures belong to the past**). The very small risk of post-splenectomy sepsis in adults can be further reduced by patient education and vaccination (anti-*Pneumococcus*, anti-*Meningococcus* and anti-*Haemophilus influenzae*).

There is a range of opinions regarding the trigger for abandoning conservative management. Some believe that untreated hypotension alone (from a presumed splenic source) justifies intervention; others are prepared to transfuse up to a maximum of 2 units of blood before changing course. **The message is clear: do not persevere with multiple blood transfusions to treat ongoing splenic bleeding**. The initial CT scan may reveal a contrast 'blush' in the splenic parenchyma pointing to active bleeding; there is evidence to suggest that routine **angioembolization of these bleeding vessels, in the stable patient, increases the success rate of non-operative management**.

Liver

The intra-operative control of hepatic bleeding is difficult. The loss of the tamponade effect at laparotomy followed by mobilization of the liver can result in renewed hemorrhage, sometimes torrential. **In tackling a bleeding liver, there is no equivalent simple procedure like a splenectomy. Therefore, more diligence is called for in the pursuit of conservative management, as well as a greater reliance on aggressive transfusions of blood products and factors.** There has been increasing recourse to angioembolization in attempts (often successful) to avoid surgery. **With hepatic injuries treated non-operatively, there is a higher complication rate than with splenic injuries.** Increasing right upper quadrant pain, jaundice, melena or sepsis should prompt specialized investigations (repeat CT scan, endoscopic retrograde cholangiopancreatography [ERCP], angiography). Most of these complications can be treated by interventional radiology (see also ➲ Chapter 23).

When to operate in blunt trauma?

The most common indications for surgery in blunt trauma are:

- The **hemodynamically unstable patient** with a significant hemoperitoneum preferably demonstrated by DPL or FAST; these investigations may be omitted when other extra-abdominal injuries are confidently ruled out in a hypotensive patient with a tense, distended abdomen.
- The patient with an acute post-traumatic **diaphragmatic hernia** demonstrated on chest X-ray or CT scan.
- The patient with or without peritoneal signs but with **free intraperitoneal air** demonstrated on an upright chest X-ray or abdominal CT scan.
- The patient with a **hollow viscus injury** (bowel, gallbladder, intraperitoneal urinary bladder) demonstrated clinically or on a CT scan.
- The patient with CT evidence of a **significant pancreatic injury**.
- The patient with a significant **hemoperitoneum in the absence, on CT scan, of solid organ injury**; think of a severe mesenteric injury with a potential for bowel ischemia.
- The patient with **signs of sepsis or a persistently tender abdomen** in the presence of equivocal CT images.
- The patient in whom **conservative management of a hepatic or splenic injury (identified initially by CT scan) has failed**.

(For the operative management of these specific injuries see the next section.)

To summarize

Clinical evaluation is often unreliable in the management of blunt abdominal trauma. Great reliance is placed on the abdominal CT scan in stable patients, and on DPL or FAST in hypotensive patients. The results of these investigations always need interpretation in the overall clinical context.

Things have changed since it was stated more than 100 years ago:

> *Exploratory laparotomy offers, in our judgment, the quickest and the safest method of positive diagnosis. The emergency warrants a decisive step.*
>
> **Albert Miles**

3 Operative management of individual organ injuries

> *It is judgment not genital insufficiency driving a surgeon to pack his patient's abdomen.*
>
> **David J. Richardson**

You have decided to perform a laparotomy. Nowadays, this is more likely for penetrating than for blunt trauma as **most solid visceral injuries in blunt trauma can be managed conservatively: often doing 'less' is 'better', with limited blood loss and the avoidance of unnecessary tissue injury**. The incision and assessment of the damage are described elsewhere in this book (➲ Chapters 10 and 11).

Diaphragm

A through-and-through diaphragmatic laceration requires suture-repair with interrupted (or running) heavy (0 or 2-0 non-absorbable monofilament such as Prolene®) suture material. Lacerations with substantial tissue loss are very rare and need repair with a synthetic mesh. A prosthesis may not be necessary when the tissue loss is at the periphery; instead, the diaphragm can be reimplanted to the ribs more cephalad. This is of particular benefit in the presence of extensive contamination. **Remember that even in the absence of a pre-operative pneumothorax, an ipsilateral chest tube must be inserted at some stage of the procedure**. It is often said that minor diaphragmatic tears can be ignored on the right side because the bulk of the liver prevents future bowel herniation. However, large right-sided lacerations (seen usually in blunt trauma) must be repaired because the liver itself can, in time, be 'sucked up' into the chest.

Liver and biliary tree (see also ➲ Chapter 23)

An irreverent classification of hepatic injuries is shown in ■ Table 30.1.

Table 30.1. Classification of hepatic injuries.
■ Grade I: Nothing should be done (treat conservatively).
■ Grade II: Something should be done (local hemostasis).
■ Grade III: Too much should not be done (packing only).
■ Grade IV: Only God can do something (heroic measures).

The following are some practical management principles:

- Bleeding from small, superficial capsular tears can be controlled by cautery, individual vessel ligation or clipping, or by atraumatic suture-repair of the fragile hepatic capsule.
- More severe bleeding from a deep or craggy hepatic laceration constitutes a surgical challenge requiring a stepwise approach. After a quick glance, bimanual compression of the hepatic parenchyma will control the bleeding temporarily, allowing the anesthesiologist to catch up with the blood loss. **This must be followed by rapid mobilization of the liver by division of the falciform, left and right triangular ligaments — the liver can be literally dislocated into the abdominal incision**. Additional exposure via a median sternotomy or right thoracotomy is rarely indicated. The *Pringle maneuver* (inflow occlusion of the undissected triad of the portal vein, hepatic artery and common bile duct) is sometimes useful and safe for up to 60 minutes. Deep parenchymal bleeding is controlled as well as possible by clipping visible bleeding vessels and by *conservative resectional debridement*. This rarely controls the hemorrhage completely — **supplementary packing is necessary**. Packs must be judiciously placed around (not into) the liver. The aim is to close the laceration by tight packing and thereby tamponade the bleeding. Excessive packing

must be avoided because it can result in inferior vena cava compression or abdominal compartment syndrome with aggravation of the hypotension. **And always leave the abdomen open after packing**. A return to the OR will be necessary in 36-72 hours for pack removal. **There is always a danger of losing sight of time and the amount of blood loss that is incurred while trying to achieve an elusive 'perfect' result. More bleeding will require more transfusions and aggravate the coagulopathy in a well-known vicious cycle. We strongly advise you to look at the clock before you tackle a nasty liver laceration: you should achieve both vessel control and packing, ideally within 45 minutes**.

- **Retrohepatic caval injuries** are characterized by exsanguinating hemorrhage despite inflow occlusion. **There are probably more techniques described for immediate hemostasis than there are survivors**. It is perhaps best to resort to damage control with packing and come back to fight another day. However, the presence of an experienced hepatic-biliary surgeon may change the approach — and the fate of the patient.
- Injuries to the **porta hepatis** require a wide *Kocher maneuver* for exposure. The injured portal vein should be repaired, or ligated as a last resort. Hepatic artery ligation is better tolerated than portal vein ligation. Suture-repair or Roux-en-Y biliary enteric anastomoses are the treatment options for an injured common bile duct; the latter can be performed either at the initial operation or at the reconstruction phase of a damage control strategy. Unilateral lobar bile duct injuries should be managed initially by ligation (or drainage); biliary-enteric reconstruction can be undertaken at a later stage.
- An injured gallbladder should be resected.

Spleen

The treatment at laparotomy of an actively bleeding spleen in the adult is splenectomy. **Again: acrobatic surgical splenic conservation procedures belong to expensive surgical textbooks; they have no place in the OR**. The risk of post-splenectomy sepsis is small and can be further reduced by vaccination, vigilance and appropriate prophylaxis, as discussed in the previous section.

Pancreas

The state of the main pancreatic duct and the site of the presumed injury (proximal versus distal) are crucial determinants of the operative

strategy in the injured pancreas. In blunt trauma, fracture of the pancreatic parenchyma opposite the vertebral column is typically seen on the pre-operative CT scan. It usually involves disruption of the main duct. **Confirmation in the stable patient may require endoscopic (ERCP) or magnetic resonance cholangiopancreatography (MRCP) if these investigations can be carried out immediately.**

The question of duct integrity is often posed during the trauma laparotomy. The anterior aspect of the pancreas is exposed through the lesser sac by division of the gastrocolic omentum; the posterior aspect of the head is exposed by a Kocher maneuver, while the posterior aspect of the tail is achieved by splenic mobilization. Intra-operative pancreatography (through a duodenotomy and cannulation of the ampulla of Vater) is described, **but it is rarely performed in practice.** In superficial pancreatic wounds, the main duct may be presumed to be intact and drainage alone is sufficient. In deeper parenchymal wounds of the body or tail, ductal transection is likely and a distal pancreatectomy (with splenectomy) is warranted. For deeper injuries of the head, wide drainage is indicated; the management of the inevitable pancreatic fistula in a stable patient is simpler than treating a leaking anastomosis after Roux-en-Y pancreaticojejunostomy. **The Whipple procedure is reserved for massive injuries of the pancreatic head, with biliary ductal and duodenal**

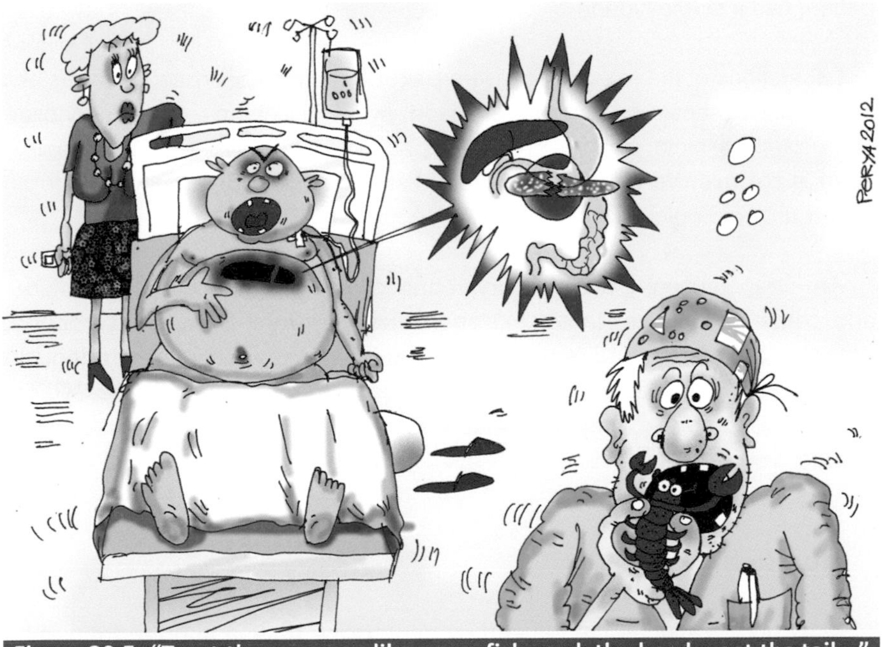

Figure 30.5. "Treat the pancreas like a crayfish, suck the head... eat the tail..."

disruption. This procedure is attended by a high mortality; it should be preferably 'staged', with the definitive reconstruction performed only after the patient has been stabilized.

The following aphorism captures very graphically the management of this injury (see ■ Figure 30.5):

> ***For pancreatic trauma, treat the pancreas like a crawfish: suck the head, eat the tail.***
>
> **Timothy Fabian**

Kidney, ureter and bladder (see also ➲ Chapter 35)

The intra-operative discovery of a perinephric hematoma is usually indicative of renal injury. A large proportion of these are self-limiting. **Renal exploration is indicated in the presence of an expanding or pulsatile hematoma, or when a hilar injury is suspected**. Moderate severity injuries can be controlled usually by cortical renorrhaphy and drainage; occasionally, a polar nephrectomy may be indicated. A shattered kidney or a vascular hilar injury are treated by nephrectomy; **preliminary control of the renal artery and vein should not be attempted in the presence of hemodynamic instability**. Attempts at saving a kidney, in these situations, are not warranted, unless the patient has a single kidney.

Lacerations of the renal pelvis are repaired with fine absorbable sutures. An injured ureter should be carefully exposed, avoiding ischemic damage by over-enthusiastic skeletonization. Primary repair with absorbable material over a stent is the rule. Very proximal or very distal ureteric injuries may require an expert urologic opinion.

An intraperitoneal bladder injury requires repair with absorbable sutures and catheter drainage. **In an extraperitoneal rupture from blunt trauma, catheter drainage alone is sufficient**. A urethral Foley catheter is adequate in most cases. In severe, complex bladder injuries or significant bleeding, suprapubic drainage may be added to allow for efficient, postoperative bladder irrigation.

Stomach

Most gastric injuries are caused by penetrating trauma and are treated by simple, one-layer suture-repair. **The posterior gastric wall should always be checked by opening the lesser sac**. In penetrating trauma of the upper abdomen, a bloody nasogastric tube aspirate is often indicative of a gastric injury: search for it diligently and remember that some areas of the stomach are difficult to assess: the gastroesophageal junction, the fundus and the uppermost parts of the lesser curve and posterior wall. Blunt injuries are rare (unless the patient is kicked in the bar on his full stomach) and gastric resection is required only in exceptional cases.

Duodenum

Intramural duodenal hematomas do not require evacuation; nasogastric decompression, fluid replacement and adequate nutrition (usually parenteral) need to be instituted for up to 3-4 weeks.

Small, clean-cut lacerations can be safely repaired primarily. Extensive lacerations, the presence of significant tissue contusion (usually inflicted by blunt trauma), the involvement of the common bile duct or high-velocity gunshot injuries should be treated by **duodenal repair and pyloric exclusion**. This procedure consists of closure of the pylorus (by stapling or suture from inside the stomach) and re-establishment of gastrointestinal continuity by a gastrojejunostomy; the addition of a truncal vagotomy is not warranted. A feeding jejunostomy is a useful adjunct for the provision of enteral feeding.

However, there is currently a feeling that this procedure (i.e. 'exclusion') is overused. Instead, we often prefer primary repair supplemented by tube duodenostomy. A Foley catheter is inserted through the corner of the duodenal suture line and suction drainage to pick up the leakage around the repair is provided. The aim is to decompress the duodenal lumen through a controlled fistula. We do not advise a duodenostomy through an intact duodenal wall.

Small bowel

Most lacerations can be treated with one-layer suture-repair. Occasionally a segmental resection may be required in injuries involving the mesenteric side of the intestine or for the treatment of multiple lacerations in close proximity. **Neglected, longstanding lacerations (more than 24 hours) with an established peritonitis may require the fashioning of a temporary stoma rather than primary repair**. Rarely, an extensive mesenteric laceration may endanger a very large segment of bowel which, if resected, would result in a short-gut syndrome; at least 100cm of small bowel in the absence of the ileocecal valve (or 75cm with preservation of the ileocecal junction) are deemed necessary for adequate enteral nutrition.

Colon

Right- or left-sided simple colonic lacerations can be safely treated by suture-repair in most cases. If the severity of the laceration warrants a resection, an ileocolic anastomosis (after a right hemicolectomy) is usually safe. A colocolic anastomosis (after a more distal resection) may not be as safe. **In any case, a colostomy rather than repair is recommended in the presence of massive peritoneal contamination, severe associated injuries or gross hemodynamic instability.** In borderline cases, we advise you to err on the side of performing a colostomy; the stubborn resort to primary repair may turn out to be a costly act of surgical bravado: **more trauma patients die from a leaking primary anastomosis than from a subsequent closure of a colostomy gone wrong.** Large mesocolic hematomas are best treated by segmental colectomy. Extensive deserosalization (typical in seat-belt injuries of the cecum or sigmoid colon) should be treated by serosal repair rather than resection.

Rectum

In the absence of gross fecal contamination, minor lacerations can be treated by simple suture-repair. **In all other cases, a proximal diverting colostomy must be added**; a loop sigmoid colostomy is usually adequate. Small lacerations of the extraperitoneal rectal segment require neither extensive mobilization of the rectum nor suture-repair; a diverting colostomy alone is sufficient. **Wash-out of the distal rectal stump and presacral drainage are unnecessary except in very extensive injuries with wide dissection and soiling of the perirectal spaces.**

Intra-abdominal vascular injuries

- **Aorta.** A most important step in the management of aortic injuries is exposure in order to achieve proximal and distal control. Depending on the level, this 'medial visceral rotation' maneuver begins either lateral to the spleen or, lower down, by incising the white line of Toldt lateral to the left colon. The viscera, including the spleen, pancreatic tail, left colon and, if necessary, the left kidney are gradually mobilized medially. The suprarenal aorta can be approached through the gastrohepatic omentum (via the lesser sac) with retraction of the stomach and esophagus to the left. For injuries of the supraceliac aorta, a left thoracotomy may be required. Aortic injuries are repaired with 3-0 or 4-0 sutures of polypropylene monofilament.

- **Infrahepatic vena cava**. The exposure is achieved by incision of the white line of Toldt lateral to the right colon with medial reflection of the right colon, duodenum and, if necessary, the right kidney. The bleeding site must be occluded by direct finger or sponge-stick pressure; vascular clamps may be used but no attempt should be made to encircle the vessel. Venorrhaphy can be achieved with 4-0 or 5-0 monofilament vascular sutures. The presence of a posterior laceration should be checked for: if present, it can be repaired by gentle rotation of the vena cava or from inside the lumen. In massive disruptions, a synthetic graft may be used, but more commonly the inferior vena cava is ligated. **Ligation above the renal veins is not well tolerated**.
- **Common or external iliac artery**. Suture-repair or, if necessary, use a graft. A synthetic graft may be used even in the presence of peritoneal soiling. In this case polytetrafluoroethylene (PTFE) is the preferred material. If gross contamination is present, consideration should be given to arterial ligation and restoration of the circulation by means of an extra-anatomical femorofemoral bypass. The internal iliac artery may be ligated with impunity.
- The exposure of the **iliac veins** is notoriously difficult and may require the division of the ipsilateral internal iliac artery or even a temporary transection of the common iliac artery. Iliac veins may be ligated with acceptable morbidity; compression stockings and limb elevation are indicated postoperatively.
- The **celiac artery** and the **inferior mesenteric artery (IMA)** may be ligated. In desperate situations, to control life-threatening bleeding, the proximal (retropancreatic) superior mesenteric artery (SMA) can be ligated as well (with preservation of blood flow through collaterals); but in general, repair or shunting is the preferred strategy.
- **The infrapancreatic portion of the SMA should be repaired**. The **superior mesenteric vein** should be repaired if possible, since its ligation may cause bowel infarction, severe postoperative intestinal congestion and intestinal varices. The **inferior mesenteric vein** may be ligated without risk.
- Heroic attempts at restoring flow by repairing a vessel in a patient *in extremis* are to be avoided. At times, ligation with later revascularization may be possible. A better approach is a temporary shunt across the injury with definitive grafting over the subsequent 24 hours.

Retroperitoneal hematomas

The main issue is whether to explore such a hematoma discovered in the course of a trauma laparotomy.

As a general rule, all retroperitoneal hematomas in **penetrating trauma** should be explored, irrespective of size or location. In **blunt trauma** a more selective policy can be applied depending mainly on the location of the hematoma — as follows.

- **A central abdominal location** (Zone I) including the main abdominal vessels and the duodenopancreatic complex always warrants exploration.
- **Lateral hematomas** (Zone II) including the kidneys and retroperitoneal colonic wall can be left alone unless they are very large, pulsating or expanding.
- **Blunt (unlike penetrating) traumatic pelvic hematomas** (Zone III) should not be explored. Breaching the intact retroperitoneum may result in a loss of the tamponade effect with catastrophic intraperitoneal hemorrhage (see ■ Table 30.2).

Table 30.2. Approach to traumatic retroperitoneal hematoma.

Type of hematoma	Penetrating injury	Blunt injury
Central (Zone I)	Explore	Explore
Lateral (Zone II)	Usually explore	Usually do not explore
Pelvic (Zone III)	Explore	Do not explore

Management of blunt traumatic pelvic hematomas

With the exception of isolated fractures of the iliac crest, fractures involving the pelvic or obturator rings and/or sacrum have the potential for significant bleeding leading to shock and death. The pelvis is always imaged in severe blunt trauma, either by CT scanning (in stable patients) or by a simple anteroposterior radiograph (in unstable patients). Bleeding from a pelvic fracture arises from disrupted pelvic veins, from lacerated branches of the internal iliac arteries and from cancellous bone, in various combinations.

In an unstable patient with a significant pelvic fracture who does not respond or responds partially to resuscitation, one must assume that the source of bleeding is pelvic in origin, once an extra-abdominal source of hemorrhage has been ruled out. **The first step is then to minimize the pelvic blood loss by increasing the tamponade effect of the pelvic retroperitoneum: this is best achieved by the application of a specially designed pelvic sling or binder (every emergency department should have one); otherwise a sheet should be tightly wrapped around the iliac crests, criss-crossed anteriorly and tied down**.

This temporary stabilization of the pelvic bony fragments may result in hemodynamic improvement; if this succeeds, an abdominal CT scan may be obtained and will enable one to differentiate definitively between abdominal visceral bleeding and pelvic bleeding. The former warrants an emergency laparotomy. **If the latter is present alone, a laparotomy should be avoided because it may increase the bleeding by loss of the tamponade effect. In that scenario, transfer of the patient to the angiography suite for attempts at angioembolization of pelvic arterial bleeding is the best strategy; throughout the procedure, resuscitation must be pursued by the trauma team (the radiology staff, while excellent at what they do, have difficulty in spelling the word 'resuscitation' — if any radiologist is reading this we are just joking of course!)**. If angiography facilities are not available, the application of an external pelvic fixator by the orthopedic team may be beneficial (it works best when the bleeding arises from a venous or bony source but may fail to make a difference in arterial bleeding).

A grossly unstable patient, unresponsive to resuscitation, is fit only for transfer to the OR. In order to control pelvic bleeding, a low vertical midline incision can be used to both evacuate the pelvic hematoma (which has displaced the intraperitoneal viscera upwards) and **pack this extraperitoneal space**. If access is required for a concomitant intraperitoneal hemorrhage from another source, it is advisable to enter the abdominal cavity through a transverse incision higher up. Mortality remains extremely high in that scenario. (In some trauma centers preperitoneal packing takes precedence, and is performed in the ER/trauma room.)

The abbreviated trauma laparotomy (damage control)

When physiology is severely compromised, attempts at restoring anatomy are counterproductive.

In a small minority of patients, time-consuming organ repair cannot be undertaken safely when the physiological status is critically impaired. A bailout procedure consisting of the temporary control of bleeding and contamination is the only viable option. **These cases can be recognized either by a set of physiological criteria or by an anatomical pattern of injuries**. In the former model, the presence of coagulopathy, hypothermia and acidosis are indicators of impending physiological exhaustion. Each one of these amplifies the other two in a vicious cycle that is aptly referred to as the 'triad of death'. In that scenario, a dogged determination to spend the time it takes to achieve definitive organ repair may result in the patient's demise. If the latter model is applied, the surgeon takes the decision for a bailout procedure by a flash assessment of the injury pattern. For example, an injury to a major intra-abdominal vessel associated with a severe duodenopancreatic disruption is recognized immediately as a potential for massive blood loss should a prolonged, definitive, reconstructive procedure be undertaken. **In these circumstances, there is only a place for a combination of packing, vessel shunting, tube drainage and the simplest means of preventing peritoneal contamination** (by stapling or tying off injured intestine with tapes). Abdominal closure consists of expeditious cutaneous approximation or is better avoided altogether — preventing the commonly associated abdominal compartment syndrome (➲ Chapter 31). The patient is then treated in the surgical intensive care unit where secondary stabilization is conducted over the next 24-48 hours. Delayed definitive organ repair (or resection) and abdominal closure are undertaken only in a patient who is hemodynamically more stable, rewarmed and who has an improved clotting profile.

To sum up...

Injured organs must be surgically repaired or resected as soon as possible. This being said, the surgeon should be able to recognize the potential for spontaneous healing of even severe visceral injuries (as in some cases of blunt trauma). **Furthermore, he should know to temper his enthusiasm for immediately restoring the anatomy in the face of severely impaired physiology**.

Oops: we almost forgot to mention another form of human-induced trauma — that of hanging. So here is some important advice:

"In a case of hanging: cut the rope holding the victim and immediately loosen it from around the neck, unless the body is perfectly stiff — rigor mortis."

American Red Cross First Aid Text-Book, 1933

Chapter 31

The abdominal compartment syndrome

Ari Leppäniemi and Rifat Latifi

Abdominal compartment syndrome is a whole body disease.
Thomas Scalea

Abdominal compartment syndrome (ACS) is more common than we think. **It comprises a conglomerate of symptoms and signs that follow an increase in intra-abdominal pressure (IAP), causing intra-abdominal hypertension (IAH), due to trauma or any other major catastrophe. Irrespective of the cause, treatment consists of decompression and dealing with the source.**

ACS can be primary, secondary or recurrent:

- **Primary IAH or ACS**: caused by a condition developing within the abdomen and pelvis. Think about abdominal trauma, pelvic fracture, ruptured abdominal aortic aneurysm, or any other abdominal catastrophe causing an acute increase in intra-abdominal volume.
- **Secondary IAH or ACS**: where the primary cause of IAH is outside the abdomen or pelvis. For example, massive fluid resuscitation for trauma, sepsis or burns causing swelling of the viscera. **Of course, secondary IAH can develop simultaneously with primary IAH** — think about the swollen gut you find during laparotomy for, say, a ruptured spleen (after more than a few liters of lactated Ringer's given during transportation…).
- **Recurrent IAH or ACS**: developing following previous surgical or medical treatment of primary or secondary IAH or ACS. Usually the initial cause has not been adequately eradicated. **Even patients**

having some form of temporary abdominal closure (TAC) can have recurrent ACS!

Although not as rigid as the intracranial, intracervical, intrathoracic or extremity fascial spaces, **the abdominal cavity is a contained space with clear boundaries**. This relative lack of rigidity is why some of us are fat or become pregnant and still do not develop ACS. As in all confined spaces with rigid or semi-rigid boundaries, any attempt to increase the volume contained in such a space, particularly acutely, will lead to a rise in intracavity pressure. Such acute increases in pressure are never healthy for the physiology!

There are many causes of increased intra-abdominal 'volume' and the progression from normal pressure to IAH and then to ACS depends on the cause and the acuity of such an increase. But let's first look at some of the definitions:

- **IAP — intra-abdominal pressure** is the steady-state pressure within the abdominal cavity, expressed in mmHg and is normally 0-5mmHg. If you sneeze or try to defecate, or if your anesthesiologist wakes your patient violently (so you can watch for wound dehiscence starting right at the end of the case...), it may temporarily be much higher — but don't worry, that is not ACS...
- **IAH — intra-abdominal hypertension** is a sustained or repeated pathological elevation of the IAP >12mmHg.
- **ACS — abdominal compartment syndrome is defined as sustained IAP >20mmHg that is associated with new organ dysfunction or failure**.
- **APP — abdominal perfusion pressure** is the mean arterial pressure (MAP) minus IAP. In sick patients in the ICU try to keep APP above 60mmHg!

(For those of you who still use cmH_2O (you shouldn't), remember that 1mmHg = $1.36cmH_2O$.)

<u>Remember</u>: IAH — whatever the IAP — is not ACS unless the patient also has the typical manifestations of the syndrome:

- Increased airway pressure (respiratory distress, difficult ventilating).
- Decreased cardiac output (hypotension despite adequate volume status).
- Decreased or abrupt cessation of urinary output (renal dysfunction despite optimal hydration)
- Increasing abdominal distension.

■ Table 31.1. shows the grading of ACS.

Table 31.1. Grading of intra-abdominal hypertension (IAH).

- ■ **Grade I:** IAP 12-15mmHg.
- ■ **Grade II:** IAP 16-20mmHg.
- ■ **Grade III:** IAP 21-25mmHg.
- ■ **Grade IV:** IAP >25mmHg.

So, while IAH refers to a continuous variable (like arterial hypertension), ACS is like pregnancy, either you are or you are not pregnant!

Risk factors for IAH and ACS

There are many conditions that can lead to IAH, for example, abdominal trauma — especially with over-resuscitation with crystalloids. Remember how our patients in the 80s and 90s looked like a Michelin man — requiring opening of the abdomen in the SICU and then keeping it open? Other examples: severe acute pancreatitis or ruptured abdominal aortic aneurysm (even patients who have undergone endovascular repair can develop ACS).

In order to better characterize the risk factors it is useful to group them according to the main pathophysiological problem. Some of the people who put this list together are intensivists, so have some patience, and be nice to them...

- **Increased intra-abdominal contents**: hemoperitoneum or pneumoperitoneum or intraperitoneal fluid collections or abscesses, liver dysfunction with tense ascites, peritoneal dialysis, intraperitoneal or retroperitoneal tumors, acute pancreatitis, laparoscopy with excessive insufflation pressures, packing during damage control surgery. Note that even normal pregnancy causes sustained IAH!
- **Increased intraluminal contents**: gastric dilatation, ileus, colonic pseudo-obstruction (■ Figure 31.1), volvulus.
- **Diminished abdominal wall compliance**: major burn to the abdominal wall, abdominal wall edema due to massive resuscitation, prone position.

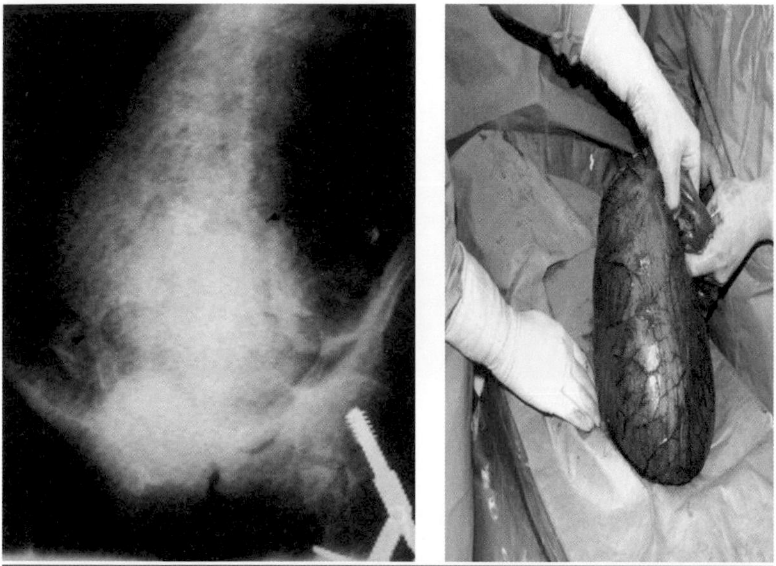

Figure 31.1. Abdominal X-ray showing a massively dilated rectosigmoid — causing IAH and ACS — and the corresponding findings at operation.

- **Capillary leak/fluid resuscitation**: acidosis, damage control laparotomy, hypothermia, massive fluid resuscitation, polytransfusion.
- **Others**: coagulopathy, bacteremia, age, massive ventral hernia repair, obesity or increased body mass index, peritonitis, pneumonia, sepsis, shock or hypotension, mechanical ventilation, positive end-expiratory pressure (PEEP) >15-20mmHg.

As you can see from the list above, almost all of your patients — including those who did not undergo any abdominal operation — or even those who do not suffer from any intra-abdominal pathology (particularly burns) — can develop IAH! So, for example, if your patient is morbidly obese with a huge omentum nestling within the abdomen, this means that the patient suffers from a chronic IAH and is susceptible to ACS.

Pathophysiology of IAH and ACS

Almost all organ systems are affected by IAH: some more than others. The most easily detected signs are renal and respiratory dysfunction but do not overlook the effects on the cardiovascular and gastrointestinal systems, or on intracranial pressure (■ Figure 31.2).

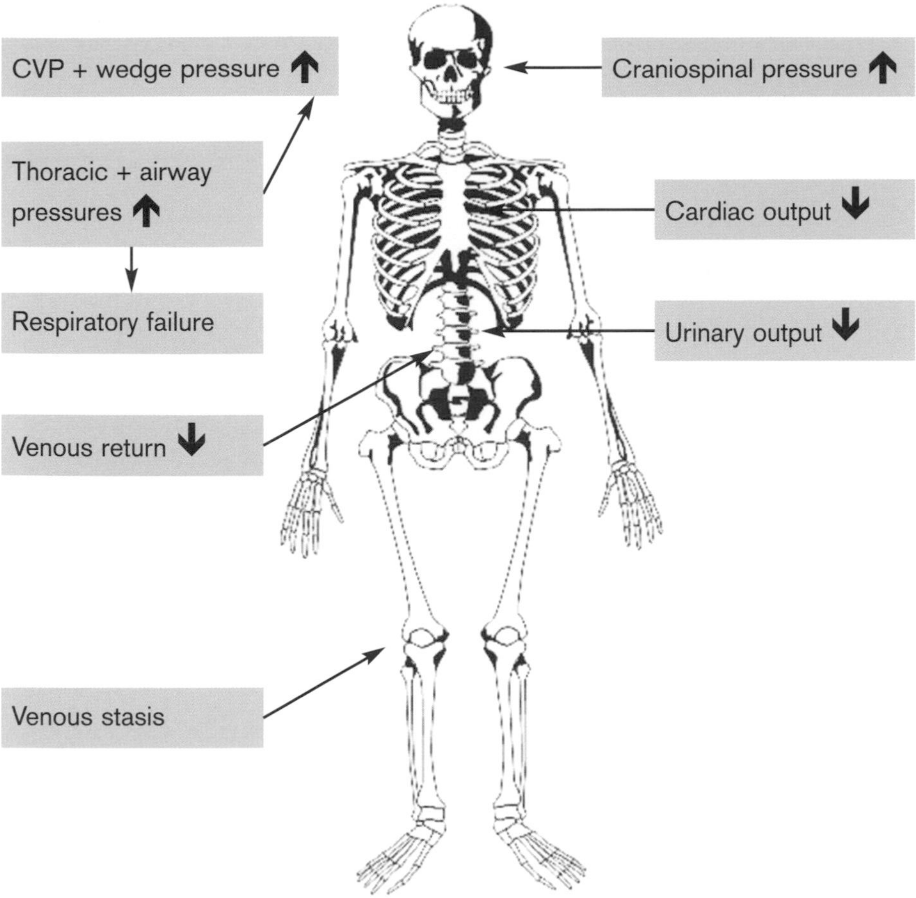

Figure 31.2. The abdominal compartment syndrome.

■ Table 31.2 summarizes the physiological consequences of IAH. For those of you who are not intensivists, here is a list of the consequences of IAH that surgeons understand:

- Increased <u>airway</u> pressure.
- Decreased <u>cardiac</u> output.
- Decreased <u>urinary</u> output.
- Decreased <u>intestinal</u> blood flow.
- Increased <u>intracerebral</u> pressure.
- Decreased blood flow to the <u>abdominal wall</u>.

Table 31.2. Physiological consequences of intra-abdominal hypertension.

	Increased	Decreased	No change
Mean blood pressure	✓	✓	✓
Heart rate	✓	-	-
Peak airway pressure	✓	-	-
Thoracic/pleural pressure	✓	-	-
Central venous pressure	✓	-	-
Pulmonary capillary wedge pressure	✓	-	-
Inferior vena cava pressure	✓	-	-
Renal vein pressure	✓	-	-
Systemic vascular resistance	✓	-	-
Cardiac output	-	✓	-
Venous return	-	✓	-
Visceral blood flow	-	✓	-
Gastric mucosal pH	-	✓	-
Renal blood flow	-	✓	-
Glomerular filtration rate	-	✓	-
Cerebrospinal fluid pressure	✓	-	-
Abdominal wall compliance	-	✓	-

These abnormalities are often present despite apparently normal cardiac filling pressures because transmission of increased IAP to the thorax elevates central venous pressure (CVP), right atrial pressure and pulmonary capillary wedge pressure.

Cardiovascular, respiratory and renal functions deteriorate and become progressively more difficult to manage unless IAP is reduced dramatically. Rarer consequences of ACS have been described, such as intestinal ischemia following laparoscopic cholecystectomy or spinal cord infarction in the setting of IAH following perforation of a gastric ulcer.

It is easy to understand why the effects of IAH are not limited to the abdominal cavity but also affect the chest cavity and even the intracranial space. **When two or more anatomical compartments have elevated compartmental pressures, it is called a polycompartment syndrome.** These are more common in polytrauma and you can miss them easily unless you re-examine the patient continuously.

When to suspect IAH?

Seeing a patient with a massively distended abdomen might be a hint (■ Figure 31.3) but realizing that physical examination (palpation) is highly inaccurate in determining IAP, we stopped using that as a criterion, especially since measuring IAP is so simple that even surgeons can do it. **So, all you need to do is to suspect and measure IAP, especially when the patient has**:

- A tense, distended abdomen (ask the patient or family — is this distension a baseline?).
- Acute respiratory failure or deterioration of ventilator settings.
- Diminished cardiac output as measured by low blood pressure and/or oliguria non-responsive to conventional management.
- Acidosis.

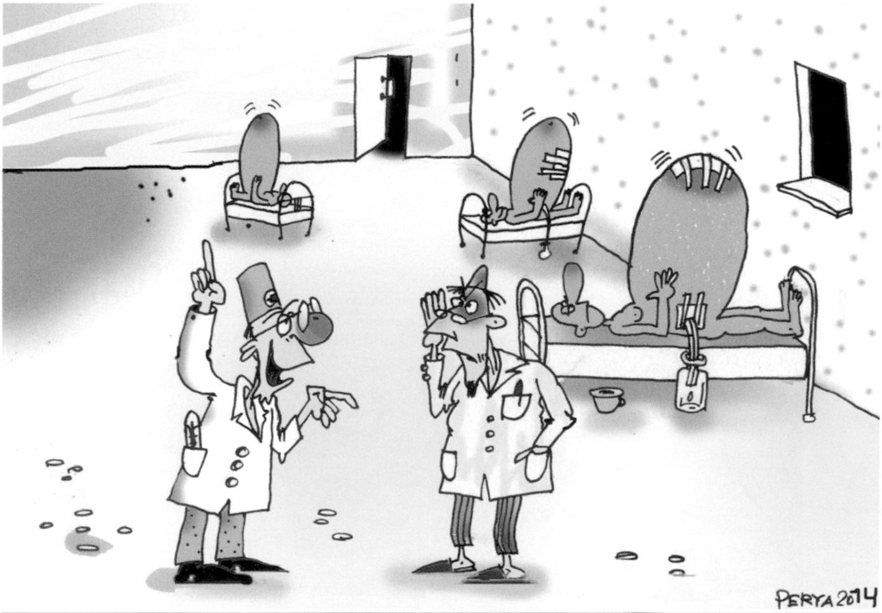

Figure 31.3. "What? Abdominal compartment syndrome? Never heard of it!"

Diagnosis of IAH

If you don't take a temperature, you can't find a fever.
So, if you do not think of ACS you will miss it.

Why guess? Just measure the IAP! You don't need fancy equipment, just a Foley catheter and a tube system that costs a few dollars (■ Figure 31.4). However, you need to be aware of the principles of IAP measurement as stated by the 2013 consensus definition of the World Society of the Abdominal Compartment Syndrome:

2013 consensus definition of the World Society of the Abdominal Compartment Syndrome: "The reference standard for intermittent IAP measurements is via the urinary bladder with a maximal instillation volume of 25ml of sterile saline. IAP should be expressed in mmHg and measured at end-expiration in the supine position after ensuring that abdominal muscle contractions are absent and with the transducer zeroed at the level of the mid-axillary line." (Mark the mid-axillary line in the pelvic area with a pen so that you use the same zero-level next time you measure the pressure.)

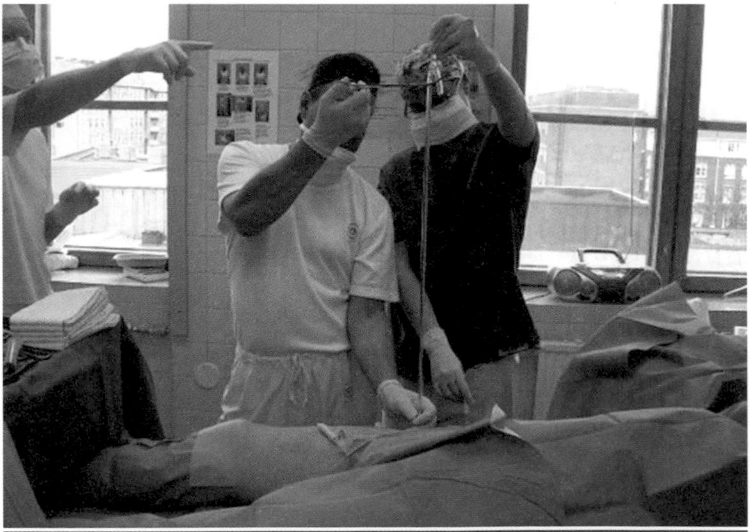

Figure 31.4. Ari measuring IAP.

So basically, **all you need to measure IAP is to have the patient quiet, and a Foley catheter**: disconnect it from the urine bag; instill 25ml saline into the bladder and elevate the disconnected catheter perpendicular to the supine patient and his bed. If you don't have a transducer in your allegedly 'cutting edge' institution — the height of the water-urine column in the catheter is the IAP in cmH_2O (1cm H_2O=0.735mmHg). The level will fluctuate with the patient's respiratory cycle — up during inspiration, down during expiration — following the movements of the diaphragm. **A neurogenic or small contracted bladder, or after bladder surgery for bladder rupture, may render the measurements invalid**. Errors can also occur if the catheter is blocked or if a pelvic hematoma selectively compresses the bladder. (In the case of a suprapubic catheter and a transurethral Foley, make sure you close the suprapubic one when you measure the pressure.) Because the Trendelenburg position (or its reverse) may affect intra-bladder pressure, accurate measurements are best achieved in the supine position. **The trend of the IAP, measured periodically, is sometimes more important than an isolated measurement**.

How common is IAH?

Very common. We can still remember the time when patients with severe acute pancreatitis developed 'early' multiple organ failure and then just died in spite of 'adequate' fluid resuscitation. **Some of them probably had unrecognized and untreated ACS**. Some 20 years ago, when we started routinely measuring the IAP of all pancreatitis patients in the ICU in Helsinki, we found that about 40% of them had IAH and about 10% developed ACS. **Of course, since that time we have learned; we now know to avoid excessive fluid resuscitation leading to IAH!**

In a general ICU with mixed medical and surgical patients, the incidence of IAH used to be about 50% and ACS about 10%. **However, with increasing awareness, and better prevention and treatment of IAH, the incidence of full-blown ACS has decreased dramatically**. **Leaving the abdomen open after damage control surgery for trauma or other surgical emergencies (see below) has also had a major effect in reducing this, mostly iatrogenic, disease.**

Prevention

It is always better to prevent than treat and here are some simple rules for surgeons on how to avoid ACS.

Consider leaving the abdomen open:

- After any damage control surgery — not only after trauma.
- If massive visceral edema is present.
- After prolonged operations — usually for abdominal catastrophes.
- If massive resuscitation with crystalloids (less with blood transfusion) has been given.

Decrease the risk of ACS by avoiding:

- **Massive crystalloid resuscitation**. By now you should understand that over-resuscitation is a common producer of IAH and ACS. It is very easy to 'overlook' liters of fluid being infused in your patient...
- **Too tight abdominal closure**.

Consider avoiding closing the abdomen by using temporary abdominal closure (TAC), or closing the skin only, in high-risk situations as described in ➲ **Chapters 37 and 44**.

Treatment

Non-operative management

Unless the patient seems to be dying on you, try non-operative management first. **The aim is to reduce the intra-abdominal volume and improve abdominal wall compliance**. Inserting nasogastric and rectal tubes, temporarily stopping enteral nutrition, using gastro- and colo-prokinetic agents and performing colonoscopic decompression will reduce the volume of gastrointestinal content and consequently IAP. Utilizing percutaneous drainage of ascites or large localized fluid collections is also helpful, at least temporarily.

What often happens is this: a sick patient with elevated IAP, and not in need of immediate surgery, is transferred to the ICU. After adequate sedation, pain management and optimization of haemodynamics, IAP decreases significantly. In addition, avoiding the prone position, not elevating the head of the bed above 30°, and removing constricting bandages (check that the abdominal/pelvic binder is not applied too tight and it is not kept on for long!) improves abdominal compliance and decreases IAP.

Using **neuromuscular blockade** is controversial but we use it occasionally for short periods. **More significant results can be achieved by aiming for a negative fluid balance by increasing diuresis**. The last resort (before surgery) is hemodialysis-ultrafiltration to remove excess fluids and thus alleviate tissue swelling.

Surgical management

In true ACS, if medical management fails, surgery usually doesn't (unless the patient is already too sick to survive). Obviously, a patient with full-blown, life-threatening ACS needs surgical decompression — even in the ICU in the most urgent cases. This will be the most satisfactory laparotomy you have ever done...

The dramatic improvements in ventilation and urine output are instantaneous and will convince even the most hardline skeptic that ACS is for real (we've seen this 'conversion' many times).

However, again, the decision to decompress the abdomen should not be taken based on isolated measurements of IAP without taking into account the whole clinical picture.

A good guideline is the abdominal perfusion pressure (remember APP = MAP – IAP). If APP is >60mmHg, and there are no signs of significant organ dysfunction (check urine output, lactate, liver function, cardiovascular and respiratory parameters), it is usually safe to continue with non-operative management.

To prevent hemodynamic decompensation during the decompressive laparotomy, intravascular volume should be restored, oxygen delivery maximized, and hypothermia and coagulation defects corrected. Following decompression, the abdominal skin and fascial edges are left open using one of the temporary abdominal closure (TAC) methods described in ➲ Chapter 44.

Technique of surgical decompression

A full-length (OK, leave a couple of centimeters of fascia on both ends to facilitate later closure) midline abdominal incision is the standard

approach for abdominal decompression. There are other techniques such as a transverse bilateral subcostal incision (sometimes used in patients with severe pancreatitis who might need necrosectomy later) or less aggressive methods such as the subcutaneous linea alba fasciotomy that leaves the skin (except three short transverse skin incisions to do the fasciotomy) and peritoneum intact.

The '**non-invasive fasciotomy**' can be used for borderline cases; it avoids the morbidity of an open abdomen and can easily be extended to a full-thickness laparostomy if necessary. The downside is the unavoidable hernia that can be fixed later on with the component separation technique.

So...

IAH is yet another factor to consider in the overall management of the emergency abdominal surgery patient. It may be obvious — 'crying' for abdominal decompression. More commonly, however, it is relatively silent but contributing to your patient's acute illness, organ dysfunction and death. Be as aware of intra-abdominal hypertension as you are of arterial hypertension. It is much more common and clinically relevant than you have suspected hitherto.

"At the end of an emergency laparotomy don't ask only 'how should I close the abdomen?' Ask also 'should I close it?'"

Chapter 32

Abdominal aortic emergencies

Paul N. Rogers

Abdominal/back pain and hypotension = a ruptured AAA, unless proven otherwise.

Urological and orthopedic wards are a cemetery for ruptured AAA cases.

The editors wondered if there was still a need to include this chapter in the fifth edition. In many places vascular surgery has completely separated from general surgery and furthermore has become "vascular and endovascular surgery", a distinct and not entirely *surgical* specialty. We decided, however, to continue for two reasons: specialist vascular services are not available all over the world; and, even in those places with a vascular service, abdominal aortic emergencies often present to the workhorse general surgeon. So here we go again...

Ruptured abdominal aortic aneurysm: presentation

It is usually easy to make the diagnosis of a leaking abdominal aortic aneurysm (AAA). **Typically the patient presents with a sudden onset of acute lumbar backache, abdominal pain and collapse associated with hypotension. On examination the presence of a pulsatile abdominal mass confirms the diagnosis**. In this situation the patient proceeds directly to the operating room with a delay only to allow cross-matched blood to become available, if the patient is stable.

Ruptured abdominal aortic aneurysm: atypical presentation

Not infrequently, however, the diagnosis can be problematic. There may be no history of collapse and the patient may be normotensive on admission. **The only clue may be non-specific back or abdominal pain. A pulsatile mass may not be palpable**. Ruptured AAA patients are frequently obese; thinner patients tend to notice their AAA and present early for an elective repair.

A leaking AAA may be mislabeled as "ureteric colic" but the absence of microscopic hematuria should alert one to the possibility that a leaking aneurysm is responsible for the symptoms. Similarly we have seen patients present with acute scrotal pain, diagnosed as epididymo-orchitis and then cured by insertion of an aortic tube graft. **Always keep the diagnosis of a leaking AAA in your mind; otherwise you may overlook it**. In appropriate individuals, particularly men in late-middle and old age, if significant and unexplained abdominal or back pain causes the patient to present acutely, abdominal aneurysms should be excluded by means of ultrasound or CT.

The diagnostic dilemma: a known AAA but is it leaking?

A different diagnostic problem occurs in the patient who is known to have an aneurysm and who presents with abdominal or back pain, which may or may not be related to the aneurysm. The difficulty here is that a small, contained, 'herald' leak from an aneurysm might produce pain without any hemodynamic instability. Examination in these patients may be unhelpful in that the aneurysm may not be tender. **These patients are at high risk of a further bleed from the aneurysm and this could be sudden and catastrophic**. For this reason it is important that they are identified appropriately and have an operation before a major, possibly fatal, hemorrhage occurs. The difficulty of course is that such a patient might easily have another cause for the symptoms, mechanical backache for example, which is unrelated to the aneurysm. Here, an operation is clearly not in the patient's best interests, particularly if his or her general health is poor.

This dilemma, of operating without delay in patients who require it yet avoiding operation in those in whom it is not necessary, is a difficult one, sometimes even for experienced clinicians to resolve. An emergency CT scan (with i.v. contrast) is indicated in this situation to delineate the AAA and the presence of any associated leak — usually into the retroperitoneum. **In general, however, in this situation it is safer to err on the side of operating on too many rather than too few patients.**

Who should have an operation?

A useful rule of thumb is that the chances of survival in a patient with a ruptured AAA are directly proportional to the blood pressure on admission.

Profoundly shocked patients rarely survive; sure, they may make it through the operation but usually do not leave hospital by the front door. Consequently, it has been proposed that operating on shocked ruptured AAA patients is futile and a waste of resources.

Another view is that you should proceed with the operation unless the patient is clearly 'agonal' or known to suffer from an incurable disease. You may be able to save the occasional patient and gain additional experience, which may help you to save the next rupture patient. These issues of philosophy of care are for the individual surgeon to resolve with his God, his patients and their families. **It is always worth ensuring — this seems self-evident but is often overlooked — that the patient himself is really up for a big operation, even when the alternative is death.** More than 20 years ago a scoring system was proposed to help with this decision-making. The so-called Hardman criteria relate the presence of several easily determined variables to the likelihood of survival after surgery for a ruptured aneurysm.

The Hardman criteria [1] (■ Table 32.1)

Perhaps not surprisingly, since these criteria were published, other workers have demonstrated that it is possible to operate on patients with three

Table 32.1. The Hardman criteria [1].

- Age >76.
- History of unconsciousness.
- Hemoglobin <9.0g/dL.
- Creatinine >190μmol/L (2.1mg%).
- ECG evidence of ischemia.

Results from the original study showed that:

If three or more criteria are present the mortality is 100%

If two are present the mortality is 72%

If one, 37%

1 Hardman DT, Fisher CM, Patel MI, *et al.* Ruptured abdominal aortic aneurysms: who should be offered surgery? *J Vasc Surg* 1996; 23: 123-9.

Hardman criteria successfully (confirming the rule of "never say never"). The waters have been further muddied by reports from several series of endovascular repair showing that the peri-operative mortality for all categories of patients is lower than for open repair. Nevertheless, the criteria remain a useful adjunct to the decision-making process in these patients.

The operation

Resuscitation in ruptured AAA means only one thing: a clamp placed above at the neck of the aneurysm!

Once the diagnosis of aortic rupture has been established, or strongly suspected, the patient should be rushed to the operating theatre without delay. Do not even bother with additional lines and intravenous fluids as what you pour in will pour out, and increasing the blood pressure will only increase the bleeding. **Aim for stable hypotension in resuscitation — the so-called permissive hypotension.**

Preparation

'Prep and drape' (including both groins in case aortofemoral bypass is necessary) for surgery while the anesthetic team establishes the appropriate monitoring lines. Do not allow them, however, to waste time by inserting unnecessary gimmicks such as the pulmonary arterial catheter. Administer prophylactic antibiotics. **Anesthesia *should not* be induced until you are ready to make the skin incision**; not infrequently, the administration of muscle relaxants at induction, and the subsequent relaxation of the abdominal wall, is sufficient to permit a further bleed from the aneurysm with an immediate hemodynamic collapse. **Remember: your clamp on the aorta proximal to the aneurysm is more important than anything else.**

Incision

Open the abdomen through a long midline incision extending from the xiphisternum to a point mid way between the umbilicus and the symphysis pubis. Occasionally, if the distal iliac arteries are to be approached, the incision must be extended. In most cases, however, for the insertion of a simple aortic tube graft, an incision as described is adequate.

Proximal control

Upon entering the peritoneal cavity, the diagnosis is immediately confirmed by the presence of a large retroperitoneal hematoma. The first priority is to obtain control of the aorta proximal to the aneurysm. **In the majority of patients who are stable at this stage (with a contained retroperitoneal leak), there is time to approach the aorta above the aneurysm and just below the level of the renal arteries**. In patients who are unstable, rapid control of aortic bleeding may be obtained by approaching the aorta just under the diaphragm and temporarily applying a clamp there until the infrarenal aorta can be dissected.

Other approaches to unstable patients, or those who become unstable during dissection, include blunt compression of the proximal aorta by 'a swab on a stick' (gauze held in a Rampley forceps) and insertion of a large Foley catheter through the aortic defect if this is encountered during dissection of the AAA neck; balloon occlusion of the aorta may then allow you a few extra minutes to gain control:

- **Subdiaphragmatic aortic control: remember how you do truncal vagotomy?** Of course you don't! So pay attention. Incise the phrenoesophageal ligament overlying the esophagus (feel the nasogastric tube underneath). With your index finger bluntly mobilize the esophagus to the right; forget about hemostasis at this stage. Now feel the aorta pulsating to the left of the esophagus, dissect with your index finger on both sides of the aorta until you feel the spine. Apply a straight aortic clamp, pushing it 'onto' the spine. Leave a few packs to provide hemostasis and proceed as below. An alternative approach is to go through the lesser sac, elevate the stomach and apply a clamp on the aorta immediately above the pancreas.
- **Infrarenal aortic control**. Returning to the matter of isolation of the aortic neck, note that **the main principle to be observed is to avoid disturbing the retroperitoneal hematoma while gaining control of the proximal aorta**. Once you enter the retroperitoneum at the neck's level, dissect bluntly using your finger or the tip of the suction apparatus, to identify and isolate the neck of the aneurysm. Once the neck is identified carry on backwards on either side of the aorta until the vertebral bodies are reached. Do not attempt to encircle the aorta with a tape. **Apply a straight aortic clamp in an anteroposterior direction with the tips of the jaws of the clamp resting against the vertebral bodies**. Placement of this clamp is facilitated by placing the index and middle fingers of your non-dominant hand on either side of the aorta so that the vertebral bodies can be palpated. The jaws of the open clamp are then slid along the backs of the fingers until the clamp

lies in the appropriate position. During this maneuver an 'extra' length of aorta can often be isolated by retracting the aneurysm gently downwards with your hand. Now you can remove the subdiaphragmatic clamp. You want the kidneys and the bowel to be perfused, right?

- **Juxtarenal neck**. Occasionally the aneurysm extends close to the origin of the renal arteries. If this is the case then the neck of the aneurysm will be obscured by the left renal vein, which may be stretched anteriorly. Care must be taken that the vein is not damaged. It may be divided to facilitate access to the aneurysm neck. This is done by very gently mobilizing the vein from the underlying aorta. It should be ligated securely as close to the vena cava as prudence permits. If this is done then the vein may be ligated with impunity and the kidney will not be endangered, because collateral venous drainage will take place via the adrenal and gonadal anastomoses. **How do you know that effective proximal control has been achieved? Simple — the retroperitoneal hematoma stops pulsating. If it pulsates your clamp is not properly placed. Reapply it!**

Distal control

The next part of the dissection, to identify the common iliac arteries, is often more difficult. Under normal circumstances the pelvis is the site of accumulation of much of the retroperitoneal hematoma and the iliac arteries are buried within this. The arteries are difficult to locate not only because they are buried in hematoma but because with the aorta clamped proximally, there is no pulsation to guide the operator. **In most patients, however, the presence of atheroma in the vessels makes palpation in the depths of the hematoma possible**. Again, use of the suction apparatus facilitates isolation of the iliac vessels. Otherwise, dig with your fingers within the hematoma and 'fish' the iliacs out. **As with the aorta, no attempt should be made to encircle the iliac vessels with tapes. This invariably produces damage to the iliac veins, which is a disaster**. It is sufficient to clear the anterior and lateral aspects of the iliac vessels and apply clamps in an anteroposterior manner as before.

An alternative — balloon control

After proximal control has been achieved and when the iliacs are immersed within a huge hematoma you may also rapidly open the aneurysm sac and shove a Foley or large Fogarty catheter into each iliac artery, inflating the balloons to produce temporary distal control. Advance occlusion of the lumen of any catheter used in such a way is an obvious necessity.

Aortic replacement

Once the proximal and distal arterial tree is controlled, incise the aneurysm sac in a longitudinal fashion; stay slightly to the right of the midline to avoid the origin of the inferior mesenteric artery. Evacuate the clot and control back bleeding from any patent lumbar arteries and the inferior mesenteric artery with sutures within the aneurysm sac. This can be done in a controlled way firstly by packing the upper and lower ends of the lumen with gauze swabs and then tackling each part of the aneurysm in turn. **A small self-retaining retractor placed within the aneurysm sac to retract its cut edges facilitates this and the next few stages of the procedure; a hinged laminectomy retractor is best**.

The proportion of patients in whom aortic replacement with a simple tube graft can be achieved varies widely from surgeon to surgeon and center to center. **We believe that in the majority of patients insertion of a tube graft can be achieved quite satisfactorily**. The advantages of this are that limitation of dissection in the pelvis minimizes the risk of damage to the iliac veins and to the autonomic nerves in the pelvis. Furthermore, there seems little point in extending the length of what is already a difficult operation by inserting a bifurcation graft unnecessarily. **Obviously there are circumstances when a tube graft is not acceptable** — namely when the patient has occlusive aorto-iliac disease, when the iliac arteries are also significantly aneurysmal, or in some situations when the bifurcation is widely splayed so that the orifices of the common iliac arteries are far apart. In the latter two situations it may be possible to insert a bifurcated prosthesis and still remain inside the abdomen by anastomosing to the origins of the common or external iliac arteries. **Avoidance of groin incisions, which are notoriously prone to infection, is a good thing**.

Take care when fashioning the aorta to receive the graft. The longitudinal incision in the aortic sac should be terminated at both ends by a transverse incision so that the incision becomes T-shaped at each end. The limbs of the 'T' at either end should not extend more than 50% of the circumference of the normal aorta.

Suture the graft in place using monofilament material so that a *parachute technique* can be used. This allows you to visualize clearly the placement of the individual posterior sutures. Large bites of the posterior aortic wall should be taken because the tissues in this situation are often very poor. Furthermore, leaks that occur after completion of the anastomosis are difficult to repair if they are situated at the back wall. Once the upper anastomosis has been completed, a clamp is applied to the graft just below the anastomosis and the clamp on the aorta then released.

Assuming there are no significant leaks at the upper end, attention is turned to the distal anastomosis. This is completed in a similar fashion to the proximal anastomosis. Back-bleeding from the iliac vessels should be checked before the distal anastomosis is completed. Likewise, the graft should be flushed with saline and one or two 'strokes' of the patient's own cardiac output to clear it of thrombotic junk. If there is no back-bleeding it may be necessary to pass balloon embolectomy catheters into the iliac systems to check that there has been no intra-arterial thrombus formation.

Once the distal anastomosis has been completed and found to be secure, the iliac clamps should be released individually allowing time for any hypotension to recover before the second clamp is removed. The anesthesia team will appreciate a warning from you that the time is approaching for removal of the clamps, allowing them to be well ahead with fluid replacement. Inadequate fluid replacement at this stage will result in significant hypotension when the iliac clamps are released.

A word about heparin

It is clearly not sensible to administer systemic heparin prior to cross-clamping in patients who are bleeding to death from an aortic rupture. In patients in whom surgery has been carried out for suspected rupture, however, and in whom no rupture is found at operation, systemic heparinization according to the surgeon's normal practice should be carried out. It is permissible, however, to heparinize locally the iliac vessels once the aneurysm sac has been opened and back-bleeding from the small vessels has been controlled. Heparinized saline may be flushed down each of the iliac vessels in turn before reapplying the iliac cross-clamps. No consensus on the need for this practice has been reached and in most patients it appears to be unnecessary.

Abdominal closure

The large retroperitoneal hematoma and visceral swelling resulting from shock, resuscitation, reperfusion and exposure, commonly produce severe intra-abdominal hypertension, which becomes manifest after closure of the abdomen. Rather than closing under excessive tension use temporary abdominal closure as discussed in ➲ Chapters 31 and 44, and come back to close the abdomen later.

The avoidance of abdominal compartment syndrome is crucial in these physiologically compromised patients in whom any further derangement may be the straw that breaks the camel's back.

In emergency operations for AAA, simplicity of the operation is the key to survival: rapid and atraumatic control, avoidance of injury to large veins, tube graft, minimal blood loss, and rapid surgery.

Many patients who reach the operating table will survive the operation only to die in its aftermath, usually from associated medical illnesses such as myocardial infarction. A successful outcome therefore requires excellent postoperative ICU care as well as competent surgery. **The operation is only half the battle**.

In ruptured AAA, the operation is commonly the beginning of the end — the end arriving postoperatively (■ Figure 32.1).

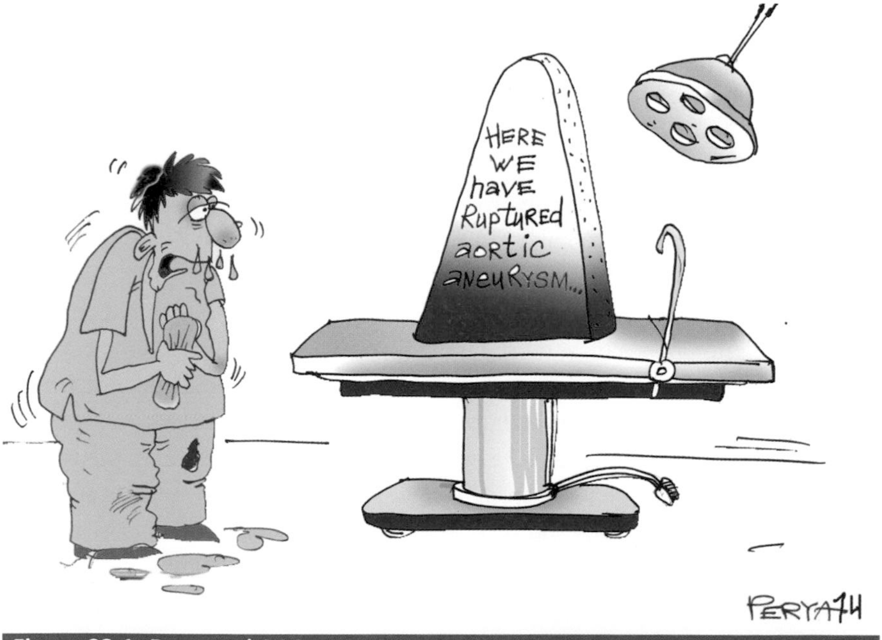

Figure 32.1. Ruptured AAA: common outcome...

Endovascular repair

As aortic stent-grafting has become an established treatment for AAA in the elective patient, interest has gradually increased in the use of the same techniques in ruptured AAA patients in the hope of reducing the operative mortality from the current 40-50%.

Emergency endovascular aneurysm repair (eEVAR) is confined to major centers but is becoming more commonplace as familiarity with the necessary arrangements increases. The limitations of this treatment are the need for rapid pre-op CT, an expensive stock of modular prostheses and immediate availability of appropriately skilled surgeons and radiologists (or endovascular surgeons — the new breed). **The patient needs to be stable enough to cope with the delay to obtain the CT images that are required to assess measurements for the stent-graft**.

This procedure is gaining acceptance in the centers where it can be carried out safely and it appears that the proposed benefits in terms of reduced mortality are being realized. It should be obvious that if you work in such a center then involving the vascular team immediately is essential.

Free intraperitoneal hemorrhage (see ■ Table 11.1)

Most AAA patients with a free intraperitoneal rupture will not reach surgery. In the few who do, rapid proximal control is even more crucial.

Other causes of non-traumatic intraperitoneal bleeding are rare and include **ruptured visceral artery aneurysms**. If this is encountered then the common sense principle of first stopping the bleeding by suture ligation or packing is followed by an assessment of the need for revascularization. **Splenic artery aneurysms** are the commonest of these lesions; they occur most often in women and rupture is a disaster particularly associated with pregnancy. **When exposure and thus proximal and distal control are difficult do not forget the option of *endoaneurysmorrhaphy***: open the sac of the aneurysm, control the bleeding with finger pressure and/or balloon catheters, and suture the proximal and distal openings from within. Currently, more and more such aneurysms are diagnosed on CT and managed angiographically by the radiologist — in stable patients of course.

Aortic occlusion

This emergency is characterized by acute ischaemia of the legs with mottling of the skin of the lower trunk. It occurs for three reasons:

- **Saddle embolus**. A large clot originating from the heart occludes the aortic bifurcation. The patient most likely will have signs of atrial fibrillation or a recent history of acute myocardial infarction.
- **Aortic thrombosis**. The patient probably has a history of pre-existing arterial disease suggestive of aorto-iliac involvement. Occasionally this disaster will occur unannounced in a patient who is desperately ill for some other reason. Extreme dehydration, for example, may cause 'sludging' of major vessels if there has been some pre-existing atheroma. Malignancy may produce intra-arterial thrombosis.
- **Aortic dissection**. Suspect this if there is a history of interscapular pain associated with obvious hypertension. Look for evidence of other pulse deficits or signs of visceral ischemia suggesting involvement of other aortic branches.

Management

This depends on the etiology and the presence of any relevant underlying pathology. **Embolism may often be dealt with easily by bilateral transfemoral embolectomy under local anesthetic**. Thrombosis on pre-existing atheroma is a more difficult problem. Catheter thrombectomy is unlikely to be successful either in the short or long term. If the patient is very fit (unlikely), aortofemoral bypass may be indicated. More likely an **extra-anatomic bypass** (axillofemoral) may be feasible, always assuming that any underlying illness is not likely to cause the patient's demise in the immediate future. Often these patients are not fit for any intervention and the aortic thrombosis is an indication that the end is near.

Aortic dissection is a complex illness and its management is variable. The mainstay is control of hypertension and relief of major vessel occlusion by endovascular 'fenestration' of the dissection. The details of this therapy are beyond the scope of this little book.

> **"To refuse to treat any aneurysm... is unwise; but it is also dangerous to operate upon all of them."**
>
> **Antyllus, second century A.D.**

"The entire gastrointestinal system to vascular surgeons is an incidental finding on the way to the aorta!"

Leo A. Gordon

"Why vascular surgeons do not like bowel surgery? Because blood don't smell and st don't clot."**

Chapter 33

Gynecological emergencies

The Editors

Have you ever seen a surgeon who is convinced that the 'pelvic acute abdomen' in a woman is surgical and not due to a gynecological affliction?

B. Cristalli

We respect the quotation above but have you ever seen a gynecologist who is convinced that the 'acute abdomen' is gynecological in origin, and not due to acute appendicitis?

In most locales, general surgeons are not expected to undertake practical obstetrics, but it is certain you'll face a gynecological emergency at some stage. This would commonly involve evaluation of low abdominal pain in a woman or unexpected gynaecological pathology in the OR. Acute abdominal pain is common in women during their reproductive years when such pain is as likely to be *gynecological* as it is to be *surgical*. Your gynecological colleagues, talented as they are, often possess a vision limited by the boundaries of the bony pelvis (■ Figure 33.1). **Consequently, they are often reluctant to diagnose any acute condition as 'gynecological' unless you have ruled out acute appendicitis**. On the other hand, occasionally you operate for what you think is acute appendicitis, and the findings are gynecological (it could happen only if you didn't read ➲ Chapter 21...). Another situation which provides you with the opportunity of interacting with gynecologists/obstetricians, is the **pregnant patient**. As you know, complications of pregnancy itself may be the cause of abdominal pain while in addition it may modify the presentation of common surgical disorders, making diagnosis difficult. It can also present real problems in the injured patient.

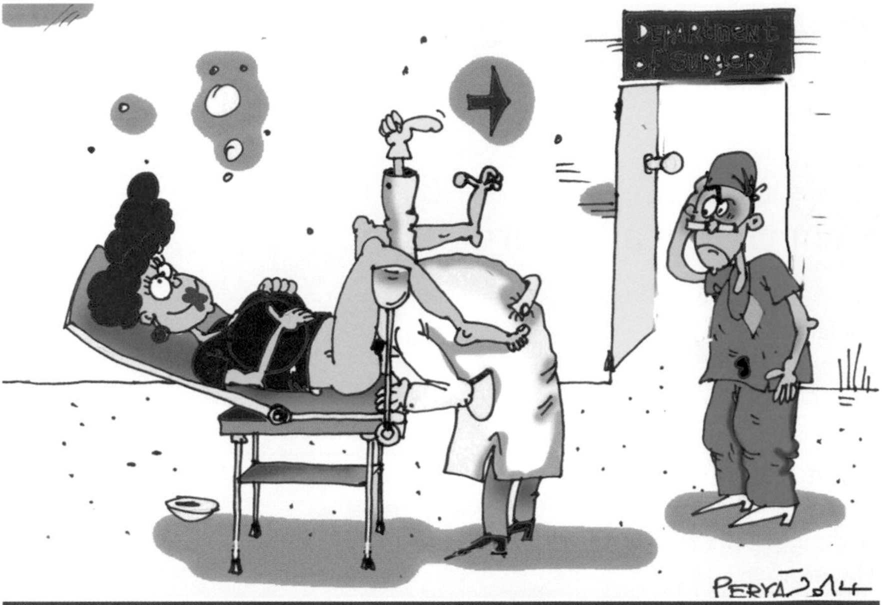

Figure 33.1. "Call the general surgeon."

If you happen to be on call and see women, whether referred directly or via your local gynecologist, **you'll encounter mainly two kinds of syndromes: pain and bleeding**. These two conditions may present alone or be associated with other symptoms such as fever, vaginal discharge, etc. We're not going to address painless bleeding, which is the bread and butter of gynecological practice.

The **age of the patient** is an important consideration since the gynecological pathology you are likely to encounter differs markedly among the following groups: premenstrual, menstrual-fertile, pregnant, menopausal — each group having its own disease profile and associated, different, clinical approach. **This chapter deals with problems encountered in women of child-bearing potential and those who are already pregnant since these are the two groups that most frequently produce dilemmas.**

Acute abdominal pain in the fertile woman

Assessment

As a sweeping generalization, all women should be considered fertile (and potentially pregnant) until proven otherwise. In these days of ovum

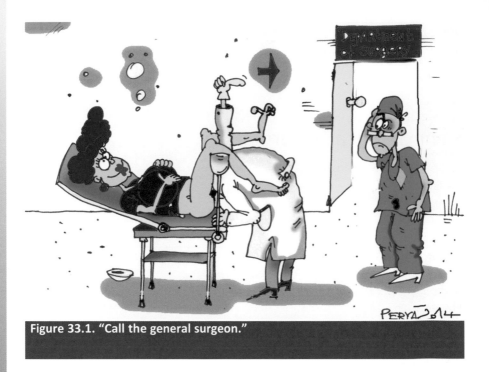

donation IVF, pregnancy in women in their late fifties is no longer a great rarity!

We do not have to remind you to take a history concerning *menstruation*, *sexual activity* and *contraception*. **Pregnancy, whether uterine or *ectopic*, should always be ruled out; this is done in most hospitals with a rapid pregnancy test**. Any history of pain which occurs during the first days of the menstrual period, hints at underlying *endometriosis*. Acute pain developing mid-cycle (*mittelschmerz*) may be due to rupture of the Graafian follicle at ovulation. **Pain referred to the shoulder raises the possibility of *free intraperitoneal blood* irritating the diaphragm, with a likely source of bleeding being a *ruptured ovarian cyst* or an *ectopic pregnancy*.**

We do not want to talk to you about physical examination. You surely know that the conditions to be discussed below can produce signs of peritoneal irritation, often indistinguishable from those of acute appendicitis. However, the **site of pain and local findings on examination** are helpful in narrowing the differential diagnosis (➲ Chapter 3). When bilateral, consider *pelvic inflammatory disease (PID)*; when on the right think about *acute appendicitis*; when on the left, in an older lady, consider *acute diverticulitis*. Bimanual vaginal examination performed by your gynecological colleague (or by you) is an essential part of the assessment of these patients. You are palpating for masses or fullness in the cul-de-sac (pouch of Douglas) and looking for *excitation tenderness* — when moving the cervix produces a lot of pain (PID, ectopic pregnancy).

Ultrasound (we hope your gynecologist is armed with a **transvaginal ultrasound**) is the key investigation, allowing visualization of any free fluid, the uterus and adnexae.

Many acutely painful gynecological conditions can be treated non-operatively. With all the above information at hand, your job, together with the gynecologist, is to classify the patient into one of the following groups:

- 'Benign' abdominal examination — most probably a gynecological condition. Get an US. Treat conservatively.
- 'Impressive' abdominal examination with no apparent gynecological pathology. Get a CT. For some this perhaps is the best indication for diagnostic/therapeutic laparoscopy.
- 'Not sure'. Get a CT +/- admit and observe.

Ectopic pregnancy

The great French surgeon Henri Mondor said: "**When faced with an acute abdomen, consider ectopic pregnancy, think always about it, always. Just thinking about it again is not enough, keep thinking about it**."

Ectopic means that the fertilized ovum has implanted somewhere outside the usual location (i.e. the body of the uterus). **The most common site for an ectopic is the tubes**, but implantation may occur in the ovary, cervix and peritoneal cavity. The latter (**abdominal ectopic pregnancy**) is rare and associated with a higher maternal mortality rate than ectopic pregnancies in general. **Heterotopic pregnancy** (intra-uterine and ectopic pregnancy at the same time) is so rare that if a normal pregnancy is seen on ultrasound, an ectopic can be ruled out.

Although the presentation of these patients varies tremendously, typically they have abdominal pain and vaginal bleeding. Many women do not even know about the pregnancy, ignoring associated symptoms of pregnancy such as a missed menstrual period. Some elements of history may be considered risk factors: previous history of ectopic pregnancy, PID, endometriosis and tubal surgery — **including previous tubal ligation!** Contraception with an intra-uterine device (IUD) is not a risk factor in itself but an **early pregnancy with an IUD *in situ* has to be considered ectopic until proven otherwise**. An IUD prevents intra-uterine pregnancies, but not ectopics! IVF is a risk factor.

The diagnosis rests on a tripod of pregnancy, pain and vaginal (and intra-abdominal) bleeding. Typically, the patient arrives with a sharp and sudden unilateral pelvic pain, mild brownish vaginal bleeding and a positive pregnancy test — with an empty uterus at ultrasound. The diagnosis comes easily when the woman knows she's pregnant and has vaginal bleeding. It can be a lot more difficult when pain is the only sign and the pregnancy is yet to be discovered. **Cataclysmic hemorrhage is very rare nowadays, but any internal hemorrhage syndrome in a woman is a ruptured ectopic pregnancy until proven otherwise**.

Physical findings include signs of hypovolemic shock and peritoneal irritation that are proportional to the amount of blood loss. On pelvic examination you may find a para-uterine painful mass or at least a 'little something' next to the uterus. The pouch of Douglas is tender and may contain a boggy mass (hematocele).

Ultrasound is the imaging of choice to show the ectopic gestational sac and free intraperitoneal bleeding.

Management

Although some ectopic pregnancies may resolve and absorb spontaneously over time, the standard of care is an operative approach in all cases. As a general surgeon you are most likely to be involved with the more dramatic scenario of a ruptured tubal ectopic (usually affecting the distal segment of the tube) which may occur as early as the 4th week of gestation.

The sudden development of acute peritonitis and hypovolemic shock will force you to proceed without the gynecologist. Whether you have time to obtain imaging in order to confirm the diagnosis — while the patient is being resuscitated — depends on the urgency of the situation. Most patients will become stable enough to allow a laparoscopic approach. However, if you need to rush, do not hesitate to enter the abdomen through a midline incision or a Pfannenstiel incision — depending on the situation and the build of the patient. Salpingectomy is usually the safest option. Control the bleeding sites with suture-ligatures and preserve the ovary.

If the patient is not 'bleeding to death' (which commonly is the case) then the procedure should be preferably performed laparoscopically. In early cases, the uterus is normal or mildly enlarged and the ectopic pregnancy can be seen as a tube swollen by a blue 'tumor' and there is a small to moderate amount of black blood in the pouch of Douglas. Just suck out the free blood and achieve hemostasis by evacuating the pregnancy; this is usually achieved with **salphingectomy, as in most cases the tube is unsalvageable.** If you know how to do laparoscopic appendectomy then removing the salpinx is a piece of cake; use whatever you have — clips, bipolar diathermy, endoloops, LigaSure™... However, in the presence of known or observed contralateral tubal disease and the desire for future fertility, *salpingotomy* should be considered instead. When the ovaries are left intact, the patient can still undergo *in vitro* fertilization even after bilateral salpingectomies.

Ovarian cysts

Ovarian cysts are common in young women — they are usually *'functional' cysts* (follicular or corpus luteum) and mostly asymptomatic. However, when cysts develop in postmenopausal women ovarian cancer must be suspected and excluded. **Only complicated ovarian cysts, regardless of etiology, present as surgical emergencies.**

Acute pain develops when a cyst bleeds or undergoes torsion or rupture. The intensity of pain and abdominal signs of peritoneal irritation are proportional to the amount of bleeding. Pain is severe in the case of torsion. **In women of childbearing age, complications of ovarian cyst may mimic acute appendicitis, so to prevent an unnecessary operation you must image the abdomen**.

Imaging

Typically, functional cysts are solitary, simple and small (<8cm). Free fluid in the pouch of Douglas suggests rupture and bleeding. Larger and more complex cysts suggest pathology such as a dermoid cyst. **Absence of blood flow on ultrasound strongly indicates torsion**. Most such patients initially undergo a CT examination to exclude acute appendicitis, which in addition to showing a normal appendix may document the free pelvic fluid and the ovarian pathology. If this is the case, we would follow up with a transvaginal ultrasound which is more accurate in delineating the pelvic pathology.

Management

Small (<8cm) simple ruptured cysts with minimal local and systemic findings should be treated conservatively. If, however, the rupture results in significant intraperitoneal hemorrhage and when another pathology cannot be ruled out (e.g. larger or complex cysts), surgical intervention is indicated. **Laparoscopy is preferable for smaller cysts and when malignancy is not suspected, but for very large cysts (>10cm) laparotomy allows removal of the intact ovarian mass without disrupting it**. Whether you can do this through a Pfannenstiel incision depends on the build of the patient, but anyway you better leave this job to your gynecologist.

Torsion is usually associated with more severe and persistent pain and more dramatic abdominal findings together with systemic manifestations; it is an indication for urgent operation. At operation if there is active bleeding from the cyst, obtain local hemostasis by whichever means. **There is no need to aspirate or resect the cyst and please, do not even think of removing the ovary**. If viable, the tube and ovary can be detorted and conserved; only if clearly non-viable is the ovary resected. Dermoid cysts are resected. Ovarian malignancies are beyond the scope of this little book.

Pelvic inflammatory disease (PID)

Pelvic inflammatory disease is seldom a surgical emergency nowadays, but it remains a frequent reason to visit the emergency room. It is an infective syndrome which involves, to a greater or lesser extent, the endometrium, tubes and ovaries. The patient is commonly young and sexually active. The clinical spectrum of infection is wide, ranging from minimal pain, dyspareunia, fever, and vaginal discharge, associated with mild endometritis/salpingitis, to severe peritonitis and septic shock due to a ruptured tubo-ovarian abscess. Likewise, physical findings depend on the disease process and vary from localized abdominal tenderness to generalized tenderness and rebound. Note that the pain and tenderness are commonly *bilateral*. Pelvic examination reveals a purulent discharge with cervical motion tenderness. Ovarian or pelvic abscesses may be palpated or seen on ultrasound or CT.

Treatment

Without treatment the infection may develop into a tubal abscess and then spread intrapelvically and result in a true peritonitis. The late risk is tubal obstruction and pelvic adhesions leading to infertility and chronic pelvic pain. **Most mild cases should be treated with antibiotics**. Outpatient treatment is appropriate for patients who can tolerate an oral diet. Patients with severe abdominal and systemic manifestation should be admitted for intravenous antibiotic therapy. Antibiotic treatment is empiric, targeting the common causative organisms which are, in isolation or combination, *Chlamydia trachomatis*, *Neisseria gonorrhoeae*, *Escherichia coli* and *Haemophilus influenzae*. Many oral and i.v. agents are available for you to choose from (e.g. doxycycline or amoxycillin/clavulanic acid orally, ampicillin/sulbactam or cefoxitin intravenously).

Patients who do not respond to the above regimen or in whom the diagnosis is uncertain are subjected to laparoscopy. This should be left to the gynecologist. **The typical case you will be involved with is the ruptured tubo-ovarian abscess, causing severe pelvic or diffuse peritonitis**. During laparotomy or laparoscopy you'll find pus. The abscess should be drained; whether to remove the uterus and ovaries depends on the age of the patient, the operative findings and your gynecologist.

When talking about PID, textbooks usually mention the *Fitz-Hugh-Curtis syndrome* or 'perihepatitis' as a late sequel — ascending from the pelvis. Although originally associated with *gonococcal* infection, nearly all present-day cases are associated with *C. trachomatis* infection. It may produce non-specific abdominal complaints and has been reported to mimic acute cholecystitis, but in our experience it has never represented a specific entity warranting operative measures. We have seen it, however, as an incidental finding of perihepatic 'piano-string' adhesions at laparoscopy or laparotomy for other conditions.

Vaginal tears

Vaginal tears are rare but may cause severe hemorrhage representing a true gynecological emergency. A vaginal tear can occur in young females at their first intercourse — the 'bloody defloration'. It can affect women of any age who experience violent or peculiar sexual relations, alone or with a partner. **Always suspect that rape may have been a causative factor**. Clinically, the bleeding is obvious. Diagnosis is by speculum examination: there is a lateral laceration, beginning at the hymen and extending upwards and the edges are rather neat. In some cases, the tear is transmural and involves the cul-de-sac. Treatment consists of hemorrhage control and repair of the laceration with an absorbable continuous stitch in the lithotomy position; whether to do it under local or regional or general anesthesia depends on the extent of the laceration and the individual patient.

Acute abdominal pain in the pregnant woman

In men nine out of ten abdominal tumors are malignant; in women nine out of ten abdominal swellings are the pregnant uterus.

Rutherford Morrison

General considerations

A consultation about abdominal pain in a pregnant or immediately postpartum woman is frequently an anxiety-provoking experience for the general surgeon. We think that the following few paragraphs will help you to approach these difficult problems with a new understanding and confidence based on some simple concepts.

Abdominal emergencies in pregnant women pose a great challenge for the following reasons:

- The growing uterus gradually distorts the normal abdominal anatomy, displacing organs and thus changing the typical clinical scenario.
- Physiologically, the pregnant woman is different; nausea and vomiting are common during the first trimester; thereafter, tachycardia, mild elevation of temperature and leukocytosis (and even C-reactive protein [CRP]) are considered 'normal'.
- To a certain degree, abdominal 'aches and pains' are common during pregnancy.

- When dealing with a sick pregnant woman you automatically have two patients — the life and wellbeing of the fetus must also be considered.

When it comes to treatment, there may be a conflict of interest between the mother and fetus. Early in pregnancy, the risk is of miscarriage, while at the end it is premature labor, and in both cases it is hard to determine which is more risky — surgery or non-operative management.

In general, acute abdominal conditions during pregnancy are either 'because' or 'regardless' of pregnancy.

Abdominal emergencies specific to pregnancy

These are either:

- **Obstetric** — such as ectopic pregnancy (see above), abortion and septic abortion (a septic uterus may present with an impressive 'acute abdomen'), 'red degeneration' of a fibroid, placental abruption, rupture of uterus, and pre-eclampsia. These conditions won't be further discussed. Hey, we didn't promise you a manual of obstetrics.
- **General** — such as acute pyelonephritis, which is more common in pregnant women, or rupture of a visceral aneurysm (e.g. splenic artery), which is rare but 'typically' occurs during pregnancy. Another condition, which may be associated with pregnancy, is **spontaneous hematoma of the rectus abdominis muscle** (this condition may also develop in non-pregnant men and women, particularly in anticoagulated patients). The hematoma originates from a ruptured branch of the inferior epigastric artery and develops deep to the muscle. On examination a tender abdominal wall mass is often felt; it won't disappear when the patient tenses his or her abdominal wall (Fothergill's sign). Ultrasound or a CT can confirm the diagnosis. Treatment is conservative.

Abdominal emergencies randomly developing during pregnancy

Any abdominal emergency may occur during pregnancy. Here are a few basic considerations:

- **'Think in trimesters'**: during the *first trimester* the fetus is most susceptible to the potentially damaging effects of drugs and X-rays. **Abdominal operations at this stage may precipitate an abortion.** Operations during the *third trimester* are more likely to induce

premature labor, posing additional risk to the mother and fetus. Thus, **surgery is best tolerated during the *second trimester*** — if you have the luxury of choice.

- **The wellbeing of the mother overrides that of the fetus**. If maternal and fetal distress are present simultaneously on presentation, all therapeutic efforts should be for the benefit of the mother. A Cesarean section is considered only if the fetus is more than 24 weeks old and in persistent distress despite maximal therapy to the mother.
- **Pregnant women suffer from a chronic abdominal compartment syndrome** (➲ Chapter 31). The abdominal emergency (e.g. perforated appendicitis or intestinal obstruction) will further increase the intra-abdominal pressure, reducing venous return and cardiac output. Place such patients in a *left lateral decubitus position* in order to shift the gravid uterus away from the compressed inferior vena cava.

You should be aware of acute appendicitis, acute cholecystitis and intestinal obstruction.

Acute appendicitis

You are commonly called to 'exclude acute appendicitis' in a pregnant woman. Address the problem as discussed in ➲ Chapter 21. Remember that although the cecum is usually fixed in place it may be displaced by the gravid uterus. Similarly, the omentum is 'lifted' away and thus may not provide 'walling-off' protection to the perforated appendix — making free perforation more likely. An **ultrasound** may help in excluding acute cholecystitis and ovarian or uterine causes of pain and may document an enlarged appendix. CT is not advisable because of the risks of irradiation of the fetus. **However, MRI has emerged as a reasonable diagnostic alternative — use it if it is available as it may help to avoid an unnecessary operation**.

Diagnostic laparoscopy and/or laparoscopic appendectomy during pregnancy have been reported as safe to both mother and fetus, yet remain somewhat controversial — particularly in late pregnancy. **And, as in acute appendicitis in general, nothing is wrong with open appendectomy** — in that case place a muscle-splitting incision directly over the point of maximal tenderness, wherever it is (it may be higher than usual). And of course do not forget to tilt the table to the left. **Also remember: treatment of acute appendicitis occurring early in pregnancy may be non-operative — with antibiotics. We don't hesitate to offer this to the patient!**

Acute cholecystitis

This is easily recognized clinically and ultrasonographically (➲ Chapter 18) during pregnancy. **During the first trimester try conservative management,**

delaying the operation until the second trimester. If it occurs during the third trimester try to postpone the operation, if possible, until after delivery.

Laparoscopic cholecystectomy (LC) appears to be safe during pregnancy. Inflate the abdomen with the lowest pressure possible and rotate the table well to the left to decrease compression of the IVC by the uterus. When cholecystectomy is (very rarely) required late in pregnancy, when the uterus fills the entire abdominal cavity, an open approach through a small subcostal incision may be simpler... However, no one will condemn you for proceeding with LC.

This is perhaps the place to mention a few relatively rare syndromes which can be confused with gallbladder disease during pregnancy:

- **Intrahepatic cholestasis of pregnancy**. This typically develops in the third trimester, presenting with itching and dark urine and fatigue. Right upper quadrant pain is possible. Liver enzymes are elevated and so are bile acid levels. The syndrome — which is thought to be caused by the surge in hormones and genetic predisposition — subsides spontaneously after delivery.
- **HELLP syndrome** (Hemolysis, Elevated Liver enzymes, and Low Platelet count). This syndrome may develop in a pre-eclamptic, pre-term patient and may be confused with acute biliary disease (even a 'mild' HELLP may stretch the liver capsule producing severe RUQ pain). Liver hemorrhage and hematoma and even liver rupture are serious complications of the HELLP syndrome and represent a surgical emergency; the child should be promptly delivered, and the liver managed based on trauma principles. In the unstable, coagulopathic patient the liver should be packed.
- **Acute fatty liver of pregnancy**. This rare but potentially life-threatening syndrome occurs in the third trimester but can develop also after delivery. It presents with jaundice and progressive liver failure. Google it up...

Intestinal obstruction

Sigmoid or *cecal volvulus* is more common during late pregnancy. The displacement of abdominal structures during pregnancy may also shift longstanding adhesions, producing small bowel obstruction or volvulus. Pregnancy tends to cloud presenting features and impedes early diagnosis. Note that a few plain abdominal X-rays, with or without *Gastrografin®*, are entirely safe even in early pregnancy. So, if you suspect a large or small bowel obstruction, do not hesitate. **Remember that intestinal strangulation threatens the life of the mother and her child. This is no time for timidity**.

Trauma in pregnancy

The management of abdominal trauma in pregnancy is identical to the management in the non-pregnant woman (➲ Chapter 30), except that in pregnancy there is concern for two patients — the mother and the fetus. **Remember that the pregnant woman has a marked increase in blood volume, a fact which tends to mask or delay clinical features of hypovolemic shock**. Assessment of the fetal status either by Doppler or by continuous cardiotocography is mandatory when the clinical circumstances permit.

The major specific clinical concerns in the injured pregnant female are **uterine rupture** and **abruptio placentae**. The former condition is suggested by abdominal tenderness and signs of peritoneal irritation, sometimes in conjunction with palpable fetal parts or an inability to palpate the fundus. The latter is suggested by vaginal bleeding and uterine contractions. **When the fetus is in jeopardy, a rapid Cesarean section is usually in the best interests of both the mother and fetus**.

The 'postpartum' period

Abdominal emergencies are notoriously difficult to diagnose during the early postpartum or post-Cesarean section period. Abdominal pain and gastrointestinal symptoms are commonly attributed to 'after pain', and fever or systemic malaise to 'residual endometritis'. In addition, at this stage the abdominal wall is maximally stretched out and redundant, such that guarding and other peritoneal signs may be missing. 'Things move around' the abdomen during delivery and a loop of bowel may be twisted or caught. We have treated perforated acute appendicitis, perforated peptic ulcer and acute cholecystitis during the early postpartum days; we even did a splenectomy for spontaneous rupture of the spleen following an uneventful vaginal delivery!

Diagnosis is usually delayed and so is the treatment. **Be aware, suspect and use imaging liberally!**

> **"A male gynecologist is like an auto mechanic who has never owned a car."**
>
> **Carry P. Snow**
>
> **(Yes, but what about a female urologist?)**

Chapter 34

Abdominal emergencies in infancy and childhood

Wojciech J. Górecki

Children are not small adults.

The dictum that children are not small adults is not only because of differences in physiology and metabolism, but also because of a different clinical spectrum of abdominal emergencies, their presentation and management.

The first principle to remember is that you are less likely to commit an error if you consider an atypical presentation of a common condition than a typical presentation of a rare condition. In other words, a pediatric acute abdomen is intussusception in infancy or appendicitis in childhood — until proven otherwise. Another (seemingly forgotten) principle is that, much as with adults, watchful waiting is a prudent strategy in children.

General approach to pediatric abdominal pain

The philosophy of classifying the multiple etiologies of the acute abdomen into several well-defined clinical patterns (see ➲ Chapter 3) works for children as well.

But let's start with some basics...

- **Timing**: children with abdominal pain present at varying stages of disease because the timing of presentation depends on the parents. Some parents delay, while others rush their darlings to the ER at the slightest sign of trouble. Parents' attitudes to emergencies could be described like this: when their first child swallows a coin they rush to the ER; when that happens to the second child, they search for the coin in the child's feces; the third child has the coin deducted from his pocket money. **As a general rule — as originally stated by Sir Zachary Cope — consider any abdominal pain lasting more than 6 hours as a potential surgical problem**.

- **History**: younger children do not give you a history, but listen to the parents because they know their kids so well. A classic example is intussusception, where a description of the child's behavior and a glance at the stool (see below) can point you to the diagnosis even before the physical examination.
- **Examination**: the importance of gentleness during abdominal palpation cannot be over-emphasized. Most children with a sore tummy object to abdominal palpation. Sometimes a toy provides a temporary distraction that will allow you to examine the abdomen, but it is pointless to persist if the child is antagonized. Instead of the usual 'head-to-toe' sequence of the physical exam in adults, take advantage of a spell of sleep or inattention to sneak a warm gentle hand underneath the blanket to palpate the abdomen. **Gentle abdominal percussion or bed shaking with your knees, while watching the child's face, will get you the sense of peritoneal irritation without provoking an intentional pain**.
- **An infant** who will not allow a gentle attempt even when held in his mother's lap should be sedated, because sedation does not affect muscle guarding. Our preference is intranasal midazolam spray 0.1-0.2mg/kg given or assisted by mom.
- **Examination of the scrotum** is essential for two reasons. First, an acute condition in the right testicle, such as torsion, can present with pain in the groin and iliac fossa. Secondly, perforated appendicitis occasionally presents with a painful scrotal swelling, because pus enters the patent processus vaginalis, causing acute funiculitis.
- **Rectal examination** is best left to the end of physical examination, after looking at the throat and ears, and is not needed if there is a clear indication for surgery.

Clinical patterns of the acute abdomen in children (see also ➲ Chapter 3)

Here are a few key points:

- **The combination of acute abdominal pain and shock is rare in children**, and should make you think of occult abdominal trauma with rupture of an enlarged solid organ or intra-abdominal malignancy. **Ruptured ectopic pregnancy is possible in an adolescent girl.**

- **Generalized peritonitis in children is most commonly due to appendicitis.** Do not try to elicit rebound tenderness, as you will lose the confidence and cooperation of your patient. (This applies to adults too!). The good habit of measuring the serum amylase as described elsewhere in this book would prevent an exploratory laparotomy for **acute pancreatitis** in children as well.
- **Localized peritonitis** in the left lower quadrant can be due to acute constipation, whereas right or left upper quadrant tenderness is commonly due to acute distension of the liver or spleen, respectively. **Please note that constipation is the second most frequent diagnosis found on emergency discharge records for missed pediatric abdominal catastrophes in court cases** (e.g. neglected massive colonic distension causing abdominal compartment syndrome).
- **Intestinal obstruction in a virgin abdomen is caused by intussusception or appendicitis.** One of ten children with complicated rotational anomalies of the midgut presents after the neonatal period. The critical concern with malrotation is midgut volvulus with acute extensive bowel ischemia. This life-threatening condition carries the risk of rapid transmural intestinal necrosis. Your surgical intervention should be prompt because simple counter-clockwise detorsion of the bowel may save it. Don't put the baby at risk of a miserable life with a short bowel, yielding to the anesthesiologist "because the blood is not ready".
- **A surgical scar** signifies adhesion-related small bowel obstruction until proven otherwise. In doubtful cases, the *Gastrografin®* challenge test (pediatric dose is 2ml/kg up to 100ml) described in ➲ Chapter 19 is safe and effective in children.
- **A word of caution for 21st century surgeons relating to the scarless abdomen.** Sutureless plastic closure of gastroschisis and transendorectal pull-through for Hirschsprung's disease may present you with patients after major intra-abdominal manipulations but with absolutely no scars.
- **The two major pitfalls in pediatric small bowel obstruction are:** missing an incarcerated inguinal hernia and waiting too long with conservative management before surgery.

A wide spectrum of non-surgical conditions may mimic abdominal emergencies. Particularly in infants, any acute systemic disease may present with apathy, vomiting and stool abnormalities. The converse is also true. A child with an acute abdomen may present with a wide array of seemingly unrelated symptoms suggesting early meningitis, a neurological disorder or poisoning. **Although gastroenteritis is common in children and typically presents with acute abdominal complaints, for a surgeon it should only be a diagnosis of exclusion. Remember, it is the first common erroneous diagnosis in court cases**.

Specific pediatric emergencies

The relative incidence of various conditions in different age groups is depicted in ■ Figure 34.1.

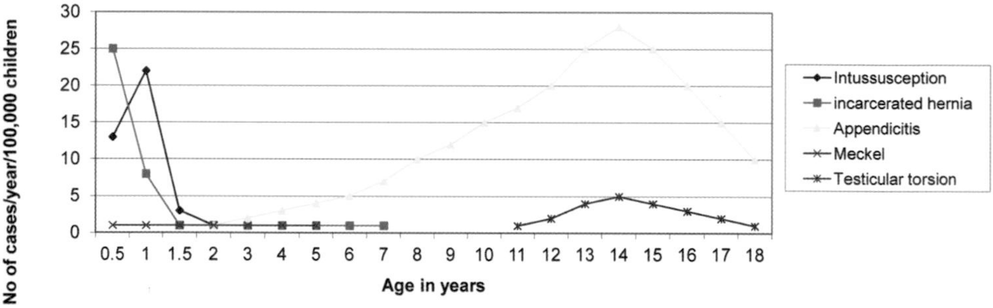

Figure 34.1. Pediatric abdominal emergencies.

Acute appendicitis (AA) (see also ➲ Chapter 21)

AA is rare during the first year of life and is uncommon during the second. **Thereafter, the incidence rises and peaks between the age of 12 and 20. AA in infancy typically presents as generalized peritonitis due to perforation**. The infant looks unwell, with fever, tachycardia and tachypnea. The abdomen is distended and diffusely tender with guarding. Diarrhea is more common than constipation. Pay attention to the useful 'hunger sign'; it's rare to see a hungry child who turns out to have AA. **Consider AA in the second place on your list of differential diagnoses for an infant with an**

acute abdomen, and in the first three places in a child. Admitting children with equivocal signs for observation is a safe option, as the chance of rupture under observation in a pediatric surgical ward is negligible.

A limited helical CT with rectal contrast is highly accurate in diagnosing AA in children, but clinical examination by an experienced pediatric surgeon is just as good. Even if the CT scan is positive, appendectomy is not indicated if the child improves clinically. In our institution, children with early appendicitis receive antibiotics and undergo appendectomy during daytime hours. Evidence suggests that perforation and complication rates are not increased for patients who undergo appendectomy more than 6 hours versus less than 6 hours after diagnosis.

What is the role of laparoscopy in the doubtful case? While it offers the advantage of a diagnostic modality that can be immediately followed by appendectomy, it will subject some children to an unnecessary operation. If you can get the child into a CT scanner without general anesthesia, this should be your preferred choice instead of diagnostic laparoscopy

However, I agree that it is important to minimize exposure to radiation at such an early age; thus, if local expertise is available, **ultrasound examination is a valuable alternative to CT to confirm the diagnosis**.

Although a valid alternative to the open technique, the value of laparoscopic pediatric appendectomy remains controversial because there are no good data to suggest that it confers an advantage. Like adult patients, children after laparoscopic appendectomy have significantly fewer wound infections and a shorter duration of hospital stay, but higher rates of readmission, intra-abdominal abscess formation, and higher hospital costs. **Good evidence to support decreased postoperative pain and earlier return to normal activities after laparoscopic appendectomy in children is lacking**.

The short distances involved and the thin abdominal wall of children allow a '**port-exteriorization appendectomy**', performed via two ports, where the appendix is exteriorized by pulling it out of the right iliac fossa port and then the entire appendectomy is performed outside the abdomen, or the appendix can be pulled out of the umbilical port. If you have a laparoscope with a working channel, you can perform a single-port appendectomy using the same technique.

...which would be equivalent to a conventional 'no-port appendectomy' through a 2cm incision. **The Editors**

There is no point in culturing the peritoneal fluid in cases of obvious AA because the results are predictable, and antibiotics have usually been stopped by the time the culture results become available. Decide on the duration of postoperative antibiotics according to the degree of contamination/infection found in the peritoneal cavity (see ➲ Chapter 40).

Peritoneal drains are not necessary. They do not reduce the incidence of wound infection or abscess after appendectomy for perforated appendicitis in children; instead they increase cost, and a child is subjected to stress and pain at the removal (➲ Chapter 36).

Finally, not all children with acute appendicitis must be operated upon. The indications for a non-operative approach are similar to those described in adults (➲ Chapter 21).

Intussusception

Telescoping of one portion of the intestine into another can turn a healthy baby into a critically ill patient within a few hours. **This problem typically occurs between the ages of 5 and 7 months, and the etiology is idiopathic. In children older than 2 years, look for an underlying pathology, the most common being a Meckel's diverticulum**. Early intussusception is generally a benign condition, although it is a strangulating obstruction eventually, if not treated promptly, leading to vascular compromise. **Most cases start in the ileum as an ileo-ileal intussusception and then progress through the ileocecal valve to become ileocolic intussusception**.

The diagnosis is straightforward if the infant exhibits the classic clinical syndrome: a previously healthy infant suddenly starts to scream, pulls up its legs and perhaps clutches the abdomen. The pain is then relieved, and the child may relax for a while only to have a similar bout 15-30 minutes later. This leaves the infant pale and ill. Vomiting and passing of 'redcurrant jelly' stools is also characteristic, although salmonellosis may show a similar clinical picture.

Atypical presentations are common, however, and lead to diagnostic errors. The infant may be fretful and restless without either pain or vomiting. Pallor and peripheral coolness due to vasoconstriction, lethargy and seizures may also confuse the picture. **The crucial physical sign is palpation of an abdominal mass**. The ultrasonographic findings of a 'target' sign on cross-section and a 'pseudo-kidney' sign in a longitudinal view are important adjuncts to the clinical diagnosis (■ Figure 34.2).

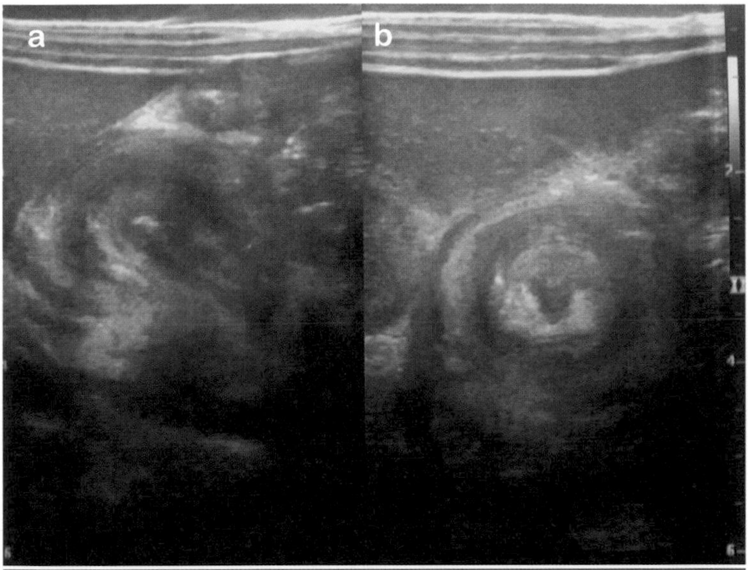

Figure 34.2. Sonographic images of intussusception: a) in a longitudinal plane showing a 'pseudo-kidney' sign; b) in a transverse plane showing a 'target' sign.

With regard to the management, children with diffuse peritonitis, perforation, progressive sepsis and possible gangrenous bowel should undergo an urgent laparotomy. Early intussusception without peritonitis is reduced non-operatively with hydrostatic or pneumatic pressure, under radiographic (for contrast and air) or ultrasonic (for saline) guidance (■ Figure 34.3). Ultrasonic guidance is preferred, if available, to reduce radiation exposure. Barium is better avoided in cases of suspected perforation, but is hardly available, anyway. Water-soluble contrast and saline for ultrasound are much safer than barium in cases of suspected perforation. Reduction is successful in most cases but requires close collaboration between the surgeon and radiologist. In a good environment comprising prompt presentation of a symptomatic child, instant diagnosis with ultrasound followed by hydrostatic decompression, 97% of cases can be managed this way. It is not unusual to complete residency in pediatric surgery without seeing a surgery for intussusception. After successful non-operative pressure reduction, a child may be discharged home safely directly from the emergency

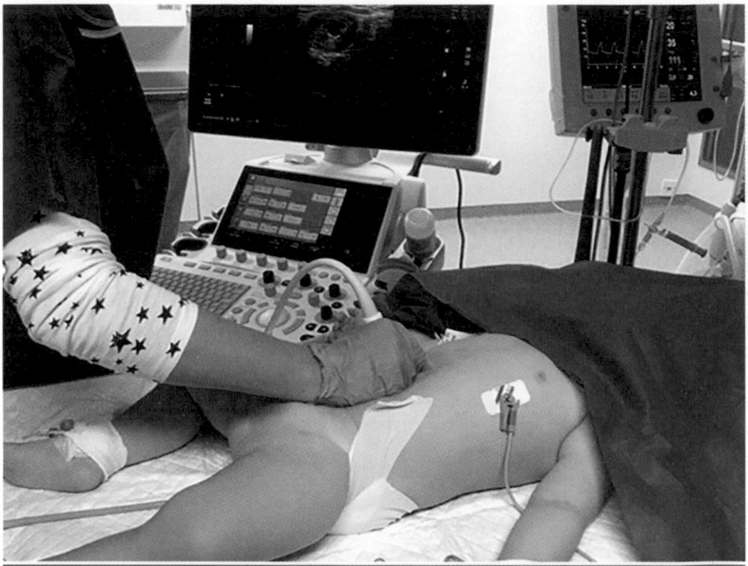

Figure 34.3. Hydrostatic reduction of intussusception (Foley catheter wedged in the rectum) under ultrasonic guidance.

room. However, one in ten children may come back with a recurrence within 72 hours. **Unless the aforementioned contraindications are present, repetitive attempts at non-operative pressure reduction are justified. And, again, beware of anatomical abnormalities at the leading point, especially if the child is older. Do not repeat pressure decompression after the third or fourth presentation but explore — CT may not show you a Meckel's diverticulum or an intraluminal polyp.**

During operative reduction of an early intussusception (in an open procedure), squeeze on the apex of the intussusceptum while the bowel is still within the abdomen so that the intussuscepted segment begins to slide proximally. When the reduction reaches the region of the hepatic flexure it may become more difficult, but after you eviscerate the cecum the reduction can be completed under direct vision by gentle pulling of the telescoped loop.

After achieving complete reduction remember to examine the entire bowel for any pathology serving as a lead point. **If the intussusception is truly irreducible or if the bowel has suffered a serious vascular compromise — resect it.**

Meckel's diverticulum

Two-thirds of Meckel's diverticula encountered by surgeons are incidental findings while the remaining one-third will present with a complication. Pediatric surgeons encounter more such cases, as the incidence of these complications is maximal during the first 2 years of life. These complications include bowel obstruction (adhesive obstruction, volvulus or intussusception), complications of peptic ulceration in ectopic gastric mucosa (stricture, hemorrhage, or perforation), or acute inflammation ('second appendicitis'). There is also a distinct tendency for foreign bodies to penetrate and perforate a diverticulum. We have seen a 5-year-old girl with complete bowel obstruction caused by a Meckel's diverticulum filled with excessively ingested gummy bear candies. *Littré's* inguinal hernia contains a strangulated Meckel's diverticulum and, like *Richter's* hernia, may not produce typical signs of intestinal obstruction.

The treatment of a symptomatic diverticulum is resection. Diverticulectomy is possible if the base is wide and non-inflamed, but remember to check the base of the diverticulum and the adjacent ileum for ectopic mucosa because a bleeding source may lie within it. **If in doubt, or if there is any technical difficulty, resect the involved segment of ileum.**

What should you do with an incidentally found Meckel's diverticulum during emergency surgery for another indication? Consider the degree of peritoneal infection (caused by the primary indication for laparotomy), the patient's age and the shape of the diverticulum. **On balance, the arguments against removing an asymptomatic Meckel's diverticulum are a little stronger than those in favor, and the strength of the argument increases with the age of the patient.** Thin-walled, wide-mouthed, mobile (without a fibrous band to the umbilicus or mesentery) diverticula should be left alone.

Irreducible inguinal hernia

This emergency occurs primarily in boys during their first year of life. The fundamental difference between an irreducible inguinal hernia in an infant and an adult is that the former presents a danger to the viability of the testis, whereas with the latter the major concern is the potential for bowel strangulation. Neonates with symptoms lasting for more than 24 hours and with intestinal obstruction are at the greatest risk of testicular infarction. **Necrosis of incarcerated bowel is extremely rare in pediatric hernias.**

The diagnosis is straightforward because the baby cries and vomits and the parents have usually noticed a tender lump in the groin. Major differential diagnoses include torsion of a maldescended testicle, acute inguinal lymphadenitis and a hydrocele of the cord ('funiculocele').

The treatment, after making the diagnosis, is to sedate the infant and place him in a head-down position. In most babies, with the addition of gentle manual pressure, or even spontaneously, this will result in reduction. If the hernia has not reduced within 1-2 hours, then take the patient to the OR for an emergency operation. If, however, reduction was successful then let the tissue swelling subside for a day or two and schedule the child for an elective herniotomy on the next available operative list.

The operation for an irreducible inguinal hernia in an infant is fraught with danger and should be undertaken only by a surgeon with previous experience in pediatric surgery. The hernia sac is edematous and extremely fragile, and the ductus deferens is almost invisible. A simple herniotomy at the level of the neck of the sac is all that is required. Always make sure that the testicle is safely replaced in the lower part of the scrotum. **In a female infant, a movable tender lump may be an irreducible ovary**. The child may be almost asymptomatic yet require emergency herniotomy because of the risk of ovarian ischemia. The boy after inguinal hernia incarceration should be followed up for ischemic testicular damage and testis positioning. Disorders of sex differentiation may present as bilateral, gonad-containing inguinal hernias.

Testicular torsion (see also ➲ Chapter 35)

The key to successful treatment of testicular torsion is speedy detorsion, within 6 hours of the onset of symptoms. The incidence of torsion rises sharply around the age of 12, with two of every three cases occurring between the ages of 12 and 18. **Some boys present with lower abdominal and inguinal pain so you will miss the diagnosis if you fail to examine the scrotum**. The testis may be localized low in the inguinal canal or high in the scrotum and the pain not precisely localized by a child or projected higher. **I have seen children who previously had a negative appendectomy with atrophy of the right testis!** No clinical sign or test is foolproof!

Color Doppler US is the test of choice to differentiate testicular torsion from other acute scrotal conditions. However, a "normal testicular blood flow" result does not absolutely exclude testicular torsion and is operator-dependent! Last night I explored the scrotum of a child for suspected testicular torsion, finding a completely necrotic, twisted testis. He had been seen a day previously in the emergency department and had been released home because the US scan had detected testicular blood flow. What shall we now tell the parents? That the child should have had a 10-minute surgical procedure via a 1cm scrotal incision that would have saved his testicle?

Thus, common sense dictates that we have a low threshold for exploring an 'acute scrotum'.

If prompt access to the operating room is not available, **manual detorsion** in a lateral direction under sedation or local anesthetic infiltration of the cord may restore testicular blood flow, but is not a substitute for surgery. The degree of twisting of the testis may range from 180 to 720°, requiring multiple rounds of detorsion.

Surgical exploration is necessary even after clinically successful manual detorsion (i.e. relief of pain, correction of the transverse lie of the testis to a longitudinal orientation, lower positioning of the testis in the scrotum, return of normal arterial pulsations in a color Doppler study). Residual torsion may be present that can be further relieved and anyway orchidopexy (fixing the testicle to the scrotal wall) must be performed to prevent recurrence. **Fixation of both the involved testis and the contralateral uninvolved testis should be done since inadequate gubernacular fixation is usually a bilateral defect.**

The window of time to save the testis is narrow and a delay in detorsion of a few hours leads to progressively higher rates of non-viability of the testis. The time to presentation is the most important factor affecting the salvage rate.

At operation, after induction of anesthesia, first examine the scrotum to rule out incarcerated hernia or testicular tumor, both requiring an inguinal incision. Then proceed with a scrotal exploration via a vertical incision in the median raphae of the scrotum or, alternatively, two transverse incisions on each side. Enter the serosal compartment of the scrotum to deliver and detort the testis. Place it in a warm moist sponge while exploring the opposite hemiscrotum. If the affected testis remains necrotic, remove it. **Orchidopexy** of the viable testis is performed by suturing, with non-absorbable sutures, the tunica vaginalis (after it has been wrapped-everted around the testicle) to the wall of the scrotum, at four points. If you find torsion of the testicular appendage, simply excise it.

Ovarian torsion

Should you encounter pediatric ovarian torsion, whether anticipated or as a surprise finding during an operation for suspected appendicitis, the adolescent girl will be fortunate in having you as the surgeon if you detort the 'non-viable' adnexa and leave it alone. The macroscopic appearance of the ovary is not a reliable predictor of necrosis or of the potential for gonad recovery. If an underlying lesion is found, then cystectomy, tumorectomy (even in cases with a very large teratomata, there is a rim of normal ovary at the hilum that can be preserved), or cyst aspiration, with possible oophoropexy should be considered. If you are not comfortable with this situation, just detort the ovary and close the abdomen — or remove the laparoscope. **Remember the key principle: you are more likely to preserve functional ovarian tissue than cause any morbidity by leaving *in situ* what appears to you a non-viable ovary in little girls.**

There is some controversy regarding fixation of the detorted ovary (oophoropexy). Spontaneous ovarian torsion (no underlying ovarian pathology), recurrence of torsion and torsion of the only ovary are arguments in favor. Should you be faced with such circumstances, suture the ovary to the uterus, pelvic wall or simply plicate the round ligament.

Pediatric abdominal injuries (see ➲ Chapter 30)

Trauma is the chief cause of death among children older than one year, and is responsible for more deaths than all other causes combined. In one out of seven injured children, the abdominal injury is dominant. The patterns of blunt abdominal trauma and the clinical pictures are similar to those in adults, with injuries to the kidneys, spleen, liver and the intestines being the most common. Most cases can be treated conservatively and laparotomy is required in only one child in four. The major deterrents to an operative approach to abdominal trauma in children are the risks of non-therapeutic laparotomy and overwhelming post-splenectomy infection.

Even children with hemodynamic instability on admission often quickly improve with crystalloid administration and remain hemodynamically stable thereafter. If the situation stabilizes after three infusions of 20ml/kg of fluid, then it is safe to observe the child in an intensive care unit. If the child continues to bleed and no other source of hemorrhage is apparent, a prompt laparotomy is indicated.

The Achilles' heel of this conservative approach is the possibility of missed injuries to hollow organs. Thus, if the child develops increasing abdominal tenderness or peritonitis, this too is an indication for laparotomy. A useful clinical marker of blunt bowel trauma is the triad of a fastened lap belt, a seat belt sign on the abdominal wall, and fracture of a lumbar vertebra.

No discussion of pediatric trauma can be complete without emphasizing the need for always suspecting child abuse. While isolated abdominal trauma is a rare presentation of child abuse, unusually shaped or multiple bruises, associated long bone fractures or inexplicable genital lesions should always raise the suspicion of this tragic and potentially life-threatening condition.

Special situations

I would like to emphasize three specific situations:

- **The neurologically impaired child**. In patients with spinal cord dysfunction, the history is crucial as physical examination may not be reliable. Close observation and complementary imaging studies are necessary.
- **The immunologically compromised child**. **Here, perityphlitis is the first diagnosis until proven otherwise — diagnosed and monitored by CT**. Perforation, uncontrolled bleeding and clinical deterioration require surgical intervention.
- **The adolescent girl**. Here, menstrual history, a pregnancy test and ultrasound are the first-line approach. A low threshold for diagnostic laparoscopy in the presence of an adnexal mass is justified to exclude torsion.

Now you know that... Most children with acute abdominal pain do not require surgery, and one-third of them get no specific diagnosis. Consider the most common causes of surgical abdominal pain, the most common misdiagnoses for the surgical pediatric abdomen, be careful in special situations and look out for child abuse (■ Table 34.1). And you understand that children are not small adults but... (■ Figure 34.4).

Table 34.1. Common sense approach to pediatric abdominal emergencies.

Most common causes of pediatric acute abdomen	Most serious erroneous diagnosis	Special situations	Traps in diagnosis/timing
Intussusception <2 y.	Constipation	Neurologically impaired patient	Ischemic bowel obstruction
		Immunocompromised patient	Missed incarcerated inguinal hernia
Appendicitis >2 y.	Gastroenterocolitis	Adolescent girl	Testicular torsion
			Diabetic ketoacidosis
			Pancreatitis
Child abuse			

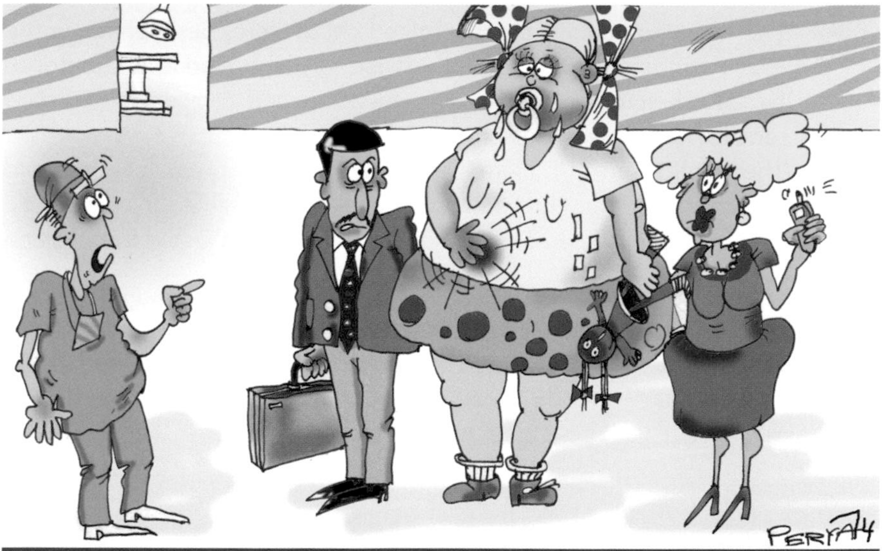

Figure 34.4. "But... but I'm a pediatric surgeon..."

"Pediatric surgery: screaming kids, difficult parents but easy exposure!"

Chapter 35

Urological emergencies

Jack Baniel

Has the patient renal stones
Painful, brittle, broken bones
Complaints of thirst and constipation
Next to peptic ulceration
And you doubt his mental state
Determine calcium and phosphate
Sure the underlying mechanism
Might be hyperparathyroidism.

Hajo A. Bruining

Urology is not associated with many emergencies. Actually one of the main advantages enjoyed by the senior urologist is that most of our surgery is elective, and unlike his fellow general surgeon, his nights may be spent out of the OR and in a warm bed. Most acute urological problems are managed in the ER with the help of other disciplines. **I shall discuss here those common scenarios that a general surgeon may encounter, and solve, while the urologist slumbers.**

Acute renal colic

Renal colic is quite easy to diagnose and usually involves intrinsic obstruction of the renal pelvis or ureter, by a stone. **The classic complaint is of acute flank pain in a restless patient.** The pain radiates from the back forwards, is spasmodic and recurrent. It is often associated with nausea and, less frequently, vomiting. The pain is caused by the dilatation of the urinary tract proximal to the stone. As the stone travels down the ureter by force of the forward pressure caused by the urine flow, the location of the pain changes, radiating toward the lower abdomen, inguinal area and then to the genitalia. As the stone reaches the lower ureter the patient will complain of frequency and urgency and then all abates as the stone is expelled into the bladder. **Thus, one may trace the advancement of the stone by the patient's complaints**. Stones need to pass three narrow spots in the collecting system on their way to the bladder: the ureteropelvic junction, the iliac vessels and the vesico-ureteral junction. These points are where calculi usually get stuck.

The most important factors to assess in this situation are the stone's size and its location within the urinary system. **Most stones less than 5mm in size and those in the lower ureter (beyond the iliac vessels) should be expelled spontaneously (80-90%) and thus are managed expectantly. Larger stones and those higher in the ureter need to be manipulated out. Most stones that pass spontaneously do so within 3-4 weeks**.

Diagnosis

Most stones are radiopaque and thus a regular plain abdominal X-ray is the initial diagnostic step. (If you have ever wondered why sometimes a plain abdominal film is called KUB — 'Kidney-Ureter-Bladder' — it's the urologists' fault, looking for stones...). Looking at the X-ray we use the four Ss rule:

When searching for **S**tones check that the **S**ide corresponds to the pain, that the **S**keleton does not hold surprises (*metastasis*) and that there are no suspicious **S**ilhouettes (tumor).

Non-contrast CT (NCCT) is the gold standard in the diagnosis of stones in the ER setting. NCCT may diagnose all stones regardless of their composition (uric acid, etc.). Ultrasound is helpful in the assessment of hydronephrosis and obstruction — urine flow into the bladder is visualized by urine jets in the bladder; its absence is a surrogate marker of obstruction.

Management

The pain of ureteric colic is mediated by prostaglandins and therefore intramuscular NSAIDs are the drug of choice in the management of pain. Fluids are given to increase diuresis and force the stone down the ureter, and smooth muscle relaxants (e.g. papaverine i.v.) also have merit in alleviating acute pain. Steroids and calcium channel blockers have been tried in the past with minimal value. Lately, tamsulosin (Flomax®, Omnic®), an α-adrenergic blocker used for prostatism, has been found to facilitate stone expulsion.

Remember: on initial assessment of the patient, look for signs of *infection* or *renal dysfunction*. These, along with intractable pain, are indications for hospitalization.

Laboratory tests should include a complete blood count, creatinine and electrolytes. Some patients presenting with renal colic will be septic or in severe renal failure (beware of patients with a single kidney). **These patients must be admitted to hospital and have emergency decompression of the collecting system, as the penalty for a delay in treatment may be death from sepsis.** Decompression may be done by insertion of a self-retaining stent (JJ) (now you'll have to call your urologist) or by percutaneous nephrostomy by the radiologist. The available options to get rid of the obstructing ureteral stone disease are (usually) to insert a stent and fragment the stone later (shock wave lithotripsy), or to perform immediate ureteroscopy and stone fragmentation with laser. **Ureteroscopy is the definitive solution for most lower ureteral stones. Stones in the upper ureter or in the renal pelvis are usually fragmented by external shock wave lithotripsy (ESWL).** Open nephrolithotomy belongs to the history books in most places, but may still be practiced in under-privileged parts of the world.

Torsion of testis (see also ➲ Chapter 34)

As a general surgeon you will see most 'acute scrotal conditions' well before the urologist — some may present as depicted in ■ Figure 35.1. Torsion of the spermatic cord is the most dramatic 'acute scrotum'; it requires emergency management and if missed the testis will be lost. It commonly occurs in young boys but may appear at all ages, even in the neonate.

As the testis descends through the inguinal canal it pushes ahead of it a sliver of peritoneum. When the testis reaches the scrotum the peritoneum is sealed off and only the part attached to the lower pole of the testis is left — this actually fixes the lower testicular pole to the scrotal wall. But the peritoneum may adhere higher around the spermatic cord and wrap the entire testis within an isolated peritoneal sac. In this situation the testis may rotate, twist itself around its vessels within the *tunica vaginalis* (the retained part of the peritoneum) and cause acute ischemia. **This anomaly occurs equally on both sides of the scrotum.**

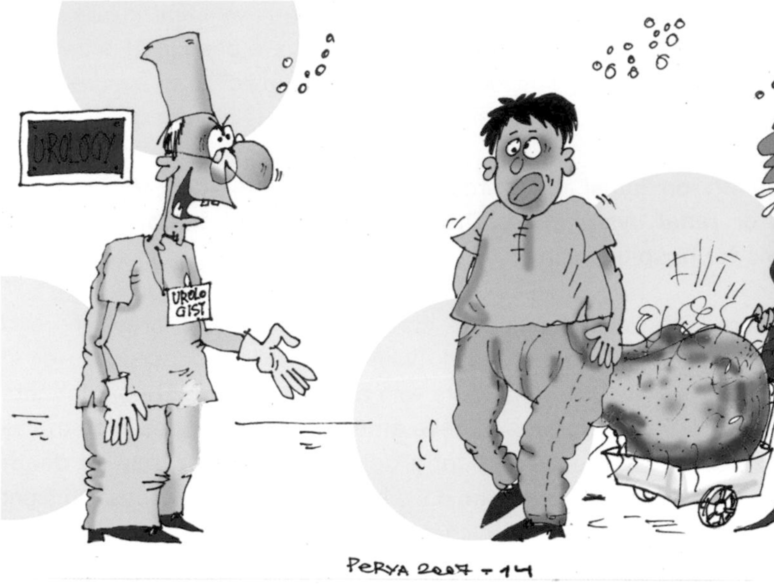

Figure 35.1. "What's that? A water melon?"

Medical literature from the 1960s observed a high frequency of delay in diagnosis and a very high orchiectomy rate. But with more attention paid to the clinical symptoms, and the adoption of an aggressive operative approach, most torted testes can be saved.

The classic symptoms are acute unilateral scrotal pain, swelling, nausea and vomiting, without fever or urinary symptoms. Usually there are difficulties in gait as the patient wishes to keep his legs apart to avoid pressure on the scrotum. Often the presentation is not so clear, and pain and swelling are the only signs. **The most common differential diagnoses are inflammatory intrascrotal conditions (e.g. epididymitis, orchitis), but in the young patient torsion is more frequent than inflammation**.

Torsion of a *testicular appendage* may also occur and confuse the examining physician. The testis has two appendages, one emanating from the testis itself at the upper pole; another from the epididymis (■ Figure 35.2).

If they twist around their origin, a large scrotal swelling occurs which is very painful. **In this case the testis itself is normal**. On examination one may see a local enlargement called a 'blue dot'.

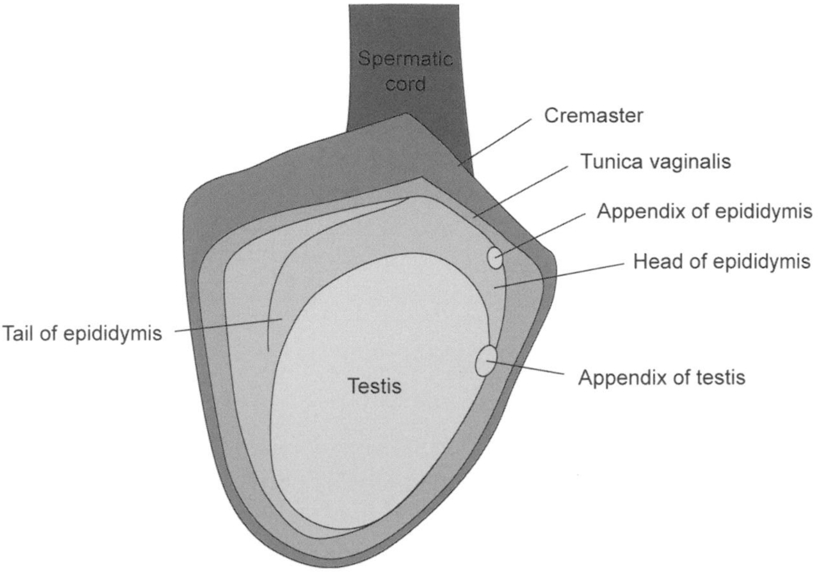

Figure 35.2. Testicular appendages.

> Signs of testicular torsion on examination include: a high riding testis, transverse lie, a negative dartos sign (normally, stroking the thigh elevates the testis), and local pain and sensitivity.

The diagnosis is assisted by a Doppler ultrasound that shows reduced testicular perfusion — an indication for exploration! Note that also **equivocal ultrasound results along with indicative signs and symptoms warrant surgical exploration. The testis may withstand 4-6 hours of ischemia, after which there are irreversible changes resulting in atrophy**. Practically, accurate assessment of time of onset of the torsion is usually difficult and thus the recommendation is to explore the affected testis whenever signs are significant.

Exploration is performed trans-scrotally. I prefer to place a separate incision on each side. In my hands a vertical incision works better, since it may be extended to the inguinal area should you want to explore the cord. So if you need to 'pexy' the other testis (and you need to if it's there!), use a separate contralateral vertical one. The exposed testis is 'untorted' and wrapped in warm pads. If blood flow returns, as seen by a pinkish color, the testis is fixed with non-absorbable sutures to the scrotal wall in at least three places. If blood flow does not return, the testis must be removed. If left *in situ*, the atrophic testis may produce autoantibodies, damaging the contralateral testis, and causing infertility. **At the same procedure, the contralateral testis must be explored as well and fixed to the scrotal wall as a prophylactic measure**. Being 'aggressive enough' one may expect a negative exploration in up to one-third of patients — (exactly what was true for the appendix a few decades ago...).

Acute retention of urine

You will often have to deal with acute urinary retention in the ER or in your postoperative patients. Most patients with retention are men suffering from benign prostatic hypertrophy (BPH) who give a history of 'lower urinary tract symptoms' (LUTS) such as urgency, nocturia, double micturition, hesitancy, etc. Other possible etiologies include urethral stricture and neurological disease (e.g. multiple sclerosis). In some BPH patients, retention is precipitated by sympathomimetic drugs (ephedrine for flu) or anticholinergics (psychiatric drugs). As you know, **anesthesia combined with vigorous intra-operative fluid administration predisposes patients to this complication**; so, for example, if you chose to repair an inguinal hernia under local anesthesia, rather than a general or spinal, you are likely to spare your patient that kind of urinary *tzures* [1].

Retention is manifested by severe lower abdominal pain, inability to void and (not surprisingly) agitation.

Management

Relief of this situation is by simple insertion of a urethral (Foley) catheter. **The rule in this case is to insert a catheter with a moderate caliber but not too large as it may have to stay in place for some time**. A good choice is a 16Fr Foley catheter. Bladder neck stenosis, a large prostate or urethral stricture may make it difficult to pass through the urethra. If insertion of a regular Foley fails, one may use a 14Fr Tiemann catheter that has a special tip and an angle with a better chance of negotiating the bends and curves of the urethra. **Third-line catheters are tougher and transparent with a Tiemann tip and no balloon, and of different calibers**.

1 In Yiddish: suffering; trouble; misery.

Failure of all these measures would necessitate the insertion of a cystostomy tube (suprapubic catheter). In most cases we would first insert a large-bore needle in the midline above the pubic bone and when urine pours out we thread the cystostomy kit *de jour* into the bladder. **Caution must be practiced if the patient has had prior surgery in the area; in which case cystostomy is best done under ultrasound guidance.** Of course, renal function must be assessed, as some patients may have chronic retention causing renal failure.

It is very important to measure urine output for 2-3 hours after insertion of a catheter. A common occurrence is **post-obstruction diuresis** with production of very large amounts of urine. The pathophysiological basis for the polyuria is an acute washout of solutes that due to retention were not excreted properly, as in a hyperosmolar state. Other reasons are: an inability of the medulla to conserve water due to loss of urea; or pseudo diabetes insipidus — a temporary incapacity of ADH receptors in the distal nephron. **This situation is life-threatening especially in older patients due to a fluid and electrolyte imbalance.**

A patient with post-obstruction diuresis (>200cc/hr) must be hospitalized. Urine output is measured every hour and i.v. fluids (0.45% saline) are given. In order to avoid 'chasing your tail', initially 80% of the voided volume is replaced; as urine output decreases replacement is given at 50% of the voided volume. Usually this is a self-limiting situation that resolves within 24 hours.

Urological trauma

Kidney

Renal injuries may be blunt or penetrating and they are commonly associated with motor vehicle accidents, falls from heights and assaults. An important consideration is to check whether a deceleration injury is involved (fall from height especially), as this may cause an **arterial intimal tear leading to renal artery thrombosis which is a real emergency. Otherwise a tendency towards conservative management has emerged over the years in all renal injuries.**

The conservative approach for stab and low-velocity gunshot wounds emerged in South Africa. It was there that physicians managing masses of injured patients in cramped ERs noticed that many of those with extensive renal injuries waiting for their turn for surgery survived without surgical exploration. **The kidney has a good recuperation potential and most injuries heal with minor sequelae**. Associated urine leaks are easily managed with drainage which may be either internal via a stent, diverting urine from the kidney to the bladder; or by a percutaneous nephrostomy tube. Obviously, penetrating injuries are commonly associated with injuries to other nearby structures according to the site of entry.

The hallmark of renal injury is hematuria. Microhematuria is defined as >5 red blood cells/high power field (RBC/HPF). We do not need to tell you what's gross, macroscopic hematuria, right?

Which patients need renal imaging?

- **Blunt trauma with gross hematuria**.
- **Blunt trauma with microscopic hematuria and shock** (blood pressure <90mmHg measured at any time since the trauma occurred).

> This does not mean that you should send a hemodynamically unstable patient with microscopic hematuria to the CT! **The Editors**

- **Penetrating trauma**: all patients with penetrating wounds in the anatomical vicinity of the kidneys.
- **Pediatric patients**: use imaging more liberally because children are more susceptible to significant renal trauma.

The preferred imaging study is contrast-enhanced CT. Most spiral CTs are performed in a 2-3-minute sequence, which reveals both an arterial and a venous phase. Urine excretion and possible injury to the collecting system may be seen only at 10 minutes, thus a delayed image must be taken at 10 minutes as well.

Important CT findings are:

- Medial perinephric hematoma — suggesting vascular injury.
- Medial extravasation of urine — ureteropelvic junction avulsion.
- Lack of contrast enhancement of the kidney — arterial injury.

The intravenous pyelogram (IVP) has been abandoned and is used for only one indication — a 'single-shot' intra-operative IVP. If at laparotomy, and without prior imaging, a surgeon encounters an unexpected retroperitoneal, perinephric hematoma he may get an IVP to assess the kidney.

A single film is obtained 10 minutes after an i.v. push of 2ml/kg contrast media. A kidney that looks normal may be left alone. Similarly, when there is a need for an emergency nephrectomy it is always comforting to know that the contralateral kidney is intact. (Of course, in some developing regions IVP continues to play the role of the poor man's CT.)

However, these days even intra-op IVP is infrequently used. The common practice is: for an expanding hematoma or a suspected hilar injury — explore; otherwise — leave alone. See Chapter 30. **The Editors**

Grading of injury

As in most organs, there is a tendency to grade renal trauma and act according to the severity of injury. The system commonly used in urology is the American Association for the Surgery of Trauma Organ Injury Scale for the kidney. Basically, Grades I-III describe the magnitude of perirenal hematoma and laceration of the renal parenchyma. Stage IV entails either a laceration extending throughout the kidney from the cortex to the collecting system or a vascular injury. Stage V includes a shattered kidney or avulsion of the renal hilum.

Managing the renal injury patient

These are the principles:

- **Grade I-III** injuries may be managed non-operatively. Patients must be carefully followed in an ICU/HDU setting with frequent hemoglobin assessment.
- **Grade IV and V** injuries often require surgical exploration.
- **If bleeding occurs** on expectant management, angioembolization may be therapeutic.
- **Renal artery occlusion** by an intimal tear (deceleration injury) must be repaired (or stented) within 6-8 hours before the kidney dies.
- **Experience shows that when in doubt it is better to explore and repair the injury rather than treat the complications**.
- **Absolute indications for operative management** include persistent renal bleeding, expanding perirenal hematoma and a pulsatile renal hematoma denoting arterial renal injury. **Relative indications** include

incomplete pre-op imaging and major urinary extravasation (with a medial urinoma — a high probability of an ureteropelvic junction tear which will not heal spontaneously).

The operation for renal injury

Exploration of an isolated renal injury is usually done for bleeding in an unstable patient or, rarely, for delayed complications. **The appropriate incision is *midline* from the xyphoid to below the umbilicus**. Although the classic access for elective nephrectomy is retroperitoneal, through the flank, in trauma one may need to approach the major vessels, and this is easier through a long midline incision.

The old dogma maintained that the renal vessels have to be controlled at their origin prior to exploring a perirenal hematoma, but this is easier said than done. Today we know that there is no real advantage for early vascular control. In practice, the perirenal hematoma 'dissects' all the planes around the kidney. The surgeon opens the retroperitoneum lateral to or above the injured kidney and evacuates the clots. **The immediate aims are to mobilize the kidney — lifting it forward and medially into the wound, and to identify the hilum in order to control the renal pedicle and assess the parenchymal damage**.

Parenchymal tears are repaired, closing the collecting system with delicate absorbable sutures and then approximating the parenchyma — over bolsters of *Surgicel®*, or even better, pieces of Teflon® felt to prevent sutures cutting through — using blunt atraumatic liver needles (absorbable sutures again). Following repair of a major tear in the collecting system, or a large partial/hemi-nephrectomy, a double J stent may be best inserted retrogradely through the bladder into the collecting system, to prevent urinary leak.

For a shattered kidney, or when the major vessels are not amenable to repair — nephrectomy is the best option. Nephrectomy is also recommended if there is major trauma to adjacent organs such as the pancreas or bowel, since urinary leak from an ill-performed partial repair may promote local septic complications. Studies in animals show that one can survive without dialysis on 33-50% of one kidney. **Thus, a safe rule of thumb is that if one can save half or more of the kidney, it is worthwhile**.

Ureter

Ureteric injuries are rare, and frequently are recognized late when urine comes out of a drain after exploration for trauma. The ureter travels in the retroperitoneum covered on all sides by fat and is very evasive. Thus, it takes a lot of bad luck to have a ureter transected by a bullet or cut by a knife. Some of the injuries are partial tears due to a high-velocity missile traveling in the vicinity, injuring the ureter wall and causing a leak.

The hallmark of ureteric injury is leakage of urine and this is what appears on IVP or contrast CT. In the setting of penetrating trauma, suspect damage to the ureter if the injury is in the lateral retroperitoneal areas or in the pelvis. **Traumatic ureteral injuries must be carefully searched for, otherwise they will be missed**.

Iatrogenic ureteric injuries may occur during C-sections and colorectal procedures. If diagnosed intra-operatively they should be repaired immediately. Some accidental injuries occur during laparoscopic surgery and they are usually missed and diagnosed late. Sometimes the ureter is obstructed by a stitch or a clip; the patient may complain of flank pain or develop asymptomatic hydronephrosis, detected on imaging.

Managing the injured ureter

The ureter must be carefully examined and any necrotic segment should be debrided although this may compromise its length. **Always stent the anastomosis to secure urine drainage and augment local tissue apposition**. Urine always finds its way out through an imperfect anastomosis; this is why you see so many different types of stents and tubes in urology and why some urologists consider themselves plumbers.

Lower ureteral injuries (distal to the iliac vessels) are more common and are easier to fix. Usually one sacrifices the distal part of the ureter and reimplants the ureter directly into the bladder. In this situation, if the ureter is too short one may pull up the bladder by suturing it to the psoas — a psoas hitch; or use a flap fashioned from the bladder — the Boari flap.

Mid and upper ureteral injuries of less than 2cm in length are fixed by an end-to-end (spatulated) anastomosis with optimal apposition using fine absorbable sutures. Longer injuries may necessitate mobilization of the ipsilateral kidney and downward positioning which may offer another couple of centimeters. If there is a large gap, several options exist: one is to connect one ureter to the other by tunneling it behind the peritoneum — *transuretero-ureterostomy*; another option, when a large gap is present, is to bridge it with small bowel — an *ileal ureter*. An extreme measure would be to autotransplant a kidney in the ipsilateral pelvis thus bridging a large gap of missing ureter. In experienced hands these measures are all done with a high rate of success.

Two important notes:

- If one encounters ureteral injury while dealing with an extensive and unstable trauma case, an easy solution is to clip the ureter above the injury. When the patient is stabilized and within 24 hours, one may insert a nephrostomy tube and secure drainage of the kidney. Further repair is delayed to a more appropriate time.
- Another point which is often overlooked: if a ureteral injury is very extensive necessitating a complex reconstruction, or diagnosed late, or when a complex urinary fistula already exists, then, if the contralateral kidney has good function, nephrectomy may be the best option.

Bladder

Bladder injuries are usually associated with pelvic trauma. Isolated bladder rupture occurs especially on holidays when a patient with a full bladder from overdrinking gets hit in the lower abdomen. Penetrating bladder injuries also are often associated with trauma to other organs. **Iatrogenic injuries are common, and obstetricians and gynecologists are the main offenders**.

Bladder rupture presents with suprapubic pain and tenderness with gross hematuria. **A cystogram is diagnostic in nearly all cases. Care must be taken to fill the bladder appropriately. In an unconscious patient a minimum of 300cc of contrast is instilled through a catheter. In a conscious patient, filling may be terminated when the patient complains of discomfort**.

Bladder tears may be extraperitoneal (lateral flame-shaped) or intraperitoneal (contrast outlines the small bowel contour). **Extraperitoneal tears are managed by draining the bladder with a large-bore Foley catheter** (20-22Fr) left *in situ* for 10-14 days until healing takes place. A cystogram should be performed prior to catheter extraction. **All intraperitoneal injuries need to be explored and sutured primarily with absorbable sutures**. Injury adjacent to the bladder neck needs careful assessment of the ureteral orifices.

Scrotum

Blunt injury of any etiology may cause rupture of the tunica albuginea of the testis. Blunt injury usually involves a single testis but penetrating trauma affects both sides of the scrotum in one-third of cases. Scrotal hematoma is a common clinical finding but may not correlate with the extent of damage to the testis itself, as bleeding may originate from any of the other structures in the scrotum. Also, failure to feel the testis does not mean that it is damaged. **Severe testicular pain radiating to the abdomen is suggestive that the testis has been injured**. We have treated patients screaming with pain, and resistant to narcotics, who had almost no scrotal swelling or hematoma on examination; at operation, however, their tunica albuginea was found to be ruptured. **Although ultrasound is the best imaging modality to assess the scrotum and testis, an unequivocal report doesn't rule out testicular trauma. When in doubt it is best to explore the scrotum**.

Management

Early exploration and repair of the testis injury is the rule. Early repair is associated with increased testicular salvage, quicker convalescence and preservation of testicular function. Explore the scrotum through a transverse incision; pass through the various layers (like cutting an onion) until reaching the tunica albuginea. When the tunica has been breached you will see the *seminiferous tubules* flowing out like tiny *spaghettini*. Damaged tissues should be debrided and the tunica albuginea repaired. Even simple clot evacuation from a large hematocele will hasten recovery.

> **"Urologists are just glorified plumbers..."**

Chapter 36

Abdominal drainage

The Editors

The more imperfect the technique of the surgeon the greater the necessity for drainage.

William Stewart Halsted

The history of abdominal drainage is as old as the history of surgery. However, abdominal drainage was always a subject of controversy, practiced in confusion and subjected to local dogmas. One hundred years ago there were ardent enthusiasts of drainage, like Robert Lawson Tait, who stated: "When in doubt drain!" Then there were the sceptics, like J. L. Yates, who understood that "Drainage of the general peritoneal cavity is a physical and physiological impossibility." And, as always, there were the undecided, such as Joseph Price: "There are those who ardently advocate it, there are those who in great part reject it, there are those who are lukewarm concerning it, and finally, some who, without convictions, are either for or against it... as chance or whim, not logic may determine."

A century has passed, during which operative surgery and supporting care have progressed astonishingly; but, looking around us, it seems that not much has changed concerning the use of drains — the same old chaos. So please forget for a moment the local dogma, dictated by your boss or mentor and listen to us.

In this chapter we will discuss when and how to use drains after emergency abdominal operations. **Percutaneous drainage** of primary and postoperative abdominal abscesses and collections is discussed in ➲ Chapter 42. **Wound drains** are mentioned in ➲ Chapter 46.

Let us start with the classification of drains:

Surgeons may give the following reasons for draining the abdomen.

Therapeutic:

- **To provide** egress for established intra-abdominal contamination or infection (e.g. peri-appendicular abscess, diffuse fecal peritonitis).
- **To control** a source of infection that cannot be controlled by other means, by creating a 'controlled' external fistula (e.g. leaking duodenal suture line).

Prophylactic:

- **To prevent** recurrent infection (e.g. hoping that by evacuating residual serum and blood they will prevent abscess formation).
- **To control** 'prospective' or 'expected' leakage from a suture line (e.g. drainage of a colonic anastomosis, duodenal closure, or cystic duct closure).
- **To warn** about complications (believing that drains would sound the warning bell about postoperative bleeding or anastomotic leakage).

Many surgeons around the world that we have seen leaving drains in the abdomen do so for no reason other than: "Why not? What's the harm?"

But rather than dwell on the subject using rigid classifications let us deal with it through the eyes of a general surgeon: **what should the current practice be for drainage after common abdominal procedures?**

Drainage in acute appendicitis (➲ Chapter 21)

Should you place a drain after an appendectomy for gangrenous or perforated appendicitis?

No. The evidence shows that drainage in these situations does not reduce postoperative complications. Even when the perforated appendix is associated with a local pus collection there is no need to leave a drain. Such abscesses are never 'non-collapsible'; thus, after you break down the walls, and evacuate the pus, the potential space for the abscess is filled up by adjacent bowel, mesentery and omentum. And even if the ruptured appendix resulted in diffuse peritonitis, drainage would be useless: drainage in this situation — **after the source control of infection has been achieved** — is an exercise in futility!

So, the source of infection has been removed, the peritoneum has been cleansed by 'peritoneal toilet'; now — for God's sake — let the superb peritoneal defense mechanisms, supported by a short course of systemic antibiotics, complete the eradication of bacteria, without being disturbed by a foreign body — the silly drain.

Insecure closure of the appendix stump as a justification for drainage sounds anachronistic: secure closure is possible (even in the event when the appendix is perforated at its base) by including in the suture or stapler line a 'disk' of adjacent cecal wall.

Drainage after cholecystectomy for acute cholecystitis (➲ Chapter 18)

Would you place a drain following an open or laparoscopic cholecystectomy for severe acute cholecystitis?

From studies performed during the era of open cholecystectomy, we have learned that **routine drainage is not beneficial**. Ultrasonographic studies showed that most post-cholecystectomy collections, whether composed of bile, serum or blood, remain asymptomatic and are absorbed by the peritoneum.

However, drains are much more effective in draining bile than evacuating feces or pus. So it makes sense to leave a drain if the surgeon has a reason to worry about an unsolved or potential bile leak; for example, if the cystic duct opening cannot securely be controlled in subtotal cholecystectomy; or there is some bile staining in the lavage fluid or in the gallbladder bed — hinting at the possibility that a duct of Luschka has been missed; or when one suspects a non-perfect closure of the cystic duct for whatever reason.

The key word is — SELECTIVE. Most patients do not need a drain after cholecystectomy, but if you are worried about the possibility of bile leak, then leave a drain!

Most drains produce almost nothing; only rarely would the prophylactic drain become therapeutic by draining a large and persisting amount of bile. **It**

is very important that drains be removed as soon as possible. A dry drain after 24-48 hours indicates that it has served its limited role. A final comment, Howard Kelly said: "Drainage is a confession of imperfect surgery." Don't justify this statement in your own practice; it may be better to suture an ultra-short cystic duct safely (and convert, if needed) than rely on faulty clip closure and a drain.

Drainage after omentopexy for perforated ulcer (➲ Chapter 16.1)

You have just repaired a perforated duodenal ulcer with a patch of omentum. Would you leave a drain?

The literature dealing specifically with this issue is scanty but does not support drainage. Omental patch repair, if correctly performed, and tested, should be leak-proof. In addition, the presence of drains when a leak occurs is usually not life-saving (➲ Chapter 43). Futile reliance on the drain when a leak develops simply postpones a necessary reoperation and hastens death.

But what about laparoscopic omental patch repair? Should it change the (non) indication for drainage? With leaks after omentopexy being so rare and large series comparing open to laparoscopic repair so scanty, it is difficult to know whether leaks are more common after laparoscopic repairs. However, those of us used to open omentopexy should be alarmed to see the reported leakage following laparoscopic repairs. It may be that the 'learning curves', the inability to feel the tension placed on the sutures to tie down the omental patch, or the reliance on suture closure rather than using the omentum, make the laparoscopic approach more prone to leakage. So if you know how to do a proper and safe omental repair, draining it would be superfluous. But if you are still climbing on your learning curve (with the declining incidence of peptic ulceration you may never reach its top...), you may want to leave a drain. In most cases it will not avoid the need for reoperation should a leak develop but it may warn you early that this is the case.

Drainage after emergency left colon resection with or without anastomosis

The two questions, about drainage after emergency resection of perforated sigmoid colon, without, or with, primary anastomosis, can be discussed together. In both situations **source control has been achieved by the colectomy**. Thus, the rationale for drainage would be either 'therapeutic' — to help treat the associated intraperitoneal infection, or 'prophylactic' — to prevent collections or to 'control' potential leakage from a suture line (e.g. the anastomosis or rectal stump closure).

The topic of drainage after colonic resection has been subjected to intensive debate for many years; proponents claim that drains would avoid reoperation if anastomotic leaks develop, while critics contend that drains actually contribute to leaks.

The reasons given by those in favor of drains are varied:

- The first is to **help combat residual, or prevent recurrent, intra-abdominal infection**, by draining the pericolic abscess found and already drained during operation or by removing secretions. However, the futility of peritoneal drainage in achieving such goals has been discussed above (see acute appendicitis) and will be re-emphasized below (see next section).
- The second is to **drain the anastomosis should it leak**. But, surely, high-risk, leak-prone anastomoses should not be constructed in the emergency situation anyway. Furthermore, as the literature points out, drains do not help much if leakage does develop — to say nothing about the false sense of security it tends to provide.
- The third reason given is to **provide drainage to the rectal closure** (Hartmann's pouch) — should it leak. But a solid stapler or hand closure of the healthy rectum away from the colonic inflammation should provide a leak-proof closure. When, however, the closure is deemed 'too difficult', then the rectal stump should be left partially open as advocated by the late John Goligher of Leeds (and consider leaving a rectal tube — see ➲ Chapter 24). In any event, only **a pathological optimist could hope that feces will climb up the drain and out of the pelvis, that is, if the drain is not already clogged by fibrin, clots or feces**.

In conclusion: drains after emergency colonic resection are a waste of time and possibly harmful!

Drainage in generalized peritonitis (➲ Chapter 13)

No comparative studies of drainage versus non-drainage in patients with diffuse peritonitis have ever been conducted, because the futility of drainage in this situation was perceived long ago by experts in surgical infections. The modern view, endorsed by those who understand surgical infections maintains the following:

It is impossible to drain the peritoneal cavity in patients with diffuse peritonitis. Therefore, the use of drains in these patients is not indicated unless: (a) the drain is placed into a well-defined abscess cavity; (b) the drain is used to establish a controlled fistula.

We recall, when we were junior residents, postoperative patients with multiple rubber drains sticking out of every quadrant of their distended bellies — like porcupines. Those drains produced some old blood, or perhaps a little pus or foul-smelling fluid. Then the patient would die with his death blamed on 'pneumonia'. How stupid we were — believing that these drains were useful! We gradually understood how worthless it is — all intraperitoneal drains seal off by adjacent tissue within 24-48 hours, unless 'perfused' by liquid effluent such as bile. So in peritonitis, if you use a suction drain it drains almost nothing, and if you leave a wicking rubber drain (e.g. Penrose, 'corrugated'), **it simply drains the infected tract it has created**.

The *only* indication to use a drain in general peritonitis is to control an uncontrollable source of infection such as a leaking duodenal suture line or a leaking gastroesophageal anastomosis. As pointed out above, we are skeptical about the term 'well defined' or 'formed' abscess as an indication for peritoneal drainage. Such 'abscesses' are pus collections which are part of the spectrum of peritonitis; after evacuation they should be treated like the rest of the infected peritoneum. Let peritoneal defenses and antibiotics do the job. **In conclusion: drains in diffuse peritonitis are senseless. Recurrent or persistent intra-abdominal infection can develop, however, and may need percutaneous drainage (➲ Chapter 42), or a reoperation (➲ Chapter 44). Drains will not change this.**

In ■ Table 36.1 you will find a summary of the situations which would or could indicate drainage. But what about leaving drains because of bleeding?

Well, about drainage for **expected bleeding** it has been said: "**If you have to use drains to take care of postoperative hemorrhage, then you did not finish the operation**." In most cases in which you leave drains for bleeding or oozing, they are unnecessary and produce little; they also produce little even when severe bleeding develops — showing only the tip of the iceberg. Having said that, if leaving a suction drain for 24 hours in an oozy gallbladder fossa makes you happy, then be our guest. As long as you know that it may not always reflect the actual magnitude of bleeding.

Table 36.1. When to drain?

Here are the situations considered by experienced surgeons (like us...) as a 'reasonable reason' for drainage:

High probability of leakage of bile or pancreatic juice. A drain placed for a biliary or pancreatic leak may be life-saving and curative.	This is the number one indication, and rightly so.	Bile and pancreatic juice are well collected and evacuated by drains.
Established pus-containing abscess. This means that the abscess is 'non-collapsible' or 'thick-walled'.	This is the number two indication. Most surgeons believe that a well-formed collection of pus deserves a drain.	Pus collections associated with acute peritonitis are a different 'animal'. No drains are needed!
Not satisfied with 'source control'	This indication overlaps with other indications such as bile leak, urinary leak or the impossibility of exteriorizing a leaking proximal jejunum or duodenum.	
'Difficult' duodenal suture line	The 'difficult' duodenal stump after Billroth II gastrectomy is a reasonable indication for prophylactic drainage.	The retroperitoneal duodenum is more susceptible to leakage and thus draining it would make sense (e.g. after duodenotomy to control post-endoscopic retrograde cholangiopancreatography hemorrhage).
The urinary tract	Drain when urine leak is expected...	After repair of kidney, ureter or bladder injury...
High-risk UGI anastomoses	After esophageal or bariatric procedures that are high risk for leakage.	However, it is unlikely that you will construct any such anastomoses in the emergency situation...
Expected bleeding	Be selective. Almost never.	See the text above.

The 'optimal' drain

Preferably, all drains should be soft and malleable to minimize the *real* dangers of pressure necrosis and erosion of bowel and blood vessels. Drains are either 'active' or 'passive':

- **Active drains are connected to a source of suction**. They tend to be clogged by tissue or clots which are 'sucked in' — the higher the sucking pressure, the more prone to blockage the drain is. 'Sump' suction drains (double-lumen system) are more resistant to blockage but usually are of rigid construction and thus not considered safe for a prolonged stay in the peritoneal cavity.
- **Passive drains** work by capillary action, gravity or overflow caused by slight pressure differences. They are considered to be an 'open system', proven to be associated with contamination of the drain tract by retrograde spread of skin bacteria ("drains drain both ways!"). Theoretically, applying a sterile colostomy bag over a drain site should convert the open system to a closed one, but we doubt that this remains 'closed' for more than a day. Whether, as some claim, passive drains are relatively inefficient in the upper abdomen because of the negative, inward sucking pressures generated during respiration, is controversial. **Evidently, the larger the drain, the wider the exit opening in the skin — the more effective is the drainage but also the more it is prone to complications**.

But practically:

- The flat and soft 'active' JP (or the Blake® drain) is the only intraperitoneal drain that we use these days in routine practice (e.g. after 'difficult' cholecystectomy). This is the drain we would also use for indications such as a potential duodenal or pancreatic fistula.
- **If you are one of those who drain *peritonitis* remember that your suction drain will be plugged with fibrin and pus within a few hours, and your open passive drain would serve mostly as a one-way *autobahn* for skin bacteria**.
- **Those who place drains adjacent to *colonic anastomoses* — do you really believe that suction drains will evacuate feces?** To form a channel capable of transferring fecal material to the outside, one must use a large passive drain (e.g. corrugated) through a generous two-finger opening in the skin and abdominal wall. By doing so we would go back to the old days of drain-site hernias, intestinal obstruction, bleeding and drain-site abscess formation.

For a list of **complications of drains** look at ■ Table 36.2. These complications are *real*; some are rare, but we have experienced each of them in the dark ages of excessive drainage. Such complications can be prevented by the correct placement and management of drains (see ■ Table 36.3) or, better, avoiding drains when not indicated. **The glory days of drains are over for several reasons**:

- With improved surgical techniques, antibiotic administration, and better imaging, the results of emergency abdominal procedures are improving. Thus, surgeons are noticing fewer complications that could allegedly be prevented by drains. This has provided surgeons with a new sense of confidence — why should they leave drains if the drains seem mostly unnecessary?
- Readily available CT scanning has added to the surgeon's confidence. Now the mysterious postoperative abdominal cavity is no longer a black box. We do not need a drain to warn us that there is an abscess — we can see it on the CT.
- The immense success of image-guided percutaneous drainage of intra-abdominal collections and abscesses has obviously added to that confidence. And it has also taught us much about the methodology of drainage itself — **that you do not need huge tubes, for many days, to get rid of an abscess — the elaborate rituals surrounding the management of drains are evaporating as well**.

Table 36.2. Complications of intraperitoneal drains.
■ Drain 'fever'.
■ Drain tract infection.
■ Drain tract hernia.
■ Drain tract bleeding.
■ Intestinal obstruction.
■ Erosion of bowel.
■ Erosion of vessels.
■ Contamination of sterile tissues.
■ Prevention of healing of fistulas.
■ Failure to retrieve: caught by fascial sutures, torn, knotted or tissue sucked in/growing into drain.
■ 'Lost' drain: migration into the abdomen or breakage.

Table 36.3. The placement and management of drains.

Insertion:

- Choose a suitable drain for the specific job but in general go with the softest and smallest.
- Place the drain carefully in the desired region, trim it to remove excessive length but leave some 'slack'.
- Place it away from bowel wall or vessels.
- Try to bring omentum between the drain and vital structures to prevent erosion.
- Bring the drain out through the skin, away from the main wound to prevent wound infection.
- Plan the shortest track possible and depending on the indication for drainage and type of drain try to exit it in a dependent location.
- When closing the main wound be careful not to catch the adjacent drain with your fascial sutures.
- Secure the drain to the skin with sutures and tape.

Management:

- Use a closed system whenever possible.
- Use low suction to prevent sucking adjacent tissue into the drain's holes.
- To keep small-caliber tube drains patent they can be flushed twice daily with small amounts of saline under sterile conditions.
- When a fistula is established (e.g. biliary), suction can be disconnected and the drain connected to a dependent bag, draining on gravity.
- Be careful that the drain's tip is not abutting the visceral defect it is draining — this would prevent the closure of the defect: check for drain position with a sinogram.

Removal:

- Remove as soon as the drain is not productive or seems to have outlived its prophylactic task.
- Long-term drains should be removed in stages to prevent abscess formation in the deep tract.
- Removal and shortening of drains could be guided (selectively) with sinograms and/or CTs.
- When shortening the drain — refix it to the skin to prevent proximal migration.

- So modern surgeons have found out that they do not need drains to 'prevent or treat' persistent or recurrent infection after, say, perforated appendicitis. They have learned that most patients do well with source control (appendectomy) and antibiotics. And if not, they CT scan them, and if necessary, drain whatever is there under CT guidance.

Let us then repeat William Stewart Halsted's motto: "**No drainage is better than the ignorant employment of it**."

Final words...

The use of routine drainage in contaminated and infected abdominal surgery is declining but still practiced in some regions of the world. Drains should be used very selectively: when their placement is the only way to control the source of infection, to provide escape for highly predicted leaking fluids (bile, pancreatic juice, urine), to drain a non-collapsible abscess (a rare animal!), or to drain, for a short while, a very oozy surface. **Prophylactic drainage of the general peritoneal cavity is senseless** (■ Figure 36.1).

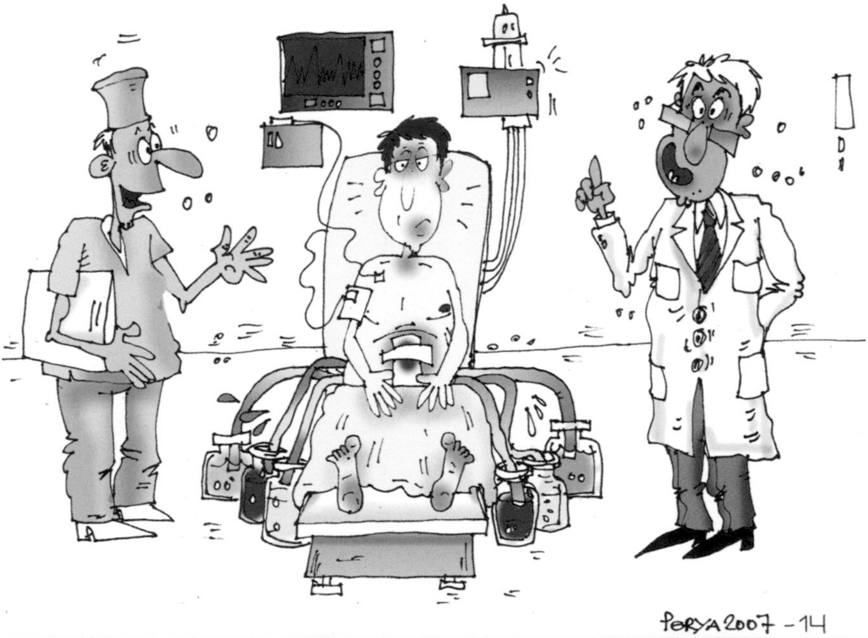

Figure 36.1. Confused resident: "Boss, he's still sick." Old-fashioned surgeon: "Perhaps we should have placed more drains..."

> **"Although more than five million surgical drains are used each year in the United States, their effectiveness, therapeutic indications, and efficiency remains an unsolved controversy."**
>
> **J. P. Moss**

Chapter 37

Abdominal closure

The Editors

> *Big bites, with a continuous monofilament suture and — above all — avoiding tension — this is how to avoid dehiscence and herniation.*

This is how we used to start this chapter in the previous editions. But as you will see below, part of this aphorism is considered now anachronistic.

It has been said that wherever three Jews meet — they immediately form five opposing political parties. The same applies to abdominal closure. If you ask 50 surgeons how they close the abdomen (we did ask) you will get 55 different versions. Your jaw will drop hearing some suggestions. Anyway, here we will share with you how we think it should be done. If you want to continue doing what your old boss has been teaching you — it is your choice.

So, finally, it is time to "get the hell out of here". You have been working all night and it is tempting to finish hastily. Impatience, however, is inadvisable since correct abdominal closure protects the patient from abdominal wound dehiscence (and later, from the development of a hernia) and it spares you a potential humiliation ('everybody knows'). **Yes, you are tired but, before closing, stop and think; ask your assistants: "Did we forget to do anything?" See the checklist in the next chapter**.

Generally, an abdominal closure fails because of poor quality of the tissues, increased intra-abdominal pressure, faulty technique, or a combination of these factors. Very rarely, a suture knot comes undone, or a damaged suture breaks, but more typically, the fault lies with the tissue and not the suture. In order to achieve secure closure, keep in mind (and hands) the following.

Suture material

Use slowly absorbable monofilament sutures (e.g. PDS® or Maxon®), but non-absorbable monofilament (e.g. nylon or Prolene®) would do as well. Rapidly absorbed material such as Vicryl® is still widely used even though its use is suboptimal in view of wound-repair kinetics. Those who fancy such suture material produce the hernias for the rest of us to repair. **Slowly absorbable or non-absorbable suture material, on the other hand, keeps the edges of the wound together until its own tensile strength takes over**.

Monofilament sutures are advantageous because they slide better, inflicting less 'saw injury' to the tissues and, when used in the preferred continuous fashion, distribute the tension evenly along the length of the wound. **The continued use by many surgeons of braided non-absorbable material (e.g. silk) — when so many better alternatives are available — is hard to understand. These sutures are associated with a tendency to produce chronic infected sinuses; they are highly reactive, and thus (when used intra-abdominally) promote fibrosis and adhesions. So stop using them for God's sake. Why are you so dogmatic?!**

The size of the suture matters. The heavier the suture — the more bulky becomes the knot. Such heavy knots tend to behave as foreign bodies in the depths of contaminated abdominal wounds — feeding an infected sinus. We observed this happening with PDS® as well. The sinuses did not close until the knots had been removed (it takes 200 days for the PDS® to be completely absorbed).

Monofilament material is not prone to breakage but damage to the suture during insertion can make this more likely. **It is therefore important to avoid grasping the suture material itself with forceps because this can damage its integrity and weaken it**.

> **Closing an abdomen is like catching a big fish** — the rules are the same: attach a line of good quality and the correct size to the hook with perfect knots; do not damage the line and keep it under optimal tension; if the fish fights then play with it for a while — if the patient starts waking up, wait for him to get 'deeper' — take your time and be patient. **If you don't follow the rules you will end up with postop dehiscence... or a hernia... and lose the fish**.

Closure of midline laparotomies: 'mass closure' vs. 'small-bite' closure

Until recently, mass closure has been the preferred technique. Many surgeons are still committed to it.

Mass closure entails single-layer suturing, using a heavy suture material, of ALL structures of the abdominal wall in a continuous manner to provide 'one strong scar'. The dogma here is to take large bites of tissue, at least 1cm away from the wound's edges; the bites closely spaced so as not to create gaps greater than 1cm. The intervening muscle is included in the bites.

However, over the last decade repeated randomized studies started emerging from Europe. They claimed that a 'small-bite closure' is advantageous over the above mentioned 'mass closure'.

The 'small-bite' method advocates **using lighter suture material (e.g. PDS®, 2-0) on smaller needles, taking 0.5cm bites in the medial edges of the fascia, closely spaced (0.5cm), and avoiding the muscle altogether. Results of such studies showed a lower incidence of dehiscence and hernia formation than when mass closure was used.** In one study, even the rate of wound infection was lower with small bites. The theoretical explanations for such surprising results include: less tissue damage/inflammation; a higher suture-to-wound ratio required to insert minimally spaced 'bites' translates to a better 'spring' effect which allows the tissues to 'breathe'; better force distribution along the fascial edge (■ Figure 37.1).

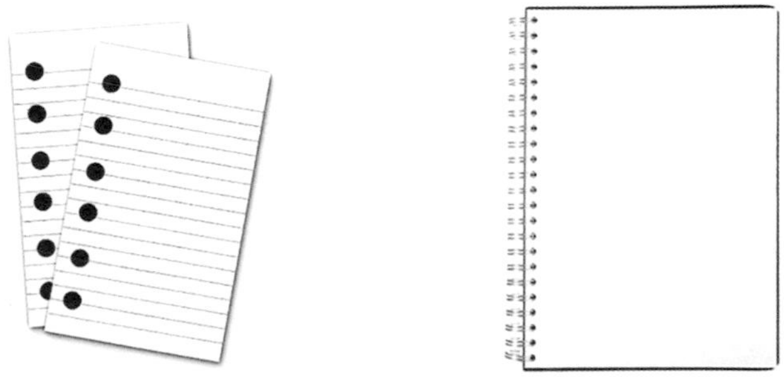

Figure 37.1. Try to rip a page from a 'mass closure' six-ring binder, compared to a page from a 'small bite' spring notebook. Kapisch?

As is often the case surgeons were (some still are) rather mistrustful: what about fat patients? What about distended ones? Would the 'small bites' be adequate? However, with experience came the confidence; after all — experienced fishermen are able to catch a 50-pound fish on a 5-pound test line☺.

Even the Editors differ in the way they close midline abdominal incisions: Paul still prefers the 'mass closure', albeit modified to avoid too much muscle if possible; Moshe is now committed to the '2-0 PDS® small bites' (his impression is that postoperative pain is diminished with this technique — no wonder: less tissue strangulation); and Danny prefers to avoid a midline laparotomy altogether...

But here are some additional points, which apply to any closure technique you decide to use:

- **The correct tension to be set on the suture is important** (■ Figure 37.2). If you pull the suture **too tight** the tissue is strangulated and necrosed, which may cause the sutures to cut through the tissue — the source of the so-called 'buttonhole hernias'. But if you keep the suture **too loose** the wound edges gape. Bear in mind that the muscles are

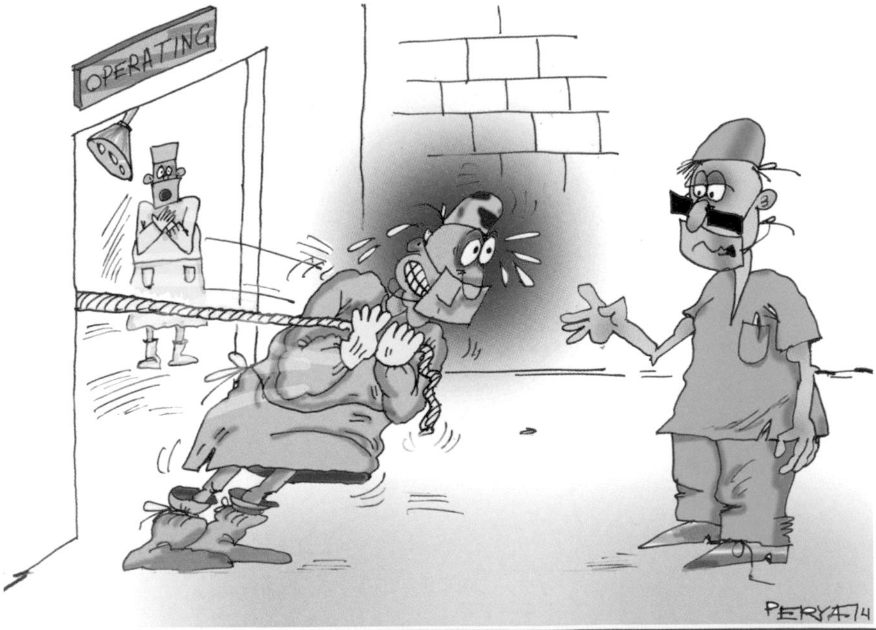

Figure 37.2. "Jack, what are you doing?"... "The boss told me to close it tight..."

relaxed as you close (or should be) and that postoperatively they will acquire their normal tone, the tissues in the wound will swell and abdominal girth will increase. All of these changes make the wound closure tighter; if it is tight when you put the sutures in then something must give way when these changes take place — the tissue tears. **A suture-length to wound-length ratio of at least 4:1 will ensure a moderate but secure tension of closure** (well, one always needs some excess to tie the knot… and since we usually start from both ends we have to use more suture length… so we are not too obsessed about measuring the exact length of suture…).

- **The corners (ends) of the incision** are the Achilles' heel of closure, especially the corner that is closed last. Do not compromise complete closure of the corner because you are afraid of injuring the underlying bowel; there are good tricks to accomplish this endeavor — learn them from one of your mentors. (If you don't have a mentor just e-mail us.) A good way to avoid difficult 'corners' is to start closing from both ends and tie the two sutures in the middle of the wound. If one uses a single suture then the final (corner) knot in our hands would be the 'Aberdeen' one — you can learn it on YouTube. We cut it long — about 5mm — and bury it deep in the subcutaneous space with any thin absorbable suture. Be careful with the knots. Our friend Berni Cristalli of Paris said: "I once asked my boss why he tied his knots seven times? 'Last time I did six, it didn't hold', was his reply."
- **Do not harm the underlying bowel**, which frequently bulges towards your needle. At the end of the operation the anesthetist always swears to God that the patient is 'maximally relaxed'; he often lies. Make him relax the patient again — do not concede. Protect the bowel by whichever instrument is available, the best, in our experience, being the commercially available rubber Fish® retractor. The assistant's hand also may be useful for this purpose but with all the hepatitis and HIV around we do not find many volunteers willing to offer a retracting hand, except our own.
- What about the 'looped' monofilament sutures which were so popular for abdominal closure? Well, with the drift toward 'small-bite' closure, using two heavy strands of suture (and the huge knot it creates) no longer makes sense to us. Dump it!

Closure of 'transverse' laparotomies

Most surgeons, including us, prefer a layered closure. For example, to close a subcostal incision we would run a PDS® 2-0 (here even heavy Vicryl® is OK) from the midline laterally — taking the posterior sheath together with the peritoneum. Next the anterior fascia is closed with a running suture starting at the lateral corner, tying the knot at the medial corner of the incision. There is no need to approximate the muscles.

The subcutaneous space

Now when the fascia is closed what to do with the subcutis? Some people (we did too) would say 'nothing', stating that there is no evidence that the so-called dead space reduction using subcutaneous fat approximation reduces wound complications; that subcutaneous sutures act like a foreign body and strangulate viable fat while not producing a more satisfactory wound. However, over the years we have realized that careful approximation of the subcutaneous layer (we use interrupted Vicryl® 3-0) produces 'healthier' and better-looking wounds. The subcut sutures support the skin closure. From time to time we see patients returning with gaping dehisced wounds a few hours after their skin sutures (or stapler) were removed. We know immediately that their surgeon ignored the subcut layer. In addition, if fascial dehiscence develops, the proper closure of the subcut-skin complex prevents 'complete dehiscence' and the need for immediate reoperation, as discussed in ➲ Chapter 45. A hernia is better than the gut falling out. Eh?

Subcutaneous drains increase the rate of infection and are indicated only in selective situations — see below and in ➲ Chapter 46. If you are unfortunate to have a boss who is forcing you to use such drains routinely, then remove them within 24-48 hours — sucking out moist fat has no real value.

Plain *saline irrigation* has been shown to be useless, but you can irrigate the wound liberally, telling the nurse "bring the Holy Water!" Making the OR team happy is almost as important as preventing wound complications... if not more. We suppose you could even try educating the OR team about the futility of dogmas...

The use of topical antibiotics (solution or powder) has been demonstrated to further decrease wound infection rates in contaminated wounds in patients who have already received systemic antibiotic prophylaxis. One of the editors (guess who?) is still a believer...

'Delayed primary' or 'secondary' closure

What about the ritual of delayed primary or secondary closure after contaminated or infected laparotomies?

We believe that these techniques are only rarely indicated. Despite surgeons' obsession with tradition, lessons learned years ago under certain circumstances are not necessarily true today. These days, with proper surgical technique and modern antibiotic administration, primary closure of the wound can be undertaken uneventfully in almost all emergency laparotomy cases. When a wound infection develops it usually responds to local measures. **Leaving all contaminated wounds gaping open — awaiting spontaneous or secondary closure — produces unnecessary physical and financial morbidity**.

Only rarely do we decide to leave a wound open, mostly in patients with planned reoperations or in the relaparotomized abdomen. In most patients — including those with established purulent or even fecal peritonitis — we irrigate the subcutaneous tissues and close them and the skin with interrupted sutures.

Studies show that early evacuation of exudate forming in the depths of fresh contaminated incisions prevents the development of infections. Therefore, in the high-risk-for-infection patients, including for example the "fat guy with a badly perforated appendix" we use a **'middle of the road' option**. This involves inserting 'wicks' (like candle wicks) between the sutures into the depths of the wound; the 'wicks' — which you can create by cutting strips from a patch of Telfa™ gauze — are removed on the third postoperative day. A simpler alternative is to leave a **Penrose drain** in the depths of the wound (below the layered closure) for 48-72 hours. We use these techniques quite often — and only very rarely do we have a wound infection despite skin closure. Believe us.

An occasional wound infection is not a disaster and is simple to treat (➲ Chapter 46).

Of course, after uncomplicated procedures, with no or limited contamination, **modern surgeons are happy to close most wounds with a subcuticular stitch of absorbable material**. This obviates the discomfort and expense of arranging staple or suture removal and gives a much neater scar. (This is the only part of your handiwork that the family and the patient can see, and you'd be surprised to discover how much this little thing matters to most patients!). A layer of *Dermabond®* (or your favourite cyanoacrylate-based glue) applied over the wound tends to protect it from 'minor problems' and from leakage from adjacent stomas. However, nothing is perfect in life, and even beautifully placed subcuticular absorbable monofilament can start 'spitting' from the wound weeks after the operation.

The high-risk abdominal closure

Classically, in patients with systemic (e.g. cancer) or local (e.g. abdominal distension) factors predisposing to abdominal dehiscence (➲ Chapter 45), 'retention' sutures were used (and still are) by surgeons. Those heavy 'through-and-through', interrupted sutures take bites of at least 2cm through all abdominal-wall layers — including the skin — preventing evisceration but not the occurrence of late hernia formation.

We don't appreciate these classic *retention* sutures, which cut through the skin and produce parietal damage (e.g. tissue necrosis, abdominal wall infection) and ugly skin wounds and scars. **Moreover, the use of retention sutures, together with abdominal distension, results in intra-abdominal hypertension**. Forceful closure under excessive tension may result in an abdominal compartment syndrome with its deleterious physiological consequences (➲ Chapter 31). Thus, when the fascia is destroyed as is often the case after multiple abdominal re-entries, or when closure may produce excessive intra-abdominal pressure, **we suggest that you do not**

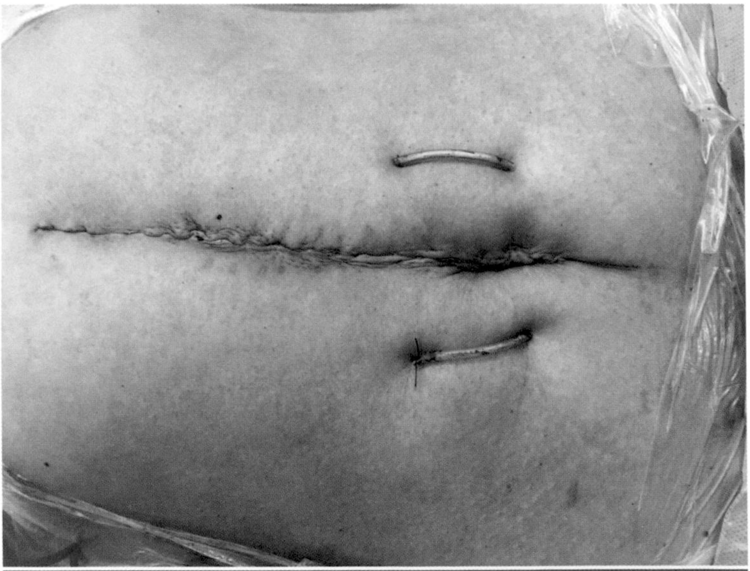

Figure 37.3. A single horizontal mattress retention suture was added to reinforce the closure where a tumor was resected from the abdominal wall. The suture is tied without excessive tension, but will add force to the closure if abdominal tension increases postoperatively. Its configuration leaves the abdominal wound exposed, allowing for wound care as needed. It also results in a better cosmetic result, preventing the long ugly scars across the incision.

close the abdomen but cover it with a temporary abdominal closure device (TACD — 'laparostomy') (➲ Chapter 44).

However, in indeterminate/intermediate cases, when a high risk for dehiscence exists without immediate abdominal hypertension, a few retention sutures may prevent evisceration and the need to return to the OR. Placing them as horizontal mattress sutures, without crossing the skin, will cause less disfiguring scarring, and allows for appropriate wound care (■ Figure 37.3).

Closing the skin only

Occasionally, in situations when we wish to avoid fascial closure — or it is deemed impossible — but do not want to condemn the patient to the not insignificant morbidity associated with *laparostomy*, **we leave the fascia unsutured but close the skin**.

Scenarios ideal for such an approach would be when you feel that no reoperation would be necessary but visceral 'bulging' prevents fascial closure without excessive tension.

> **A classic example**: a morbidly obese patient with a strangulated giant incisional hernia, necessitating bowel resection. One has to be almost crazy to insist on closure of the fascia... (oh, there are enough crazies around...).

Of course, all surviving patients will develop (or continue to have) a large incisional hernia; the very old and infirm will live with the hernia for the rest of their lives. In others, an elective repair of the hernia is associated with lower morbidity than the staged management of laparostomy. **How to do it**: always spread the omentum, if available, over the viscera; the skin is closed with 2-0 nylon interrupted mattress sutures, taking bites of at least 1cm from the skin edge. We advise to add a generous subcutaneus layer to make it watertight and 'stronger'. **And please, please, do not let anyone remove these sutures until you approve — usually not before 3 weeks**. We hope that you understand why...

Remember — the patient's own normal skin is better than the VAC system or skin grafts.

P.S.: Some, obsessed with the need to 'close the fascia' — even if it is unfeasible — would bridge the defect with one of those mega $ 'bioprostheses' — the brand and composition of which seem to change from one conference to the next. They believe that in doing so they prevent a hernia. **Let them believe.**

In conclusion: if old dogs like us can learn new tricks, you can too. Try the 'small bites' closure. Don't leave wounds open unnecessarily!

Closure of laparoscopic ports

However small they are, trocar site wounds are not devoid of complications, and trocar site hernia is a real entity. While in children even 5mm incisions may be significant, in adults these small holes are left alone, closing the skin only. **But 10mm and larger wounds may (rarely) cause acute postoperative bowel incarceration or lead to later development of small and not-so-small hernias.**

Closing the fascial defect is such a hassle, especially in obese patients, that many surgeons elect to avoid it. Some surgeons intentionally place the trocars *obliquely*, hoping that the transabdominal 'canal' will collapse and close. Some just leave them open, trusting that the resultant hernia will be fixed by a hernia surgeon… and indeed — why would the patient return to her gynecologist?

But we trust you that you would not like to leave an abdominal wall defect that may ruin your perfect laparoscopy, forcing you to return in the middle of the night to release the stuck bowel (or God forbid resect it — ■ Figure 37.4). And surely you would not like the pretty patient with the scar well hidden in the umbilicus (were you tempted to try single-trocar surgery?) to come back with an unsightly umbilical bulge.

So how to do it? In most cases a pair of small retractors will help you expose the fascia and simply close it with a figure-of-8 absorbable suture — it should be enough. In more challenging conditions you can use a **suture-passer** to close the fascia under laparoscopic vision, placing the scope through another port. If budget allows, there are some more sophisticated port closure devices on the market, which make it a snap. You may consider adding them to the patient's bill if you are a busy bariatric surgeon. Time is money!

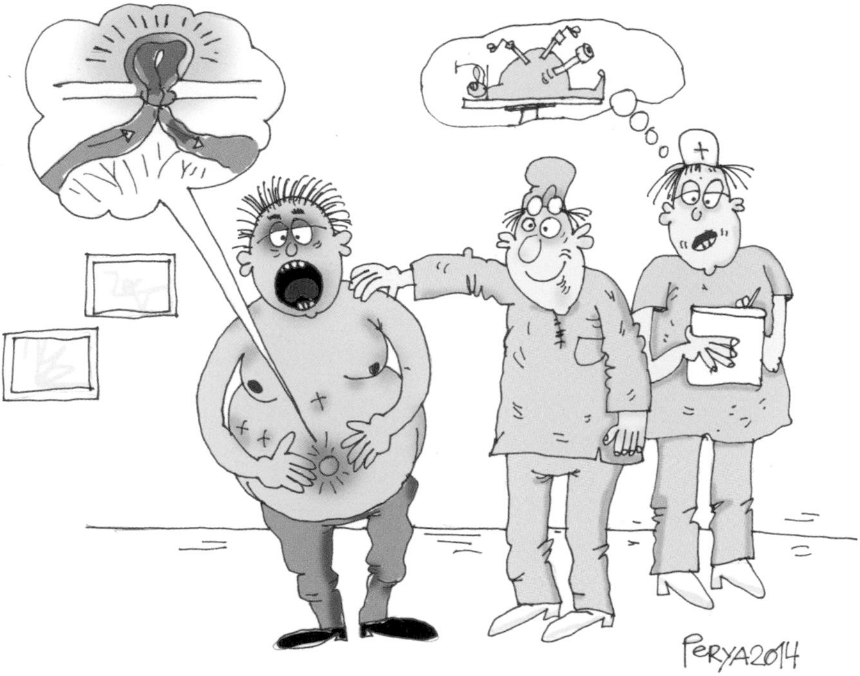

Figure 37.4. Resident: "Sir, last week this patient underwent a lap chole for biliary dyskinesia..." Surgeon: "The good news is that the dyskinesia has been cured..."

Abdominal binder

At the end of the procedure, before the patient is rolled off the table, we apply a *Velcro* abdominal binder (over the dressing) to 'support' the abdominal closure. The binder provides a counter-pressure to the intra-abdominal pressure thus negating bursting forces. With the binder applied, the patient may develop an incisional hernia but you will never see a free dehiscence. Don't laugh at the binder before you see how it helps patients to ambulate early, with reduced discomfort. Of course, the binders come in all sizes and should not be applied so tightly as to produce an abdominal compartment syndrome. They should be opened when the patient lies in bed.

Final point: close up by yourself! If you have residents, then be present and teach them how to do it correctly. An unsupervised second-year resident closing the abdomen, an unsupervised first-year registrar closing the skin — this is a good way to produce a nice series of abdominal dehiscence and increase the rate of wound complications.

"Abdominal closure: if it looks all right, it's too tight — if it looks too loose, it's all right."

Matt Oliver

Chapter 38

Before landing

The Editors

> *Take-offs are optional. Landings are mandatory.*
>
> *Pilots may have more incentive than surgeons to be perfect, right or wrong. When they botch a landing, it's usually their last. Fortunately, modern day aircraft are a lot more predictable and reliable than any of our patients.*
>
> **Tim Eldridge**

[Obviously, this quote was coined before the Boeing 737 Max affair...]

Everyone knows that a 'good landing' is one from which you can walk away. But very few know the definition of a 'great landing'. **It's one after which you can use the airplane another time**. Yes, we know that you are tired; you may have worked all night, and this may be the last of many long cases. But any landing must be perfect and even this last operation must succeed.

Before closing the abdomen you must be absolutely happy with what you did. You don't want to spend the next week with guilt and worry as your patient fails to recover promptly. Prevent 'guilt-worry'. Always ask yourself "Am I totally satisfied with my procedure?" (■ Figure 38.1).

Don't silence the little voice within you that informs you that the anastomosis is somewhat dusky, or it needs another stitch. A little paranoia makes you a better surgeon, and your patients have fewer complications. You must be absolutely convinced, at this stage, that you have done the best that your patient deserves.

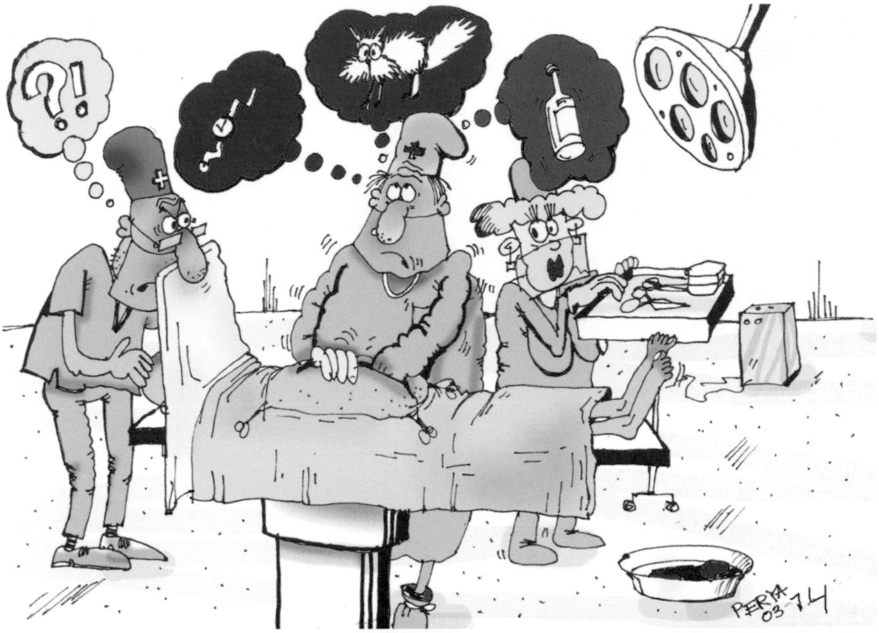

Figure 38.1. "Am I satisfied?"

If not, swallow your pride, summon the last vestige of your patience, do it again, or call for help. Hiding a potential problem will not solve it. And you will go back to sleep so much better. However, bear in mind that — to paraphrase Voltaire — **better is the enemy of good**. You must be sure that any attempts to improve a less-than-perfect situation are justified. (Remember the philosophy of the abbreviated laparotomy.) There's a thin line separating healthy perfectionism from pathological OCD.

You may want to go over a pre-closure checklist — see ■ Table 38.1.

Do not compromise. Keep looking around; there's always something you've missed. **Remember: when the abdomen is open you control it, when closed it controls you!**

And then, even if everything seems perfect, you will start worrying — nay, you have to worry. The more experience you gain the more you will worry, going over in your mind everything that, from now on, may go wrong within that abdominal 'black box'.

Table 38.1. Pre-closure checklist.

- ■ **Hemostasis perfect?** This does not mean that you have to run after each red blood corpuscle...
- ■ **Source control** achieved?
- ■ **Peritoneal 'toilet'** completed? All fluid sucked out?
- ■ **Anastomosis:** Viable? Not under tension, lying well?
- ■ Potential sites for **internal herniation** dealt with?
- ■ **Small bowel** comfortably arranged in place below the transverse colon? (Remember that jejunum belongs to the upper part of the abdomen and ileum to the lower part... ☺)
- ■ **Omentum** placed between intestine and incision; and if possible covering the anastomosis?
- ■ All additional **fascial defects** (e.g. trocar sites) closed?
- ■ **Nasogastric tube** in position (if needed)?
- ■ **Drains** (only if indicated!) in place?
- ■ **Instrument and sponge count OK?** (Is everybody sure?)
- ■ Need a **feeding jejunostomy?**
- ■ **Should I close** the abdomen at all? Or leave it open?

Happy landing!

> **"I have many colleagues of varying levels of knowledge and skill. But the ones I trust most are the ones that worry. You can see the concern, sometimes even anguish on their faces. Then, there are the sociopaths..."**
>
> **Tom Gilas**
>
> **"There are old pilots, and there are reckless pilots, but there are no old, reckless pilots! There are however old, reckless surgeons — but their patients do not live long..."**
>
> **Moshe**

PART IV

After the operation

Chapter 39

Postoperative care

The Editors

> *When is a surgeon... nervous? Not during operations. But basically a surgeon's nervousness begins after the operations, when for some reason the patient's temperature refuses to drop or a stomach remains bloated and one has to open it not with a knife, but in one's mind, to see what had happened, to understand and put it right. When time is slipping away, you have to grab it by the tail.*
>
> **Alexander Solzhenitsyn *(Cancer Ward)***

> *We repeat: As long as the abdomen is open you control it. Once closed it controls you.*

The long operation is finished, leaving you to savor the sweet postoperative 'high' and elation. But very soon, when your serum levels of endorphins decline, you start worrying about the outcome. And worry you must, for the cocksure, macho attitude is a recipe for disaster. We do not intend to bring here a detailed discussion of postoperative care or to write a new surgical intensive care manual. (For an in-depth discussion on how to prevent and treat postoperative complications look at our *Schein's Common Sense Prevention and Management of Surgical Complications.*) We only wish to share with you some basic precepts, which may have been forgotten, drowned in a sea of fancy technology and gimmicks (and endless electronic paperwork). **The following are a few practical commandments for postoperative care**.

Know your patient

This is no joke! How often do we encounter a postoperative patient looked after by someone who has no clue about the patient's pre-operative and intra-operative details? The emerging 'shift mentality', the ever increasing clutter of the EMR, and the increasing reliance on physicians who call themselves 'hospitalists' are depriving the modern surgical patient of direct contact with his surgeon! Mistakes in management are more commonly made by those who 'temporarily adopt' the case. **Once you operate on a patient, he or she is yours forever...!**

Shared responsibility often means that no one is responsible! (See more in the section "Be the leader and take responsibility".)

Touch/examine your patient

Not only from the foot of the bed. Examining the chart — or browsing the EMR from your laptop at home — or even looking at the ICU monitor is not enough. **Look at the patient, smell and palpate him at least twice a day**. Wouldn't it be embarrassing to load your patient with intravenous antibiotics or CT scan his abdomen, while an unsuspected abscess is cooking under the wound dressing, begging to be simply drained at the bedside?

> Leo Tolstoy wrote in *War and Peace*:
>
> *When he came to himself the splintered portions of his thigh bone had been extracted, the torn flesh cut away and the wound bandaged. Water was being sprinkled on his face. As soon as Prince Andrei opened his eyes the doctor bent down, kissed him on the lips with not a word and hurried away.*

We do not ask you to kiss your patients — just touch them! And you may hug their elderly wives (but please be careful with the young ones...).

Treat the pain

You know the different drugs, and their modes of administration. Sure, you always prescribe postoperative analgesia, but ordering is not nearly enough. Most randomly questioned postoperative patients complain that they are under-treated for pain. Nurses tend to be stingy with analgesia. You are the man on the spot; see that your patient does not suffer unnecessarily. Find the correct balance between effective analgesia and narcotic overuse. There are many alternatives on the market, but don't be afraid of morphine, when this cheap and effective drug is needed.

Do not 'crucify' your patient in the horizontal position

Typically, the modern patient is 'crucified' horizontally, tethered by a spaghetti of monitoring cables, nasogastric tubes, venous lines, drains, leg pumps and urinary catheters. **Free the patient from these paraphernalia as soon as possible; the nurses won't do it without your order. The earlier your patient is out of bed, sitting or walking about, the faster he will be going home**. Conversely, keeping the patient in the supine position increases the incidence of atelectasis/pneumonia, deep vein thrombosis, decubitus ulcers, and prolongs paralytic ileus, all adding fuel to the inflammatory fire. **Have your patient out of bed ASAP and this often means only a few hours after the operation. If the nurses are reluctant or 'too busy', lift the patient out of bed by yourself — lead by example!**

Decrease the plastic and rubber load

The monitoring of vital signs functions as an early warning system to detect physiological disturbances so that prompt corrective therapy can be instituted. **The invasiveness of monitoring employed in the individual patient should be proportionate to the severity of the disease: the sicker the patient, the greater the number of monitoring tubes used, the higher the likely morbidity and mortality**.

Complete discussion of the continuously growing number of monitoring methods available today is beyond the scope of this chapter. However, please note:

- In order to be able to respond to monitor-generated warning signs you must fully understand the technology being employed. **You should be able to distinguish between real acute physiological changes and electrical or mechanical artifacts of observation**.
- Understand that all methods of monitoring are liable to a myriad of potential errors, specific to the technique or caused by patient-related variables. Alertness and sound clinical judgment are paramount!
- Because of improving technology, monitoring is becoming more and more sophisticated (and expensive). Furthermore, monitoring techniques are responsible for a significant number of iatrogenic

complications in the surgical intensive care unit. **Use monitoring discriminatingly and do not succumb to the *Everest syndrome*: "I climb it because it is there.**" Before embarking on invasive monitoring ask yourself "Does this patient really need it?" Remember there are safer and cheaper alternatives to invasive monitoring: for example, in a stable patient, remove the arterial line, as the blood pressure can be measured with a conventional sphygmomanometer, PO_2 determined transcutaneously, and blood tests drawn by phlebotomy. **Each time you see your patient ask yourself which of the following can be removed**: nasogastric tube, Swan-Ganz catheter, central venous line, arterial line, peripheral venous line, Foley catheter?

Nasogastric (NG) tubes. Prolonged postoperative NG decompression to combat gastric and intestinal ileus is a common ritual. The concept that the NG tube 'protects' distally-placed bowel anastomoses is ridiculous, as liters of juices are secreted each day below the decompressed stomach. Nasogastric tubes are extremely irritating to the patient, interfere with breathing, cause esophageal erosions and promote gastroesophageal reflux. Traditionally, surgeons keep the tube until the daily output drops below a certain volume (e.g. 400ml); such a policy often results in unnecessary torture. It has been repeatedly demonstrated that most post-laparotomy patients do not need nasogastric decompression — not even following upper gastrointestinal procedures — or need it for a day or two at most. **In fully conscious patients, who are able to protect their airway from aspiration, NG tubes can be safely omitted in most patients. However, following an emergency abdominal operation, nasogastric decompression is compulsory in mechanically ventilated patients, in obtunded patients, and after operations for intestinal obstruction**. In all other cases, consider removing the NG tube on the morning after surgery. If in doubt you may want to cap or clamp the tube for 12 hours and observe how this is tolerated by the patient before removing it. A small percentage of patients will need the tube to be reinserted because of persistent ileus or early postoperative small bowel obstruction (➲ Chapter 41).

Drains. Despite the widely publicized dictum that it is impossible to drain the free peritoneal cavity effectively, drains are still commonly used and misused. As you read already in ➲ Chapter 36, we suggest that you limit the use of drains to the evacuation of an established abscess, to allow escape of potential visceral secretions (e.g. biliary, pancreatic) and to establish a controlled intestinal fistula when the bowel cannot be exteriorized. **Remove drains as soon as they have fulfilled their purpose.**

Obtain postoperative tests selectively

***Unnecessary* diagnostic procedures or *interpretative* errors in *indicated* diagnostic procedures commonly result in *false-positive* findings, leading in turn to an increasingly invasive escalation of diagnostic or therapeutic measures.** Added morbidity is the invariable price. If the results of a test are not going to affect your management, don't order the test. **Those who order routine daily serial blood counts or CRP prove their clinical immaturity.**

Realize that the problem usually lies at the operative site

The cause of fever or a 'septic state' in the surgical patient is usually at the primary site of operation unless proven otherwise. Do not become a 'surgical ostrich' by treating your patient for 'pneumonia' while he is slowly sinking in multiple organ failure from an intra-abdominal abscess (■ Figure 39.1).

Remember: In the postoperative patient everything is related to the operation unless proven otherwise — so your patient is tachypneic after his laparotomy not only due to exacerbation of his COPD, but mainly because you closed his tummy too tight!

Temperature is not a disease; do not treat it as such

Postoperative fever represents the patient's inflammatory response to different insults including infection as well as surgical trauma, atelectasis, transfusion and others. Fever does not equal sepsis **and therefore should not be treated automatically with antibiotics. Also, it should not be stifled with**

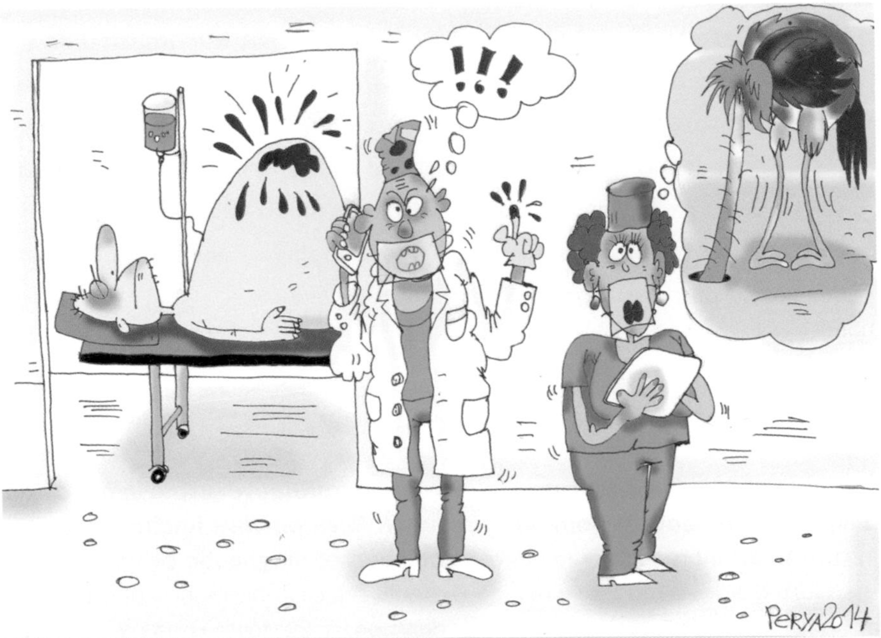

Figure 39.1. "Are you a surgical ostrich?"

antipyretics, as the febrile response has been shown to be beneficial to the host's defenses. You will have to argue with your nurses about this. "The patient will be more comfortable, he'll convulse, we always give Tylenol®," they will claim. **The absolute level of temperature is of less importance than its trend and it's difficult to assess this important sign when you are artificially suppressing it**. You know, fever is not a disease caused by the absence of antibiotics.

> *Fever is, in a measure, a beneficial process operating to protect the economy.*
>
> **Augustus Charles Bernays**

(This was said by that German surgeon in the 19th century…).

Avoid poisoning your patient with antibiotics

Tailor antibiotic administration to the patient. Avoid the common practice of administering antibiotics for as long as the patient is in the hospital and beyond (➲ Chapter 40).

Be frugal with blood-product transfusions

Generally, the amount of blood or derived products transfused inversely and independently correlates with the outcome of the acute surgical disease. Donated blood is immunosuppressive and is associated with an increased risk of infection, sepsis and organ failure, not to mention the other well-known hazards. Cancer patients in particular fare worse in the long term if they receive a transfusion. **Transfuse your patient only if absolutely necessary**. A patient 'requiring' only one unit of blood may not require any at all, but if needed, the second unit should not follow automatically. **For the vast majority of patients, a hematocrit of 30% is more than satisfactory. We would rarely transfuse a postoperative patient with a hemoglobin above 8g/dL unless he is critically ill or suffers from an underlying cardiorespiratory disease**. Those at risk of recurrent hemorrhage, from upper GI bleeding, for example, may need a higher baseline.

Do not drown your patient in salty water

Excessive postoperative fluid administration provides too much water and salt, resulting in obligatory weight gain and swelling of tissues. **And edematous tissues do not function well nor do they heal well — causing a higher rate of medical and surgical complications** (see ➲ Chapter 6). All your patient needs is enough water to replace insensible losses (500-1000ml) and to provide for urinary flow of 0.5ml/kg per hour. Additional losses (e.g. NG tube) should be replaced selectively on an ad hoc basis, but carelessly writing an order for 150ml/hour of saline and going to sleep will result in a swollen patient.

According to Tim Fabian: "**Patients never die of fluid overload on the medical service or dehydration on the surgical one**." **But the opposite may be true. You need to fine tune the fluid balance in real time and that means doing it more than once a day...** We do not hesitate adding a drop of *Lasix®* (furosemide) early on, to overcome the 'antidiuretic response' typical to the postoperative state (and the obligatory overhydration by anesthesia...) — this is especially of value in patients who have been receiving diuretics before the operation. **And get rid of the intravenous line as soon as possible!**

> *Fluids given intravenously bypass all the defenses set up by the body to protect itself against excess of any constituent, against bacterial entry... they give the patient what the surgeon thinks his tissues need and what they are damned well going to get.*
>
> **William Heneage Ogilvie**

Do not starve or over-feed your patient

Read more about postoperative nutrition at the end of this chapter.

Recognize and treat postoperative intra-abdominal hypertension

This is so important that we have dedicated an entire chapter to it. Please read ➲ Chapter 31 — "The abdominal compartment syndrome". Don't be lazy!

Prevent deep vein thrombosis (DVT) and pulmonary embolism

It is easy to forget DVT prophylaxis in the pre-operative chaos of emergency surgery. As a pilot goes over a checklist prior to any flight — you should be the one to inject the subcutaneous heparin and place the anti-DVT pneumatic device — *before* the operation. DVT prophylaxis should be continued *postoperatively* as long as the patient continues to be at high risk of thrombosis. **Selected patients (e.g. after operations for cancer) may need to continue DVT prophylaxis at home**. Do remember however that anticoagulation is not good for patients at risk of bleeding to death...

Be the leader and take responsibility

Many people tend to dance around your postoperative patient, giving consults and advice. But remember, this is not their patient; he or she is yours. At the Morbidity and Mortality meeting (or in court), the others will say "I just gave a consult — it was his patient..." (➲ Chapter 47). **The ultimate responsibility for all aspects of your patient's management falls squarely on your shoulders**.

Know when you need help and request it, preferably from one of your mentors. As Francis D. Moore said: "**Seek consultation even if it is not sure to help; never be a lone wolf**." But solicit advice judiciously and apply it selectively. **Relinquishing blindly the care of your postoperative patient to anesthesiologists, medical intensivists, hospitalists, or other modern 'experts' may be a recipe for disaster — oh, how common it is and how often we have had to relearn this message from sad experience**.

It is much better in this era to form close working relationships with colleagues who share your philosophy of care and who have expertise in areas beyond your own. We all need help with patients suffering multi-system failure;

while we can take care of the abdominal problem we do need assistance and advice to manage cardiac, respiratory and renal failure appropriately. As Mark M. Ravitch said: **"The problem with calling in a consultant is that you may feel obliged to take his advice"** (■ Figure 39.2).

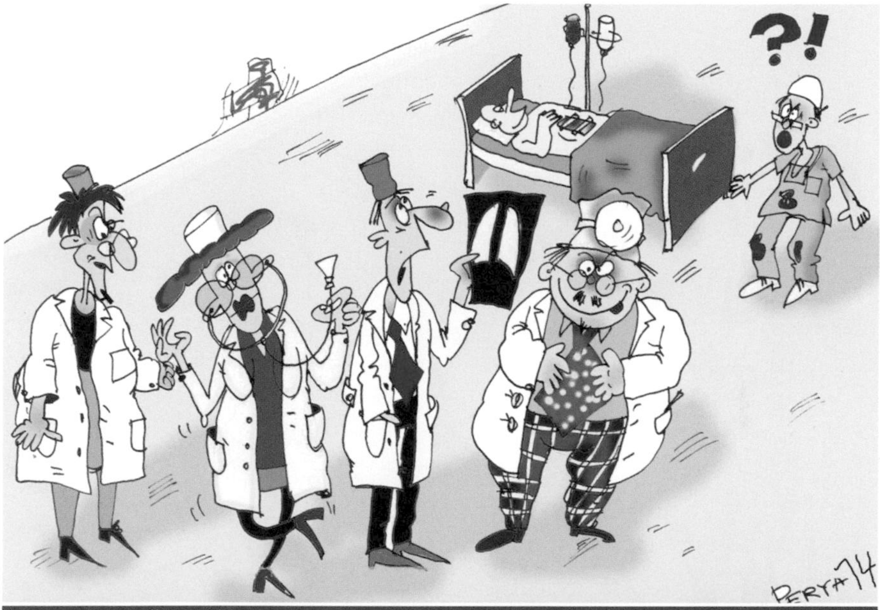

Figure 39.2. "Who is missing, guys? Where is the podiatrist?"

Another thing: if what the consultant advises seems clear nonsense, change the consultant. Or ignore him!

Analyze your care

When all is said and done, step back and assess your management. Ask yourself "What did I do well?", "What could I do better the next time I'm confronted with a situation like this?" How else will you get any better?

Oops, what about ERAS (enhanced recovery after surgery), you may ask — why didn't they mention this catchphrase? Well, despite the ever-growing number of guidelines and protocols, and abstracts and publications, there is nothing new here. It is all 'common sense' and discussed above and depicted in ■ Figure 39.3.

The operation is over when the patient is eating a cheeseburger and can't remember your name.

Leo A. Gordon

Big surgeons are those who are not too big to deal with the small things!

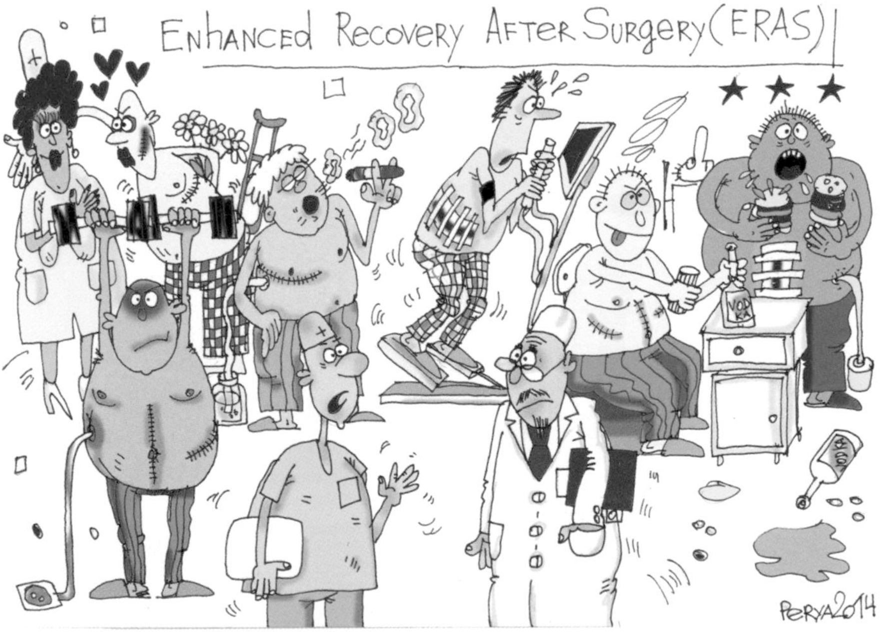

Figure 39.3. A surgeon to a visiting professor: "Sir, we have implemented an ERAS protocol."

Postoperative nutrition[1]

In every disease it is a good sign when the patient's intellect is sound, and he is disposed to take whatever food is offered to him; but the contrary is bad.

Hippocrates

God created man with a mouth, a stomach and gut — not a TPN line.

1 Dr. James Rucinski, MD FACS, contributed to this section in previous editions.

Use the enteral route whenever possible. Keep the enterocytes happy, start oral feeding on day 1, let the patient decide how much he wants to drink/eat, and stop only if the patient vomits. Perhaps this is all one needs to know. However, a few of you may want to hear more…

Starvation

Starvation results in a state of adaptation. After hepatic glycogen stores are consumed in 24-48 hours, the liver synthesizes glucose, using amino acids derived from protein breakdown. This 'auto-cannibalization' of functional protein stores is ameliorated, to some degree, by conversion to ketone metabolism of the two major 'obligate' glucose users: the central nervous system and the kidney. Fat stores help by providing ketones and, through glycerol metabolism, adding a small amount of glucose. **Injury, illness or operation greatly increases the demand for glucose to answer the consequent hyper-metabolic demands and to provide energy for wound repair and for the bone marrow and its offspring, the leukocytes. The end result is the breakdown of protein leading to a general debility, impaired reparative processes, attenuated immune function and respiratory muscle weakness that in turn may cause atelectasis, pneumonia, ventilator-dependence and death**.

The need for nutritional support is based on:

- Your physical and laboratory assessment of the patient's *nutritional reserves*.
- An estimate of the *associated stress of the underlying illness*.
- An estimate of the *time interval* that will pass before the patient can resume a normal diet.

Assessment of need for nutritional support

You must ask patients how long they have felt sick, when did they last eat and how much weight they have lost, if any. **A loss of more than 10% is associated with a higher rate of complications and death after abdominal surgery**.

Serum albumin level reflects the balance of synthesis and degradation of one of the products of hepatic metabolism. In the emergency setting, the albumin level and total lymphocyte count will be the only obtainable laboratory parameters for you to estimate *available reserves.* **A serum albumin level of <3mg/dL and a total lymphocyte count <1500 cells/µl predict increased postoperative morbidity and mortality.**

The predicted time interval that will pass before the patient can resume a normal diet is important. For example, a person with 'simple' acute appendicitis will experience cessation of normal feeding for a period of 24-72 hours; a person with perforated diverticulitis and generalized peritonitis may experience cessation of feeding for a period of perhaps 5-7 days. But patients who develop complications, such as an anastomotic leak or ileus may be deprived of normal oral food intake for as long as 10-14 days — or even longer.

With the above information you can decide which patients will be most likely to benefit from nutritional support:

- At one end of the spectrum, the patient with normal reserves by history and examination, with minimal to moderate associated stress, and with less than 7-10 days estimated before resumption of a normal diet, is unlikely to benefit from nutritional support.
- At the other end of the spectrum, the patient with depleted available reserves, moderate to severe stress, and with more than 7-10 days estimated before resumption of a normal diet, is likely to benefit from nutritional support.

Enteral versus parenteral nutrition

Nutritional support may be provided by *enteral* (through the alimentary tract) or *parenteral* (intravenous) routes. **The advantage of enteral nutrition is that it is associated with reduced rates of infection, sepsis, length of hospital stay and costs.** Moreover, **almost all outcome studies of acutely ill adults with functioning GI tracts fail to document improved outcomes from parenteral nutrition.** The only advantage of parenteral nutrition is that it can be used when the gastrointestinal tract is not functional.

This is no longer controversial; when the gut functions, use it! Clearly, *enteral* feeding is safer, cheaper, and more physiologic than *parenteral* nutrition.

Alexander Solzhenitsyn (if this name doesn't mean anything to you please Google it up) knew this more than 50 years ago, writing in *Cancer Ward*: "If I need grape sugar, give it to me through the mouth! Why this 20th century gimmick? Why should every medicine be given by injection? You do not see anything similar in nature or among animals, do you? In a hundred years' time they'll laugh at us and call us savages..."

Enteral nutrition

Tasty food given by mouth is the ideal. Oral feeding requires the cooperation of the patient, a normal swallowing mechanism and normal gastric motility. Unconscious and intubated patients obviously cannot swallow, but the main problem following abdominal operations is that the stomach is lazier than the intestine. In other words, after laparotomy the small bowel recovers motility before the stomach. In most cases the gut is ready to absorb nutrients in the first postoperative day, whereas the stomach may have delayed emptying for a few days (➲ Chapter 41). **Therefore, when early postoperative feeding is deemed necessary, or when oral intake is inadequate, the food should be instilled distally — beyond the esophagus and the stomach**.

Routes for enteral nutrition

In general, when the mouth is not available, the following feeding routes are options:

- **Nasogastric and nasoenteric**. The former is of course not usable when the stomach is not functioning. The latter delivers the nutrients directly into the duodenum and jejunum. **Transnasal intubation** in conscious patients is only tolerated with narrow-bore and soft tubes. Rare complications include nasal trauma, sinus infection and even (very rarely) misplacement into the bronchial tree with inadvertent instillation of the feeding solution into the lungs.
- **Gastrostomy and transgastric jejunal tube**. The feeding tube is operatively placed directly into the stomach, and may be advanced through the pylorus into the jejunum. The chief complication is leakage at the insertion site: outside and around the tube — which is not uncommon — or into the peritoneal cavity — which is rare but potentially fatal.
- **Jejunostomy tube**. The feeding tube (or a catheter) is inserted directly into the proximal jejunum as discussed below.

Feeding directly into the jejunum, as opposed to gastric feeding, has been associated with less risk of aspiration, better delivery of nutrients and fewer problems with gastric retention.

Should I place a jejunal feeding tube?

This is the question you should ask yourself at the end of the emergency laparotomy. It is much more convenient to do it at this stage as opposed to doing it postoperatively. You should consider the three questions mentioned above: What is the likelihood that this patient will be eating in 7-10 days? Are they malnourished or not? What is the magnitude of this illness?

A malnourished alcoholic patient who requires a total gastrectomy with esophagojejunal anastomosis for massive upper gastrointestinal bleeding represents a classic indication for a jejunal (J) feeding tube. A case of multi-trauma involving the thorax, pelvis and long bones, who undergoes a laparotomy for hepatic injury, could also benefit from immediate J-tube feedings. On the other hand, after a partial gastrectomy in a previously well-nourished patient, J-tube placement is not indicated as the potential risks override the assumed benefits.

There are three methods to place the J-tube during the operation:

- **Transnasally (no, not transanally)** — into the stomach from which you can manipulate it by palpation into the proximal jejunum. The advantage is that it does not require a gastrotomy or enterotomy; disadvantages are its nasal presence and risk of accidental dislodgment. In addition, in a patient with peritonitis and edematous viscera, it is difficult to advance the tube all the way to the jejunum.
- **Transgastric** — combined gastrostomy/jejunostomy tubes are available to allow gastric aspiration and jejunal feeding at the same time. Obviously, gastrostomy has its own complications — mainly leakage around the tube, leakage into the peritoneal cavity and abdominal wall cellulitis. **A meticulous fixation of the stomach onto the abdominal wall is mandatory.**
- **Jejunostomy** — a 14Fr or larger tube may be placed through a purse-string controlled enterotomy and then suture-tunneled with serosa over the site of entry extending 5-7cm proximally (*Witzel technique*). Alternatively, a 12- or 14-gauge catheter may be tunneled into the jejunal lumen through a needle ('needle catheter technique'). **Both techniques require suture fixation of the bowel to the site of catheter entry in the abdominal wall in order to prevent intra-abdominal leakage of small bowel contents** — or leakage of feed, if the tube is accidentally removed before an enterocutaneous tract has developed (in 7 to 10 days). Additional useful tricks include suturing the efferent and afferent portions of the loop to the abdominal wall to prevent kinking and obstruction at the site of the jejunostomy.

Also, the needle and catheter should pierce the abdominal wall *obliquely* in line with the bowel-wall tunnel; this will prevent kinking — followed by breaking — of the fine tube at the bowel-abdominal wall junction.

Continuous J-feeding may be instituted immediately following operation in most cases. Diarrhea is a common problem requiring adjustment of the volume and concentration of the specific solution you prefer to use. Be aware that nasojejunal tube feeding can be instilled proximal to enteric suture lines. As P. O. Nyström of Sweden said: "There is no way a patient is going to eat a hole in the anastomosis."

Note that cases of massive intestinal infarction have been reported in critically ill patients receiving early postoperative jejunal feeding. This is possibly due to increased metabolic demands on an already poorly perfused gut — especially if you use large volumes of enteral feeding, exceeding 60ml/hour. **Therefore, hold J-feedings in unstable patients and those on vasopressors!**

Small bowel ileus can prevent adequate J-feeding; always consider that behind the non-resolving or reappearing ileus there may be a treatable cause (➲ Chapter 41).

Postoperative placement of a transnasal J-tube

You can also place a transnasal J-tube after the operation — if indicated. This, however, is not easy and requires prolonged manipulation under fluoroscopy. An alternative is to use a gastroscope, with a long tube (e.g. nasobiliary) placed into the distal duodenum or even farther into the jejunum with the help of the scope and under vision. **Clearly, intra-operative placement is much easier. Please do not forget this option before closing the abdomen**.

Parenteral nutrition

Patients who cannot eat and won't tolerate enteral feeding may need parenteral nutritional support and in that circumstance it may be life-saving. Parenteral nutrition comes in three 'flavors':

- **Protein-sparing hydration** takes advantage of the fact that 100g of glucose a day suppresses hepatic gluconeogenesis by supplying much of the obligate daily glucose need. Two liters of dextrose 5% provide this amount of sugar. **For the average 'not so stressed' patient this is more than enough for the first 7 postoperative days**.

- **Peripheral parenteral nutrition (PPN)** contains amino acids in addition to a low concentration of glucose and may provide an additional protein-sparing effect when 'stress' is added to starvation. It is useful in the maintenance of nutrition for an intermediate period of postoperative starvation, 7-14 days, or as long as the patient's peripheral veins last. This is because PPN is a 'vein destroyer', which often requires frequent change of the venous access. If you can wait a few more days to get a proper access for TPN we recommend you save your patient the agony of unavoidable phlebitis.
- **Total parenteral nutrition (TPN)** contains amino acids and a concentrated dextrose solution, into which a lipid solution is usually added. This can provide the total amount of nutritional requirements, even in the face of maximal stress, for an indefinite period. As usual, bypassing physiology has a price — TPN is associated with a long list of mechanical, catheter-related, infectious and metabolic complications and is rather expensive. **These days we prefer to administer TPN through a PICC (peripherally inserted central catheter) line thus avoiding the complications associated with insertion of central lines**.

Do not forget that replenishing electrolytes (e.g. magnesium, phosphorus), trace elements and vitamins is crucial in patients in need of parenteral nutrition and may help to prevent the development of the 'refeeding syndrome' — potentially fatal shifts in fluids and electrolytes that may be seen in malnourished patients receiving artificial nutrition (enteral or parenteral).

Control of hyperglycemia

Data derived in the last 5-10 years suggest that optimal control of blood glucose is far more important than the route of nutrition in critical illness. **Maintenance of the blood glucose below 180mg/dL, aiming for a range of 140 to 180 (7.8-10.0mmol/L), has been shown to decrease morbidity and to decrease the rate of mortality among critically ill patients**. This is in contrast to previous evidence suggesting the need for tighter (80 to 110mg/dL, 4.4-6.2mmol/L) control. Tight maintenance is easier to accomplish with enteral, rather than parenteral, nutritional support. Wide swings in serum glucose resulting in either hypoglycemia or hyperglycemia should be avoided.

'Routine' oral feeding

Fortunately, most of your emergency abdominal patients recover from the ileus, induced by the underlying disease and its surgical treatment, within a few days. **Traditionally, resumption of oral intake was completed in stages.** First there was the nasogastric tube, which was kept *in situ* for variable periods; then the tube was removed (according to the rules established by the local dogma guru). After the patient professed the blessed sounds of flatus he was started on 'sips'; thereafter gradually being advanced from 'clear fluids' to 'full fluids' to 'soft diet', until the great day when 'regular diet' was allowed, usually indicating that discharge home was imminent.

Now we know that this is an outdated and silly practice — that patients can tolerate solid food as soon as their GI tract is ready.

Final words...

On the other side of the coin, there are surgeons who maintain that a patient who devours a beefsteak a day after a colectomy is a testimony to their superb surgical skills. This attitude is probably wrong as well — what's the point of force-feeding a patient who does not have an appetite? Interventions to hasten the resolution of postoperative ileus have been promoted (such as μ-opioid receptor antagonists and early postoperative chewing gum use), but the

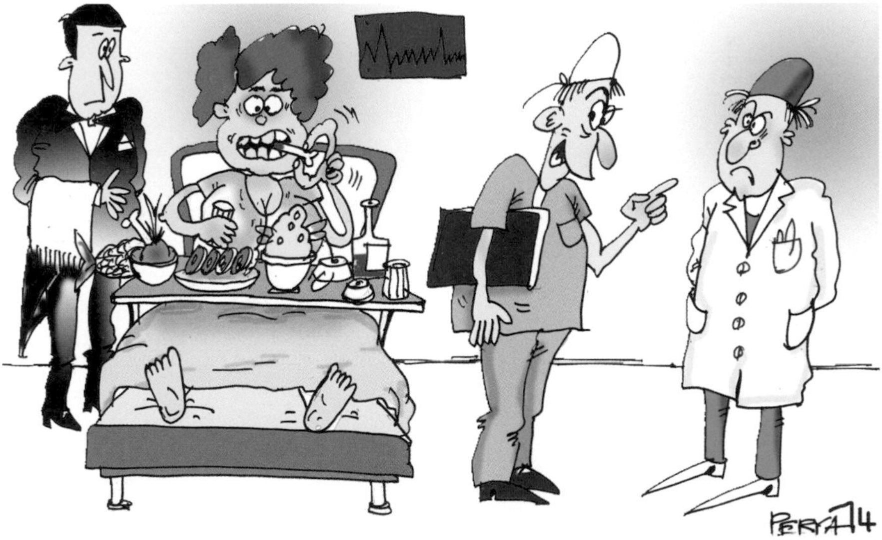

Figure 39.4. Postoperative day 1: "Let her eat as much as she wants..."

physiological postoperative ileus is a response that must have some purpose; appetite and desire to eat return when intestinal motility recovers. **Our approach is, therefore, to let the patient decide when to eat, what to eat and how much; they'll tell you when their stomach is ready for a steak or the cornmeal** (■ Figure 39.4).

> **"Some people never seem able to allow their patients to use the channels designed by nature to receive nourishment... food and fluids given by the alimentary canal allow the tissues to select and keep what they want, and to reject what is harmful or surplus to requirements."**
>
> **William Heneage Ogilvie**
>
> **"In most conditions, foods that agree with the patients may be eaten, those which do not, should not be eaten."**
>
> **Mark M. Ravitch**

Chapter 40

Postoperative antibiotics

The Editors

No amount of postoperative antibiotics can compensate for intra-operative mishaps and faulty technique, nor can they abort postoperative suppuration necessitating drainage.

The issue

Perhaps an issue as apparently banal as postoperative antibiotics does not deserve a separate chapter. Already in ➲ Chapter 7 you read about pre-operative antibiotics and which agents to use; and in ➲ Chapter 13 you were introduced to the concepts of contamination and infection and their therapeutic implications.

You may ask: why not just administer postoperative antibiotics routinely for any emergency abdominal operation until the patient is 'well'? In fact, this is not an uncommon practice in some 'surgical communities' around the world — patients receiving postoperative antibiotics for many days, many of them are even discharged home on oral agents 'just in case'. What is wrong with this approach?

One important problem with this approach is that thoughtless antibiotic administration has complications including antibiotic-associated diarrhea, colitis and the emergence of resistant strains (methicillin-resistant *Staphylococcus aureus* [MRSA] and *Clostridium difficile* colitis are major, worldwide health problems). The other problem is cost — not only of the drugs themselves but also the expense of administration and the treatment of complications. Our aim is to convince you that indiscriminate postoperative antimicrobial administration is **wrong** and to provide guidelines in order to approach this issue in a more rational way.

Only over the last decade or two (oh, how slowly are old dogmas eradicated) has the topic of *duration* of administration been addressed in the literature; for years we endured the common laconic recommendation that antibiotics should be continued until all signs of infection, including fever, leukocytosis, and even ileus subside, and the patient is clinically well. **No evidence existed, however, to prove that the continuation of antibiotics along these lines could abort an infection-in-evolution, or cure an existing one** (■ Figure 40.1).

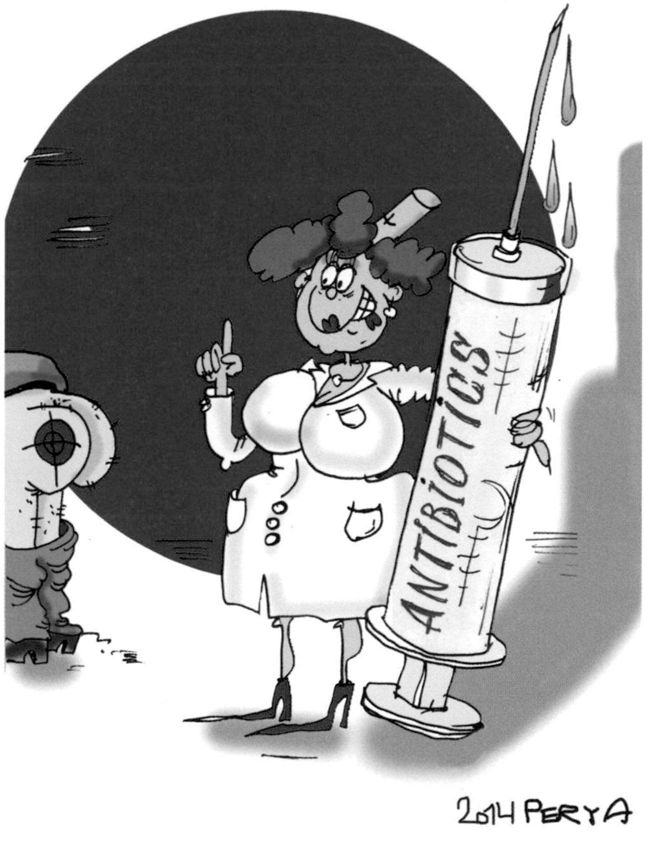

Figure 40.1. "This will cure your fever..."

Duration of postoperative administration

In the 1990s, we learned that fever and white cell response are part of the patient's inflammatory response to a variety of infective and non-infective causes. **We realized that *sterile inflammation* may manifest to some extent and for a variable duration (with fever, elevated WBC or CRP) after any operation. Is there a need to administer antibiotics after the bacteria are already dead?**

The evolving policy of **limited duration of antibiotic administration** (strongly supported by the Surgical Infection Society [SIS] — see Mazuski JE, *et al*, 2017[1] — https://www.ncbi.nlm.nih.gov/pubmed/28085573), represents a trend away from the use of postoperative therapeutic courses of fixed and often long duration. **Rather, you should attempt to stratify the infective processes into grades of risk, and to tailor the duration of administration to the severity of infection.**

The way we do things is summarized in ■ Table 40.1. It is based on the following arguments:

- **Conditions representing contamination** (e.g. early managed gunshot wound of the colon) **do not require postoperative administration** since the infectious source has been dealt with at operation; bacteria and adjuvants of infection are effectively removed by the host's defenses supplemented by peritoneal toilet, and adequate tissue levels of pre- and intra-operative prophylactic antibiotics. **By definition, prophylaxis should not be continued beyond the immediate operative phase.** Having said this, we won't send you to the guillotine for giving a few more doses, especially in high-risk patients (e.g. immunosuppressed, morbidly obese, etc).
- In processes limited to an organ amenable to excision (we call it '**resectable infection**' — for example, gangrenous appendicitis), the residual bacterial inoculum is minimal. **A postoperative antimicrobial course of 24 hours should suffice to sterilize the surrounding inflammatory reaction and deal with gut bacteria, which may have escaped across the necrotic bowel wall by translocation.** But again, we won't ridicule you at the M & M meeting for continuing antibiotics for another day...
- **'Non-resectable infections'** with a significant spread beyond the confines of the involved organ (e.g. perforated appendicitis) should be stratified according to their severity. **A therapeutic postoperative**

1 Mazuski JE, Tessier JM, May AK, *et al.* The Surgical Infection Society revised guidelines on the management of intra-abdominal infection. *Surg Infect* 2017; 18: 1-76.

Table 40.1. Suggested duration of postoperative antibiotic therapy.*

Contamination: no postoperative antibiotics (assuming appropriate pre-operative prophylaxis administered)

- Gastroduodenal peptic perforations operated within 12 hours.
- Traumatic enteric perforations operated within 12 hours.
- Peritoneal contamination with bowel contents during elective or emergency procedures.
- Appendectomy for early or phlegmonous appendicitis.
- Cholecystectomy for early or phlegmonous cholecystitis.

'Resectable' infection: 24-hour postoperative antibiotic course

- Appendectomy for gangrenous appendicitis.
- Cholecystectomy for gangrenous cholecystitis.
- Bowel resection for ischemic or strangulated necrotic bowel without frank perforation.

'Mild/moderate' infection: 2-5 days postoperative antibiotic course

- Intra-abdominal infection from diverse sources with localized pus formation.
- 'Late' (>12 hours) traumatic bowel lacerations and gastroduodenal perforation with no established intra-abdominal infection.
- Diffuse, established intra-abdominal infection from any source.

'Severe' infection: more than 5 days of postoperative antibiotics

- Severe intra-abdominal infection with a source not easily controllable (e.g. infected pancreatic necrosis).
- Postoperative intra-abdominal infection.

* These are what we recommend in general. It is not written in stone — so use your clinical judgment in the individual patient. These days you also have to think about the lawyer who may be, sooner or later, evaluating what you did. Keep the lawyer in mind and write for him a brief note in the chart or the EMR. For example: after removing a non-perforated appendix we write: "No postop antibiotics are indicated because..." And when discharging a patient a day after removing a gangrenous appendix we would write: "The patient received a 24-hour course of antibiotics which is sufficient..." It shows that you are a careful surgeon and know what you are doing...

course of more than 5 days is usually not necessary. However, certain complex situations may need **extended** courses of postoperative antibiotics. A typical example is infected pancreatic necrosis where the nidus of infection is not readily eradicated in a once-and-for-all surgical procedure. **Similarly, patients with postoperative peritonitis, where the control of the source of infection is questionable, should be considered for prolonged antibiotic therapy**. (But even in this situation the SIS doesn't recommend courses of more than 5-7 days.)

Remember that once the postop patient can eat, the course of antibiotics could be completed orally — at home if possible.

By now you should understand that the persistence of inflammation beyond the appropriate therapeutic course is not an indication to continue, restart or change antibiotics.

What should instead be done, first, is to stop the antibiotics. The fever may subside spontaneously in most patients within a day or two, with little more than chest physiotherapy. **At the same time, a directed search is undertaken for a treatable source of intraperitoneal or extraperitoneal infection**. You know how to do it: clinical examination, imaging…

We hope that you realize that unnecessary antibiotics are wrong because anything unnecessary in medicine is bad medicine. In addition, the price to be paid is high, not only financially. Antibiotics are associated with patient-specific adverse effects (the list is long, think of the gravity of *C. difficile* colitis) and ecological repercussions such as drug-resistant nosocomial infections in your hospital.

Are you convinced?

"Start antibiotics prior to any emergency laparotomy; whether to continue administration after the operation depends on your findings. Know the target flora and use the cheapest and simplest regimen. The bacteria cannot be confused, nor should you be."

Chapter 41

Postoperative ileus vs. intestinal obstruction

The Editors

> *In ileus the belly becomes hard, there are no motions, the whole abdomen is painful, there are fever and thirst and sometimes the patient is so tormented that he vomits bile... Medicines are not retained and enemas do not penetrate. It is an acute and dangerous disease.*
>
> **Hippocrates**

Five days ago you removed this patient's perforated appendix laparoscopically; you gave him antibiotics for 2-3 days, and by today you expected him to eat and go home. Instead, your patient lies in bed with a long face and a distended abdomen, vomiting bile from time to time. The wife looks at you suspiciously/accusingly and says: "our son had his appendix out in Minneapolis... he went home on the same day... the old surgeon did it without the video camera..." The daughter refuses to meet your eyes; you overhear her whispering to her mother: "we shouldn't have let him have the operation in this provincial s**thole." **So what is the problem? And what now?**

Definitions and mechanisms

The term 'ileus' as used in this book, and in daily practice, signifies a 'paralytic ileus' — as distinct from *mechanical* ileus, which is a synonym for intestinal obstruction. In essence, the latter consists of a mechanical stoppage to the normal transit along the intestine whereas the former denotes hindered transit because the intestines are 'lazy'.

In previous chapters you noted that ileus of the small bowel, colon or both, can be secondary to a variety of intra-abdominal (e.g. acute appendicitis), retroperitoneal (e.g. hematoma) or extra-abdominal (e.g. hypokalemia) causes, which adversely affect normal intestinal motility. **Following abdominal operations, however, ileus is a 'normal' physiologic phenomenon.**

Ileus

Unlike mechanical intestinal obstruction, which involves a segment of the (small or large) bowel, **postoperative ileus concerns the whole length of the gut**, from the stomach to the rectum. The physiological postoperative ileus resolves gradually: the small bowel resumes activity almost immediately, followed, a day or so later, by the stomach, and then the colon, being the laziest, is the last to start moving.

The magnitude of postoperative ileus correlates to some extent with that of the operation performed and the specific underlying condition. The more you do, the more you get. Major dissections, prolonged intestinal displacement and exposure, denuded and inflamed peritoneum, residual intraperitoneal or retroperitoneal pus or clots, are all associated with a prolonged ileus. Thus, for example, after simple appendectomy for non-perforated appendicitis, ileus should be almost non-existent, whereas after a laparotomy for a ruptured abdominal aortic aneurysm expect the ileus to be prolonged. **Common postoperative factors that can aggravate ileus are the administration of opiates and an electrolyte imbalance**. In general, laparoscopic abdominal procedures are followed with a lesser magnitude of ileus than their 'open' counterparts.

While the physiological postoperative ileus is diffuse, ileus due to some complications may be local. A classic example is a postoperative abscess that may 'paralyze' an adjacent segment of bowel. Other examples include a localized leak from an ileo-transverse anastomosis after right hemicolectomy that may paralyze the adjacent duodenum, mimicking a picture of gastric outlet obstruction, or a pancreatic phlegmon paralyzing the adjacent stomach.

Early postoperative small bowel obstruction (EPSBO)

A common postoperative question: are we dealing with an ileus or mechanical intestinal obstruction?

You have become familiar with small bowel obstruction (SBO) in ➲ Chapter 19. **Early postoperative small bowel obstruction (EPSBO) is**

defined as one developing from the early days after the operation or within 4 weeks. Two primary mechanisms are responsible: **adhesions** and **internal hernia**.

Early post-laparotomy **adhesions** are immature, inflammatory, poor in collagen — thus 'soft' — and vascular. **Such characteristics indicate that early adhesions may resolve spontaneously, and that surgical lysis may be difficult, traumatic to involved viscera, and bloody**.

Postoperative adhesions may be diffuse, involving the whole length of the small bowel at multiple sites, as is occasionally seen following extensive lysis of adhesions. Localized obstructing adhesions may also develop at the operative site with the bowel adherent, for instance, to exposed mesh or raw peritoneal surfaces.

The recent operation may also have created new potential spaces in which the bowel can become trapped and obstructed — forming internal hernias. Typical examples are the partially closed pelvic peritoneum after abdominoperineal resection, the space behind an emerging colostomy, or an incidental peritoneal defect created during preperitoneal laparoscopic inguinal hernia repair. The narrower the opening into the space, the more likely the bowel is to be trapped. **And let us not forget laparoscopic trocar sites!**

Diagnosis

Failure of your patient to eat, pass flatus or evacuate his bowel within 5 days after the abdominal procedure signifies a persistent ileus or a possible EPSBO. This does not mean that you do not start worrying much earlier — it depends on the individual case. So, for example, you would be much more concerned about a patient developing vomiting and abdominal distension, a day after a repair of his umbilical hernia than after undergoing a total colectomy.

In **ileus**, the abdomen is usually distended and silent to auscultation. Plain abdominal X-ray typically shows significant gaseous distension of both the small bowel and the colon (➲ Chapters 4 and 5). However, the diagnosis of **EPSBO** in the recently operated abdomen is much subtler. Textbooks teach you that on abdominal auscultation "ileus is silent and SBO noisy" — this may be theoretically true but almost impossible to assess in the recently operated upon belly.

If your patient has already passed flatus or defecated and then ceases to manifest these comforting features, SBO is the most likely diagnosis. However, the truth is that in most instances the patient will improve spontaneously without you ever knowing whether it was an EPSBO or *just* an ileus.

The natural tendency of the operating surgeon is to attribute the 'failure to progress' to an ileus rather than SBO, and not to suspect a potentially treatable cause of the ileus — and to procrastinate. Procrastination is not a good idea, however. A distended and non-eating patient is prone to the iatrogenic hazards of nasogastric tubes, intravenous lines, parenteral nutrition, and bed rest (➲ Chapter 39).

You must be alert, active and proceed with diagnostic steps in parallel to therapy.

Management

There is no need to remind you that optimal peri-operative management (e.g. avoiding overhydration and consequent tissue swelling) and a perfect operation can help prevent ileus or decrease its severity. Correct postoperative management (your cliché-ridden managers would use the term 'ERAS' or 'goal-directed'...) would have beneficial effects as well.

What else should you do?

- **Reduce the dose and duration of opiates which are the most common promoters of ileus**. Pain should be controlled but not excessively nor for too long. Consider the use of alternative medications (e.g. NSAIDs).
- Measure and correct **electrolyte imbalances**, especially potassium!
- When the ileus/EPSBO is prolonged consider **parenteral nutrition** as described in ➲ Chapter 39.
- There is some evidence that **early ambulation, positional changes, manual abdominal massage** and/or **chewing gum** hasten the resolution of ileus. So let the patients chew gum — even if it does not alleviate ileus it will surely promote salivary flow and oral hygiene and improve his or her mood.
- **Gimmicks?** It does not seem that **prokinetic agents** like metoclopramide or erythromycin alleviate or shorten ileus. Patients receiving **laxatives** (e.g. bisacodyl suppositories) were shown to

defecate a little earlier but to stay just as long in the hospital. What about *alvimopan* — a peripherally acting μ-opioid receptor agonist shown to accelerate the time to GI recovery after elective surgery in a few randomized trials? We have no personal experience with this very expensive agent and do not know anyone who has been using it after emergency abdominal operations. Finally, the use of **epidural anesthesia** doesn't have much influence.

A management algorithm is presented in ■ Figure 41.1. **Pass an NG tube** — if not already *in situ* — to decompress the stomach, prevent aerophagia, relieve nausea and vomiting, and measure gastric residue. **Now carefully**

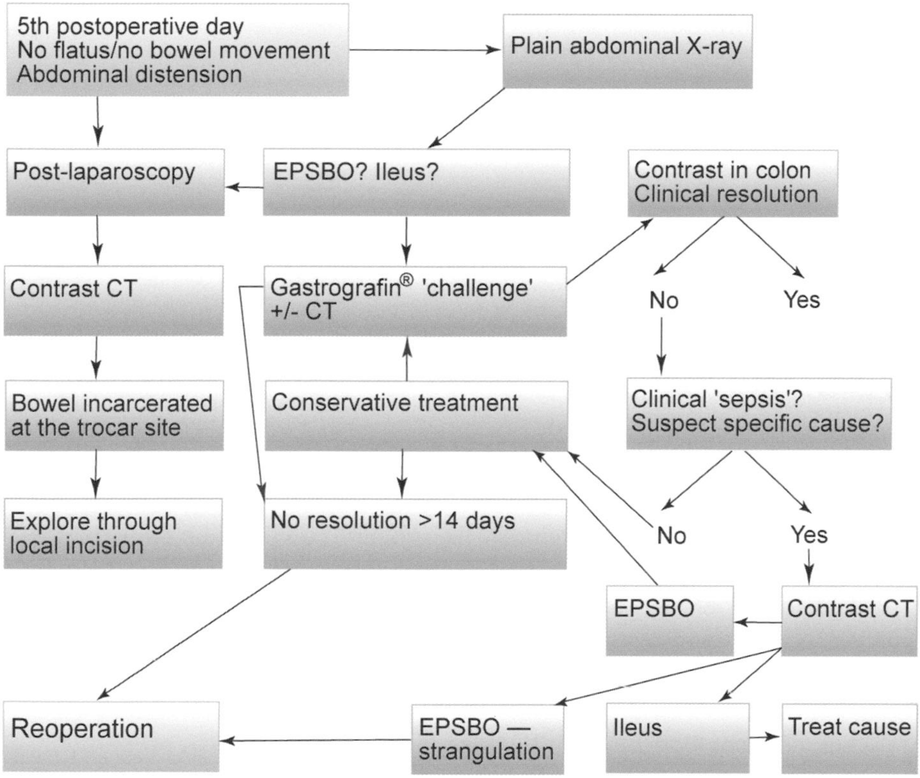

Figure 41.1. Management algorithm for ileus and EPSBO.

search (with abdominal imaging) for any potential manageable causes of prolonged ileus: a hematoma, an abscess, an anastomotic leak, postoperative pancreatitis, postoperative acalculous cholecystitis — all can produce ileus or mimic EPSBO.

And do not forget that significant *hypoalbuminemia* leads to generalized edema, involving the bowel too. Edematous and swollen bowel does not move well; this is called '**hypoalbuminemic enteropathy**' and should be considered.

Practically speaking, if on the fifth post-laparotomy day your patient still has features of ileus/EPSBO, we recommend a CT scan. If the latter suggests an ileus or EPSBO, a Gastrografin® challenge, as described in ➲ Chapter 19, may be useful in relieving both conditions and pinpoint the problem. We often order a CT with oral contrast — a single imaging study which achieves all the above goals in one shot.

In the absence of intra-abdominal or extra-abdominal causes for ileus, and when the 'ileus' does not respond to the Gastrografin® challenge (i.e. failure of the contrast to arrive at the colon) — the most likely diagnosis is EPSBO.

In the early postoperative phase this is NOT an indication for a reoperation as intestinal strangulation almost never occurs in adhesive EPSBO. Evidence and experience show that most such cases will resolve spontaneously within up to 2 weeks.

So as long as you have excluded (by imaging) obstruction caused by a loop of bowel 'caught' in a well-defined anatomical space (see below), rushing to reoperate would be a grave mistake. Treat conservatively while providing parenteral nutritional support and improving the patient's general condition.

Lack of resolution beyond 2 weeks is an indication for a reoperation, which may be difficult and hazardous because of the typical early, dense and vascular adhesions cementing the bowel at many points. **When you experience reoperating on one of these cases you will understand why avoiding reoperation for EPSBO is such a good idea...**

EPSBO following laparoscopy

EPSBO developing after laparoscopic procedures deserves specific consideration. As adhesions are less common, a correctable cause should be looked for more actively. Cholecystectomy, appendectomy and the various laparoscopic hernia repairs and gynecologic laparoscopies are the most common procedures associated with post-laparoscopic EPSBO. **Despite their rarity, adhesions are still the culprit in half of the patients and small bowel incarceration at the port site in the other half**. Practically, all port-site herniations involve the use of 10 or 12mm trocars and the umbilical port is the commonest site. **Adequate fascial closure was either not attempted or thought to have been achieved at the initial operation**. Even with fascial closure, a strangulated hernia may develop, with the bowel caught in the preperitoneal space behind the closed defect. As mentioned above, laparoscopic repair of inguinal hernias (be it transabdominal [TAPP] or totally extraperitoneal [TEP]) can leave behind peritoneal defects through which a loop of bowel may migrate into the preperitoneal space. Another cause for EPSBO following laparoscopic cholecystectomy are **spilled gallstones**, which can lead to the development of an inflammatory mass to which the bowel adheres.

Therefore, when EPSBO follows laparoscopy, CT examination of the abdomen is recommended to provide an early and specific diagnosis.

Physical findings suggestive of these conditions (such as a mass or exceptional tenderness at the trocar site) may be missing and CT identification of the conditions responsible for the EPSBO allows immediate operation to relieve the obstruction. When a trocar site hernia occurs, surgery can be carried out through the (extended) original incision, or by laparoscopy, to release the stuck bowel and close the defect under vision.

Remember: unlike EPSBO following open procedures, post-laparoscopy obstruction usually won't resolve without a reoperation. You must understand that post-laparoscopy EPSBO is a specific entity which calls for immediate action. (See also ➲ Chapters 12 and 37.)

Additional considerations

The 'hostile' abdomen (see also ➲ Chapter 19)

Any mixed series of patients with EPSBO includes a subgroup of patients in whom the index operation has disclosed a 'hostile' peritoneal cavity suggesting that any further surgery to relieve the obstructive process would be hazardous and futile. To this group belong patients with **extensive radiation enteritis** in whom persisting obstruction can be defined as 'intestinal failure' and who are best managed with long-term parenteral nutrition. **Indiscriminate reoperation in such patients often leads to massive bowel resection, multiple fistulas and death, and should be avoided**. Patients with evidence of **peritoneal carcinomatosis** at the index operation also belong to this group. **In general, only one-third of patients with 'malignant' bowel obstruction from peritoneal carcinomatosis will have prolonged postoperative palliation**. Thus, EPSBO in such patients is an ominous sign; abdominal reoperation should be avoided, and future palliative treatment planned, based on the individual patient's functional status and the burden of cancer.

Finally, every surgeon has some personal experience with a little reported entity, the **frozen abdomen**, in which intractable SBO is caused by dense, vascular and inseparable adhesions — fixing the bowel at many points. **The astute surgeon knows when to abort early from a futile dissection before multiple enterotomies — necessitating massive bowel resection — are created**. He also knows not to reoperate on such patients even if persisting EPSBO develops after what appeared to be a successful adhesiolysis. Prolonged parenteral nutrition over a period of months, with complete gastrointestinal rest, may allow the adhesions to mature — with resolution of the SBO, or at least allowing a safer reoperation.

Anastomotic obstruction

A bowel anastomosis at any level may cause early postoperative upper gastrointestinal, small bowel or colonic obstruction. 'Edema' is usually blamed, but faulty technique (➲ Chapter 14) is sometimes the cause. A self-limiting 'mini' anastomotic leak is often responsible but is under-diagnosed (➲ Chapter 43). Diagnosis is reached with a contrast study (water-soluble please!) and/or CT. **Most of these early postoperative anastomotic obstructions are 'soft' and edematous, resolving spontaneously within a week or two. Do not rush to reoperate**; gentle passage of an endoscope — if practical — may confirm the diagnosis and 'dilate' the lumen.

Delayed gastric emptying

Often the stomach fails to empty following a partial gastrectomy or a gastrojejunostomy performed for any indication. This is more common when a vagotomy has been added or when a Roux-en-Y loop has been constructed. A contrast study will show that the contrast persistently sits in the stomach. **The differential diagnosis is between a gastric ileus (gastroparesis) and mechanical obstruction at the gastrojejunostomy or *below* it** (yes, do not miss the mechanical obstruction in the small bowel just 'below' the stomach!). A complete discussion of the various post-gastrectomy syndromes is beyond the scope of this modest volume but remember this fundamental principle — **postoperative gastric paresis is self-limiting — it will always resolve spontaneously but may take as long as 6 weeks to do so. Exclude mechanical stomal obstruction with an endoscope and contrast study and then treat conservatively with nasogastric suction and nutritional support.** Try to pass a feeding tube distal to the stomach. Parenteral *erythromycin* has been shown to enhance gastric motility and is always worth a trial in this situation. **Resist the devil within you — tempting you to reoperate for gastric paresis — for it will eventually resolve, while reoperation may only make things worse.**

Acute gastric dilatation

This chapter gives us an opportunity to mention the entity of **acute gastric dilatation** — well known and feared by previous generations of surgeons — but for some reason vanishing from our collective awareness. It can develop after any operation or following trauma but may occur spontaneously as well — especially in debilitated and immobilized patients. It has been described in patients with eating disorders such as bulimia.

Acute gastric dilatation manifests itself with abdominal distension, pain, nausea and vomiting, and if not treated promptly can result in aspiration, abdominal compartment syndrome and even gastric necrosis.

The waning use of nasogastric tubes may explain why we still occasionally see these cases in the postoperative phase. Here are two cases to ponder...

A young lady underwent repair of an umbilical hernia with mesh under local anesthesia and i.v. sedataion. An hour after the operation she complained about severe, diffuse abdominal pain. Her heart rate was 120/min and the abdomen was diffusely tender. "Did I injure her intestines?," the anxious surgeon asked himself. Abdominal X-ray showed a huge stomach. A nasogastric tube, left *in situ* for a few hours, cured the acute gastric dilatation.

A middle-aged man underwent an uneventful laparoscopic cholecystectomy. An orogastric tube was inserted by the anesthetist during the procedure and removed at its end. An hour after being discharged from the recovery room the patient complained about severe abdominal pain, which persisted despite repeated doses of opiates. He developed tachycardia despite adequate hydration. The abdomen was diffusely tender. These worrying features of possible injury to intestine or an early bile leak, which persisted for a few hours, promoted the surgeon to take the patient back to the OR for relaparoscopy — which proved to be normal, except for massive distension of the stomach. An NG tube was inserted, and the patient went home the next morning.

Message: if you don't think about it, you may miss the option of a simple, safe and effective treatment, in the form of an NG tube.

Prevention

As anywhere in life "An ounce of prevention is worth a pound of cure" (a cliché', we know).

It is imperative to emphasize that you can, and ought to, prevent prolonged postoperative ileus or SBO by sound operative technique and attention to detail. Gentle dissection and handling of tissues, careful hemostasis to avoid hematoma formation, not using the cautery like a blowtorch, leaving as little foreign material as possible (e.g. large silk knots, spilled gallstones during laparoscopic cholecystectomy), not denuding the peritoneum unnecessarily, not creating orifices for internal hernias, folding back the bowel loops into a nice gently-curved position, carefully closing large port sites, and not catching loops of bowel during abdominal closure, are self-explanatory essentials. We are not yet too impressed with the evidence supporting the expensive commercial products that allegedly 'prevent adhesions'. It seems that nobody is...

In summary, diagnose and treat causes of persistent ileus, treat EPSBO conservatively as long as indicated, think about specific causes of SBO (e.g. herniation at a laparoscopic trocar site) and reoperate when necessary. **In most instances, ileus/EPSBO will resolve spontaneously** without you being able to know whether it was 'mechanical' or 'paralytic'... (■ Figure 41.2).

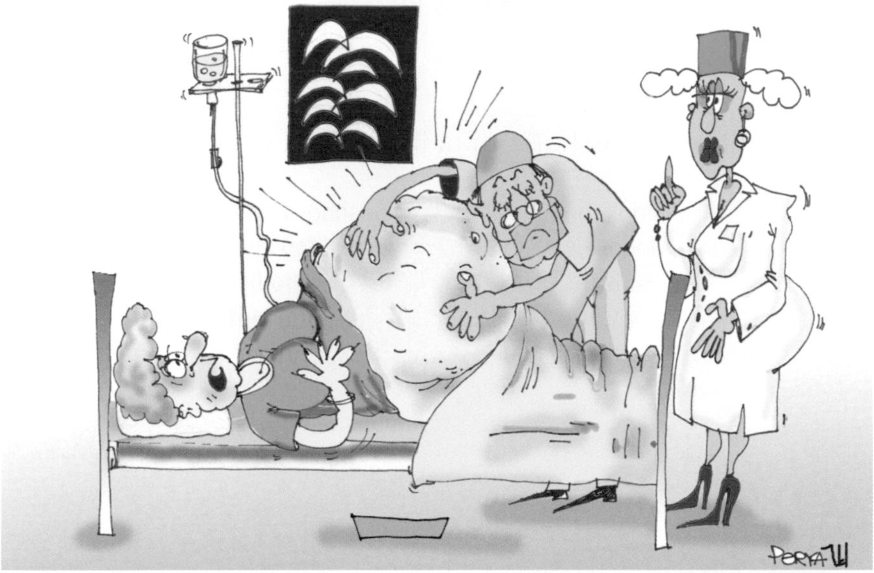

Figure 41.2. "Doctor, is it mechanical obstruction or ileus?"..."Shh... let me hear..."

Look also at Chapter 8, *Schein's Common Sense Prevention and Management of Surgical Complications*.

"Better to leave a piece of peritoneum on the bowel than a piece of bowel on the peritoneum."

"The postoperative fart is the best music to the surgeon's ears..."

Chapter 42

Intra-abdominal abscesses

The Editors

Signs of pus somewhere, signs of pus nowhere else, signs of pus there — under the diaphragm (this was 100% true when we were students, 50% true when we were residents. Today it is irrelevant...).

The contents of this chapter could have been summarized in a sentence: an abscess is a pus-containing, confined structure, which requires drainage by whichever means available. The ancients said it even more aptly — *Ubi pus, ibi evacua*. We believe, however, that you want us to elaborate.

Abscesses may develop anywhere within the abdomen, resulting from numerous conditions. Specific types such as diverticular or peri-appendicular abscesses are covered elsewhere in this book; this chapter will introduce you to general concepts — with emphasis on what is probably the commonest abscess in your practice — the **postoperative abscess**.

Definition and significance

Erroneously, the term 'intra-abdominal abscess' has been and still is used as a synonym for secondary peritonitis (➲ Chapter 13). **This is not true as abscesses develop as a result of effective host defenses and represent a relatively successful outcome of peritonitis**. The term 'collection' (as seen on CT) is commonly used, but not every collection is infected and not every collection is an abscess — as discussed below.

To be termed an abscess, the confined structure must be contained by an inflammatory wall and possess a viscous interior. In contrast, free-flowing, contaminated peritoneal fluid or loculated collections, which are deprived of a wall, represent a phase in the spectrum of peritoneal infection and not an abscess.

Pathogenesis and classification

All abscesses signify an intermediate natural outcome of infection. At one end of the spectrum infection persists, spreads and kills; at the other, the process is entirely cleared by host defenses — assisted by your therapy. **Abscesses lie in no-man's land, where the peritoneal defenses are only partially effective** — being disturbed by an overwhelming number of bacteria, micro-environmental hypoxemia or acidosis, and adjuvants of infection such as necrotic debris, hemoglobin, fibrin and (God forbid) barium sulphate. **An untreated abdominal abscess won't kill your patient immediately, but if neglected and undrained, it will become gradually lethal, unless spontaneous drainage occurs**.

The myriad forms of intra-abdominal abscesses make their classification complex (■ Table 42.1), but practically, abscesses are **visceral** (e.g. intrahepatic or splenic) or **non-visceral** (e.g. subphrenic, pelvic), **intraperitoneal** or **extraperitoneal**.

Visceral abscesses are usually caused by hematogenous or lymphatic dissemination of bacteria to a solid organ; but a direct invasion is also possible, like in hepatic abscess secondary to posterior wall perforation of a gallbladder, or a splenic abscess in continuity with a perforation of the splenic flexure of the colon due to cancer or acute diverticulitis.

Non-visceral abscesses arise following the resolution of diffuse peritonitis during which loculated areas of infection and suppuration are 'walled off' and persist; or arise after a perforation of a viscus, which is effectively localized by peritoneal defenses.

Retroperitoneal abscesses may result from perforation of a hollow viscus into the retroperitoneum as well as by hematogenous or lymphatic spread.

Another distinction is between the **postoperative abscess** — for the development of which we surgeons feel responsible — and **spontaneous abscesses**, unassociated with a previous operation.

Table 42.1. Classification of abdominal abscesses.

Classification	Examples
Visceral vs. non-visceral	Hepatic vs. subphrenic
Primary vs. secondary	Splenic vs. appendiceal
Spontaneous vs. postoperative	Diverticular vs. peri-anastomotic
Intraperitoneal vs. retroperitoneal	Tubo-ovarian vs. psoas
Simple vs. complex	Complex: • Multiple (liver) • Multiloculated • Communication with bowel (leaking anastomosis) • Associated with necrotic tissue (pancreatic) • Associated with cancer
Anatomical	Subphrenic, subhepatic, lesser sac, paracolic, pelvic, interloop, perinephric, psoas

A further clinically significant separation is between **simple abscesses vs. complex abscesses (e.g. multiple; multiloculated; or associated with tissue necrosis, enteric communication or tumor) — the latter mentioned require more aggressive therapy and carry a poorer prognosis**.

The traditional **anatomical classification**, based on the specific anatomical location of an abscess — which typically develops in one of the few constant potential spaces — has diminished in significance since the advent of readily available modern imaging and percutaneous drainage techniques.

Microbiology

Generally speaking, abdominal abscesses are polymicrobial. Abscesses that develop in the aftermath of secondary peritonitis (e.g. appendiceal or diverticular abscess) possess the mixed aerobic-anaerobic flora of secondary peritonitis (➲ Chapters 7 and 13).

It appears that while endotoxin-generating facultative anaerobes, such as *Escherichia coli*, are responsible for the phase of acute peritonitis, the obligate anaerobes, such as *Bacteroides fragilis*, are responsible for late abscess formation. These bacteria act in **synergy**; both are necessary to produce an abscess, and the obligate anaerobe can increase the lethality of an otherwise non-lethal inoculum of the facultative micro-organisms. The vast majority of visceral abscesses (e.g. hepatic and splenic) are polymicrobial — aerobic, anaerobic, Gram-negative and -positive. This is also true for retroperitoneal abscesses. **Primary abscesses** (e.g. psoas abscess) are often monobacterial, with *Staphylococci* predominating. **Postoperative abscesses are often characterized by the flora typical of nosocomial infection — representing superinfection with yeasts and other opportunists** (➲ Chapter 13). The low virulence of these organisms reflects the global immunodepression of the affected patients.

Clinical features

The clinical presentation of abdominal abscesses is as heterogeneous and multifaceted as the abscesses themselves. **The spectrum is vast; systemic repercussions of the infection vary from frank septic shock to nothing at all when suppressed by immunoparesis and antibiotics**. Locally, the abscess may be felt through the abdominal wall, the rectum or vagina; in most instances, however, it remains physically occult.

In our modern times, when any fever is an alleged indication for antibiotics, some abscesses are initially partially treated or masked — presenting as a systemic inflammation with variable organ dysfunction. **Ileus is another notable presentation of abdominal abscess**; in the postoperative situation it is an 'ileus that fails to resolve' (➲ Chapter 41).

In this age of instant and repeated imaging, of obsessive wielding of needles and knives, we tend to forget the *real* natural history of intra-abdominal abscesses. The following case will serve as an example.

An 88-year-old lady presented with massive *fecaluria*. Imaging showed a phlegmon/abscess involving the sigmoid colon with a large colovesical fistula. The family refused our recommendation to proceed with an emergency sigmoidectomy or a diverting colostomy plus percutaneous drainage of the abscess. "Let her die in peace", they pleaded and summoned her Priest. The patient returned to her nursing home but refused to die. Instead she continued to flourish while draining feces into her urine. Six months later she developed a subcutaneous abscess on the lower abdominal wall. We drained it under local anesthesia — it produced feces. A colostomy bag was placed on the drainage wound — voilà, a *spontaneous* colostomy. The urine became clear. A year later the patient continued to thrive. She passed away at the age of 90.

Just makes you stop and ponder...

Diagnosis

Life has become simple! Modern abdominal imaging has revolutionized the diagnosis of abdominal abscesses. Yes, you still need to suspect the abscess and carefully examine your patient but the definitive diagnosis (and usually the treatment) depends on imaging techniques. Computed tomography (CT), ultrasound (US) and even radioisotope-scanning techniques are available. Which is the best?

Both US and CT provide good anatomical definition including the site of the abscess, its size and structure (■ Figure 42.1). Both can guide PC drainage. US is portable, cheaper, and more accurate at detecting abscesses in the right upper abdomen and pelvis. It is, however, extremely operator-dependent. **We surgeons are better trained to read CT scans rather than US; hence, we prefer CT, which allows us to visualize the entire abdomen, independently assess the anatomy of the abscess, and plan its optimal management. CT, enhanced with intravenous and intraluminal contrast, is also helpful in classifying the abscess either as simple or complex** (■ Table 42.1).

Do understand that imaging during the first postoperative week cannot distinguish between a sterile fluid collection (e.g. residual lavage fluid) and an infected fluid collection before the development of a frank, mature abscess. The only way to document the infective nature of any visualized fluid is a **diagnostic aspiration** — subjecting the aspirate to a Gram stain and culture.

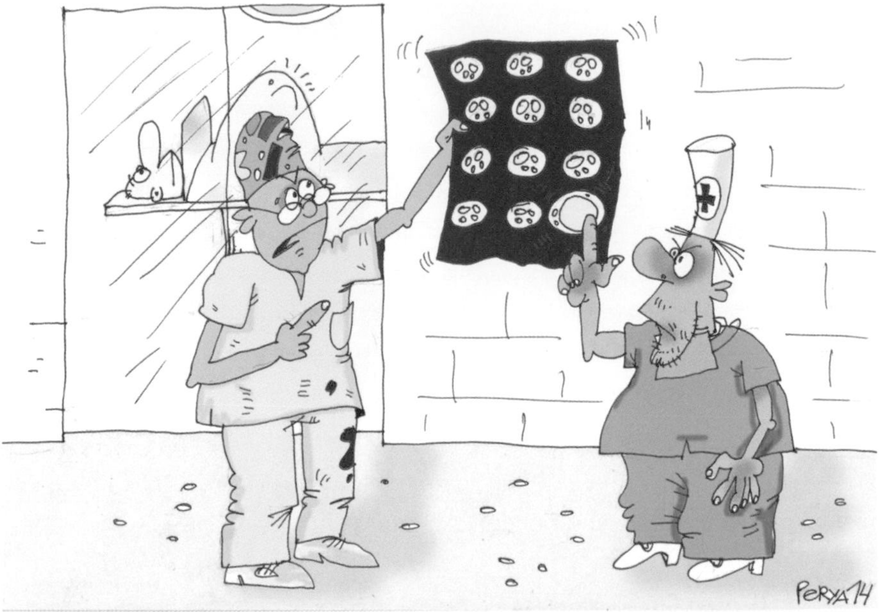

Figure 42.1. "You call that an abscess? THIS is an abscess!"

CT features suggestive of a proper abscess are a contrast-enhancing, well-defined rim, and the presence of gas bubbles.

Hence, bear in mind that not all fluid collections that are detected in the postoperative abdomen require active management; be guided by the patient's clinical condition at all times. Be resistant to the offers of aggressive radiologists to drain all accessible collections, particularly in the early postop period.

Antibiotics

Abdominal abscesses should be drained. When an 'active' source of the abscess exists, it should be dealt with. Antibiotic treatment is of secondary importance.

The truth is that no real evidence exists to prove that antimicrobial agents, which penetrate poorly into established abscesses anyway, are necessary as an adjunct to the complete evacuation of pus. Think about the good old days, not many years ago, when pelvic abscesses were observed until reaching 'maturity' and then drained through the rectum or the vagina; no antibiotics were used, and the recovery was immediate and complete. (But then again who cares about the 'truth' and 'evidence' — we follow the trends...).

The prevalent standard of care, although lacking evidence, maintains that when an abscess is strongly suspected or diagnosed, then antibiotic therapy should be initiated. The latter should initially be empirically targeted against the usual expected polymicrobial spectrum of bacteria; when the causative bacteria are identified the coverage can be changed or reduced as indicated.

How long to administer antibiotics? Again, there are no scientific data to formulate logical guidelines. Common sense dictates that prolonged administration after effective drainage is unnecessary. Theoretically, antibiotics may combat bacteremia during drainage and eradicate locally spilled micro-organisms; **but after the pus has been evacuated, leading to a clinical response, antibiotics should be discontinued**. The presence of a drain is not an indication to continue with administration.

Conservative treatment

Traditionally, **multiple hepatic abscesses**, as a consequence of portal pyemia, which are not amenable to drainage, are treated with antibiotics, with a variable response rate.

There are those who claim that non-operative treatment, with prolonged administration of antibiotics, is also effective in **children who develop abdominal abscesses following appendectomy** for acute appendicitis. The problem with such 'success stories' is that the alleged 'abscesses', which were imaged on US or CT, were never proven as such. Instead, they probably represented sterile collections — the majority requiring no therapy at all — or early, unwalled, infected fluid collections into which antibiotics do penetrate. In addition, small (<5cm) pericolic 'diverticular' abscesses can resolve with antibiotics only — without the need for drainage.

Drainage

With regard to the general philosophy and timing of drainage, the current prevailing paradigm, when an abscess is suspected on a CT or US, is to hit the patient with antibiotics and rush to drainage. In this hysterical hurry to 'do something', clinical lessons learned over centuries are often ignored. Only a few generations ago, a patient who spiked a temperature after an appendectomy was patiently but carefully observed without antibiotics (which did not exist); usually the temperature — signifying a residual inflammatory response — subsided spontaneously. In a minority of patients, 'septic' fever persisted reflecting maturing local suppuration. The latter was eventually drained through the rectum when assessed as 'mature'. Today, on the other hand, antibiotics are immediately given to mask the clinical picture, and imaging techniques are instantly ordered, only to diagnose 'red herrings', which in turn promote unnecessary invasive procedures.

Remember, in a stable patient, fever is a *symptom* of effective host defenses — not an indication to be aggressively invasive.

For balance, we cannot forget that patients were dying from appendicitis and its complications in the pre-antibiotic era... and that it's difficult to defend in court a septic complication that was not treated with antibiotics. We just urge you to be reasonable.

Practical approach

When an abscess is suspected, a few dilemmas arise and should be dealt with stepwise:

- **Is it an abscess or a sterile collection?** The CT features mentioned above may be helpful, but the clinical scenario is as important — especially when postoperative abscesses are concerned. **Abscesses are rarely ready for drainage in the first postoperative week. At 3 weeks after the operation, the cause of 'sepsis' is rarely within the abdomen.** When in doubt, image-guided diagnostic aspiration is indicated.
- **Percutaneous (PC) versus open surgical drainage?** During the 1980s it was said by some that, paradoxically, despite the attractiveness of PC techniques for abscess drainage in the most ill patients, a better chance of survival is achieved with surgical treatment, and that surgical treatment should not be avoided because the patient is considered to be too ill. We now believe no more in such a theory. **Instead we think that pus has to be drained by the least invasive method, which can spare the patient the unpleasantness and obvious risks of yet another open abdominal operation. So, if the abscess appears to be amenable to image-guided drainage — this is the way to proceed.**

- **The concept of a complex abscess is clinically useful. Abscesses that are multiple, multiloculated, associated with tissue necrosis, enteric communication or tumor, are defined as complex and are less likely to respond to PC drainage**, whereas most **simple** abscesses do. However, in gravely ill patients with **complex** abscesses, PC drainage may offer significant **temporizing** therapeutic benefits — allowing a definitive semi-elective operation in better-stabilized patients.
- **PC drainage and surgical drainage techniques should not be considered competitive but rather complementary.** If an abscess is accessible by PC techniques, it is reasonable to consider a non-operative approach to the problem. You, the surgeon, should consider each abscess individually together with the radiologist, taking into consideration the pros and cons presented in ■ Table 42.2.
- **Percutaneous aspiration only versus catheter drainage?** A single PC needle aspiration may successfully eradicate an abscess — especially when it is small and contains low-viscosity fluid or when it is located within a solid organ such as the liver or spleen. **There is good evidence, however, that PC catheter drainage is more effective.**
- **Size of PC catheters/drains?** Some claim advantage for large-bore trocar catheters for PC drainage but the evidence indicates that size 7Fr PC sump drains are as effective as size 14Fr. When needed, a small size catheter can be changed into a bigger one with percutaneous techniques.
- **Management of PC drains.** There is not much science here; these are small tubes and should be regularly flushed with saline to remain patent. PC drains are notoriously prone to falling (prematurely) out. Radiologists are superb in placing them but useless in securing them to the skin. Help them! The drain site should be regularly cleaned and observed; there are single case reports of **necrotizing fasciitis** of the abdominal wall around a PC drain site. PC drains are removed when clinical inflammation has resolved and the daily output (minus the saline injected) is below 25ml. **On average, after PC drainage of a simple abdominal abscess, the drain is removed after 5-7 days.**
- **Reimaging.** Clinical improvement should be seen within 24 to 72 hours following PC drainage. Persistent fever and leukocytosis on the fourth day after PC drainage correlates with management failure. **Non-responders should be reimaged with CT. Water-soluble contrast injected through the drain may help.** Depending on the findings, a decision should be taken as to the next appropriate course of action: a repeat PC drain or an operation. Persistence of high-output drainage in a patient who is clinically well can be better investigated with a tube sinogram to delineate the size of the residual abscess cavity. **Abscess cavities which do not collapse tend to recur.**

Table 42.2. Intra-abdominal abscesses: percutaneous (PC) versus open surgical drainage. Considerations in selecting the approach.*

	Prefer PC drainage	Prefer open drainage
Surgical accessibility	Hostile abdomen	Accessible
PC accessibility	Yes	No
Source controlled	Yes	No
Location	Visceral	Interloop
Number	Single	Multiple
Loculation	No	Yes
Communication with bowel	No	Yes
Associated necrosis	No	Yes
Associated malignancy	No	Yes
Viscosity	Thin	Thick debris
Invasive radiologist	Available	Not available
Severity of illness	'Stable'	Critically ill — cannot tolerate delay
Failed PC drainage	No	Yes

* These factors are not 'written in stone' and should be considered together with the specific clinical situation.

Failure of PC drainage: when to 'switch over' to surgical drainage?

Patients who deteriorate after the initial attempts at PC drainage should be operated upon promptly; further procrastination may be disastrous.

In stable non-responders to the initial PC drainage, a second attempt may be appropriate, according to the considerations mentioned in ■ Table 42.2. An inability to effect the second PC drainage successfully, or its clinical failure, mandates an open procedure.

Surgical management of intra-abdominal abscesses

At least in modern environments it is unusual that an intra-abdominal abscess is not suitable for PC drainage and requires an open operation. But if this does happen a few practical dilemmas exist:

- **Exploratory laparotomy vs. direct surgical approach.** A 'blind' exploratory laparotomy to search for an abscess 'somewhere', so common less than 30 years ago, is currently very rarely necessary. **A direct approach is obviously more 'benign', sparing the previously uninvolved peritoneal spaces and avoiding bowel injury and wound complications.** It is almost always possible in spontaneous abscesses, which are so well defined on CT (but those are also the kind of abscesses that usually respond to PC drainage). Nowadays, although postoperative abscesses are anatomically well localized on CT, those that fail PC drainage are usually 'complex', and therefore often not amenable to a direct approach (e.g. interloop abscess) or they require additional procedures to control the intestinal source. Criteria for choosing the correct approach are summarized in ■ Table 42.3. And by the way, if you already have a PC drain in place but it does not drain sufficiently, open exploration is easier when you 'follow the drain'.
- **Direct approach: extraperitoneal versus transperitoneal?** There are no significant differences in overall mortality and morbidity between the two approaches; however, the transperitoneal route is associated with a higher incidence of injury to the bowel. It is logical to suggest that the extraperitoneal approach should be used whenever anatomically possible. Subphrenic and subhepatic abscesses can be approached extraperitoneally through a subcostal incision or — if posterior — through the bed of the 12th rib. Old-timers are still familiar with these techniques, which are currently rarely utilized — having been replaced by PC drainage. Pericolic, appendicular and all sorts of retroperitoneal abscesses are best approached through a loin incision. Late-appearing pancreatic abscesses too can be drained extraperitoneally — through the flank — but occasionally need a bilateral approach. Pelvic abscesses are best drained through the rectum or vagina.
- **Drains?** Classically, at the end of the open procedure a drain was placed within the abscess cavity — brought to the skin away from the main incision. The type, size and number of drains used depended more on local traditions and preferences than on science. Similarly, the postoperative management of drains involved cumbersome rituals with the drains sequentially shortened, based on serial contrast sinograms, to ascertain the gradual collapse of the cavities and drain-tracks. House surgeons and nurses forever changed dressings and irrigated the drains — again according to the locally prevailing ritual. **Our experience is that these elaborate rituals should belong to history. With adequate surgical drainage, when the source of**

Table 42.3. Exploratory laparotomy vs. 'direct' open drainage of abdominal abscesses.

	Prefer exploratory laparotomy	Prefer direct open drainage
Abscess accurately localized on CT	–	✓
Early postoperative phase	✓	–
Late postoperative phase	✓	–
Single abscess	–	✓
Multiple abscesses	✓	–
Lesser sac abscess	✓	–
Interloop abscess	✓	–
Source of infection uncontrolled	✓	–
Subphrenic/subhepatic	–	✓
Gutter abscess	–	✓
Pelvic abscess	–	✓

infection has been controlled, when the abscess cavity is 'filled' with omentum or adjacent structures, and prophylactic peri-operative antibiotics are administered — no drains are necessary. Trust the peritoneal cavity to deal with the residual bacteria better in the absence of a foreign body — the drain. For a more detailed discussion of drains go to ➲ Chapter 36.

And to sum up...

Tailor your approach to the anatomy of the abscess, the physiology of the patient, and the local facilities available to you. Do not procrastinate, do not forget to deal with the source, do not over-rely on antibiotics, and get rid of the pus. Sepsis, the host-generated systemic inflammatory response to the abscess may persist, and progress to organ failure, even after the abscess has been adequately managed. Try not to be too late.

> **"No drainage is better than the ignorant employment of it... A drain invariably produces some necrosis of the tissue with which it comes in contact, and enfeebles the power of resistance of the tissues toward organisms."**
>
> **William Stewart Halsted**

Chapter 43

Anastomotic leaks and fistulas

The Editors

> *Anastomotic leakage is a completely avoidable complication; providing you don't perform an anastomosis.*
>
> **Brendan Moran**

> *If there is a possibility of several things going wrong, the one that will cause the most damage will be the one to go wrong.*
>
> **Murphy's Law, Arthur Bloch**

> *And if things do go wrong, there is no limit to how bad they can get...*
>
> **Ari Leppäniemi**

In this chapter we will focus on leaks originating from the small bowel.

For a comprehensive treatise on how to deal with all types of leaks (from the esophagus to the colon and rectum) we recommend that you study Chapter 6 in *Schein's Common Sense Prevention and Management of Surgical Complications*. (Or simply email a request for this chapter to mosheschein@gmail.com or drosin@mac.com and we will send you a free PDF ☺.)

Here we offer an abbreviated version, looking at the basics from a different perspective.

There are two chief clinical patterns of postoperative intestinal leak:

- **The leak is obvious** — you see intestinal contents draining from the operative wound (or from the drain, but we are sure you rarely use these…).
- **The leak is suspected** — you do not see it…

Scenario 1: the obvious leak

It is postoperative day 6 after a laparotomy for small bowel obstruction (➲ Chapter 19). The procedure was uneventful, except for two accidental enterotomies, which were closed with interrupted Vicryl® 3-0 in one layer. During morning rounds the patient complains: "Look, doctor, my bed is full of this green stuff." You uncover the patient's abdomen to see bile-stained intestinal juice pouring through the incision! Now you are very upset — *why did this happen to me?! I did a perfect operation…* True, the patient's recovery was not smooth; he was running a fever and a high white cell count. And now this terrible disaster! It is a disaster indeed, for the morbidity of this complication is horrendous and the mortality significant.

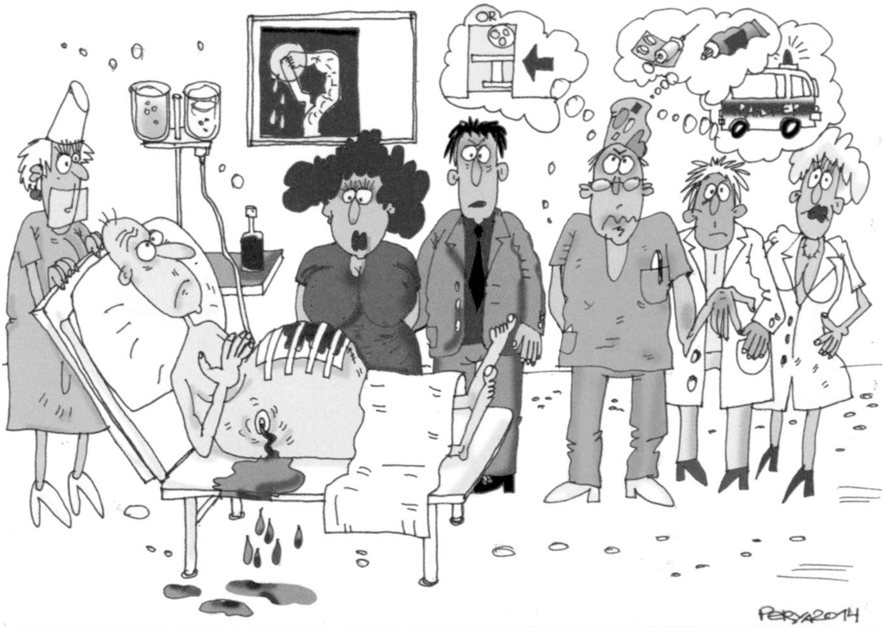

Figure 43.1. What's in their minds? "Reoperate?" "Treat as fistula?" "Transfer?" "Why is this happening to me?"

Your first reaction is: *let's get him immediately to the operating room and fix this mess...* Or perhaps treat conservatively? And what about shipping him out — let the guys in the ivory tower deal with it...?

What to do with such a nightmare (■ Figure 43.1)?

The controversy

There is little controversy that established postoperative external enterocutaneous fistulas, which usually result from leaking anastomoses or incidental enterotomies, should initially be managed, if possible, *conservatively*. As noted in previous chapters, there is also little controversy that acute gastrointestinal perforation, be it spontaneous or traumatic, is an indication for an emergency laparotomy to deal with the source of contamination/infection (➲ Chapter 13).

So, what about the early postoperative small bowel leakage? Is it like a 'simple perforation' requiring an immediate operation, or like a 'fistula' to be managed conservatively?

We contend that this scenario represents both conditions and should therefore be managed selectively in the individual patient.

The role of non-operative management

With proper supportive management, and in the absence of distal obstruction or loss of bowel continuity (i.e. it is a 'side-fistula', not an 'end-fistula'), a large percentage of postoperative **small bowel fistulas** will close spontaneously within 6 weeks. Those which fail to close by this time will require *elective* reoperation. **This, when performed on an anabolic, non-septic, non-'inflamed' patient, in a less hostile peritoneal environment, will restore the integrity of the gastrointestinal tract with an acceptable risk of complications.**

A crucial issue when deciding on a trial of conservative management is the presence or absence of significant peritonitis and sepsis — their presence being an indication for an immediate source control, usually by operation or, if possible, with percutaneous drainage. Even when clinical peritonitis is not present, evidence of sepsis should trigger an aggressive search for drainable intra-abdominal pus. This is best done with a CT scan; associated abscesses should be drained (➲ Chapter 42).

Remember: The chief cause of death in patients who develop anastomotic leaks is neglected intra-abdominal infection.

The role of early operative management

As stated above, diffuse peritonitis or complex intra-abdominal abscesses not suitable for — or not responding to — PC drainage, are indications for laparotomy (sometimes laparoscopy) to achieve source control. **But why not operate on all such patients?** Why not just surrender to the temptation buzzing in your brain: "I know where this leak is coming from; let me just return to that abdomen and fix this frustrating problem with a few more sutures… and abort this bad dream?"

Why not? Because — almost always — resuturing the leak won't solve the problem!

Primary closure of a disrupted intestinal suture line is doomed to fail.

Each of us can remember an isolated success in closing an intestinal leak (see below for specific indications to do so), but the collective experience points to an overwhelmingly high rate of failure. Attempts to close an intestinal leak, even after only a day or two days, in an infected peritoneal cavity are seldom successful. Similarly, redoing an intestinal anastomosis in the presence of postoperative peritonitis is an exercise in futility. (This, by the way, is true for any leaking suture line — in the esophagus, stomach, duodenum or colon.)

Obviously, if successful, the surgeon is a hero who either saves his patient's life, or at least prevents prolonged hospitalization and morbidity. **If, however, a leak redevelops, as it usually does, it produces a tremendous 'second hit' — added to the insult of the reoperation — which strikes an already primed, susceptible and compromised host. Sepsis and death are then almost inevitable.**

Suggested approach to early leaks/postoperative intestinal fistulas

A trial of conservative management is warranted when the leak is controlled:

- There is no clinical peritonitis.
- There are no associated abscesses on CT.

An immediate relaparotomy is warranted when the leak is not controlled:

- There is evidence of clinical peritonitis.
- There is systemic sepsis with proven or suspected intraperitoneal abscesses which cannot be drained percutaneously.

What to do during an emergency relaparotomy?

There are three things to consider:

- **The condition of the bowel.**
- **The condition of the peritoneal cavity.**
- **The condition of the patient.**

Very rarely — in a stable, minimally compromised patient, when peritonitis appears minimal, when the bowel appears of 'good quality' (meaning the consistency of thick slices of *prosciutto* — not *mortadella*), when the patient's serum albumin levels are reasonable — we would resect the involved segment of small bowel and reanastomose. Such a sequence of events is possible only when the leak presents within a day or two after the operation (usually caused by a technical mishap). An immediate reoperation before local and systemic adverse repercussions develop may thus provide a definitive cure. Other circumstances when attempts at repair of the leak are reasonable would be during early reoperations for upper gastrointestinal leaks (e.g. following omentopexy for perforated peptic ulcer, or gastric leaks after bariatric surgery), where exteriorization of the leaking part is impossible. **So one tries to patch and to achieve adequate drainage. And if the leak redevelops — and usually it does — one hopes to establish a controlled fistula.**

In all other circumstances, the less heroic but logical and life-saving option of exteriorization (if technically possible) of the leaking point as an enterostomy should be carried out, and at any level — even just distal to the duodenojejunal flexure. If this seems impossible just aim to achieve a controlled, external fistula — intubate the hole with a suitable catheter and drain!

So essentially your job is: "Let the st out and keep it flowing out..." Not for nothing are surgeons compared to plumbers specializing in toilets.**

Conservative management

The principles of management are few and simple:

- Provide aggressive supportive care.
- **Restore fluid and electrolyte balance**. All the fistula's losses should be measured and replaced.
- **Treat associated infection**. This has been mentioned before and is repeated here only to emphasize that when your fistula patient dies it is usually because you were not aggressive enough in pursuing our advice. Try to do it percutaneously. If an operation is needed, try to drain the abscess through a direct, local approach, avoiding the risks of a 'complete' laparotomy (➲ Chapter 42).
- **Protect the skin** around the fistula from the corrosive intestinal juice. A well-fitting colostomy bag around the fistula often does the trick. Otherwise, place a tube connected to a continuous suction source adjacent to the fistula, place **Stomahesive®** sheets around the defect, and cover the entire field with an adhesive transparent dressing — similar to the 'sandwich' mentioned in ➲ Chapter 44. (Alternatively, you may want to support the shares of a company which produces one of the commercial vacuum-assisted closure [VAC] systems.) Make generous use of karaya gum and/or zinc paste to protect the skin around difficult-to-manage, complex fistulas. Although such wounds require lots of effort and dedication, they are almost always manageable — but only if you care. **The way the abdominal wall of your fistula patient looks is how you look!**
- **Provide nutrition**. Proximal gastrointestinal fistulas require total parenteral nutrition (TPN) initially until a nasal feeding tube is inserted beyond the leak level. Most distal small bowel and colonic fistulas will close spontaneously whether the patient is fed orally or not. As emphasized in ➲ Chapter 39, using the intestine for feeding, if

possible, is better. In proximal fistulas it is often possible, and beneficial, to collect the fistula's output and reinfuse it, together with the enteral diet, into the bowel below the fistula. This is labor-intensive, as you will surely hear from your nurses, but worthwhile.

- **Delineate anatomy.** This is best done with a sinogram — injecting water-soluble contrast into the fistula tract. This will document the level of the bowel defect and, hopefully, the absence of distal obstruction or loss of continuity — prerequisites for successful conservative management. Your modern radiologist will probably prefer a CT with oral contrast, rather than a 'messy' sinogram, but your presence during this dynamic study will help you get it, and also better understand the anatomy.
- **Strive to achieve spontaneous closure** — the likelihood of which depends on the site and anatomy of the fistula; **this should be possible in most cases provided the following factors are not present**: distal obstruction; loss of bowel continuity; undrained infection; superficial fistula with no adjacent structures to cover it; associated cancer, foreign body or necrotic tissue. Oops, we almost forgot to mention tuberculosis, irradiated bowel or actinomycosis...
- **Proceed with surgical closure when indicated**, but delay it until the patient, his abdominal wall and the peritoneal cavity are ready — **usually after at least 3 months**. In patients recovering from major abdominal catastrophes (resulting in an abdominal wall defect and complex fistulas — see below), we would often wait 6-12 months. **The longer you wait the easier will be the reoperation**.
- **Refer the patient to a specialized center** if your own set-up is unable to cope with the demanding care of fistula patients.

Gimmicks or no gimmicks

The initial output of a fistula has little prognostic implications. A fistula which drains 1000ml/day during the first week has the same chance of spontaneously sealing as one with an output of 500ml/day. **Artificially decreasing a fistula's output with total starvation and administration of a somatostatin analogue is cosmetically appealing but not proven to be beneficial**.

In patients with a well-established (and long) fistula tract (which takes a few weeks to develop), it is possible to hasten the resolution of the fistula by blocking the tract. Many 'innovative' methods have been reported as successful (usually in tiny series of patients), ranging from the injection of fibrin glue (through an endoscope) deep into the tract, to plugging the tract's orifice with chewing gum (chewed by the patient not by you...).

Endoscopic attempts to seal the early leak with clips, glue and stents are becoming increasingly popular among esophageal, bariatric and colorectal surgeons but, obviously, are not practical for small bowel leaks.

Fistulas associated with a large abdominal wall defect

Not uncommonly, the end result of intestinal leaks and reoperative surgery is an abdominal wall defect with multiple intestinal fistulas in its base. Such defects are sometimes the result of spontaneous dehiscence of the wound but with the widespread practice of open abdomen management techniques, these types of fistula are observed with increasing frequency.

The distance of the fistulous opening in the intestine from the surface of the defect and the condition of the peritoneal cavity have a crucial bearing on the treatment of this condition.

It is practical to distinguish between two clinical situations (■ Figure 43.2):

- **The 'uncontrolled' fistulas. This is a scenario occurring early after the development of the intestinal leak** (e.g. a gastric leak after a subtotal gastrectomy associated with upper abdominal wound dehiscence). Here the opening is deep and the contents spread

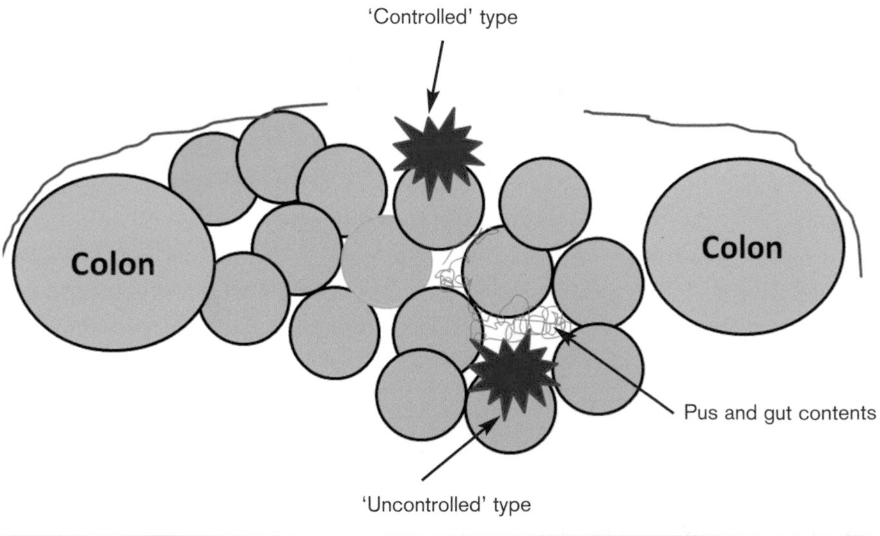

Figure 43.2. Fistulas associated with a large abdominal wall defect.

around, resulting in prolonged contact of large peritoneal surfaces with gastrointestinal contents. This increases absorption of toxic products and perpetuates local and systemic inflammatory responses and organ dysfunction. **In such instances reoperation is necessary to exteriorize or divert and/or drain the intestinal leak away from the defect**. Otherwise, the patient is doomed, as many patients with this type of postoperative fistula die!

- **The 'controlled' fistulas. This is a late phenomenon in the natural history of leakage associated with an abdominal wall defect**. These are 'exposed' fistulas near the surface of the defect. Also called '*enteroatmospheric*' or 'bud' fistulas, they result from damage to matted intestine which forms the 'bed' of the defect (the so-called 'central visceral block'). Because the peritoneal cavity is usually clean and sealed away from intestinal contents, the patient is free of sepsis but the management of such fistulas needs a lot of ingenuity.

Management

With the uncontrolled type, your aim is to exteriorise the leak or divert it. If this is technically impossible then you should 'intubate' the leak or at least drain it adequately. Once the intestinal effluent stops pouring into the general peritoneal cavity the situation is no longer immediately life-threatening.

With controlled fistulas, the immediate task is to control the output of the fistula — to facilitate nursing! Use your creative skills to construct a sealed vacuum dressing of your choice to cover the whole defect — sucking out the fistula's effluent. We use a modification of our 'sandwich' (➲ Chapter 44). Others would suture a large colostomy bag all around the rim of the fistula (bag-enterostomy), placing a suction tube into the bag. And there are all those commercial products...

Some surgeons have described 'local' attempts to close small enteroatmospheric fistulas, by suturing the bowel and covering it with glue, biological dressings, skin graft or musculocutaneous flaps. Sometimes you may be lucky and the defect is so small that you can suture the intestinal hole and mobilize healthy surrounding skin to cover the suture line and close the defect.

In most such patients, however, you will have to control the fistula, support the patient, wait for the abdominal wall defect to contract, wait for resolution of the peritoneal inflammation, wait for maturation of intra-abdominal adhesions, and only then — after at least 6 months and usually more than that

— consider 'take down' of the fistula and undertake abdominal wall reconstruction.

A simple rule of thumb is that the condition of the abdominal wall defect reflects the condition of the peritoneal cavity. A well-contracted abdominal wall defect, and fistulas that look like surgical stomas are indicators that an elective intervention is possible and safe (see also ➲ Chapter 44).

Remember: the key term in such patients is W.W.W. — wait, wait and wait!

Scenario 2: you suspect a leak but do not see one

Your patient is now a week after an uneventful right hemicolectomy for a carcinoma of the cecum. She is already at home, and eating, when a new pain develops on the right side of her abdomen, accompanied by vomiting. The patient returns to the emergency room. She is febrile, her right abdomen is tender with a questionable mass, the abdominal X-ray suggests an ileus or partial small bowel obstruction, the white cell count is elevated. You suspect an anastomotic leak.

From a clinical standpoint there are three types of intestinal leaks that 'you cannot see':

- **Free leak**. The anastomosis is disrupted, and the leak is not contained by adjacent structures. The patients usually appear 'sick', exhibiting signs of diffuse peritonitis. **An immediate laparotomy is indicated as outlined above**.
- **Contained leak**. The leak is partially contained by peri-anastomotic adhesions to the omentum and adjacent viscera. The clinical abdominal manifestations are localized. A peri-anastomotic abscess is a natural sequela.
- **A mini-leak**. This is a 'minute' anastomotic leak — usually occurring late after the operation when the anastomosis is well-sealed off. Abdominal manifestations are localized and the patient is not 'toxic'. A mini-leak is actually a **'peri-anastomositis'** — an inflammatory phlegmon around the anastomosis. Usually it is not associated with a drainable pus-containing abscess.

In the absence of diffuse peritonitis, you should document the leak and grade it, which is best done by combining a contrast study with a CT — searching for free intraperitoneal contrast or abscesses. There are a few possibilities:

- **Free leak** of contrast into the peritoneal cavity (a lot of free contrast and fluid on CT). You must reoperate. We have previously discussed what to do: it's best to take down the anastomosis, if technically feasible.
- **Contained localized leak** (a local collection or abscess on CT). The rest of the peritoneal cavity is 'dry'. This is initially treated with antibiotics and PC drainage.
- **No leak on contrast study** (a peri-anastomotic phlegmon on CT). This represents a mini-leak or 'peri-anastomositis' and usually resolves after a few days of antibiotic therapy.

A contained leak or a mini-leak may be associated with an obstruction at the anastomosis — a result of local inflammation. Such obstruction usually resolves spontaneously (within a week or so) after the pus has been drained and the inflammation has subsided.

We have tried to persuade you that an anastomotic leak is not one disease but a variety of conditions requiring customized approaches. To keep morbidity at bay, tailor your treatment to the specific leak, its severity and the condition of the affected patient. **Above all — remember that non-drained intraperitoneal bowel contents and pus are killers — often silent ones**. And read Chapter 6 in our complications book!

"We tend to remember best those patients we almost killed; we never forget those we actually managed to kill."

"Good surgeons operate well; great surgeons know how to manage their own complications."

Chapter 44

Relaparotomy and laparostomy for intra-abdominal infection

The Editors [1]

This chapter has been subdivided into the following three sections:

1. Relaparotomy.
2. Laparostomy.
3. Laparoscopic abdominal re-exploration.

It's just that as an old general surgeon, I usually reserve optimism until the day after discharge, or often until the first post-op visit. Until then I plan for the next worst potential problem.

Jerry Kaplan

You probably remember the principles of management of *intra-abdominal infection (IAI)* we discussed earlier (➲ Chapter 13). **We told you that to improve survival, in some patients, source control and peritoneal toilet must be pushed a little further; some patients need a relaparotomy and in many of these the abdomen is left open (laparostomy).** These modalities will now be discussed in greater detail. At the end of the chapter, we will discuss **laparoscopic abdominal re-exploration** after open surgery.

1 Roger Saadia, MD FRCS(Ed), contributed to this chapter in the previous editions.

1 Relaparotomy

Definitions

Before we continue you should be reintroduced to some definitions.

'On-demand' versus 'planned' relaparotomy:

- **'On-demand'**: in the aftermath of an initial laparotomy, clinical or radiological evidence of an intra-abdominal complication forces the surgeon to reoperate.
- **'Planned'** (or 'electively staged'): at the initial laparotomy, the surgeon makes the decision to reoperate within 1-3 days, irrespective of the patient's immediate postoperative course.

Both these types of relaparotomy have a place in the postoperative management of some patients following a laparotomy, but they apply in different clinical contexts.

Relaparotomy 'on demand'

The classic indication for emergency relaparotomy is generalized peritonitis due to an anastomotic leak. Leaks take place typically between the fifth and eighth postoperative days, but may occur earlier or later. If not 'controlled', or if not 'contained' and thus not amenable to percutaneous drainage, the abdomen may have to be re-explored (➲ Chapter 43).

There are many other situations calling for a reoperation: accidental intestinal injury (duodenum during lap cholecystectomy); strangulated intestinal obstruction (within a port site); ischemic bowel (people do ligate the SMA by mistake...); complete abdominal wall dehiscence (embarrassing); abdominal compartment syndrome (why did I close?); necrotizing fasciitis of the abdominal wall; retained sponge, instrument or drain (*oi vey*); retracted or necrotic stoma (why didn't I do it better?); missed diagnosis (mainly in penetrating trauma) — the list is long, use your imagination. **All such situations are discussed within the specific chapters; here we will focus on the common denominator — postoperative peritonitis**.

Postoperative peritonitis

Peritonitis complicating a laparotomy is termed 'postoperative peritonitis'. **This is one of the most lethal types of peritonitis — killing a large proportion of sufferers — for the following three reasons**:

- **The diagnosis is usually delayed**, mainly because the abdominal and systemic signs are initially masked by the expected similar signs of the normal postoperative abdomen, the analgesia and antibiotics.
- **It occurs in the postoperative phase**, when the patient is catabolic, with associated systemic inflammation and immunodepression.
- **This is a case of *nosocomial* secondary peritonitis** where the microbiology is less predictable and more noxious due to previous antibiotic administration and the prevailing hospital flora.

There are several possible clinical presentations developing within days of a laparotomy as outlined below.

Generalized peritonitis

The abdominal findings are out of proportion to the normal postoperative state (severe abdominal pain and tenderness, massive or prolonged ileus). There may be associated systemic repercussions (fever, leukocytosis) that are uncharacteristic of the expected postoperative recovery. Sometimes, the diagnosis is made easier by the additional presence of an enterocutaneous fistula (➲ Chapter 43), deep space SSI (➲ Chapter 46), or abdominal wall dehiscence (➲ Chapter 45). Obviously, any clinical feature which promotes early abdominal imaging, like persistent postoperative ileus (➲ Chapter 41), would aid in the diagnosis.

Organ dysfunction

Renal failure or incipient acute respiratory distress syndrome (ARDS) could be masquerading as atelectasis or pneumonia. Not infrequently, the surgeon seeks expert advice from medical colleagues (nephrologist, chest physician, infectious disease specialist or intensivist). Of course, renal failure or pneumonia may well occur in a postoperative patient for a variety of reasons that are unrelated to an intra-abdominal complication. **However, persistent or recurrent intra-abdominal infection may present initially as a single system dysfunction and progress, in time, to multiple organ failure (MOF).**

It is essential, firstly, to be aware of the relationship between IAI and organ dysfunction and secondly, to be humble enough to consider the possibility of a surgical complication in one's patient (➲ Chapter 39). **The diagnosis is established by careful clinical evaluation of the patient — supplemented with abdominal imaging — mainly computed tomography (CT).**

The intensive care setting

The diagnosis of IAI is considered because of the need for prolonged ventilation or aggravation of multiple organ dysfunction in a critically ill postoperative patient; for example, after massive trauma or major abdominal surgery. Intensivists are usually quick to point to the abdomen as the culprit and eager to spur the surgeon to re-explore. **In a ventilated, paralyzed patient, the abdomen cannot be evaluated clinically**. There is therefore a real dilemma in differentiating between, on the one hand, the presence of an abdominal focus of infection and, on the other hand, systemic inflammation (with no infectious focus) or an infection elsewhere.

Abdominal CT scanning is very useful but, unfortunately, less so in the first few postoperative days. After any laparotomy, tissue planes are distorted and potential spaces may contain fluid; even the best radiologist cannot be certain — on postoperative day 3 — whether the fluid is blood, serous fluid, leaking bowel contents or pus; or whether the quantity of free air is inappropriate to the index operation. In addition, transporting a critically ill patient on maximal organ support to the CT suite is not an innocuous undertaking. **Thus, the decision to reoperate during the first few postoperative days can be extremely vexing and requires good cooperation between surgeons, intensivists and radiologists. It also helps if the surgeon has big (gender-neutral) balls!**

Intra-abdominal abscesses (➲ Chapter 42)

Remember: The diagnosis of postoperative intra-abdominal 'septic' complications is extremely difficult. **Denial is a major culprit in 'missed' cases!** Surgeons hate to admit to their own failures and confront them. Consider, for a moment, your experience: haven't you seen patients fading away while their deterioration is blamed on a bad bout of pneumonia? Autopsy would have revealed unsuspected intra-abdominal complications in a good proportion of them.

Mark M. Ravitch reminds us wisely: "The last man to see the necessity for reoperation is the man who performed the operation."

The following admonition should be deeply imprinted in your surgical soul: "Look for 'pneumonia' inside the abdomen."

'Planned' (electively staged) relaparotomy

A negative relaparotomy is better than a positive autopsy but is not, nevertheless, a benign procedure.

The policy of planned relaparotomies is decided upon during, or immediately after, the initial, index, emergency operation. The surgeon decides to reoperate within 1-3 days, irrespective of the patient's immediate postoperative course. Historically, mesenteric ischemia (➲ Chapter 22) was probably the first instance when a planned relook laparotomy was advocated. In the context of IAI, the main justification for a relook is to control the source of contamination/infection (a goal which was impossible to achieve for various reasons during the index operation as described below), to anticipate the formation of new ones before they have had the time to amplify the existing sepsis and to tip the patient into irreversible multiple organ failure.

Indications for planned relaparotomies

These need to be better defined and restricted to well-selected patients. A relaparotomy is best undertaken during the first few postoperative days, a period when abdominal CT findings are 'non-specific' and CT-directed percutaneous procedures are not an option.

So this is when we may consider a planned reoperation:

- **The most appropriate indication is failure to obtain adequate source control during the initial operation**. A classic example is infected pancreatic necrosis (➲ Chapter 17). Another example is an intestinal leak which cannot be safely repaired or exteriorized (e.g. a neglected leak from the retroperitoneal duodenum).
- The necessity to **redebride or redrain poorly localized, 'stubborn' infected tissues**; for example, in diffuse retroperitoneal necrotizing infection (some call it 'retroperitoneal fasciitis') due to retroperitoneal perforation of the duodenum or colon.
- In the massive trauma situation (➲ Chapter 30), the poor shape of the patient during the initial operation may occasionally lead to an

abbreviated 'damage control' procedure, **with an obligatory subsequent planned relaparotomy to complete source control and peritoneal toilet**. In brief, the reoperation is to 'complete the job' (e.g. a deferred anastomosis) — **the first operation is for physiology, the second is for anatomy**. Obviously, when hemostatic packs have been left *in situ*, a relaparotomy is needed to remove them.

- In the past, **diffuse fecal peritonitis** was considered a relative indication, with the rationale that in the face of massive fecal contamination another laparotomy is necessary to achieve an adequate peritoneal toilet. Nowadays, we believe, most such patients can be treated with a 'single' operation — supplemented, if necessary, with percutaneous drainage or an 'on demand' reoperation.

The conduct of a relaparotomy

The key piece of advice for the surgeon who plans to re-enter a recently opened abdomen is to be gentle! The peritoneal surfaces are edematous, friable and vascular, and so is the bowel. Reoperative abdominal surgery is a situation where the dictum "first do no harm" has particular relevance. **Do not perforate the bowel, do not cause bleeding — such mishaps in an already compromised patient are often a death sentence.**

Another important tip: know your way around. Ideally, the surgeon who has performed the original procedure should either be the one to reoperate or at least be a member of the reoperating team. Think about the infected postoperative abdomen as a dense jungle; a previous journey through it renders a return easier. You will remember, for example, that the colon was 'stuck' to the lower end of the incision; your partner who did not accompany you on your first trip may instead enter the lumen of the colon, with horrendous consequences. **Even in this glorious era of 'surgical hospitalists' and 'shift mentality' we feel it is neglectful for a surgeon to expect others to fix *his* patients without being directly involved!**

The abdominal relook itself aims at draining all infected collections and controlling, if necessary, persistent sources of contamination. How thorough the exploration should be depends on the individual case. Sometimes there are several inter-loop abscesses that need to be drained and the whole bowel must be carefully unravelled. **However, particularly later in the natural course of peritonitis the intestines are matted together, forming a 'central visceral block'; it is then prudent to explore only the spaces *around* the matted bowel — subphrenic spaces, paracolic gutters, pelvis. Leave the glued intestine alone!**

The decision about the extent of exploration is important because the more extensive it is, the more dangerous it is to the viscera. As you have been told here again and again, the more you do, the more local and systemic inflammation you trigger. **The extent of the exploration depends not only on whether your operation is 'directed' or 'non-directed' but also on its timing.**

'Directed' versus 'non-directed' relook

Let the CT scan be your guide. A 'directed' reoperation implies that you know exactly where you want to go. The CT scan identifies a right subhepatic collection, with the rest of the abdomen appearing clean. You can proceed directly to where the trouble is, sparing the rest of the abdomen the potentially damaging effects of your manipulations. Conversely, a 'non-directed' relook is a blind re-exploration when you are not sure where the problem lies, for example, when the CT scan shows diffuse collections; in this instance, a thorough search is required.

Timing of the relook

When you re-explore the abdomen 24-72 hours after the index operation, the adhesions between viscera and peritoneal surfaces give way easily; you can enter any space with atraumatic dissection. At this stage total abdominal exploration is readily feasible. **However, as time goes by, the intra-abdominal structures become progressively cemented to each other with dense, vascular, immature adhesions that are troublesome to divide.** Clearly, abdominal re-entry between 1-4 weeks after the index operation may be hazardous, and will remain so until the eventual maturation of the adhesions months later.

So, dissection of the individual loops at this intermediate stage is dangerous and non-productive because significant collections are to be found only at the periphery — **above** (under the diaphragms or under the liver), **below** (in the pelvis), and on the **sides** (in the gutters). **Leave the 'central visceral block' alone!**

During re-exploration sharp tools are rarely needed. Your fingers are the safest dissecting instrument. Remember: where tissue planes are fused, forbidding admission to your gently pinching fingers, nothing is to be found. **So follow your fingers to where the pus lies.** Remember the old jingle about the Yellow Pages? "Let your fingers do the walking." **In a scarred operative field, never cut anything unless you can see through it.**

The leaking intestine

Dehisced suture lines and anastomoses must be defunctioned, ideally by the fashioning of appropriate stomas or, if this is not possible, by tube drainage. **Resuturing leaking bowel in an infected peritoneal cavity is doomed to failure and carries a prohibitive mortality**. No, we will never tire of driving home this point! (➲ Chapter 43).

Drains

The use of intraperitoneal drains is controversial in this setting. They are certainly not required if planned relaparotomies continue. The placement of a drain at the **final laparotomy** is another matter; the advantages need to be weighed against the risk of damage to viscera that are extremely friable as a result of recent re-explorations. **The use of drains in our practice is strictly limited to specific situations as discussed elsewhere** (➲ Chapter 36).

When to stop 'planned' relaparotomies (■ Figure 44.1)?

As in most vital aspects of life, too much of anything is not good, and too many relaparotomies are harmful. When to stop? In such a management

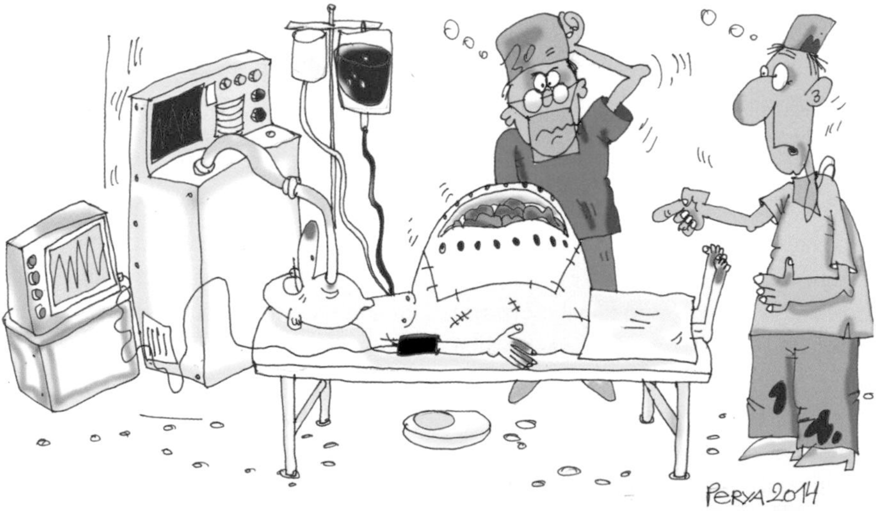

Figure 44.1. Junior surgeon to Professor: "Sir, this morning the patient underwent relaparotomy number 21. When should we stop re-exploring?" Professor: "When his C-reactive protein normalizes..."

program, the decision to quit must be based on the finding of a macroscopically clean peritoneal cavity and evidence that sources of contamination have been controlled definitively. Whether the source is controlled or not is obvious but estimation of whether the peritoneal cavity is 'clean' or not requires experience and judgment. **Thus, do not send your junior partner or senior resident to re-explore it alone**. (We bet you are familiar with this scenario: the internationally famous master of laparoscopic surgery does a beautiful operation. He is now abroad at a meeting, when on postop day 2 his Fellow has to try and fix the disaster. The outcome is predictable…).

Frequent dilemma: "take your spouse for dinner or the patient back to the OR?" (you may lose even if you make the correct choice!).

Are 'planned' relaparotomies beneficial?

What is the verdict? Do 'planned' relaparotomies reverse, prevent or aggravate sepsis and multi-organ dysfunction? Is the benefit/risk ratio favorable? There it is, at the risk of being repetitive.

Any surgical maneuver that successfully eliminates the source of infection and evacuates contaminants and pus must be beneficial; this is axiomatic. **The problem is that 'planned' relaparotomies are a double-edged sword** — they may achieve the above goal but may also injure the host. **Indeed, strict adherence to the policy of 'planned' relaparotomies is a definite overkill**. If one operates until the abdomen is clean then — in retrospect — the last operation was unnecessary. Multiple relaparotomies are attended by a high morbidity accounted for by destabilizing an ICU patient during repeated trips to the OR, iatrogenic bowel injuries and possibly the stimulation of an exaggerated inflammatory response (not to mention the late negative effects on abdominal wall integrity).

We believe that, in the long run, we serve our patients better with a low-threshold policy of postoperative *on-demand* percutaneous CT-guided drainage procedures or *on-demand* CT-directed laparotomies. One or two planned relaparotomies may still have a place in the indications listed above and only in the first postoperative week when both the imaging is less reliable and the abdomen safer to re-enter. But wholesale application of such a policy and relegating the relaparotomy performance to junior staff at the end of the OR slate are recipes for disaster.

It is our opinion that in most patients, 'on demand' is the way to go, based on the patient's clinical condition and convincing imaging. **Common sense and experience must prevail when high level evidence is lacking**.

2 Laparostomy

P. Fagniez of Paris has coined the term *laparostomie* (laparostomy) which entails leaving the abdomen open. Open management of the infected abdomen was instituted in the belief that the infected peritoneal cavity should be left open like an abscess cavity. It soon became clear, however, that many times there was still a need for thorough abdominal re-exploration in search of deep pockets of infection. **Laparostomy has become an *adjunct* to the repeated laparotomies; indeed, if the abdomen is to be reopened 48 hours later, why close it at all?**

The potential advantages of laparostomy are substantial: necrosis of the macerated abdominal midline incision closed forcefully and repeatedly in the presence of an edematous and distended bowel is avoided; better diaphragmatic excursion may be expected; and — by leaving the abdomen open — **the abdominal compartment syndrome with its renal, respiratory and hemodynamic repercussions is prevented** (➲ Chapter 31).

Indications

For practical purposes, consider **laparostomy either when the abdomen cannot be closed or should not be closed.**

The abdomen cannot be closed:

- After major loss of abdominal wall tissue following trauma or debridement for necrotizing fasciitis.
- Extreme visceral or retroperitoneal swelling after major trauma, resuscitation or major surgery (e.g. ruptured abdominal aortic aneurysm).
- Poor condition of fascia after multiple laparotomies.
- 'Burst abdomen' with elevated intra-abdominal pressure and/or necrotic fascial edges.

The abdomen should not be closed:

- Planned reoperation within a day or two — why lock the gate through which you are to re-enter very soon?
- Closure possible only under extreme tension, compromising the fascia and creating intra-abdominal hypertension (IAH).

Technical considerations of laparostomy

Now that you have decided not to close the abdomen, how should you manage it?

The option of simply covering the exposed viscera with moist gauze packs has been practiced for generations but is inadvisable: intestine, if not matted together, can eviscerate; it is also messy, requiring intensive work to keep the patient and his bed clean and dry. More importantly, it carries a significant risk of creating spontaneous, 'atmospheric' (i.e. exposed to the open air and without a track) intestinal fistulas (➲ Chapter 43). The friable, dilated bowel does not bear well the trauma of exposure and repeated dressing change, and is likely at some point to break down. **Temporary abdominal closure (TAC) devices to cover the laparostomy wound are therefore highly recommended**.

Temporary abdominal closure (TAC)

The ideal method (still to be invented) must:

- **Allow re-exploration**, offering easy access for relaparotomies, if needed.
- **Offer drainage** to the peritoneal exudate and later for possible fistulas.
- **Preserve fascia** for future abdominal closure.
- **Avoid 'loss of domain'**: when the fascial edges retract, the viscera bulge out and then cannot be returned to the peritoneal cavity.
- **Be kind to the underlying bowel** especially in the absence of an interposed omentum.

Your local guru probably has his own preferred method of TAC be it a 'Bogota bag' made of a large sterile intravenous-fluid bag, a ready-to-use transparent 'bowel bag', a synthetic mesh (absorbable or non-absorbable), a Velcro®-type material, which can be tightened like your tennis shoe ('Wittmann patch') or some 'innovation' featured in ■ Figure 44.2. We even know a guy in South America who uses discarded nylon hose for this purpose. Nowadays, there is a whole line of homemade or commercial products based on the vacuum concept.

In fact, one of the Editors (MS) was the first to introduce a vacuum-suction system for TAC (The 'sandwich technique' in the management of the open abdomen. *British Journal of Surgery* 1986; 73(5): 369-70). Subsequently, as usually is the case, the industry took over and now most of you are probably addicted to one of the commercial 'VAC' products. Thus, in this edition, we avoid a detailed discussion of the specific system.

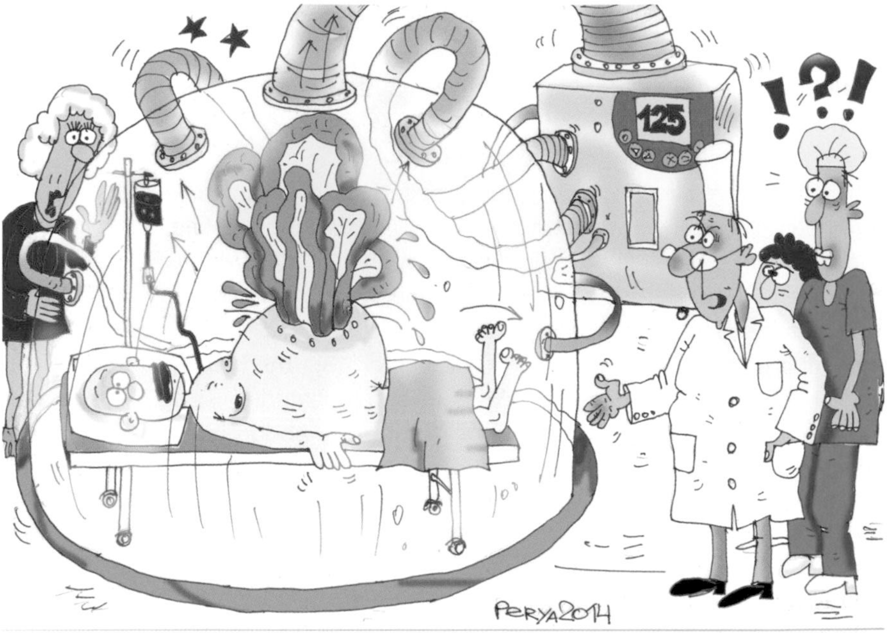

Figure 44.2. Surgeon to visitors: "This is our new temporary closure device. It allows us to apply negative pressure to the whole patient..."

Terminating the laparostomy

Once the laparostomy has outlived its usefulness, it is time to plan for abdominal closure. Two options exist, depending on both the surgeon's preference and local abdominal conditions: **early abdominal closure or delayed abdominal wall reconstruction**.

Early abdominal closure

The optimal time window is quite narrow, about a week from the last abdominal exploration. Beyond that, the fascia retracts laterally and adhesions form between intestine and abdominal wall. You will find it then impossible to mobilize and push the bulging viscera back into the abdominal cavity ('loss of domain'), to say nothing of the stubborn refusal of the fascial edges to meet in the midline. **Even within the first week, the longer the delay, the more difficult and risky this endeavor becomes**.

It goes without saying that feasibility of early closure is predicated on several factors including defect size, resolution of the ileus, absence of fistulas and negative fluid balance. In rare cases, the defect is so small that the fascial edges lend themselves to midline suturing without tension (one wonders, in such cases, whether a laparostomy was indicated in the first place!). More commonly, in small-size defects, the fascia is left open, but primary cutaneous closure is possible after undermining the skin edges. The patient is left with a ventral hernia, but **skin cover is superior to any prosthetic material** (➲ Chapter 37).

Most laparostomy wounds in the aftermath of a *real* abdominal disaster are large and present with fixed, retracted edges, and with loss of domain for the abdominal viscera. Recently developed biomaterials are being aggressively marketed (a new such product is being alleged as 'superior' almost every month...) for this setting. They are claimed to be better than synthetic meshes in resisting infection in these frequently contaminated wounds. It turns out that they are not totally immune to infection. While providing a temporary 'bridge', their other claim to fame is their purported ability to stimulate growth of site-specific cells to replace the prosthesis with new fascia (not scar). **In practice, most patients undergoing early abdominal closure with these 'wunderbioprostheses' are found, on brief follow-up, to have large ventral hernias. It seems therefore that, in many instances, these so called 'bioprostheses' are no more than a tremendously expensive TAC.**

Some surgeons advocate early reconstruction using 'component separation techniques' to approximate the fascia, occasionally buttressing the midline with an underlay of bioprosthesis. Experimentation with these novel techniques is inadvisable for the uninitiated. In our practice, most patients are treated with **delayed abdominal reconstruction.**

However you manage the abdominal wall defect, remember that your patient has just recovered from the immense stress of severe peritonitis and multiple operations — he cannot take much more at this stage.

Delayed abdominal wall reconstruction

Consider the following scenario:

> An obese patient develops a breakdown of his colorectal anastomosis with severe fecal peritonitis. The patient is now grossly distended, 'septic' and in respiratory failure. He undergoes a Hartmann's; and, obviously, his abdomen cannot be closed — so he is managed with a laparostomy. Early closure is not a realistic option. How to proceed?

At this stage, we would have used a vacuum TAC system to cover the abdomen. A couple of weeks later, a healthy layer of granulation tissue would develop over the underlying intestine/omentum. **Now, a split-skin graft can be applied onto the granulating fascial defect.** The resulting ventral hernia is usually wide-necked and well tolerated except for its cosmetic appearance. Many patients feel fortunate enough to have survived their 'surgical saga' and find the end-result acceptable with the added support from an abdominal Velcro® binder.

A detailed discussion of the delayed *elective* abdominal reconstruction of the laparostomy defect is beyond the scope of this 'emergency surgery' book. However, here are the principles involved:

- **Delay reconstruction for up to 12 months, or even more**, until the abdomen looks and feels like 'jelly': the skin graft is 'loose' and 'pinchable' away from underlying structures, the scar is soft, the stomas or fistulas, if present, are prolapsing.
- **At operation**, excise the skin graft, lyse all adhesions and use the 'component separation technique' (it seems that every day we have a new modification to this technique...) to close the fascial defect, combined, if necessary, with synthetic mesh. You should probably avoid the use of synthetic mesh in a contaminated field; for example, when the operation involves the resection of an intestinal fistula or take down of a stoma.

In summary...

***Relaparotomy* and *laparostomy* are therapeutic measures that are indicated in a small minority of patients.** They represent, for the time being, the heaviest weaponry in the surgeon's mechanical armamentarium for the treatment of severe intra-abdominal infection and other post-laparotomy abdominal catastrophes. **Remember that unnecessary relaparotomies carry significant morbidity in these patients.**

An aggressive but selective policy of directed, 'on-demand' relooks, supplemented sparingly by laparostomy, is superior to the indiscriminate use of 'blind' planned relaparotomies with routine laparostomy.

He who operates and runs away, may get to reoperate on the same patient another day.

3 Laparoscopic abdominal re-exploration

Why laparoscopy rather than relaparotomy?

The presence of a fresh abdominal wound makes it appealing to re-explore through this same incision. However, reopening of a recent incision and re-exploration by laparotomy may increase short- and long-term morbidity. Relaparotomy is associated with pain, ileus and an increased risk of abdominal infection. It may increase the risk of wound infection, and eventual wound dehiscence or later development of an incisional hernia. Overall, it may extend the recovery period of the patient, on top of the condition that prompted it, serving as a 'second hit'.

Treatment of complications after laparoscopic surgery is frequently attempted by a repeat laparoscopy — trying to avoid a formal laparotomy (see also ➲ Chapter 12). Indeed, complications such as bleeding or bile leak after laparoscopic cholecystectomy can be successfully approached by a second laparoscopy (➲ Chapter 18).

Laparoscopy is frequently performed in the presence of abdominal scars and previous operations and, thus, adhesions and moderately distended bowel are no longer considered to be contraindications for laparoscopic intervention. Given the morbidity associated with relaparotomy, and the ability of trained laparoscopic surgeons to deal with acute abdominal conditions, **it naturally follows that acute postoperative complications may be optimally handled by a minimal access approach**.

Postoperative conditions treated by laparoscopy

Mesenteric ischemia (➲ Chapter 22)

One of the earliest applications of laparoscopy after a recent laparotomy was to perform a 'second-look' operation after treating acute mesenteric ischemia. The purpose of this procedure was to ascertain the viability of potentially ischemic segments of bowel, for example, around the anastomosis after resection of gangrenous bowel. As the secondary intervention was a simple diagnostic procedure (in the absence of more ischemia), it could readily be accomplished via laparoscopy. It was even suggested that laparoscopic ports should be left in place at the end of the first operation. As explained in Chapter 22 this is no longer advisable because a relaparotomy is necessary, as bowel of questionable viability should not be anastomosed in the first place. There is however a potential role for laparoscopy in the very occasional patient who has had an anastomosis of what was believed to be perfectly viable bowel and who then deteriorates unexpectedly.

Early postoperative small bowel obstruction

Early postoperative small bowel obstruction (➲ Chapter 41) is a relatively infrequent condition, as opposed to the more common postoperative ileus. At times, it will require a second intervention. Laparoscopic management of bowel obstruction is an established procedure and we have successfully applied this approach in several cases of early postoperative obstruction after appendectomy, colectomy and laparotomy for trauma. This is especially rewarding when a single adhesion is the culprit.

Peptic ulcer perforation

Peptic ulcer perforation (➲ Chapter 16.1) is another rare postoperative complication, not directly related to the specific procedure performed but possibly related to the postoperative stress response or to ulcerogenic medications. These cases can be treated by laparoscopic omentopexy, like the standard approach to 'primary' duodenal peptic perforations. Imagine your relief when you re-explore for postoperative free air and find an intact anastomosis and a small duodenal hole. Wouldn't you be happy that you avoided a new laparotomy?

Intra-abdominal abscesses (➲ Chapters 13, 42, and earlier in this chapter)

Most postoperative abscesses are amenable to percutaneous CT-guided drainage, but a few are not accessible and mandate surgical drainage. Unless the patient is critically ill, laparoscopy can be used to access the abscess cavity, drain and irrigate it, and leave suction drainage in the area.

Anastomotic leak (➲ Chapter 43)

Laparoscopy may permit bowel exteriorization and abdominal toilet, without disturbing the original laparotomy wound. In addition, 'perianastomositis', although usually responding to antibiotic treatment, may be associated with the presence of free abdominal gas but without actual spillage of bowel contents. This is frequently treated by anastomotic takedown or a proximal diversion. However, in some patients in whom laparoscopy revealed a localized inflammatory process around a sealed-off anastomotic leak, drainage alone led to full recovery.

Technique

Access to the abdominal cavity should be established by the open technique, as the bowel may be distended and adherent to the abdominal wall. The port is placed away from the previous incision, usually laterally in the abdominal wall, to avoid the inevitable adhesions to the fresh scar.

Some of the adhesions can be separated bluntly by careful movements, as the bowel may be edematous and friable. Trocars are placed as necessary, when enough space is established, to complete the abdominal exploration. Non-traumatic instruments should be used, and bowel handling should be kept to the minimum, preferably manipulating the bowel by grasping its mesentery to avoid serosal tears and perforations. Although at times the pathology is evident, it is frequently hidden by adhesions of omentum and bowel loops. **The abdomen may initially appear 'benign', but a thorough search in spaces such as the pelvis, subphrenic areas or retroperitoneum may reveal a compartmentalized process. Previous imaging obtained by a CT scan should help you direct the exploration and prevent false-negative explorations and missed pathologies.**

To conclude, laparoscopy is a valuable tool, 'in good hands', to treat postoperative situations that were once considered as a clear indication for relaparotomy. It may serve you and the patient well, but good hands are not enough, unless there is common sense to guide them.

> **"A surgeon... is like the skipper of an ocean-going racing yacht. He knows the port he must make, but he cannot foresee the course of the journey. At every stage he must have a plan, based on a working knowledge of his present position, that will allow him to make for the best of several available harbours should things go wrong, or if none is suitable he must know where to find temporary refuge under the lee of the land till he can resume his journey."**
>
> **William Heneage Ogilvie**

Chapter 45

Abdominal wall dehiscence

The Editors [1]

There are few things more embarrassing to a surgeon than the sight of his recently operated patient, his abdomen gaping, and the gut spilling out all around...

Such a catastrophe occurs either because you did not close the tummy properly (that is because you didn't bother reading ➲ Chapter 37...), or it should not have been closed at all.

Because we are all such good surgeons, and possess superb judgment, our incidence of *complete* postoperative abdominal wound dehiscence should be negligible. Over the last 20 years we do not recall having to take a patient back to the operating room to reclose a burst abdomen. But from time to time we have had to do it for other surgeons (e.g. gynecologists) and this experience provided us with the opportunity to learn what they did wrong, and to savor the sweet-sour taste of *Schadenfreude*...

From colleagues working in the developing world (e.g. India), and from the literature, we learn that in some deprived environments dehiscence of the abdominal wound is still quite common, with some centers able to gather as many as 60 cases over 4 years. This obviously reflects the fact that they operate on neglected, undernourished patients under adverse conditions — often lacking proper suture material or even training.

1 Modified from Chapter 7, *Schein's Common Sense Prevention and Management of Surgical Complications*. Shrewsbury, UK: tfm publishing, 2013.

Let us start with some **basic definitions**; like everything in surgery (and life) so too dehiscence has a spectrum, from the annoying 'closed eventration' to the dramatic evisceration:

- **Complete dehiscence**: is full partition of the fascia and skin. Loops of small bowel — if not glued in place by adhesions — eviscerate or are completely exposed at the base of the gaping wound.
- **Partial dehiscence**: is a separation of the fascial edges of the wound without evisceration but often with exposure of the underlying omentum or viscera. The fascial gap varies in width and length — in some cases you may glimpse a loop of bowel at the bottom of the defect; in others the only sign of dehiscence would be some serosanguinous peritoneal fluid seeping through the wound.

In some series, cases of *complete* dehiscence outnumber the *partial* ones. But this is an artifact: while the true incidence of the former is known, that of the latter is not. **In an unknown number of patients, partial dehiscence remains *covert* or latent (some surgeons preferring not to be aware of it...), only to present later as incisional hernias**. So partial dehiscence is 'good news', in the short term — you do not need to reoperate; in the long term it heralds the development of an incisional hernia.

Dehiscence, be it complete or partial, is associated with significant morbidity and mortality. Obviously, local and systemic factors contribute to such outcomes, but proper management is crucial in lessening the impact of this complication.

Why does dehiscence develop?

Abdominal closure fails for one, or more, of three main reasons:

- **The patient is to blame** — this seems to be the main problem.
- **The suture breaks** — rare!
- **The surgeon is at fault**: poor surgical judgment or technique — not so rare...

Patient factors include multiple systemic and local problems (see ■ Table 45.1), presenting before the operation or developing after it, which render the tensile strength of the fascial closure inadequate. **These factors cause either *poor tissue healing* or increased *intra-abdominal pressure (IAP)* — allowing the sutures to cut through the fascia. You'll find a few of these factors in most patients who suffer dehiscence**.

Table 45.1. Factors predisposing to abdominal wall dehiscence.

PATIENT-RELATED		SURGEON-RELATED
Poor wound healing	Increased intra-abdominal pressure	Judgment
Hypoalbuminemia — poor nutrition	Ileus or early postop small bowel obstruction	To close fascia or leave open? Close the skin only?
Systemic or local infection (deep wound infection)	Obesity	Choice of **incision**: *midline incision* responsible for most cases!
	Ascites	
Shock (reduced perfusion of abdominal wall)	Chronic cough	Choice of **suture material**
Anemia	Vomiting	Inadequate **closure technique**
Hypoxia		
Uremia		Placing **stomas** or **drains** through the main wound
Malignancy		
Corticosteroids		
Uncontrolled diabetes		

How to prevent dehiscence by correct closure of the abdomen you will have read in ➲ Chapter 37. And you must remember that:

- There are situations **when the abdomen cannot be closed or should not be closed** (see ➲ Chapter 44).
- **Sometimes resorting to a 'planned hernia' (i.e. closing skin only** ➲ Chapter 37) **is much better tolerated than fascial dehiscence or laparostomy!**

After the operation

After the operation, anything which exerts excessive tension on the fascial suture line — anything elevating intra-abdominal pressure — contributes to the risk of dehiscence. Thus, severe coughing, retching, vomiting, abdominal distension and constipation should all be avoided. Letting the patient have an abdominal binder, despite your colleagues' eye-rolling, is not such a bad idea.

Some claim that wound infections predispose to fascial dehiscence. We are not sure whether this is true for superficial wound infections — a more plausible explanation for such an association would be that both such complications simply coexist because they share similar risk factors (e.g. malnutrition, emergency surgery, etc.).

However, there is no doubt that **deep SSIs** can chew up the fascial repair leading to dehiscence. It is unclear in such cases what came first, the chicken or the egg, as in some cases (those that should not have been closed — see page 618, ➲ Chapter 44) it is possible that the extra-tight fascial sutures 'strangulate' the fascia, predisposing it to necrosis and subsequent infection. **In addition, deep SSI may be associated with intra-abdominal infection; often neglected forms of the latter initially reveal themselves through dehiscence**.

Recognize the warning signs...

Educate your residents and staff (and yourself) to recognize the signs heralding fascial dehiscence: **moderate to large amounts of serosanguinous salmon-colored fluid draining from the wound during the first postoperative week**. That this is not pus but intraperitoneal fluid is often missed by non-experienced doctors, who then rush to remove 'a few sutures', believing that they are treating a wound infection. An hour later the nurse calls them back: "Hey Doc, I think his belly is open!" — "What the f...!" (■ Figure 45.1).

As a **general rule** (and this applies not only to sutures but also to staples, tubes, drains, lines): **do not allow anybody to remove anything from your patient's body that has been placed by you!** It is not easy nowadays to implement such rules within our modern, pseudodemocratic (*chaotic* would be a more accurate term) environment of healthcare, but try you must.

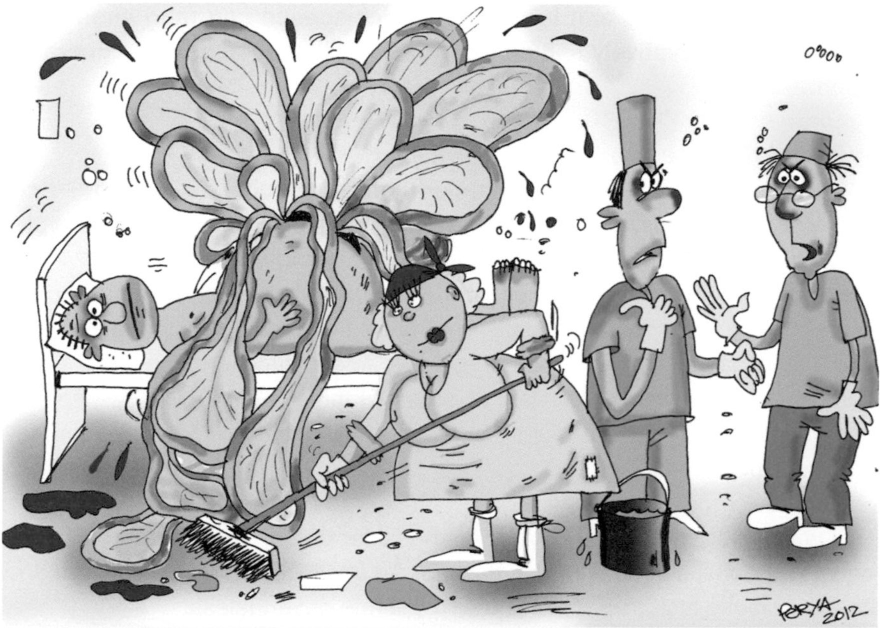

Figure 45.1. Surgeon to his buddy: "I don't understand what happened — I used PDS 2..."

Management of dehiscence

The seepage of serosanguinous fluid through a closed abdominal wound is an early sign of abdominal wound dehiscence with possible evisceration. When this occurs, the surgeon should remove one or two sutures in the skin and explore the wound manually, using a sterile glove. If there is separation of the rectus fascia, the patient should be taken to the operating room for primary closure. Wound dehiscence may or may not be associated with intestinal evisceration. When the latter complication is present, the mortality rate is dramatically increased and may reach 30%.

The above quotation is from one of many online texts of surgery. **We believe that the advice it provides is wrong!** But unfortunately, it reflects the recommendations given in other modern texts as well. Furthermore, why is the quoted mortality so high? **Because the dehiscence itself is not responsible for the high morbidity and mortality — it is the conditions predisposing to dehiscence and the emergency reoperation to correct it that contribute to poor outcomes**. Forcing the distended intestines back into a cavity of limited size may kill the patient by producing intra-abdominal hypertension with all its deleterious physiological effects.

We believe that by and large, partial dehiscence can (and should) be managed conservatively and only complete dehiscence must be operated upon.

Partial dehiscence

Partial dehiscence is best managed conservatively. The viscera are not falling out so why rush to reoperate? In our experience the natural course of a partially dehisced wound is to heal by granulation and scarring with or without the formation of an incisional hernia. On the other hand, reoperating through such a friable wound, in an ill patient, involves the additive risks of anesthesia and abdominal re-entry while not precluding an eventual hernia. If the bowel is partially exposed, we approximate (if possible) the skin to cover it. Otherwise, the wound is managed as any open wound until healed. A VAC system may be of use here…

If you manage to avoid reoperation, consider getting a CT scan to rule out an intra-abdominal cause for this mishap. An abscess should be drained, and an anastomotic leak may force you to reoperate nevertheless.

Complete dehiscence

Complete dehiscence necessitates an operation to reduce the eviscerated abdominal contents. **What to do at laparotomy after the viscera have been reduced depends on the perceived cause of the dehiscence**. You can resuture the fascia when a broken suture or faulty closure technique is the assumed cause. The use of 'onlay' mesh re-enforcement has been suggested, with 'good results', despite the risk of infection. We have not yet jumped on this wagon… But close only if local circumstances permit — the edges can be approximated without excessive tension and the fascia is viable and not grossly infected. **If this is not the case you should leave the abdomen temporarily open, using one of the temporary abdominal closure (TAC) methods** which are preferred in your center (➲ Chapter 44.2). As mentioned above, skin closure only (a 'planned hernia') is another excellent option.

In principle, avoid abdominal reclosure if the cause of the evisceration is still present, or if you predict the need to re-explore the abdomen within the next few days.

"Oops, you forgot", a few of our readers may shout, "you forgot to mention the use of 'retention sutures'!" Didn't our professor close tight a few burst abdomens, with a few heavy sutures, and the patients did all right? Look again at ➲ Chapter 37 to learn why we frown upon those ugly sutures.

We hope that after reading this chapter you will agree with us that...

- Abdominal dehiscence is a *symptom* rather than a *disease*.
- Sometimes, dehiscence of the abdomen represents a spontaneous decompression of intra-abdominal hypertension, and thus could be considered a 'beneficial' complication.
- You must operate for complete dehiscence with evisceration; resuture it or treat it as a laparostomy.
- Partial dehiscence is best treated conservatively.

"The gut bursts out either because you did not close the tummy properly or it has no place inside."

"Dehiscence of the abdominal wound represents a spontaneous decompression of intra-abdominal hypertension."

Chapter 46

Wound management

The Editors

A minor complication is one that happens to somebody else.

All that is visible to the patient of your wonderful, life-saving, emergency abdominal operation is the surgical wound (■ Figure 46.1). Wound complications, although not life-threatening, are an irritating source of painful, and often prolonged, morbidity, which bothers the patient and surgeon alike. It is no wonder then that throughout generations, surgeons have developed elaborate rituals to prevent and treat wound complications. Now that you are reading one of the last chapters of this book you are, we hope, sufficiently brain-washed to deplore elaborate gimmicks, and to demand pragmatic solutions instead.

Definitions and the spectrum

For practical purposes you do not need complicated definitions used by epidemiologists or infection-control nurses — the (usually humorless) 'authorities' who tell you not to walk out of the operating room with your scrubs on (in some countries they even force you to remove your handsome necktie and discard your groovy IWC Swiss wrist watch!).

Wounds are either uncomplicated or complicated.

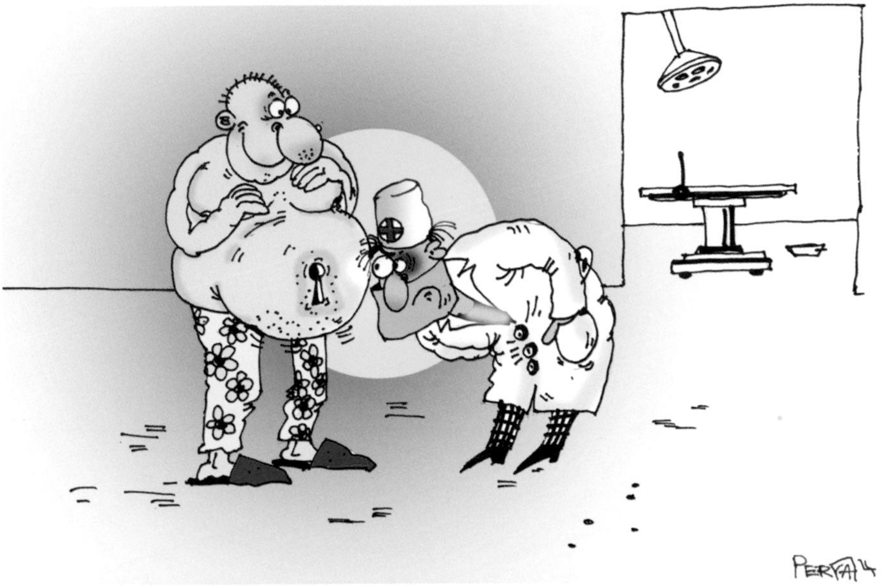

Figure 46.1. "I hope you are satisfied with the beautiful wound, eh?"

An **uncomplicated wound** is a sutured wound that heals uneventfully by primary intention. Note that following emergency abdominal surgery, an entirely uncomplicated wound is an exception! You don't believe us? Start to document from now on all your wounds and see for yourself the number of weeping or red and swollen wounds your patients have.

Complicated wounds are extremely common after emergency surgery when prospectively assessed by *independent* observers. Conversely, when 'reported' by surgeons they become 'rare' or 'minor' due to our natural tendency to suppress or ignore adverse outcomes. **Besides, most of these wound problems manifest after the patient has been discharged**. Do you know any surgeon who would run after the infection control Tzar in his hospital begging her to advertise his wound infection rate? Thus, in real life the rate of wound infections is grossly under-reported and underestimated, and the corresponding hospital statistics biased!

The spectrum of wound complications is wide and encompasses infective and non-infective complications, minor and major.

- **Minor complications** are those irritating aberrations in the process of healing that, however, do not impede primary healing of the wound: a small hematoma, a little erythema, some serous discharge, a tiny suture abscess. The distinction between an infectious and non-infectious process is difficult and also unnecessary; why take swab cultures from such a wound if it will not affect therapy?
- **Major complications** are those that interfere with the process of primary healing and require your intervention: a large hematoma or a wound abscess in need of drainage.
- **Wound infection — for practical purposes this is a wound that contains pus and requires drainage**. Usually such an infection represents a 'walled-off' wound abscess, with minimal involvement of adjacent soft tissues or underlying fascia (the term du jour for this entity is 'superficial SSI'). Sometimes, there may be significant surrounding cellulitis or involvement of the deep fascia, denoting an **invasive** infection (deep-space SSI).

Prevention

Surgical technique and overall patient care are of great importance in minimizing the incidence of wound infection. **Rarely is one aspect of management of singular importance, rather it is the sum of the parts that yields favorable results (the modern term for that is a 'bundle')**. Emergency surgery is particularly associated with wound problems for several reasons. Contamination of the wound may arise from intestinal bacteria released at the time of bowel resection or from the organisms present in the established infection that the surgery was performed to treat (➲ Chapter 13). Additionally, there is insufficient time pre-operatively to reverse all conditions which may adversely affect wound healing such as shock, diabetes and malnutrition (➲ Chapter 6).

Evidence suggests that tissue hypoxia, hypothermia and poorly controlled blood sugar predispose to wound complications. So try — the best you can in the few hours you have (if any at all) before the operation — to oxygenate the patient better (yes, give him that oxygen mask!), warm him up and administer insulin if necessary. No, cessation of smoking for a few hours is unlikely to help... ☺.

When you deal with complicated wounds you get wound complications.

Yes, this aphorism is true, and a certain rate of wound complications is obligatory and inherent in this type of surgery. **Nevertheless, you should strive to keep it as low as possible. How?**

Let us reiterate: "**The fate of the surgical wound is sealed *during* the operation; almost nothing can be done after the operation to modify the wound's outcome.**" Whether your patient develops a wound hematoma or infection depends on your patient, and on you, and is determined during the operation — not afterwards. We quote Mark Ravitch again: "**The likelihood of wound infections has been determined by the time the last stitch is inserted in the wound.**"

Meticulous technique as described in ➲ Chapter 37 is paramount. Here, a few preventive points are re-emphasized:

- Operate efficiently and carefully; avoid 'masturbating' the tissues.
- Do not strangulate the fascia with interrupted figure-of-eight sutures of wire, Ethibond® or Vicryl®; instead, use low-tension continuous, small bites, spring-like monofilament closure — letting the abdominal wall breathe (➲ Chapter 37).
- Do not 'barbecue' the skin and underlying tissues with excessive use of diathermy.
- Do not bury tons of highly irritating chromic catgut (or anything similarly obnoxious) in the subcutaneous fat. However, when the subcutaneous layer is thick try to obliterate the dead space...
- Do not close the skin with the even more noxious silk.
- Do not place contaminating colostomies in the main abdominal wound.
- Do not leave useless drains in the wound. And if you do insert a drain then remove it ASAP. **Don't forget that drains increase the risk of wound infections**.

Transfer your meticulous technique to the ward also. Nosocomial (hospital-acquired) infection is a menace to our patients. We have already mentioned the contribution that indiscriminate use of non-indicated antibiotics makes to the emergence of resistant organisms. The prevalence of these germs as colonizers of our patients is increasing, and spread from patient to patient is a big problem. Doctors are a major vector in this spread. Wash your hands every time you touch a patient. It seems astonishing that this message must be repeated nowadays, but studies have shown time and again that nurses are much more meticulous in their approach to this issue than MDs.

This act of handwashing after each patient contact should be so ingrained that you have a sense of incompleteness until it is performed. Well, with the current COVID-19 pandemic we assume that you won't stop washing your hands until the end of your career...

Antibiotics

Antibiotic prophylaxis reduces the wound infection rate; its anti-infective effects are in fact more pronounced in the surgical wound than within the peritoneal cavity (➲ Chapter 7). **Postoperative antibiotics cannot change the fate of the wound**, as they won't penetrate the area. A brief *peri-operative* antibiotic coverage is as effective in preventing wound infection as prolonged post-op administration (➲ Chapter 40).

Non-closure or delayed closure of the wound

Leaving the skin and subcutis completely or partially open following *contaminated* or *dirty* procedures is still advocated by some 'authorities'. True, it may prevent wound infection in the minority of patients who are bound to develop one but not every severely contaminated wound will become infected (indeed, you can even smear s**t on an open wound without getting an infection!). **At the same time leaving these wounds open condemns the majority, whose wounds are destined to heal more or less uneventfully, to the morbidity of open wounds, the associated problems of management, and the risk of superinfection.** Look again at ➲ Chapter 37 to learn why we very rarely would use the so called 'delayed closure'...

Management

The uncomplicated wound

Throughout history surgeons have been fascinated with the treatment of wounds because all they could do was to manage external post-traumatic wounds. For hundreds of years surgical leaders have advocated simplicity in the management of wounds:

- Felix Wurtz wrote in the 14th century: "**Keep them as neat and clean as possible, and disturb them as little as you can; so far as may be practicable, exclude the air; favor healing under the scab; and... feed it as you would a women recovering from her confinement.**"

- The great Joseph Lister said in the 19th century: "**Skin is the best dressing.**"
- The renowned physician William Osler maintained: "**Soap and water and common sense are the best disinfectants.**"

But most surgeons took literally the famous adage by war surgeon (14th century) Ambroise Paré: "**I dressed him and God healed him,**" and practiced unnecessarily elaborate wound-management policies.

The uncomplicated primarily closed surgical wound needs almost no care. A day after the operation it is well sealed away from the external environment by a layer of fibrin. It can be left exposed.

We think that it also depends on the closure method: a careful layered closure with sutures is not equivalent to stapler closure, the latter being more susceptible to contamination from the outside during the first few post-op days. Commonly, when using subcuticular skin closure, we would apply a layer of tissue glue that completely seals the wound. Be that as it may, isn't it ridiculous to see gloved and masked nurses changing sterile dressings on routine surgical wounds?

Some patients demand their wounds be covered; cheap dry gauze is more than adequate for this purpose — but in our modern commercial environment, it is more likely that your nurses would want to use fancy expensive products. **The main achievement of elaborate 'modern' dressing materials, impregnated with antibiotics, silver or whatever, is the enrichment of the medical-industrial complex**. We try to avoid them. **Patients with uncomplicated wounds can (nay, they should) shower or bathe any time**.

The complicated wound

Here the punishment should fit the crime. Minor non-specific complications should be observed — the majority will resolve spontaneously. A 'spitting' subcuticular suture may need to be fished out. Again, starting antibiotics because a wound weeps a little serous discharge is not going to change anything; if the wound is destined to develop an infection it will, with or without antibiotics! Major wound hematomas require evacuation, but this is rare following abdominal surgery — more common if your patient resumes his warfarin or Plavix® (clopidogrel) and all that you have used for abdominal closure is a fascial suture and staples for skin.

Wound infections

Wound infection following an emergency abdominal operation is usually caused by *endogenous* bacteria — the resident bacteria of the abdominal organs breached during the operation or the bacteria which caused the intra-abdominal infection in the first place. Following non-contaminated operations (e.g. blunt splenic trauma), the bugs causing wound infections are *exogenous* — skin residents, usually a *Staphylococcus*. Carriers of MRSA (methicillin-resistant *Staphylococcus aureus*) are prone to wound infections caused by this bug but this is another story. **The same goes for *Streptococcal* wound cellulitis which may develop a day (nay, even hours) after the operation with local pain (severe pain at the operative site is typical) and unexplained systemic toxicity**. Early on in this infection the wound itself is a little erythematous — the typically thin exudate lies in the deeper layers. **This is a rare but life-threatening complication; if you don't think about the treatment (wide drainage of the wound — including the deep layers and removal of mesh, if present — and appropriate antibiotics), it may arrive too late with bitter consequences** [1].

As alluded to above, wound infections also may present in your private office even weeks after the operation, skewing — underestimating — the elaborate statistics of your hospital infection control.

When in doubt, do not rush to poke in or open the wound — creating complications in wounds that would otherwise heal. Instead, be patient, wait a day or two, let the infection mature and declare itself.

Remember: a 'hot red' surgical wound with surrounding erythema does not mean 'cellulitis'. It means that there is pus within the wound that needs to be drained. As a rule, removing a few skin sutures and draining the pus treats most wound infections. There is no need to lay the whole wound open if only part of it is infected. You do not need a CT scan to diagnose a wound infection (this is not a joke... this is what 'modern medicine' is educating people to do). All you need do is to remove a few sutures or staples and probe the wound. If the cavity does not extend further up — or downwards — stop there and leave just that part open.

1 Look at Chapter 5 on wound complications in *Schein's Common Sense Prevention and Management of Surgical Complications*. Shrewsbury, UK: tfm publishing, 2013.

Aftercare

Aftercare should be simple. Open shallow wounds are covered with dry non-adherent gauze and cleaned once or twice daily with water and soap. There is nothing better for an open wound than a shower or bath! Deeper wounds are **loosely** — loosely, not plugged! — packed with gauze to afford drainage and prevent premature closure of the superficial layers. Antibiotics are usually not necessary. Do you give antibiotics after the incision and drainage of a peri-anal abscess? Of course not. So why treat wound infections with antibiotics? A short course of antimicrobials is indicated when severe cellulitis is present or the abdominal fascia is involved, indicating invasive infection.

Wound swabs? Wound cultures? Gram stains? In most cases these are unnecessary. As you know by now, the causative bacteria are mostly predictable (➲ Chapter 13) and, besides, how could the microbiological results change the therapy outlined above? The answer of course is that they don't. But some wounds will become problematic and it is then valuable to know the nature of the organism involved. Then the correct antibiotic can be administered without having to guess sensitivities or wait for the result of cultures. MRSA is currently endemic in the United States and elsewhere in the world, and is increasingly responsible for our postoperative wound infections. Early treatment of complications from these wound infections is obviously desirable. Early cultures from leaking wounds do therefore have some role to play, but be sure to prevent your junior colleagues from prescribing antibiotics just because a positive culture appears. Explain to them that even cultures taken from their own hands will grow a zoo...

Nurses and for-profit home-care agencies push elaborate and expensive wound care methods in order to justify their continued involvement. Local application of solutions or ointments of antiseptics or antibiotics destroy micro-organisms and human cells alike, induce allergy and encourage bacterial resistance.

Simple is beautiful. Use soap, water; and for our problematic wounds we are enthusiastic users of honey. Try it!

However, in selected situations the application of a **negative pressure (vacuum) wound system** can facilitate management and hasten wound closure. We would use it for deep, productive wounds — never for the simple ones.

(For a more elaborate discussion on wound complications and their management — including the use of honey, as depicted in ■ Figure 46.2 — we advise you to read the chapter referred to in the earlier footnote.)

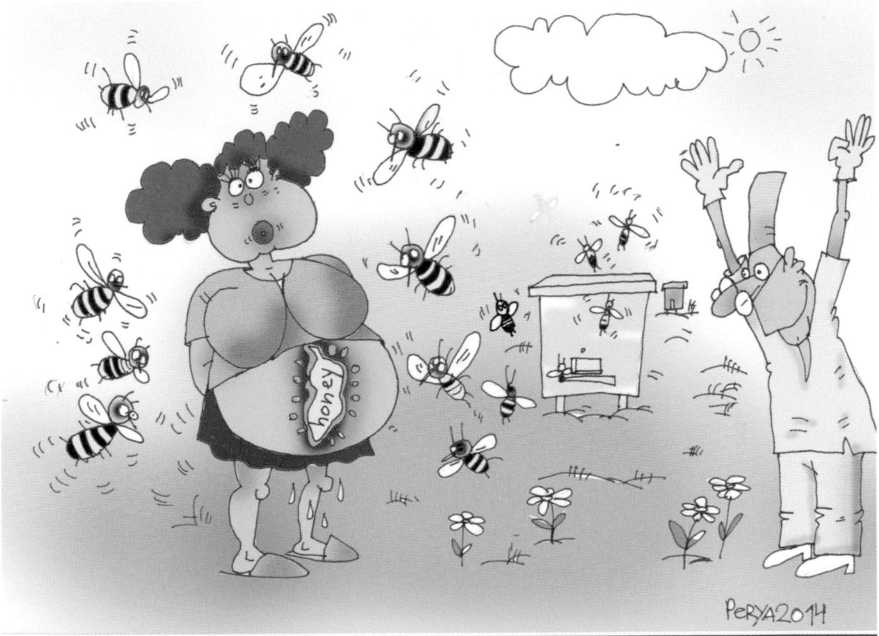

Figure 46.2. "Welcome to my honey management wound center."

Our friend Barry Alexander of Australia (also known as Baz) has summarized wound management very elegantly:

"I describe to my students what an injured animal does: it lies under a shady bush (rest, splint) by a water source (fluids, nutrition), licks the wound frequently (dressing changes) until it is clean and healing (time and patience) — and hope it makes them think past the gorgeous dressing promoted by manufacturers' reps."

"Dressings on undrained wounds serve only to hide the wound, interfere with examination, and to invite adhesive tape dermatitis."

Mark M. Ravitch

Chapter 47

In the aftermath

The Editors

Again and again I find that there are few things so quickly forgotten by the surgical system as a dead patient.

P. O. Nyström

A 'big' operation in a fit patient may be 'small'.
A 'small' operation in a sick patient may be 'big'.
A 'big' surgeon knows to tailor the operation and its trauma to the patient and his disease.

Let us hope that your patient survives his emergency abdominal operation and his postoperative course is uneventful. Unfortunately, the overall mortality of such procedures is still far from negligible and the morbidity rate is generally high. As somebody said: "you can't make a chicken salad out of chicken shit" — **shit happens!**

Now, after the storm has abated, it is time to sit down and reflect on what went wrong. As Francis D. Moore said: "**You want a surgical team that faces each error, each mishap, straight up, names it, and takes steps to prevent its recurrence.**"

Surgical audit and the morbidity & mortality meeting

The greatest pioneer (at least in the USA) in the establishment of an objective surgical audit, and the morbidity and mortality (M & M) meeting, was a surgeon who practiced a century ago — Dr. Ernest Amory Codman (1869-1940) of the Massachusetts General Hospital in Boston, who stated: "I am naturally disgusted with humbug, self-deception, hypocrisy, smugness, cupidity and injustice." About a patient in whom Codman had ligated the common hepatic duct, leading to death, he said: "I had made an error of skill of the most gross character and even [during the operation] failed to recognize that I had made it." **Codman classified errors into lack of knowledge or skill, surgical judgment, lack of care or equipment, and lack of diagnostic skill**.

At any place where a group of surgeons is working, it is crucial to conduct some form of a regular M & M meeting (MMM). This is the venue where you and your colleagues should *objectively* analyze and discuss — in retrospect — all the recent complications and mortalities.

You are familiar with the cliché that "some surgeons learn from their own mistakes, some learn from those of others, and some never learn". The aim of the MMM is to abolish the last entity.

Do you have a regular M & M meeting in your department? If you are associated, as a resident or a qualified surgeon, with a teaching department in the USA, you must have a weekly MMM, because without a routine MMM the department's residency program cannot be accredited. However, we know that in many corners around the world MMMs are not conducted; **all blunders and failures are swept under the carpet**.

Elsewhere still, MMMs are conducted in name only, being used to present 'interesting cases' or the latest 'success stories'. This is wrong! As David Dent said: "**A handful of polite show-case presentations do not make a true M & M conference**."

The MMM exists to analyze objectively your mistakes and complications — not to punish or humiliate anyone, but to educate and improve results. You do not want to repeat the same error twice. So, see to it that proper MMMs are conducted wherever you provide surgical care. Even in small rural hospitals. And if your partners are not interested, or if you are a 'solo' surgeon — then conduct your own MMM!

The optimal format for the MMM:

- A routine hour should be dedicated to the MMM each week.
- ALL interns, residents and surgeons should attend — regularly.
- ALL complications and deaths that occurred in any patient treated by any member of the department should be presented.
- A complication is a complication — irrespective of whether the outcome was a triumph or tragedy. All must be presented.
- The MMM is a democratic forum. The boss's blunder or that goof by the 'local giant' are as 'interesting', if not more, as that caused by a junior resident.

The resident-team that was involved with the case should present it. They should know all the details and rehearse the presentation in advance. The patient's chart and X-rays should be readily available. If you are the presenting resident, be objective and neutral. **Your task is to learn and facilitate the learning of others, not to defend or cover up for the involved surgeon; you are not his or her lawyer**. Understand that the majority of those who are present are not stupid — they sense immediately when the truth is deserted.

The assessment of complications

After the case has been presented, the person who presides over the meeting should initiate and encourage a discussion with the intent of arriving at a consensus. An easy way to break the commonly prevailing and embarrassing silence is to point at one of the senior surgeons and ask: "Dr. X, please tell us, had this patient been under your care from the beginning, would the outcome be the same?" This technique usually manages to break the ice, prompting a sincere and complete response.

The issues to be addressed during the discussion are:

- **Was it a 'real' complication?** Some surgeons may argue that blood loss, which required transfusion, is not a complication but a technical mishap, which simply can 'happen'.
- **Assess the cause: was it an error of judgment or a technical error?** Operating on a dying terminal cancer patient reflects poor judgment; having to reoperate for hemorrhage from the gallbladder bed marks a technical error — poor hemostasis at the first operation. **The two types of errors are often combined and inseparable**: the patient with acute bowel ischemia died because his operation was 'too late'

(poor judgment) and the stoma, which was performed, has retracted, leaking into the peritoneal cavity (poor technique). Often it is impossible to define whether a technical complication (e.g. anastomotic leak) is caused by poor technique (technical error) or patient-related factors, such as malnutrition or chronic steroid intake.

- Another possibility is to look at the error as either **an error of commission or omission**. One either operates too late or not at all (**omission**) or operates too early or unnecessarily (**commission**). One either misses the injury or resects too little (**omission**) or does too much (**commission**). After the operation one either fails to reoperate for the abscess (**omission**) or operates unnecessarily when percutaneous drainage was possible (**commission**). **Note that the surgical community tends to consider errors of omission more gravely that those of commission; the latter are looked at with understanding: "we did all we could, but we failed."**
- **Was there negligence? A certain rate of mistakes (hopefully low) is an integral part of any surgical practice as only those who never operate commit no errors — but negligence is deplorable**. The operation was delayed because the responsible surgeon did not want to be disturbed over the weekend or the surgeon operated under the influence of alcohol: this is clearly 'negligence'. When an individual

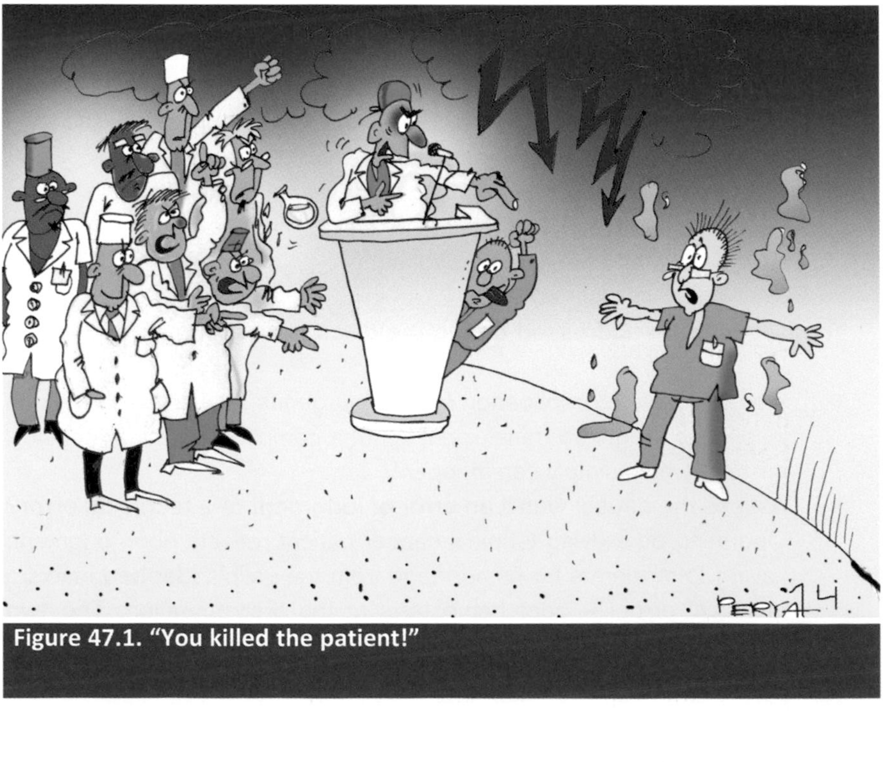

Figure 47.1. "You killed the patient!"

surgeon repeats errors over and over again, a *pattern* is exhibited, which in itself may constitute negligence.

- **Was the complication/death preventable or potentially preventable?** Each case is different and must be analyzed individually.
- **Who was responsible?** The MMM is not a court (■ Figure 47.1). **Culpability is not the issue, but at the end of the presentation it should be clear to all present how things might have been done better.** Blame is to be avoided at all costs (except in the most extreme cases, and then the MMM is not the forum to deal with them) because any system that aims to apportion blame as part of the quality control processes will fail; the truth will be hidden and confrontation avoided. Such is human nature. **The sad truth, however, is that in many instances complications and mortality are caused by 'system failure' — which in purely surgical terms means that the hospital is a cesspit with a malfunctioning chain of command, organization, supervision, education and morals.**

Here is an example...

The old man was gasping unattended for 6 hours in the emergency room before you were called to assess his acute abdomen. You decided on an emergency laparotomy, but no operating room was available for 2 hours. Because the orderlies went for dinner another half-an-hour was lost until you decided to fetch the patient yourself. Only then did you realize that the antibiotics and intravenous fluids you ordered had not been given. A clueless anesthetist then struggles with the intubation producing prolonged hypoxia... and so on and so on... how much damage can an old man take? **System failures are much more common than you think, just look around your own environment...**

- **Was the standard of care met? As you surely know, the 'standard of care' means different things to different people. ("The good thing about a standard of care is that there are so many to choose from.")** It has a spectrum, which should be well represented and assessed by a group of well-informed practicing surgeons. Take, for example, a case of perforated sigmoid diverticulitis with local peritonitis: any operation ranging from a Hartmann's procedure (the 'conservative' surgeon) to a sigmoid resection with anastomosis (the 'daring' surgeon) would fall within the accepted standard of care (oh well, the 'ultra-modern' surgeon may have elected to treat such a patient with laparoscopic lavage only...). Primary closure of the perforation would not. This would be easy to assess: "anyone who would attempt closing the perforation please raise your hand." No hand is raised; the responsible surgeon is left lonely to understand that what he did is not acceptable and is outside the practiced standard **in his community**. The responsible surgeon may, however, present published literature to support that what he did is acceptable elsewhere. And, obviously, local surgeons can be dogmatic and wrong!

- **Evidence-based surgery**. At the end of the presentation the resident should present the literature to pinpoint the 'state of the art' and associated controversies, emphasizing what could have been done, and should be done when we see a similar case in the future.
- **The surgeon in whose patient the complication arose**. At the end of the discussion the most senior surgeon involved in the care of the concerned patient should offer a statement. He or she may choose to present additional evidence from the published literature to show that what was done is acceptable elsewhere. **The most graceful way to deal with the situation is to discuss the case scenario frankly, and humbly admit any mistakes one may have made. If you had another chance with the same patient how would you manage him?** By standing up and confessing, you gain the respect of all present. When you lie, cover up and refuse to accept the verdict of the gathering, you evoke silent contempt and disdain (or perhaps sympathy from other obsessive liars). So stand up and fess up!

Conclusions and corrective measures

Finally, the person in the chair should conclude — was there an error? Was the standard of care met? And what are the future recommendations and the corrective measures? If you are that chairman, and you may be some day, don't be wishy-washy. Be objective and definitive, for the audience is not stupid. **Essentially, in any department of surgery, the face of the MMM, its objectivity and practical value, reflects the face and ethical standards of the department's chairman or director**.

> Most 'avoidable' surgical disasters and mortalities are not caused by one sentinel — horrendous, clearly evident — error which cries "I am negligent". Instead, most such avoidable catastrophes result from a chain of allegedly 'minor' hesitations, confusions, ignorance, greed, inattention, overconfidence, arrogance, stupidity — which together drive the nails into the coffin. Taken together they may whisper: "we are negligent!"

We hope that after reading this little book you will want to look at our other book dedicated to COMPLICATIONS [1] from which we want to bring here this:

As you see, definitions are not clear cut and a wide gray area exists. But let us offer a unifying concept — a practical one.

"St happens/s**t should not have happened."**

Please forgive the coarse language but this is how weathered trench-dwelling surgeons tend to consider the recurring dilemma, how they look at and analyze complications — whether their own or produced by their colleagues. Any complication is either a known/potential consequence of the procedure and/or was unpreventable ("s**t happens") or the opposite is true: "**s**t should not have happened**." Each case should be analyzed individually and in some cases the answer remains unknown.

In some cases, even if it is hard to admit that "st has happened" — it still stinks!**

So now go and read our *Schein's Common Sense Prevention and Management of Surgical Complications*, which will help you to reduce the incidence of **** happening and to deal with it when it does occur.

The SURGINET

An ideal and objective MMM as featured above is not conducted in many places because of local sociopolitical constraints. If this is the case in your neck of the woods, it may be damaging to your own surgical education; how would you know what is right or wrong? Books and journals are useful but cannot replace a thorough analysis of specific cases by a group of learned surgeons. Well, if you have a PC and email access, you can subscribe to SURGINET, an international forum of surgeons, who would openly and objectively discuss any case or complication you present to them (■ Figure 47.2). Should you want to take part in this 'international MMM' send an email message to Dr. Tom Gilas of Toronto, tgilas@sympatico.ca, or to drosin@mac.com or mosheschein@gmail.com.

1 *Schein's Common Sense Prevention and Management of Surgical Complications.* Shrewsbury, UK: tfm publishing, 2013.

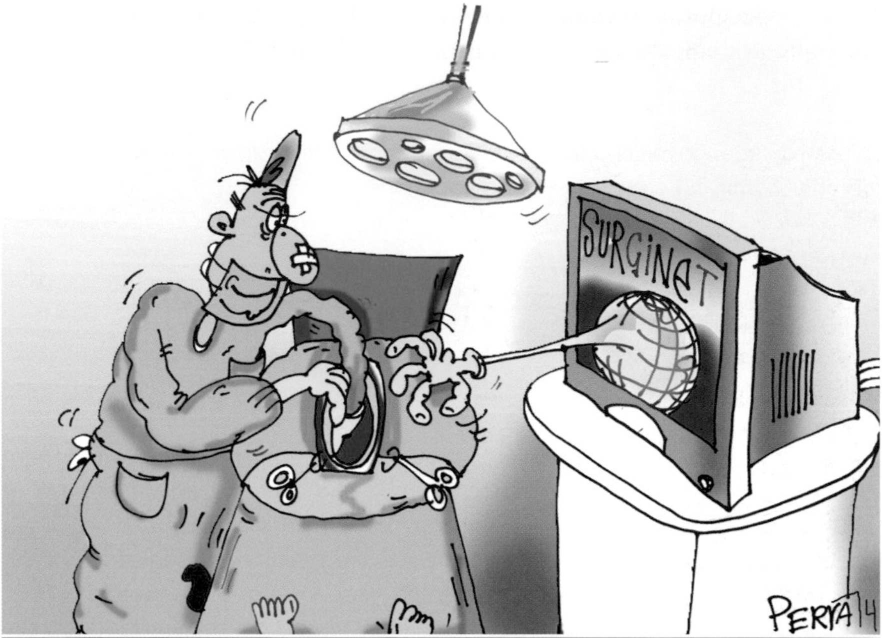

Figure 47.2. "SURGINET — please help me!"

Before we close...

As you know, there are many ways to skin a cat, and it is easy to be a smart ass looking at things through the blinding lights of the 'retrospectoscope'. Our sick patients and the events leading to the MMM are very complex. But behind this chaos there is always an instructive truth which should be and can be disclosed and announced.

Farewell

An emergency room at midnight. The same scenario in San Francisco or Mumbai or Lisbon. The same situation in 2020 as it was in 1920. The patient lies on his bed or stretcher holding his tummy in agony. Members of the family are all around. You walk in and introduce yourself: "I am the surgeon." All eyes are raised up to you with relief and hope, but also appraisal: *Finally, he has arrived, the only one who can help our father but... is he up to the job?*

You approach the patient and take his hand. Just go ahead. We know that you are up to the task — with all your training... and having just finished this book ☺. Go ahead and save yet another life. "Be strong and courageous. Do not be frightened, and do not be dismayed." **Joshua 1:9**

Thanks for reading

We hope you enjoyed our *magnum opus* ☺. Let us wish you *adieu* using this memorable quotation from Winston Churchill's broadcast (1941) to the people of conquered Europe:

"Good night then: sleep to gather strength for the morning. For the morning will come. Brightly will it shine on the brave and the true, kindly on all who suffer for the cause, glorious upon the tombs of heroes. Thus will shine the dawn."

You — the emergency surgeons — are the heroes of medicine. For you the dawn will shine!

The Editors

"It is usually the second mistake in response to the first mistake that does the patient in."

Clifford K. Meador

"The two unforgivable sins of surgery. The first great error in surgery is to — operate unnecessarily; the second, to undertake an operation for which the surgeon is not sufficiently skilled technically."

Max Thorek

Index